THE
BEST
OF
DIABETES
SELF-MANAGEMENT

THE DEFINITIVE
COMMONSENSE GUIDE TO
MANAGING YOUR DIABETES

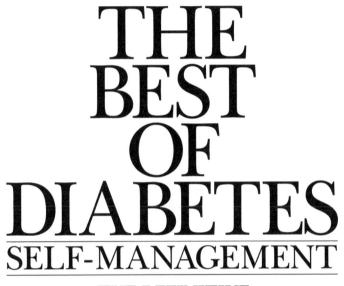

THE
BEST
OF
DIABETES
SELF-MANAGEMENT

THE DEFINITIVE
COMMONSENSE GUIDE TO
MANAGING YOUR DIABETES

DIABETES SELF-MANAGEMENT BOOKS
NEW YORK

Copyright © 2002 by Diabetes Self-Management Books.

ISBN 0-9631701-5-5

PROJECT EDITOR
RICHARD HANTULA

DESIGN AND ILLUSTRATION
RICHARD BOLAND

Diabetes Self-Management Books is an imprint of R.A. Rapaport Publishing, Inc.,
150 West 22nd Street, New York, NY 10011.

Printed in the United States of America.

10 9 8 7 6 5 4 3 2 1

Contents

PREFACE

Back in 1983, when we started publishing *Diabetes Self-Management* magazine, our aim was to give people with diabetes accessible, "how-to" information to help them achieve and maintain physical well-being and peace of mind. When you have diabetes, up-to-date, authoritative information on nutrition, the latest drugs, medical advances, self-help, exercise, and so much more is crucial to managing your health and enjoying life to its fullest.

If you subscribed to *Diabetes Self-Management* to get reliable health advice, you made a wise investment; the most important tool you can have in managing your diabetes is information. And keeping up to date with a continuous source of new and trustworthy information is important. But you also need a comprehensive reference manual sometimes—solid, reliable information on everything you need to know about managing your health, all in one book. That's the reason we put together *The Best of Diabetes Self-Management.* No other book begins to approach the wealth of information contained in this single book—expert advice in clear, easy-to-understand language on every aspect of diabetes management.

This book is not just a collection of previously published material. Each article was painstakingly updated by the author and reviewed by the editorial staff of *Diabetes Self-Management,* so you know you can trust every word. Every article was carefully chosen for its importance to diabetes treatment and self-care.

Whether you have just been diagnosed with diabetes or have been intimately involved in your own treatment for many years, *The Best of Diabetes Self-Management* will give you information that will allow you to take greater charge of your diabetes and your physical and emotional well-being. Read it in good health.

For the staff and authors who made this book possible,

James Hazlett
Editor, *Diabetes Self-Management*

CONTRIBUTORS

Jo Ann Ahern, A.P.R.N., M.S.N., C.D.E., is Coordinator of the Yale Program for Children With Diabetes in New Haven, Connecticut.

Susan L. Barlow, R.D., C.D.E., is past President of the American Association of Diabetes Educators and Diabetes Clinical Liaison for Amylin Pharmaceuticals in San Diego, California.

Neil Baum, M.D., is Associate Clinical Professor of Urology at Tulane Medical School and Louisiana State University School of Medicine in New Orleans, Louisiana.

Kim Begany, R.Ph., Pharm.D., is an Ambulatory Care Clinical Pharmacist with the Cleveland Clinic Foundation in Cleveland, Ohio.

Prudence E. Breitrose, M.A., is chief writer of health education materials for the Stanford Center for Research in Disease Prevention.

Barbara N. Campaigne, Ph.D., an exercise physiologist and a fellow of the American College of Sports Medicine, is a Scientific Communications Associate Consultant in Diabetes Care at Eli Lilly and Company in Indianapolis, Indiana.

Wayne L. Clark is a freelance medical and science writer based in Maine who has written extensively on diabetes.

Marilyn M. Clougherty, R.N., M.S.N., C.D.E., is a diabetes educator at the Children's Hospital of Pittsburgh and a certified group exercise instructor in Pittsburgh, Pennsylvania.

Nancy Cooper, R.D., C.D.E., is a diabetes nutrition specialist at the International Diabetes Center in Minneapolis, Minnesota, and a Contributing Editor of *Diabetes Self-Management*.

Ann M. Coulston, M.S., R.D., conducts research on the effects of diet on diabetes at the Stanford University Medical Center, General Clinical Research Center, in Stanford, California.

Martha Jo Dendinger, C.M.P., a convention manager for health-care organizations, has had diabetes for over 20 years.

Robert S. Dinsmoor is a freelance writer based in Massachusetts and a Contributing Editor of *Diabetes Self-Management*.

J. Shawn Faulk, M.S., R.D., C.D.E., has served as the President of the San Diego Transplant Association in California, is creator and editor of a multiorgan transplant newsletter for San Diego County, and helps coordinate a nationwide program for transplant recipients.

Orna Feldman is a freelance medical writer based in Boston, Massachusetts.

Vivian Fonseca, M.D., is Professor of Medicine, occupying the Tullis–Tulane Chair in Diabetes, at the Tulane University Medical Center in New Orleans.

Martha M. Funnell, M.S., R.N., C.D.E., is Associate Director for Administration of the Clinical Implementation Core at the University of Michigan Diabetes Research and Training Center.

Eve Gehling, M.Ed., R.D., C.D.E., is a dietitian at Health-Partners in Minneapolis, Minnesota.

Patti Bazel Geil, M.S., R.D., L.D., C.D.E., is a diabetes nutrition specialist in Lexington, Kentucky.

Susanne K. Giorgio, R.D.H., is Lecturer of Surgery at MCP Hahnemann University School of Medicine, in Philadelphia, Pennsylvania.

Joan I. Gluch, R.D.H., Ph.D., is Assistant Dean, Community Relations, and Assistant Professor, Dental Care Systems, at the University of Pennsylvania, School of Dental Medicine, in Philadelphia, Pennsylvania.

David E. Goldstein, M.D., is Professor of Pediatrics and Director of Pediatric Endocrinology and Diabetes at the University of Missouri Health Science Center in Columbia, Missouri.

Jacqueline Laks Gorman is a freelance writer and editor based in De Kalb, Illinois.

Joseph Gustaitis is a freelance writer based in New York City.

Linnea Hagberg, R.D., is a freelance writer based in Gloucester, Massachusetts.

Laura Hieronymus, R.N., M.S.Ed., C.D.E., is a diabetes health consultant in Lexington, Kentucky.

Priscilla Hollander, M.D., Ph.D., a former investigator in the Diabetes Control and Complications Trial, is an endocrinologist and Medical Director of the Ruth Collins Diabetes Center at the Baylor University Medical Center in Dallas, Texas.

Dennis J. Janisse, C.Ped., is President and C.E.O. of National Pedorthic Services, Inc., Director of Pedorthic Education for P.W. Minor & Son, former President of the Pedorthic Footwear Association, and Clinical Assistant Professor in the Department of Physical Medicine and Rehabilitation at the Medical College of Wisconsin.

LilyAnn Jeu is a pharmacy student at Long Island University in New York City and a former Editorial Assistant with *Diabetes Self-Management.*

Julia V. Johnson, M.D., is Associate Professor in the Department of Obstetrics and Gynecology at the University of Vermont in Burlington.

Diane M. Karl, M.D., is Medical Director of Diabetes Services at the Adventist Health System in Portland, Oregon, and Clinical Assistant Professor of Medicine at Oregon Health Sciences University.

Karen Kelly, R.N., B.S.N., C.D.E., is a diabetes educator who works with children and adolescents at the Children's Hospital of Pittsburgh.

Tina Kress, R.N., B.S.N., C.C.T.C., C.P.T.C., is Kidney/Pancreas Transplant Coordinator at the Sharp Memorial Hospital in San Diego,

California, and has also coordinated the procurement and placement of donated organs for San Diego's Organ and Tissue Acquisition Center.

Karmeen Kulkarni, M.S., R.D., C.D.E., is a dietitian and diabetes educator at St. Mark's Hospital in Salt Lake City, Utah.

Daniel L. Lorber, M.D., is Medical Director of the Diabetes Care and Information Center of New York in Flushing, New York.

Barbara K. Lynch, R.D., L.D., C.D.E., a clinical dietitian in Southern Illinois hospitals for 13 years, is currently in private practice, serving area doctors with individualized patient counseling.

J. Christopher Lynch, Pharm.D., is Assistant Professor of Pharmacy Practice at Northeast Louisiana University, Clinical Instructor of Medicine at Tulane University Medical School in New Orleans, and Clinical Pharmacist for the MCL-NO Diabetes Center.

Ivy D. Marcus, Ph.D., C.D.E., a licensed clinical psychologist, is codirector of The Center for Cognitive-Behavioral Psychotherapy in New York City, Consulting Staff Psychologist at the Joslin Center for Diabetes in New York City, and Consulting Staff Psychologist at Winthrop–University Hospital in Long Island, New York; she maintains a private practice in Port Washington, Long Island.

James McGuire, P.T., D.P.M., C.Ped., W.C.S., is Director of the Advanced Wound Healing Center at the Temple University School of Podiatric Medicine in Philadelphia.

Belinda O'Connell, M.S., R.D., L.D., is a diabetes nutrition specialist at the International Diabetes Center in Minneapolis, Minnesota.

Linda Pachucki-Hyde, R.N., M.S., C.D.E., a member of the Osteoporosis Task Force of the Endocrine Nurses Society, is a diabetes educator based in Milwaukee, Wisconsin.

Teresa Pearson, M.S., R.N., C.D.E., is a manager at HealthPartners in Minneapolis, Minnesota.

Virginia Peragallo-Dittko, R.N., M.A., C.D.E., is a diabetes nurse specialist and Director of the Diabetes Education Center at Winthrop–University Hospital in Mineola, New York.

William H. Polonsky, Ph.D., C.D.E., is Assistant Professor in Psychiatry at the University of California–San Diego and Head of the Health Psychology Division, Naval Medical Center, San Diego, California.

Charles A. Reasner, M.D., is Associate Professor of Medicine and Medical Director of the Texas Diabetes Institute at the University of Texas Health Science Center at San Antonio, San Antonio, Texas.

Rita Revak-Lutz, A.R.N.P., M.S.N., C.D.E., is a nurse practitioner for the Department of Obstetrics and Gynecology at the University of Florida in Gainesville, Florida.

Matthew C. Riddle, M.D., is Professor of Medicine and Head of the Section of Diabetes at Oregon Health Sciences University.

Jean Betschart Roemer, R.N., M.N., C.P.N.P., C.D.E., is a pediatric nurse practitioner at the Children's Hospital of Pittsburgh in Pittsburgh, Pennsylvania, and a Contributing Editor of *Diabetes Self-Management.*

Jeanne L. Rosenthal, M.D., is Attending Surgeon and Assistant Director of the Retinal Service, New York Eye and Ear Infirmary and Clinical Associate Professor of Ophthalmology at New York Medical College in New York City.

Helen L. Ross, M.D., is a board-certified obstetrician/gynecologist and a clinical instructor with the Department of Obstetrics and Gynecology at the University of Florida in Gainesville, Florida.

Tami Ross, R.D., L.D., C.D.E., is a diabetes nutrition specialist and certified diabetes educator in Lexington, Kentucky.

Richard R. Rubin, Ph.D., C.D.E., is Associate Professor in Medicine and in Pediatrics at the Johns Hopkins University School of Medicine and a staff member of the Diabetes Center and the Pediatric Diabetes Clinic at the Johns Hopkins Hospital in Baltimore, Maryland.

Kenneth Ruge, D.Min., a psychotherapist and pastoral counselor, is a principal of The Vocare Group in New York City, which offers seminars and counseling for people who are redirecting their lives and careers using spiritual and self-discovery tools.

Patricia M. Schaaf, M.S., R.D., conducts research on the effects of diet on diabetes at the Stanford University Medical Center, General Clinical Research Center, in Stanford, California.

Gary Scheiner, M.S., C.D.E., maintains a private practice in diabetes education, Integrated Diabetes Services, in Wynnewood, Pennsylvania.

Ingrid Strauch is Managing Editor of *Diabetes Self-Management.*

Robert Taibbi, L.C.S.W., a specialist in child and family therapy and a frequent contributor to *Diabetes Self-Management*, resides in Charlottesville, Virginia.

Virginia Valentine, R.N., M.S.N., C.D.E., is a clinical nurse specialist and CEO of a diabetes disease management company in Albuquerque, New Mexico.

Elizabeth Warren-Boulton, R.N., M.S.N., is Senior Writer for Hager Sharp, Inc., a health communications firm in Washington, D.C., and a contractor to the National Diabetes Education Program, sponsored by the U.S. National Institute of Diabetes and Digestive and Kidney Diseases and the Centers for Disease Control and Prevention.

Richard M. Weil, M.Ed., C.D.E., C.S.C.S., is an exercise physiologist and a consultant to the Naomi Berrie Diabetes Center at Columbia Presbyterian Hospital in New York City.

Ann S. Williams, M.S.N., R.N., C.D.E., a diabetes-care consultant in private practice, is former Chair of the American Association of Diabetes Educators' Visually Impaired Persons Specialty Practice Group.

Janice L. Woodrum, R.N., B.S.N., is Diabetes Education Coordinator at the Linn County Family Care Clinics in Kansas.

Tim Wysocki, Ph.D., is a pediatric psychologist at the Nemours Children's Clinic in Jacksonville, Florida.

Carol Younkin, R.N., M.Ed., C.D.E., C.H.E.S., is a senior clinical research administrator and diabetes educator for Eli Lilly and Company in Indianapolis, Indiana.

BASIC INFORMATION

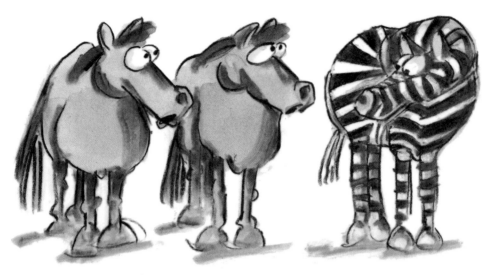

WHAT'S YOUR TYPE?
Type 1, Type 2—Or Something Else?
by Wayne L. Clark

It used to be much easier to talk about the "types" of diabetes because most of us were familiar with only two types that were quite different. The conventional wisdom was that children got one type, and adults got the other. Thin people were more likely to get one, overweight people the other. One type required insulin injections, the other didn't. It was simple.

Today we know it's not that simple. The old rules have so many exceptions that the distinction between one type and the other can sometimes be blurred. Classifications seem destined to be made even more complicated in the future, but for good and important reasons.

The difference between types is important to you and your doctor, because the right treatment requires the right diagnosis. Recent research, such as the Diabetes Control and Complications Trial, and new treatments—such as insulin "sensitizers," which include the drugs pioglitazone (brand name Actos) and rosiglitazone (Avandia)—have uncovered new ways of looking at both major types of diabetes and new ways of approaching treatment.

Diabetes primer

Let's start at the beginning. There *are* just two major types of diabetes, although there are some other, less common types (see "Typecasting" on page 16). Over the years, however, the names of the two major types have changed.

In 1979, the terms "juvenile" and "adult-onset" diabetes were changed to "insulin-dependent" and "non-insulin-dependent." In 1997, the American Diabetes Association and the World Health Organization issued new guidelines about the classification of diabetes, in part as a reaction to increasing confusion. The guidelines confirmed the two major "types," but with a distinction. What used to be called "insulin-dependent" diabetes was renamed "Type 1" diabetes. What used to be called "non-insulin-dependent" diabetes was renamed "Type 2" diabetes.

One element of the confusion leading up to the 1997 name changes was that more and more, Type 1 diabetes was found to be occurring in adults. In fact, 25% of cases of Type 1 diabetes occur in people older than 20. At the same time, the incidence of Type 2 diabetes in children was observed to be rising dramatically.

The 1997 guidelines are different from previous guidelines because they base classification on the cause, or *pathogenesis,* of the diabetes rather than the treatment. Type 1 diabetes is an autoimmune disease, in which the body's immune system attacks and destroys the insulin-producing beta cells of the pancreas. The result is "absolute insulin deficiency," because the beta cells no longer produce insulin.

Type 2 diabetes is a combination of insulin resistance and *relative* insulin deficiency. In insulin resistance, the ability of the body's tissues—such as muscle cells and the liver—to use insulin to regulate cellular activity is hampered. At the same time, there appears to be less insulin available. In some people, insulin resistance is the larger issue; in others, the relative insulin deficiency seems to be the bigger problem.

So the pathogenesis of the two types is quite different: Type 1 is an autoimmune process and Type 2 is a metabolic process.

Times still are a-changing

Don't expect the 1997 guidelines to be the last word in the classification of diabetes.

"I think it's safe to say that those will not be our last guidelines, as we're learning more about the pathogenesis," says Irl B. Hirsch, M.D., Associate Professor of Medicine at the University of Washington Medical Center. "Even within the most common type of Type 2 diabetes, when you look at different ethnic groups and even different families, there are different things going on making the diabetes different. For instance, in some groups the muscle seems to be the bigger problem for insulin resistance; in other groups it's the liver."

Type 1 diabetes also does not always follow the rules. Even the old "juvenile-onset" conventional wisdom has fallen apart.

"The classical Type 1 patient gets his diabetes in childhood," Dr. Hirsch says, "but we now understand that the autoimmune destruction of islets can occur at any age."

Clinicians and researchers have developed a designation for some of the older people who develop Type 1 diabetes. Typically, these people are not overweight, as is common in Type 2 diabetes, and they come to their doctor with the acute symptoms of diabetes: frequent urination, excessive thirst and hunger, and ketones (a by-product of fat metabolism) in their urine. Because they are adults with what used to be thought of as "juvenile-type" symptoms, and because their progression to complete insulin deficiency is

slower than that seen in children with Type 1 diabetes, their disease is called "Latent Autoimmune Diabetes of Adults," or LADA.

The advent of new laboratory tests for autoimmune "markers" has helped define yet another important subset of diabetes: people who appear to have Type 2 but in fact may have Type 1. It's not known how many people this may include, but estimates range from 5% to 25% of people thought to have Type 2 diabetes.

The tests measure two of the antibodies created by the autoimmune process of Type 1 diabetes: antibodies to glutamic acid decarboxylase, or GADA, and antibodies to islet cells, or ICA. The tests can help distinguish it from the metabolic process of Type 2 diabetes.

There has been some discussion in the medical literature that tries to fit LADA into the "Type 1" and "Type 2" nomenclature by referring to it as "Type 1.5" diabetes. However, others have used the term "Type 1.5" for those people who appear to have Type 2 diabetes yet have at least one of the immune markers of Type 1 diabetes. These classifications will need to be clarified in the future. For now, only Type 1 and Type 2 are official classifications.

"The adult patient who is thinner, who doesn't have the 'classical' phenotype for Type 2 diabetes—overweight, sedentary, a strong family history of Type 2 diabetes—is more likely to require insulin in the first couple of years after diagnosis," says Desmond A. Schatz, M.D., Professor of Pediatrics at the University of Florida. "In those patients, we encourage antibody testing. The best test is antibodies to GAD, which are probably found in about 50% to 60% of adult patients who actually have Type 1 diabetes."

Implications for treatment

A careful diagnosis is critical for determining the type of diabetes being treated, because the therapy decisions based on the diagnosis are potentially very important.

For a person with classic childhood Type 1 diabetes, there is no question about the appropriate treatment: Insulin therapy is the only choice. A person with the classic symptoms of Type 2 diabetes may have a range of options, from more conservative treatment to more aggressive treatment. The first prescription may be diet and exercise, followed by oral medicines if that is unsuccessful, and by insulin therapy if the other options do not control blood sugar levels.

It is important to know whether the person has an autoimmune process or a metabolic process—that is,

TYPECASTING

The following descriptions of the different types of diabetes are based on the 1997 guidelines of the American Diabetes Association and the World Health Organization.

TYPE 1 DIABETES
Characterized by beta cell destruction, usually leading to absolute insulin deficiency. It is an autoimmune process in which the immune system attacks the insulin-producing beta cells in the pancreas. There are also some rare forms of Type 1 that have no known cause but also result in the destruction of the beta cells.

TYPE 2 DIABETES
Diseases of insulin resistance that usually have relative (rather than absolute) insulin deficiency. It was once believed to be a disease of adulthood, but there has been an alarming increase in Type 2 in children. In fact, for children, the risk of developing Type 2 diabetes today is statistically almost equal to that of developing Type 1: 1 in 400. An increase in obesity combined with a sedentary lifestyle is usually cited as the reason for the increase.

IMPAIRED GLUCOSE HOMEOSTASIS
A metabolic stage intermediate between normal glucose homeostasis and diabetes. It is a risk factor for diabetes and cardiovascular disease and includes both an impaired fasting blood glucose level and an impaired response to glucose (glucose tolerance).

GESTATIONAL DIABETES MELLITUS
This occurs in roughly 7% of all pregnancies. It is considered a risk factor for the development of Type 2.

OTHER TYPES
Between 1% and 2% of all cases of diabetes are due to a variety of rare causes such as the genetic beta cell defects known collectively as Maturity Onset Diabetes of Youth (MODY), genetic defects in insulin action, pancreatic cancer, the effects of cystic fibrosis, and pancreas damage from drugs, chemicals, or infection.

Type 1 or Type 2 diabetes—because there is mounting evidence that the earlier a person with Type 1 diabetes begins insulin therapy, the better.

"There is recent data that suggests that the early institution of insulin therapy preserves residual beta cell function," Dr. Schatz says. "So if you were to err and not use insulin—for instance, by trying an oral agent—the patient would lose beta cell function faster. If you can preserve beta cell function, we know that diabetes management is much easier."

"We're all taught in medical school that in Type 1 diabetes, after a short time, you don't make any insulin," Dr. Hirsch concurs. "But I have patients with Type 1 diabetes who are making insulin decades after they were diagnosed. I actually have a patient with classical Type 1 diabetes diagnosed in her 20's, whose physician—fortunately for her—started her on insulin 31 years ago. She's *still* making some insulin 31 years later.

"It appears that when you start a patient with Type 1 diabetes on insulin, you are doing something positive to their immune system so that you are slowing down the attack on the beta cells."

The "honeymoon" period, during which the remaining beta cells increase their insulin output, is a well-known phenomenon in childhood Type 1 diabetes, but it seems it may also occur in adults with Type 1 diabetes and may last for much longer.

"We have to start thinking of insulin therapy not just to lower blood sugar, but to modulate the immune system," says Hirsch.

How do you tell?

The diagnosis of diabetes, particularly as to which type, requires a combination of science and observation.

The science is straightforward. "To make a diagnosis of diabetes," Dr. Schatz says, "you need one of three criteria: a fasting blood sugar on two occasions greater than 125 mg/dl; the symptoms of diabetes—excessive urination, thirst, and hunger—coupled with a blood sugar greater than 200 mg/dl; or a glucose tolerance test that produces a blood sugar level greater than 200 mg/dl in two hours."

Beyond those criteria, especially when Type 1 diabetes might be masquerading as Type 2, observation becomes important. Here are some of the factors that might go into a diagnosis:

■ Is the person overweight? Obesity and sedentary lifestyle are possible, though not foolproof, indicators for Type 2 diabetes.

■ Is there a family history of diabetes? While 90% of people who have Type 1 diabetes have no family history of diabetes, most of those with Type 2 do have a family history of the disease. The evidence for a genetic basis for Type 2 is mounting: 39% of people with Type 2 diabetes have at least one parent with

Type 2 diabetes, identical twins tend to both develop it if one does, and the lifetime risk for a first-degree relative (parent, sibling, or child) of someone with Type 2 diabetes is five to ten times higher than if there were no family history.

■ Age is certainly a consideration, but it can't be relied on for a diagnosis.

■ Darkened, velvety patches—or *acanthosis nigricans*— on the back of the neck, armpits, genital area, or groin, are a physical marker of the high insulin levels characteristic of insulin resistance and Type 2 diabetes.

■ Having had gestational diabetes (diabetes during pregnancy) is a risk factor for Type 2 diabetes.

■ High blood levels of triglycerides and low levels of HDL cholesterol (the "good" cholesterol) are stronger predictors for Type 2 diabetes, as is high blood pressure.

■ Urine ketones are a stronger indication for Type 1 diabetes.

At one time it was thought that blood levels of C-peptide (a by-product of insulin production) were helpful in distinguishing between Type 1 and Type 2.

"The old prevailing theory was that patients with Type 2 diabetes had higher C-peptides, particularly at diagnosis," Dr. Schatz says. "I don't think there's enough data to say that C-peptide will truly distinguish Type 1 from Type 2. There has been some overlap, particularly at diagnosis, and even in a Type 2 patient, the C-peptide level may not be as high as you might expect.

"Moreover, you have higher C-peptides in adults than in children, even with Type 1 diabetes."

How about "Type 3"?

It may be that Type 1 and Type 2 are not mutually exclusive, which would muddy the classification debate even further. Dr. Hirsch describes a subset of people in which both types may be present as people with "Type 3" diabetes.

"This refers to patients who come down with classical Type 1 diabetes in childhood," he explains, "but have a family history of Type 2 diabetes or a family history of the syndrome of insulin resistance. The syndrome of insulin resistance may be present in as much as 20% of the American population.

"So when someone who develops Type 1 diabetes at the age of 10 has a parent with Type 2 diabetes, a couple of aunts and uncles with high triglycerides

and low HDL, and maybe some older relatives who have premature coronary artery disease or high blood pressure, it's not surprising that this same individual begins to develop the classic obesity of Type 2 diabetes as he reaches his 40's and 50's.

"We know a lot about these people from the Diabetes Control and Complications Trial. When you looked at the top 25% of people who gained weight on intensive insulin therapy, they gained a *lot* of weight, and they have a family history of Type 2 diabetes. So you're giving these people insulin for their Type 1 diabetes, but you have to give them huge amounts of insulin, because they have a genetic predisposition to insulin resistance.

"These people have classic Type 1 diabetes *and* they have Type 2 diabetes. I call this 'Type 3' diabetes."

If both types of diabetes are in fact present, Dr. Hirsch believes there is anecdotal evidence that insulin sensitizers, which help reduce insulin resistance, might be helpful.

Need for more accurate diagnoses

The difference between Type 1 and Type 2 diabetes is very important today for treatment decisions, and Dr. Hirsch, for one, believes physicians could do much better distinguishing between the two. "I can't tell you how many patients with Type 1 diabetes—classic Type 1 diabetes—come in with pills for Type 2 diabetes," he says. "There is at least a theoretical risk that giving sulfonylureas, a common type of oral agent for Type 2 diabetes, to people with Type 1 diabetes hastens the destruction of the beta cells." [Editor's note: Sulfonylureas include chlorpropamide, glimepiride, glipizide, glyburide, tolazamide, and tolbutamide. These are sold under various brand names.]

"The clinician should strongly suspect Type 1 diabetes, particularly in younger adult patients who are not overweight and who are failing a trial of diet and exercise or oral agents," Dr. Schatz says. "Screening for islet-related antibodies should be routine when there is any reason to suspect a Type 1 diagnosis."

The next frontier of diabetes research will make the correct diagnosis absolutely critical. "Within the next 10 years," Dr. Hirsch predicts, "we're going to be able to delay the onset of both Type 1 and Type 2 diabetes. But you can't use a specific therapy unless you know what type of diabetes you're targeting." ❏

DEBUNKING THE TOP DIABETES MYTHS

by LilyAnn Jeu and Ingrid Strauch

Isn't it amazing when something you *know* to be true turns out not to be? Sometimes, this can be a big disappointment, like finding out the tooth fairy doesn't exist. Other times, it can be a big relief.

When it comes to diabetes, there are a lot of myths and false beliefs out there. While believing some of these myths may have no practical effect on your life, believing others may cause you to restrict your lifestyle unnecessarily or, worse, make controlling your blood glucose levels more difficult.

To make sure you know what's a myth and what's a fact, we checked with the experts on some of the more commonly held false beliefs about diabetes. We hope this list brings you more relief than disappointment.

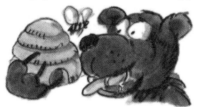

MYTH 1. Eating too much sugar causes diabetes.
FACT. Since diabetes is characterized by high blood sugar levels, it's not surprising that people once assumed that eating too much sugar leads to diabetes. However, the sugar you measure in your blood is glucose, not sucrose, or table sugar. The body produces glucose when it digests either simple sugars such as sucrose or more complex starches.

While eating too much sugar cannot be singled out as the cause of diabetes, eating too much food may well contribute to the onset of Type 2 diabetes. That's because consuming too many calories leads to weight gain, which can lead to obesity. And obesity is one of the most important risk factors for the development of Type 2 diabetes, especially in people with a genetic predisposition or other risk factors. (In contrast, most cases of Type 1 diabetes are believed to be caused by an autoimmune reaction, in which the immune system attacks and destroys the insulin-producing beta cells of the pancreas.) Excess body weight decreases the body's sensitivity to insulin and increases insulin resistance.

Researchers have found an association between Type 2 diabetes and a diet high in processed carbohydrates and low in dietary fiber. In a study reported in *The Journal of the American Medical Association* in 1997, researchers followed more than 65,000 women for six years. They found that the women who reported eating a diet high in refined starches (such as white bread, potatoes, and white rice) but low in fiber were two and a half times more likely to develop Type 2 diabetes than women who reported eating less refined starches and more fiber from whole-grain cereals.

According to the researchers, these results make sense because highly processed foods are digested and absorbed quickly, causing a surge in blood glucose and, consequently, insulin. In contrast, fiber slows the rate of digestion, preventing surges in blood glucose and insulin levels. The researchers suggest that consuming a diet high in minimally processed grains may help prevent diabetes. Other studies have suggested that such a diet may help people who already have Type 2 diabetes to better control their blood sugar levels.

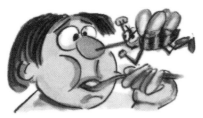

MYTH 2. People with diabetes should *never* eat sugar.
FACT. In the past, people with diabetes were told to avoid or strictly limit sugar because it was believed that any amount of sugar (including table sugar, honey, and other caloric sweeteners) would cause blood sugar levels to rise dramatically. However, studies conducted in the 1980's showed that sugary foods do not raise blood glucose any more than starchy foods (such as bread or pasta) containing the same amount of carbohydrate. In other words, the studies found that all carbohydrates, not just simple sugars, raise blood sugar.

As a result of such research, in 1994, the American Diabetes Association announced its recommendation that people with diabetes count the total amount of carbohydrate in their diet rather than just limit the amount of simple sugars. Diabetes professionals now consider sugar just another form of carbohydrate that can be enjoyed in moderation when included in a meal plan designed to keep blood glucose levels within the range recommended for an individual.

Although sugar is not the absolute diabetes no-no it once was, a diet high in simple sugars is not considered healthful. For one thing, sugar contains calories but few nutrients. Filling up on sugary foods may cause some people to skimp on nutrient-dense foods and, consequently, to consume inadequate amounts of some vitamins and minerals. In addition, high-sugar foods often tend to be high-fat foods, and consuming too many calories and too much fat can contribute to obesity and other health problems. And, of course, sugar promotes tooth decay, something we can all do without.

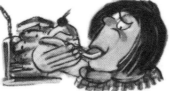

MYTH 3. It is OK for people with diabetes to eat as many "sugar-free" foods as they want.
FACT. "Sugar-free" means that a product contains no sugar or forms of sugar, such as dextrose, honey, or corn syrup. But it does not mean that a food is calorie-free or even carbohydrate-free. And anything that contains carbohydrate can raise your blood sugar level. To figure out how a sugar-free food fits into your meal plan, read the Nutrition Facts label on the package.

Some sugar-free products contain *sugar alcohols,* naturally occurring substances that are commercially produced as sugar substitutes. Examples of sugar alcohols include sorbitol, mannitol, and xylitol. These ingredients are absorbed slowly and incompletely, usually causing a smaller rise in blood sugar than glucose or sucrose and thereby not increasing a person's insulin needs. However, sugar alcohols contain 2 to 4 calories per gram, and, when eaten in large amounts, they can cause gastrointestinal problems such as bloating, stomach cramps, and diarrhea in some people.

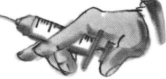

MYTH 4. Using insulin means a person has Type 1 diabetes.
FACT. It's true that all people with Type 1 diabetes must inject insulin, but it's also true that as many as 30% to 40% of people with Type 2 diabetes inject insulin, as well.

Insulin is produced by the beta cells of the pancreas. This hormone helps transport blood glucose into body cells for energy. Excess glucose is stored in the liver and released when a person's blood sugar level falls. In Type 1 diabetes, the beta cells lose their ability to produce insulin, so insulin must be injected for the body to use the energy it takes in.

In Type 2 diabetes, the beta cells remain able to produce some insulin, but other factors prevent the body from using insulin effectively, leading to high blood glucose levels. One of these factors is *insulin resistance,* a decrease in the body's ability to respond to insulin. To overcome insulin resistance and move enough glucose into tissues, the pancreas has to release more insulin.

Another cause of high blood glucose levels in Type 2 diabetes is overproduction of glucose by the liver. Insulin keeps the liver from releasing too much stored glucose between meals and during the night, when blood glucose levels normally fall. But when there is an inadequate supply of insulin to the liver, it pumps high levels of glucose into the bloodstream. Type 2 diabetes results when the pancreas is no longer able to produce enough insulin to keep up with the increased glucose load.

While some people with Type 2 diabetes are able to lower their insulin resistance and their blood glucose levels by modifying their diet, increasing their physical activity, and taking oral diabetes medicines, others need to inject insulin when these options do not provide adequate blood glucose control.

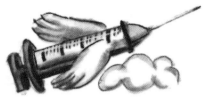

MYTH 5. Sometimes diabetes goes away.
FACT. Unfortunately, once a person develops Type 1 or Type 2 diabetes, it's here to stay. However, there are some circumstances in which it seems to go away, at least for a while.

The symptoms of Type 1 diabetes appear when about 90% of the beta cells in the pancreas have been destroyed. In some cases, when a newly diagnosed person begins taking insulin, the remaining beta cells temporarily regain the ability to produce insulin, reducing and sometimes eliminating the need for injected insulin. This period of remission is often called the "honeymoon period" because it is a temporary state, generally lasting from one month to one year. Diabetes symptoms, and the need to inject insulin, reappear after this brief period.

In Type 2 diabetes, some people are able to maintain near-normal blood glucose levels through diet and exercise alone, making it seem as though they don't have diabetes. But if these individuals were to stray from their diet and exercise regimen, the symptoms of diabetes would reappear. In addition, bodily changes, such as aging, increased insulin resistance, changes in hormone status (for women), illness, and injury, can eventually make it necessary for these people to take diabetes pills or inject insulin.

The only case in which diabetes can really disappear is *gestational diabetes,* a type of diabetes that develops in about 7% of pregnancies. During pregnancy, levels of the hormones estrogen, progesterone, and human placental lactogen rise. These hormones, along with weight gain during pregnancy, increase insulin resistance, placing greater demands on the pancreas to produce sufficient amounts of insulin. Although gestational diabetes goes away in up to 97% of the women who develop it, having this type of diabetes increases a woman's risk of developing Type 2 diabetes later in life.

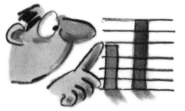

MYTH 6. There are different degrees of diabetes. Some people have a bad case of diabetes, and others have mild diabetes.

FACT. Some people refer to their diabetes as "having a touch of sugar," but the truth is that you either have diabetes or you don't. Certainly some people have an easier time controlling their blood glucose levels for reasons we don't always understand. But no matter how difficult or how easy it is to keep your blood glucose levels in the desired range, it's important to make the effort to do it. That's because chronic high blood sugar levels increase your chances of developing complications of the eyes, nerves, blood vessels, and kidneys.

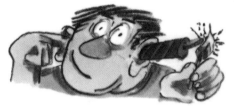

MYTH 7. Diabetes can be caused by severe stress.
FACT. While many people can trace their diagnosis of diabetes back to a particularly stressful time or event, stress does not cause diabetes. However, severe stress can unmask the symptoms of diabetes in people who are predisposed to developing diabetes.

During periods of stress, the body releases the hormones epinephrine, cortisone, and growth hormone as part of the "fight-or-flight" response. These hormones raise blood glucose levels in preparation for the brain and muscles to respond to the stressor, and they increase the body's need for insulin. In a person whose pancreas has lost the ability to produce sufficient amounts of insulin, elevated levels of these stress hormones may tax the pancreas enough to reveal diabetes as an underlying problem.

Just as stress can reveal an undiagnosed case of diabetes, it can also disrupt blood glucose control in a person already diagnosed with diabetes. So while stress management will not cure diabetes, relieving stress helps lower levels of stress hormones and helps people with diabetes maintain control of blood glucose levels.

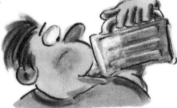

MYTH 8. People with diabetes cannot drink alcohol.
FACT. For people whose diabetes is well controlled and who do not have other health problems or take medicines that would restrict their use of alcohol, moderate alcohol intake is considered OK by most health experts. Moderate intake has been defined as no more than two drinks per day for men and no more than

one drink per day for women, according to the *2000 Dietary Guidelines for Americans* compiled by the U.S. Department of Health and Human Services.

However, before you include alcohol as part of your daily routine, keep in mind that alcohol can cause low blood sugar, especially when you drink on an empty stomach. This is because the liver, the chief organ that processes alcohol, normally releases stored glucose into the bloodstream when blood sugar levels fall. But when the liver is busy processing alcohol, it may not be able to release sufficient amounts of glucose to meet your body's needs. Eating when you drink helps slow the absorption of alcohol into the bloodstream, making it less likely to affect your liver's ability to respond to dips in blood sugar level. People who inject insulin or take sulfonylureas should drink alcohol only with meals because alcohol on an empty stomach can magnify the blood-glucose-lowering effects of these drugs.

People who take sulfonylureas also need to be on the lookout for *alcohol-intolerance reactions.* Such reactions typically cause headache, flushing or a tingling sensation in the face, nausea, and light-headedness within 10 to 30 minutes of consuming a beverage or medicine containing alcohol. Alcohol-intolerance reactions are more likely to occur in people taking older types of sulfonylureas such as chlorpropamide (brand name Diabinese) or tolbutamide (Orinase). Avoiding alcohol (or speaking with your doctor about switching to a different diabetes medicine) is the only way to avoid alcohol intolerance.

Even if alcohol intolerance isn't a problem for you, there are other reasons to drink alcohol only in moderation. Studies have shown that consuming larger amounts of alcohol with food can cause high blood glucose levels. And alcohol contains calories that must be accounted for in your meal plan. One gram of alcohol provides 7 calories, so a typical 12-ounce serving of beer, 4-ounce glass of wine, or 1½-ounce serving of distilled liquor, each of which contains about 12 grams of alcohol, provides 84 calories only from the alcohol. When incorporating alcohol into your diabetes meal plan, you can generally substitute alcohol calories for fat calories.

Alcoholic beverages can also contain significant amounts of carbohydrate. Regular beer, sweet wines, and wine coolers tend to contain more carbohydrate than light beer, dry wines, and liquors. In fact, sweeter wines and beers can contain as much as one starch exchange or carbohydrate choice (15 grams of carbohydrate) per serving. Since alcoholic beverages do not carry Nutrition Facts labels, you will need to consult a reference book such as *Encyclopedia of Food Values* by Corinne T. Netzer (published by Dell Publishing, New York, 1997) to find the carbohydrate content of your

beverage of choice. For people with access to the Internet, the Nutrient Data Laboratory Web site (www.nal.usda.gov/fnic/foodcomp) has food composition data for some 6,000 foods.

In addition to directly affecting your blood glucose level, alcohol can also impair your judgment, making it difficult to follow your diabetes-management plan and to recognize the signs of low blood sugar. So if you do decide to drink, make sure that you do not drink to the point of intoxication.

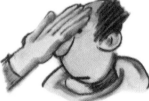

MYTH 9. A person with diabetes can tell whether blood sugar is too high or too low based on how he or she feels.

FACT. If only managing diabetes were that easy. Unfortunately, it's not. The only reliable way to know your blood sugar level at any given time is to check it on your home monitor.

While it is impossible to know your blood sugar level based on how you feel, there are certain symptoms of low and high blood glucose that should signal you to check. Some of the classic symptoms of low blood sugar (or *hypoglycemia*) are rapid heartbeat, sweating, shakiness, confusion or loss of concentration, and irritability. The symptoms of high blood glucose (or *hyperglycemia*) are more difficult to detect, but they often include increased thirst and urination and blurry vision.

When blood sugar levels fall below normal, the hormones epinephrine and cortisone are released in an attempt to raise blood sugar levels. These are the hormones that cause the symptoms of low blood sugar. When low blood sugar occurs frequently, these hormones become depleted and are no longer produced when blood sugar levels fall. This can lead to *hypoglycemia unawareness,* in which a person no longer experiences the classic early symptoms of low blood sugar. In most cases, hypoglycemia unawareness can be reversed by setting target blood glucose levels to a higher range for a short time. Your doctor can help you do this by adjusting the amount of insulin you inject.

Learning to recognize the symptoms of low or high blood glucose levels is important, but it's only the first step toward correcting a possible problem. The second step is checking your blood sugar level. Monitoring is especially important when you do not feel well or if you have recently made changes in your diabetes-care regimen. Only after you have checked are you ready to make an informed decision about what to do next.

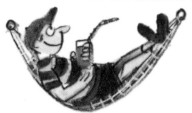

MYTH 10. People with diabetes should take it easy and not do any strenuous exercise. Being too active might make their diabetes worse.
FACT. To the contrary, exercise is an important part of diabetes treatment. Exercise can help maintain diabetes control by lowering blood glucose levels, increasing insulin sensitivity, and decreasing insulin resistance. It can help delay the onset or development of diabetes complications, and it can sometimes help a person manage the pain and discomfort of complications once they have developed. In addition, exercise can improve blood flow, strengthen the heart and bones, and improve a person's range of motion.

That said, exercising with diabetes does require some caution and planning. Before you begin any exercise program, check with your doctor about spe-cial precautions you need to take when exercising, especially if you have high blood pressure, heart disease, retinopathy, any type of neuropathy (nerve damage), or any foot problems, such as loss of sensation in the feet. Some types of exercise are not appropriate for people with certain diabetic complications. (For more information about your options, see "Exercising with Complications" on page 258.) How strenuously you should exercise depends on your current state of health and fitness, but just about everyone can benefit from exercise.

Any questions?

For those of you who were recently diagnosed with diabetes, we hope this article answered some of the questions you may have had about diabetes. For diabetes veterans, we hope you learned some useful information that will make managing your diabetes a little easier.

New information (and misinformation) about diabetes is published all the time. We encourage you to discuss what you read about or hear about with your health-care team. Your team members can help you separate fact from fiction, and getting the facts is the best way to learn how to manage your diabetes. ❏

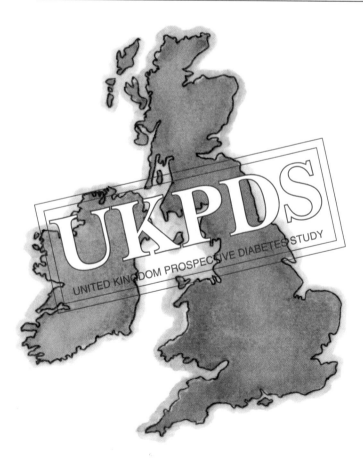

BIG NEWS FOR TYPE 2'S

by Jacqueline Laks Gorman

I n September of 1998, at the annual meeting of the European Association for the Study of Diabetes, doctors and researchers heard the results of a 20-year study—the longest and largest study ever conducted on diabetes. The results of the long-awaited study, also published in September in two prestigious medical journals, gave new insights into the treatment of Type 2 diabetes.

The study was called the United Kingdom Prospective Diabetes Study, referred to as the UKPDS. It began in 23 medical centers in Britain in 1977 and ran until 1997, involving 5,102 people with Type 2 diabetes. Doctors had hoped that the UKPDS would provide them with answers to questions they had long asked about Type 2 diabetes and the best way to treat it. Earlier research, most notably the landmark Diabetes Control and Complications Trial (DCCT), concluded in 1993, had shown the clear importance of controlling blood glucose levels in people with Type 1 diabetes. But how important was this tight control in those with Type 2 diabetes? In the long run, would it give them better health and fewer complications than the standard dietary treatment?

The UKPDS finally gave doctors the answers to some of their most important questions.

What doctors wanted to know

There are two types of diabetes. Type 1 diabetes usually appears before the age of 35. In people with Type 1 diabetes insulin is no longer produced by the pancreas, so it must be injected. Type 2 diabetes usually occurs in people over the age of 40. They have high blood glucose levels either because the pancreas does not produce enough insulin or their body tissues have lost the ability to respond to insulin or both. Most people with Type 2 diabetes control their blood glucose levels by modifying their diet, exercising, and taking oral diabetes drugs; a significant number, though, take insulin injections.

Doctors know—largely as a result of the DCCT—that intensive control of blood glucose levels in people with Type 1 diabetes dramatically reduces the risk of such diabetes-related complications as diabetic retinopathy (eye disease), diabetic nephropathy (kidney disease), and diabetic neuropathy (nerve damage). But the effects of tight blood glucose control in people with Type 2 diabetes had never been absolutely proved.

Doctors strongly suspected that the findings of the DCCT would also hold true in Type 2 diabetes—but they had no proof. And if tight control was proven beneficial in Type 2 diabetes, which drugs would be best? Would any have associated risks or dangers? In addition, doctors wanted to know, what would be the effect of controlling high blood pressure, a common and worrisome problem in many people with Type 2 diabetes? Would this also reduce the risk of diabetic complications?

The study and its parts

The UKPDS was no simple study. Rather, it had several parts to it, each of which was reported in September 1998 in separate articles in two professional publications, the *British Medical Journal* and *The Lancet*.

The UKPDS was launched in 1977 to determine whether intensive blood glucose control in people with Type 2 diabetes would reduce the risk of macrovascular complications (those such as heart attacks, involving the body's large blood vessels) and microvascular complications (those such as retinopathy, nephropathy, and neuropathy, involving smaller blood vessels). If it did, researchers wanted to know, would any particular treatment be best? This became the first part of the UKPDS, referred to as UKPDS 33.

It compared the results of conventional dietary treatment with tight blood glucose control, using either sulfonylurea drugs or insulin.

The second part, called UKPDS 34, compared the results of tight blood glucose control with either conventional treatment or the drug metformin (brand name Glucophage) in overweight people specifically. The third part, UKPDS 38, looked at tight blood pressure control and the risks of complications. The fourth part, UKPDS 39, looked at two specific blood pressure drugs and the risk of complications. (There was also a fifth report published, UKPDS 40, which examined the cost-effectiveness of improved blood pressure control in people with hypertension.)

All of the parts involved British citizens with newly diagnosed Type 2 diabetes. Let's look at the four major parts of the study.

UKPDS 33

In 1977, British researchers at 23 hospitals began recruiting volunteers for the study. Participants had to be newly diagnosed with Type 2 diabetes, between the ages of 25 and 65, with a fasting plasma glucose (FPG) level above 6 millimoles per liter (mmol/liter) measured on two mornings, one to three weeks apart; 6 mmol/liter is about the same as 108 mg/dl. None could have experienced any diabetic complications previously. Of 7,616 people referred, 5,102 were recruited. These people attended a monthly UKPDS clinic for three months and were told to follow a low-fat, high-fiber diet with half of the calories from carbohydrates. Then, their FPG levels were tested again. Those with an FPG lower than 6 mmol/liter or greater than 15 mmol/liter (about 270 mg/dl) were excluded from the study. This left 4,209 eligible subjects. Of these, 1,704 who were overweight were also included in a separate study (UKPDS 34); 342 of the 1,704 were given special treatment (described below) and were therefore not counted in UKPDS 33. This left 3,867 people in UKPDS 33. Their median age was 54, and 61% were male.

The volunteers were randomly assigned to receive conventional dietary treatment (1,138 subjects) or intensive blood glucose control treatment with either insulin (1,156 subjects) or a sulfonylurea drug (1,573 subjects). The sulfonylureas—which are commonly used oral drugs that work by stimulating the release of insulin from the beta cells of the pancreas—were chlorpropamide, glibenclamide, or glipizide. Participants attended morning clinics every three months (beginning in 1990, every four months), at which their blood glucose, blood pressure, and weight were measured. Periodically, blood samples were taken for testing triglycerides, cholesterol, and so on. Full physical exams were done every three years. The study ended in 1997.

At the end of the study, the researchers found that the group receiving intensive treatment, compared with the group receiving conventional dietary treatment, had an 11% reduction in glycosylated hemoglobin A_{1c} (HbA_{1c})—a measure of the red blood cells attached to glucose molecules, which indicates how well blood glucose levels are being controlled. Clearly, intensive treatment controlled blood glucose levels more effectively. The intensive treatment group also had a substantial reduction (25%) in the risk of microvascular complications, especially eye problems requiring a treatment called retinal photocoagulation. There was also a 16% reduction in the risk of heart attacks. Intensive treatment indeed seemed to have helped people avoid some common diabetic complications.

There were no differences found between the conventional and intensive treatment groups regarding the risk of diabetes-related mortality or overall mortality. People in the intensive treatment group did have greater weight gain and were more prone to hypoglycemia (low blood sugar). All of the drugs used in the intensive treatment group were found to be equally effective at preventing complications, and none proved dangerous. However, when oral drugs were not sufficient to control glucose levels, people were then switched over to insulin.

UKPDS 34

In UKPDS 34, 1,704 overweight people recruited for UKPDS 33 were also studied separately. Their median age was 53, and 54% were female. Overweight was defined as 120% of ideal body weight. The researchers wanted to study heavy people separately because many people with Type 2 diabetes are overweight.

These people were divided into three groups. One group (411 persons) received conventional dietary treatment, another group (951 persons) received intensive blood glucose control with a sulfonylurea (chlorpropamide or glibenclamide) or insulin, and the last group (342 persons, who were not counted in UKPDS 33) received intensive treatment with the drug metformin. Doctors were anxious to know about metformin's effects for two reasons. Classified as a biguanide drug, it acts differently from sulfonylureas, interfering with the liver's release of glucose but not affecting the pancreas. Also, sulfonylureas tend to make people gain weight and can cause hypoglycemia, while metformin does not.

And indeed, metformin proved beneficial for the overweight study volunteers. Compared with the group receiving conventional treatment, those receiving metformin had lower HbA_{1c} levels, a 32% reduc-

tion in the risk of diabetic complications, a 42% reduction in the risk of diabetes-related deaths, and a 36% reduction in the risk of deaths from all causes. Metformin also caused less weight gain and fewer episodes of hypoglycemia than the sulfonylureas or insulin and was more effective than those agents in preventing diabetes-related complications, deaths from all causes, and strokes. Based on these results, the researchers concluded that metformin could well be the recommended first-line treatment of choice in people with Type 2 diabetes who are overweight.

The only danger found was an increased risk of diabetes-related deaths if metformin was added to sulfonylureas that people were already taking—something that warranted further study, since both are often prescribed together.

UKPDS 38

In UKPDS 38, researchers looked specifically at people with Type 2 diabetes who had high blood pressure. Diabetes and hypertension are often associated, and both have significant risks for heart and kidney disease. Would tightly controlling blood pressure prevent diabetes-related macrovascular and microvascular complications?

The researchers studied 1,148 subjects who had been recruited as part of the overall UKPDS and therefore were all newly diagnosed with Type 2 diabetes. To be in this part of the study, all also had to have hypertension. Their mean age was 56, and their mean blood pressure at the beginning of the study was 160/94 mm Hg. The subjects were randomly assigned to two groups. The first group, 758 people, received tight control of blood pressure with either the drug captopril, an angiotensin-converting enzyme (ACE) inhibitor (400 people), or the drug atenolol, a beta-blocker (358 people). Both are commonly used antihypertensive drugs. The second group, of 390 people, was given less tight blood pressure control without ACE inhibitors or beta-blockers.

The study lasted for nine years. When it ended, the group receiving tight blood pressure control had significantly lower blood pressure than the group receiving less tight control—a mean of 144/82 compared with 154/87. And they had a significantly lower risk of complications. Overall, the tight control group had a 24% reduction in the risk of macrovascular disease, including heart attack, sudden death, stroke, and peripheral vascular disease. There was a 34% reduction in risk of diabetic complications, a 32% reduction in risk of deaths related to diabetes, a 44% reduction in risk of stroke, and a 56% reduction in risk of heart failure. There was also a 37% reduction in the risk of microvascular disease, especially eye problems requiring retinal photocoagulation. And subjects had a 47% reduction in the deterioration of visual sharpness. The researchers stated that as far as they knew, this was the first study to show that tight blood pressure control reduced the risk of complications from diabetic eye disease in people with Type 2 diabetes.

Since tight blood pressure control "substantially reduces the risk of death and complications due to diabetes," the researchers concluded, "the management of blood pressure should have a high priority in the treatment of Type 2 diabetes."

UKPDS 39

In UKPDS 39, the researchers examined the subjects in UKPDS 38 who received different tight blood pressure treatment—the 400 people receiving the ACE inhibitor captopril and the 358 people receiving the beta-blocker atenolol—to see if either type of drug had specific advantages or disadvantages regarding macrovascular and microvascular complications. They discovered that both drugs were equally effective in lowering blood pressure and reducing the risk of fatal and nonfatal diabetic complications, diabetes-related deaths, heart failure, and retinal problems.

What does all this mean?

What do all of these findings mean for people with Type 2 diabetes? More than likely, they mean that doctors will look closely at placing them on programs to intensively control both their blood glucose levels and high blood pressure.

Intensive treatment of high blood pressure was convincingly shown to be important in reducing diabetic complications. The specific drug used to lower blood pressure seemed to be less important than the actual act of controlling hypertension itself.

Intensive treatment of blood glucose levels may be more of a problem. The UKPDS did confirm that the results of the DCCT in people with Type 1 diabetes also hold true for Type 2 diabetes. But though it may help prevent complications, intensive treatment is not easy. It requires commitment, work, and dedication on the part of the person with diabetes—frequent self-monitoring of blood glucose levels, more visits to the doctor, and more frequent injections and/or adjustments of medication. It also carries the risk of greater weight gain and more episodes of hypoglycemia. But if the payoff is improved overall health and a longer, better life, it's clearly worth it. ❑

INSULIN RESISTANCE
AT THE ROOT OF TYPE 2 DIABETES
by Robert S. Dinsmoor

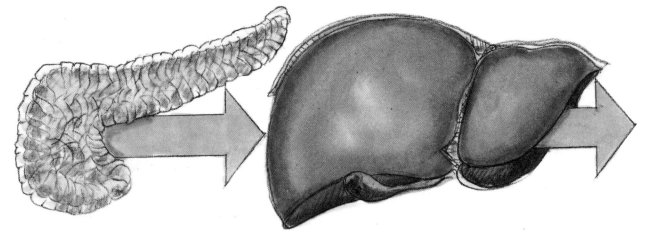

Insulin resistance is one of the most important underlying causes of high blood sugar in Type 2 diabetes. Yet many people with diabetes do not know what insulin resistance is. In fact, a nation-wide survey released by the American Association of Diabetes Educators in November of 1999 found that nearly two-thirds of the more than 1,000 people with Type 2 diabetes surveyed did not understand—or had never heard of—insulin resistance.

What is more, the survey found that the respondents who couldn't define insulin resistance had less control over their blood glucose and were less likely to be taking one of the newer diabetes drugs that specifically work against insulin resistance. These drugs, called thiazolidinediones (TZD's), include rosiglita-zone (brand name Avandia) and pioglitazone (Actos).

While the most obvious consequence of insulin resistance is high blood sugar, it is believed to have other effects on the body, as well. For example, it may play a major role in the high rate of cardiovascular disease among people who have it. As scientists learn more about insulin resistance, they also learn more about how to combat it. Among the tools already shown to reduce insulin resistance are weight loss, exercise, and a growing arsenal of drugs, including the TZD's. Since greater knowledge of insulin resistance seems to be related to improved diabetes control, let's take a look at the basics of insulin resistance and its treatment.

What is insulin resistance?

Simply stated, insulin resistance is a condition in which insulin can't do its job effectively, so a given amount of insulin lowers blood sugar less than would be expected. To understand this in more depth, it is helpful to understand what insulin normally does in the body.

Insulin is a hormone secreted by the beta cells of the pancreas that helps to regulate the way the body uses glucose. Its main job is to allow glucose in the blood to enter the cells of the body, where it can be used for energy. Insulin also controls the rate at which glucose is produced and secreted by the liver. Glucose is stored in the liver in a form called *glycogen*. When blood glucose levels drop, the liver converts glycogen to glucose and releases it into the bloodstream. When there is enough glucose in the bloodstream, insulin secreted by the pancreas signals the liver to shut down glucose production. In people who don't have diabetes, the pancreas continually measures blood glucose levels and responds by secreting just the right amount of insulin.

In a person with insulin resistance, the cells of the body are unable to take up as much glucose from the bloodstream as they should, even when there's a lot of insulin in the bloodstream. That is, the cells *resist* the insulin. On top of that, the liver may continue to secrete a lot of glucose into the bloodstream even when it isn't needed and despite the presence of lots of insulin. By some estimates, some 10% to 25% of the general population may be insulin-resistant, but there are no real statistics on how many people have the condition.

What causes insulin resistance?

The short answer is that insulin resistance appears to be a product of both our genes and our environment. Certain genes predispose certain people to develop insulin resistance, but other factors such as inactivity, weight gain, and chronically high blood sugar levels trigger insulin resistance in susceptible individuals.

Scientists are still trying to determine what causes insulin resistance on the cellular and molecular levels. Thanks to the tools of molecular biology, they have already learned a lot. Previously, considerable research focused on the insulin receptors found on muscle and fat cells throughout the body. Normally, insulin binds to these receptors, triggering a number of complex chemical reactions within cells. It used to be thought that diabetes resulted from abnormal binding to these receptors, but this is no longer believed to be the case.

Most researchers now believe that insulin resistance is caused by abnormalities in the chemical reactions that happen within the cells themselves—what are known as "postbinding abnormalities." They have identified abnormalities in a number of chemical pathways that could cause insulin resistance, as well as some of the genes that cause them. For example, researchers are now paying considerable attention to substances called *glucose transporters*, which move glucose into cells. Studies have shown that at least some insulin-resistant individuals are deficient in a glucose transporter called GLUT4, whose activity is normally regulated by the amount of insulin present.

Conditions associated with insulin resistance

Type 2 diabetes may be the most familiar condition associated with insulin resistance, but it isn't the only one. Two related conditions are impaired fasting glucose and impaired glucose tolerance. Insulin resistance is also associated with gestational diabetes, heart disease, and a condition known as polycystic ovary syndrome.

The exact role of insulin resistance in these medical conditions is unclear. While some researchers believe it to be the primary underlying cause, others believe it to be the result of some other disease process. Let's take a look at each condition individually.

Type 2 diabetes. The two main problems in Type 2 diabetes are insulin resistance and a defect in the way insulin is secreted: Specifically, the pancreas doesn't secrete enough insulin fast enough in response to meals, when large amounts of glucose enter the bloodstream. This leads to long-term high blood sugar as well as to *hyperinsulinemia* (too much insulin in the bloodstream) as the pancreas tries to compensate for the high blood sugar by churning out extra insulin.

Medical researchers disagree as to whether the underlying cause of most cases of Type 2 diabetes is insulin resistance or a defect in insulin secretion, but either condition may lead to the other, and both conditions can worsen in a vicious circle. For example, insulin resistance can lead to higher blood glucose levels, especially following meals. This causes the pancreas to secrete more insulin to compensate. At first, this may keep blood sugar levels in the normal range. But eventually, the overworked beta cells become damaged and produce less and less insulin, and high blood sugar levels ensue.

Prediabetic states. Insulin resistance is also found in two "prediabetic states" called impaired fasting glucose (IFG) and impaired glucose tolerance (IGT). Both of these conditions are defined by the American Diabetes Association in its guidelines on diagnosis and classification of diabetes mellitus.

Both conditions are defined by blood glucose levels that are too high to be considered normal, but not high enough to be considered diabetic. Impaired fasting glucose is diagnosed on the basis of a fasting plasma glucose level of greater than or equal to 110 mg/dl but less than 126 mg/dl. Impaired glucose tolerance is defined by plasma glucose levels greater than or equal to 140 mg/dl but less than 200 mg/dl two hours after ingesting 75 grams of glucose as part of an oral glucose tolerance test.

Both IFG and IGT are thought to put people at risk for Type 2 diabetes. In addition, studies suggest that people with these conditions, just like people with Type 2 diabetes, are at significantly greater risk for heart disease.

Gestational diabetes. Diabetes that starts during pregnancy is called gestational diabetes. It tends to occur in women who are already at greater risk for developing Type 2 diabetes by virtue of being overweight, having a close family member with diabetes, or being a member of a high-risk ethnic group (African-American, Asian-American, Hispanic American, Native American, or Pacific Islander).

Gestational diabetes most commonly occurs in the second or third trimester of pregnancy. Certain hormones released at that time work against the action of insulin to cause insulin resistance. According to some diabetes specialists, the hormones may serve as "the straw that breaks the camel's back," pushing these already susceptible women into the realm of diabetes. Although most women with gestational diabetes no longer have diabetes after the stress of pregnancy is over, all are at increased risk of developing Type 2 diabetes later in life.

Syndrome X. Sometimes referred to as "insulin resistance syndrome," Syndrome X refers to a cluster of conditions that all seem to run together. Those conditions are insulin resistance, hyperinsulinemia, high blood pressure, blood lipid abnormalities (increased triglyceride levels, decreased HDL cholesterol levels, and increased levels of small, dense LDL cholesterol particles), and obesity. Taken together, these conditions lead to a dramatically increased risk of heart disease.

Some researchers believe that insulin resistance is the primary problem that leads to all the others. Some also believe that insulin resistance and hyperinsulinemia, even independent of their effects on blood glucose levels, can promote heart disease through insulin's effects on blood vessel walls and the blood's tendency to clot, but this hypothesis remains somewhat controversial.

Polycystic ovary syndrome. Called PCOS for short, polycystic ovary syndrome affects only women and is characterized by elevated levels of male hormone, the absence of ovulation, irregular menstrual cycles, and infertility. About 30% of obese women with PCOS develop impaired glucose tolerance or Type 2 diabetes by age 40, and they appear to have increased risk of heart disease as well.

Traditionally, women with PCOS have been treated with oral contraceptives to lower their male hormone levels and normalize menstruation. However, recent studies have shown that reducing insulin resistance through insulin-sensitizing drugs can alleviate some of the manifestations of PCOS and restore normal menstruation.

Type 1 diabetes. Insulin resistance may also occur in Type 1 diabetes, although it is not a hallmark of the disease. In fact, it is very rare. It is most commonly due to antibodies the body makes against insulin, but this rarely occurs with the advent of more purified insulins and human insulin, which tend to provoke less of an immune response.

Treating insulin resistance

Medical researchers say it would be helpful to be able to detect insulin resistance early, so that treatment could begin before any damage is done. Scientists have several ways of evaluating insulin resistance in research subjects, but the various methods are either too complicated, too expensive, too unreliable—or all of the above—to be practical for screening people in the clinic.

What doctors can do is use fasting plasma glucose levels and the oral glucose tolerance test to screen people who are at high risk for Type 2 diabetes (those who have close relatives with diabetes, are part of a high-risk ethnic group, or are overweight). Those who turn out to have impaired glucose tolerance or impaired fasting glucose are likely to be insulin-resistant, and they may benefit from the same lifestyle changes recommended for people with Type 2 diabetes.

Exercise. While new drugs for Type 2 diabetes specifically target insulin resistance, one equally effective and inexpensive therapy with virtually no side effects is often overlooked: exercise. Physical activity has been found to increase the body's sensitivity to insulin, both during and for up to one day after the activity. In addition, over the past decade, a number of large studies carried out in the United States, Sweden, and China have shown conclusively that regular aerobic exercise (such as running, brisk walking, bicycling, and climbing stairs) can reduce a person's risk of developing diabetes by roughly one-third to one-half.

In recent years, exercise specialists have also become intrigued by the effects of resistance training. Resistance training refers to exercise such as weight lifting that uses muscle strength to work against a resistive load. As it turns out, many people with Type 2 diabetes have relatively low muscle mass for their body weight. Since it is primarily muscle tissue that burns up glucose, building muscle mass can help the body use glucose more effectively.

Diet. Two related measures are dietary changes and weight loss. Reducing one's caloric intake and losing even modest amounts of weight have clearly been shown to lower insulin resistance.

Drug therapy. Until the mid-1990's, the only drugs on the market for treating Type 2 diabetes were insulin and a class of drugs called sulfonylureas, which prod the pancreas to secrete more insulin. Both types of drug treatments work by increasing the amount of insulin in circulation, which helps compensate for insulin resistance, but neither actually addresses the problem of insulin resistance itself.

Since then, a number of new drugs for Type 2 diabetes have come on the market, some of which specifically target insulin resistance. Metformin (brand name Glucophage) targets insulin resistance in the liver, decreasing the liver's production of glucose. Rosiglitazone (Avandia) and pioglitazone (Actos) reduce insulin resistance by making muscle and fat cells more sensitive to insulin.

Because these drugs reduce insulin resistance in people with Type 2 diabetes, it is natural to wonder whether they can help treat insulin resistance that hasn't yet developed into diabetes—ideally, helping to prevent diabetes. To try to answer this question, a large study called the Diabetes Prevention Program (DPP) was undertaken. It was designed to test whether lifestyle changes, with or without insulin-sensitizing drugs, can prevent or delay Type 2 diabetes in individuals who have impaired glucose tolerance.

Originally, there were four separate study groups: one group receiving instructions on diet and exercise, aimed at weight loss; one receiving standard dietary and exercise advice and metformin; one receiving standard dietary and exercise advice and troglitazone (Rezulin); and one control group receiving standard dietary and exercise advice and an inactive placebo. However, after numerous cases of liver dysfunction and several deaths were reported among people taking troglitazone—and one person participating in the DPP died in the seventh month of taking it—researchers felt that it was unethical to continue testing a potentially harmful drug in people who don't yet have diabetes. The troglitazone group was discontinued in 1998, and Rezulin was subsequently withdrawn from the market in March 2000.

Initial findings from the DPP, announced in August 2001, clearly showed that lifestyle changes, as well as the drug metformin, could reduce the risk of developing Type 2 diabetes. During the average follow-up period of three years, 29% of people in the control group developed diabetes, whereas only 22% of people in the metformin group and only 14% of people in the intensive diet-and-exercise group developed diabetes. Put another way, people treated with lifestyle interventions reduced their risk of developing diabetes by 58% and those treated with metformin reduced their risk by 31%. In view of the increasing incidence of Type 2 diabetes in the United States, this is welcome news.

Insulin resistance and you

Now that you know about insulin resistance, what can you do about it if you have Type 2 diabetes? Well, you can't change your genetic makeup, but you can investigate ways to become more physically active and to lose weight if you are overweight. You can also speak with your doctor about trying one of the newer diabetes drugs if you find that your blood sugar levels are not being adequately controlled by your current drug regimen.

Keep in mind that there is no one-size-fits-all diabetes plan. Your plan for increased physical activity needs to be enjoyable and reasonable for you—or you won't stick with it. Your weight-loss plan also needs to be reasonable for you. And your doctor can tell you which drugs he or she thinks would be useful for you and why. (Not all of the new drugs work for or are appropriate for all people.) Changing your lifestyle and finding a drug combination that controls your blood sugar requires time, patience, and persistence. But the rewards can be great: lowered insulin resistance and a healthier you. ❑

TRAVELING WITH DIABETES
BUSINESS AS USUAL
by Martha Jo Dendinger, C.M.P.

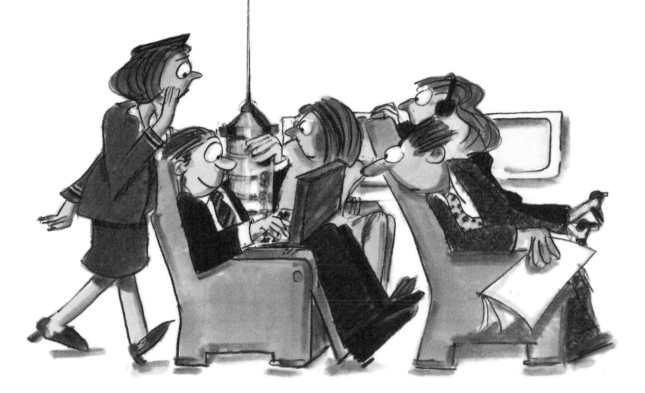

Nothing excites the soul like traveling to a new destination on a much deserved vacation, but traveling to that same place on business has a very different effect. Vacations are for relaxation, renewal, and reward and can be planned to fit your own pace and idiosyncrasies. Business trips, on the other hand, are for conducting business and are planned around schedules and meetings, with efficiency rather than personal comfort being the main goal. A trip to London may sound glamorous, but if it means that you will be working around the clock and that you will be seeing little more than the inside of your hotel room or an office, how glamorous is that?

Business travel does offer a nice break from office routines, but it hardly provides a break from office work. According to a study by Hyatt Hotels Corporation, 78% of business travelers say they work longer hours on the road than they do in the office. Survey respondents estimated that, on average, they put in up to 15 hours a day on the road, or nearly twice as many hours as they work in a day at the office.

In addition to long hours, business travel presents certain other challenges. Last-minute schedule changes, for example, are common on business trips. And coping with an unfamiliar environment can make getting the job done that much more stressful. There's no question that having diabetes compounds the challenges of business travel. The reverse is also true: The unpredictability and longer workdays that go with business travel can strain any diabetes management plan. Nonetheless, many people with diabetes have and succeed at jobs that require travel. If you are willing to do a little planning, you, too, can keep your diabetes—and your job—on track while you travel.

Pre-trip planning
The basic tenets of dealing with diabetes on the road, including carrying emergency medical information and a supply of snacks, definitely apply to business travelers. Planning ahead is paramount. The more time you have the better, but you almost always have time to buy a guidebook and load your briefcase with snacks and supplies. By being prepared, you can

accommodate unexpected changes and improve your chances of maintaining good diabetes control. Here is a list of tips to reduce the stress of traveling on business when you have diabetes:

■ Before you leave, do some homework on your destination city. Find out about customs, current events, and political and economic developments that could affect your particular industry or your diabetes control. For example, indigenous foods can affect your meal plan selections, and a traditional dinner hour that is much earlier or later than your usual dinner hour may conflict with your meal and medication schedule. Knowing about these things ahead of time allows you to make adjustments.

■ Check calendars and contact tourist organizations to find out whether businesses will be open during your stay. Holidays vary from country to country (and even from city to city), so don't be caught off guard.

■ Try to arrive the night before you are scheduled for meetings, speeches, or presentations, especially if you will be changing time zones. You will be in better emotional and physical shape, and you will have an opportunity to adapt your diabetes regimen to a different time zone and a new schedule.

■ Consider traffic patterns in your home city and in your destination when planning departure and arrival times. Try not to depart and arrive at peak traffic hours.

■ Minimize the chances for a delay in your flight by choosing nonstop flights when possible. Direct flights (which have stops but don't require you to change planes) and connections can easily delay your schedule. Ideally, you want to board the plane at the point of origin to avoid slowdowns caused by weather or mechanical problems.

■ Ask your airline how early you need to arrive at the airport for the security check. Also, be aware that airlines may vary in their rules concerning the diabetes equipment and supplies you are allowed to carry on board. As of early 2002, both the American Diabetes Association and the Federal Aviation Administration recommend that you contact your airline at least a day before your flight to confirm its policy.

■ Check the weather conditions at your destination. Major newspapers and all-weather TV channels can usually tell you at least the daytime temperature in big cities around the world. Your airline may also be able to provide some weather information. Be prepared with the proper clothing, and change your business appointments if you expect to be delayed by the weather.

■ If you travel frequently, consider joining an airline club. As a member, you have access to a lounge at the airport, which is a great setting for working, making calls, and waiting out delays. Many clubs serve food that is usually better and more nutritious than what

you find in the vending machines. Some have concierges who are as knowledgeable as any local guide. Other amenities, such as VIP check-in services and help going through customs, may be available. A locker at the lounge in airports you visit frequently is a great place to store extra supplies and snacks for emergencies or to restock your briefcase.

■ Think twice before renting a car at your destination. Car rental pickup and drop-off procedures can be time-consuming and stressful. It is often more convenient and faster to arrange to have a limousine meet you or to use a hotel shuttle service.

■ Organize appointments so that they make logistical sense. It's not practical to have one meeting at 9 AM followed by another one at 10 AM on the other side of town. Don't forget to figure in time for delays at associates' offices, meals, traffic jams, getting lost, or anything else that can make you late for your next meeting.

■ Make a list of contacts and any letters of introduction. This way, if you are delayed, you won't have to dig through your briefcase for phone numbers to let people know where you are. Also carry copies of prescriptions and pertinent medical information in case of emergency. Carry duplicates in your luggage, and leave a copy with your office and your travel agent.

You are not alone

Even if you are traveling alone, you don't have to meet all of the challenges by yourself. When you want sound advice on any subject, turn to the experts. Enlist the help of a travel agent, your diabetes support group, and anyone else who knows what you need to know. You can help yourself, too, by keeping travel journals on frequent destinations and by keeping your briefcase stocked with emergency supplies.

I use a professional travel agent when planning business itineraries. Travel agents know not just the rates and schedules, but also what services airlines, hotels, and ground transportation companies provide. Have you ever checked into a hotel and then spent the next hour fumbling under a desk and behind cabinets to find a telephone jack for your laptop, only to find that you couldn't connect to the phone line anyway? Travel agents are the experts in finding special services and amenities to help avoid these problems.

Some travel agencies specialize in business travel and can tell you where the top restaurants, business centers, and health clubs are. Try to establish a continuing relationship with one travel agent. Working with someone you know and trust every time will ease trip planning and the trip itself. My travel agent maintains a profile of my travel preferences and has copies of my prescriptions on file as a backup.

One of your best potential sources of information is your diabetes support group. Most groups have at least some members who travel on business or for pleasure and can offer tips based on their experiences. A fellow member in my group told me to check airline meal labeling after she found that meals labeled "lite" fit her meal plan better than those labeled "diabetic." Members of your group who travel often to your destination may know where to find 24-hour pharmacies, hotels and inns with special services, and restaurants with healthy menus. Group members may also be able to connect you with friends who have diabetes in cities throughout the world; such local contacts can often provide the best travel information.

Most business travelers have a specific region or territory that they cover with frequent trips to the same cities. If you visit one or a few places repeatedly, you may already keep a travel journal outlining information such as your preferred hotels and restaurants. In addition, note discoveries such as grocery stores with sugar-free items, well-stocked drug stores, and doctors and diabetes clinics that could help in an emergency.

Having spent several days at a snowed-in airport with only my briefcase, I can share with you some items you should keep in yours. A small pouch containing appropriate supplies such as pills, insulin, syringes, a blood glucose meter, and test strips will help you manage your diabetes through travel delays or lost luggage scenarios. A sandwich, packaged peanut butter and crackers, and boxed milk or juice can be literal lifesavers when the vending machines are empty and the concessions are closed. A prepaid phone card or a cell phone (remember to bring the charger) will allow you to make phone calls without a pocketful of change. A pocket flight guide, such as the *Official Airline Guide (OAG)*, can help you plan the best alternate route in case of cancellations. The *OAG* can be purchased at many airport newsstands or by subscription.

Staying in control

The time just after arrival can be the most difficult part of business travel. Delays, schedule changes, and jet lag can all upset business plans and diabetes management. Perhaps your plane landed late and you did not have time to eat lunch before your first business meeting. Is that why you feel like someone's been stuffing cotton balls into your brain all morning?

If you've been traveling across a few time zones, you would swear your symptoms are caused by jet lag. If you have diabetes, you might say your blood glucose is outside your normal range. The truth is, it could be either, or both. Jet lag can mimic the symptoms of

DOING YOUR HOMEWORK

For more tips on traveling with diabetes, consult the following resources:

THE DIABETES TRAVEL GUIDER
Davida F. Kruger
NTC/Contemporary Publishing Group
Lincolnwood, Illinois, 2000
Available from the American Diabetes Association (www.diabetes.org).

THE DIABETIC TRAVELLER'S COMPANION
Nerida Nichols
Random House New Zealand
Auckland, New Zealand, 1995

THE RESTAURANT COMPANION
Hope S. Warshaw
Surrey Books
Chicago, 1995
A guide to how and what to order in more than 20 kinds of restaurants, from fast food to upscale dining.

HEALTH INFORMATION FOR INTERNATIONAL TRAVEL 2001–2002
This biennial publication of the U.S. Centers for Disease Control and Prevention (CDC) contains vaccination requirements, advisories on potential health hazards, and general health hints. To purchase a copy, visit the Web site of the Public Health Foundation, http://bookstore.phf.org/prod159.htm, or call (877) 252-1200. The full text can also be downloaded from the CDC's Travelers' Health Web site, www.cdc.gov/travel, which in addition provides listings of disease outbreaks and emerging infections across the world.

HEALING HANDBOOK FOR PERSONS WITH DIABETES
www.umassmed.edu/diabeteshandbook
An online book by the University of Massachusetts Medical Center. Download Chapter 14, which is about travel, and tuck it into our briefcase for a handy reference.

high or low blood sugar. The only way to know for sure is to check your blood glucose regularly.

You can minimize jet lag with a few preventive measures. Before you fly, try to reduce stress, get plenty of exercise, and eat a nutritious preflight meal. Some studies suggest that the vitamins and antioxidants in green vegetables help alleviate the drowsiness and lethargy associated with jet lag, so you may want to include some greens in your meal. Get a good night's sleep before departure, and consider postponing the flight if you have a cold or any other illness that may keep you awake or affect your diabetes. Do stretching exercises on board and walk up and down the aisle every hour to prevent muscle stiffness. Drinking too much caffeine or alcohol can complicate jet lag, dehydrate you, and affect your blood glucose. By using them only in moderation or avoiding them altogether, you have one less thing to worry about.

Before you leave, talk to your doctor or diabetes educator about adjusting your diabetes management for different time zones and new schedules. On transatlantic flights, I try to leave the east coast by early evening and sleep on the plane as much as possible. When I arrive in Europe, it's breakfast time, but my body thinks it's midnight. I nibble at the breakfast served on the plane, counting it as my bedtime snack, and take my bedtime injection. When I arrive at the hotel, I sleep until noon, then get up and have lunch with my normal lunchtime injection. This works well for me, but each person's adjustment will be different, depending on his or her usual routine.

Business travel tends to have some hidden elements of exercise and energy expenditure. Sometimes you have to hurry to make tight connections or make up lost time. The extra weight you're carrying in your luggage, briefcase, and laptop makes rushing around a strenuous activity. Exercise usually comes in spurts, between long periods of inactivity. Take these different patterns of exercise into consideration when checking your blood sugar and adjusting your diabetes management routine.

Eating on the road

Sometimes it seems as if business can't be conducted without food. And when the occasion is a celebration to seal a deal, people seem to forget their normal eating habits. "What," "when," and "how much" are the major concerns in diabetes management, yet this information may seem less important or may simply be unavailable when you're faced with extravagant menus and buffets. How does one cope?

First, know your meal plan and exchanges forward and backward. Keep an abbreviated version of your meal plan with you as a reminder. Learn to swap exchanges back and forth (for example, a milk for a meat or a bread for a fruit) in case a business meal has limited options. Or have your dietitian teach you how to count carbohydrates.

If you take insulin, discuss the newer, faster-acting insulins with your doctor. These forms of insulin allow more flexibility in terms of injection timing and portion sizes. If you're ever extremely rushed or can't find a clean, private place to take your injection, you may want to consider injecting through your clothes. According to a recent study, injecting insulin through clean clothes does not raise the risk of infection or interfere with insulin absorption.

If you feel uncomfortable at business meals because you are on a diet, take a look around. These days, it seems as if everyone is on a diet. With the introduction of the food pyramid and the proliferation of other health-related meal plans, a diabetes meal plan looks like any other attempt to comply with the nutrition guidelines of balance, variety, and moderation.

When you're in charge of selecting the restaurant for a business function, learn all you can about the possible choices before deciding on one. Most good restaurants will have a staff member who can discuss how items are prepared and will fax you a menu so that you can select your meal in advance. If someone else has selected the restaurant, eat what suits your meal plan, and, if you need to, supplement the meal with snacks from your briefcase.

Introducing your diabetes

When it comes to my diabetes, my policy is, "Do ask, do tell." My medical ID bracelet is always visible. Most of my colleagues and clients know I have diabetes, and many have become more aware of their own health because of our discussions. I don't make diabetes a major topic of conversation, but if someone asks about my bracelet or wonders why I'm not eating dessert, I tell them I have diabetes. On more than one occasion I have received a response like, "Oh, really? I have diabetes, too." This newfound common ground strengthened the business relationship every time.

Unfortunately, some people feel embarrassed or uncomfortable upon learning that a person has diabetes. These people may be reacting to some misconceptions they have about diabetes. Or they may be unsure how your diabetes affects your ability to participate in the business or meal at hand. I sometimes ease a companion's worries regarding food without blowing my diet by sharing a bite of dessert and saying, "You know, the second bite tastes the same as the first." In most situations, discretion, humor, and basic manners work well, but don't let another person's discomfort interfere with your management plan. A simple "please excuse me" will allow you to go to a rest room or lounge to take a shot, test your blood glucose, or have a snack.

There may also be times when *you* feel embarrassed about your diabetes. If you find yourself hesitating to reach for a glucose tablet or a snack during a meeting or debating whether or not to excuse yourself from the room to eat in private because you don't want to disrupt the meeting, consider the alternatives. An episode of low blood sugar would cause a much larger disruption than either of these actions. Doing what you need to do in the most matter-of-fact and unobtrusive way possible will attract the least amount of unwanted attention.

Relaxing on the job

There is nothing restful about a business trip, and stress levels usually run high. Unfortunately, stress and lack of adequate rest can greatly affect diabetes control. So finding ways to unwind on the road is not selfish; it is part of good diabetes self-care.

Even on a business trip, you can carve out a little leisure time for relaxation and renewal. Here are a few suggestions:
■ Schedule either a business lunch or a business dinner, but not both. Save one meal for yourself.

■ Schedule a massage at the end of the day.
■ Take a half-hour walk each day you're on the road.
■ Invite your business associates to play tennis or golf or to go to a play or movie of their choice. Even with business associates, social activities can be refreshing.
■ Plan your trip so that you have a day or a weekend to explore the area and take a break from business.

According to an old adage, we are sure of only two things: death and taxes. In business travel you can add a third: change. Last-minute trips, transportation delays, appointment changes, and meetings that last longer than expected are almost inevitable. But they don't have to compromise diabetes management. Keeping your diabetes under control before you travel will allow you to accommodate these last-minute schedule changes.

Most travelers agree that it's best to plan for the worst. A flexible schedule buffered with leisure time, a well-equipped briefcase, and an informed staff and travel agent are not only good for business, they are also good for diabetes. ❏

PLANNING FOR A HOSPITAL STAY
by Virginia Peragallo-Dittko, R.N., M.A., C.D.E.

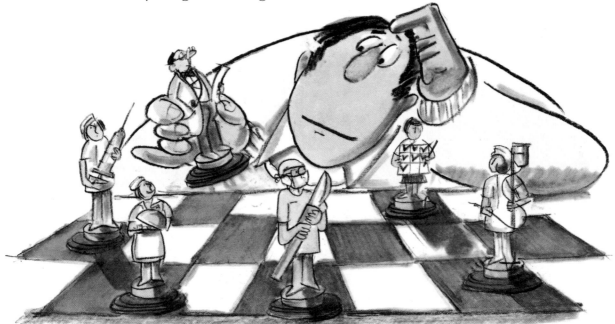

Expectant mothers pack a suitcase. They're ready to go to the hospital, full of anxious anticipation. The rest of us aren't usually so keen, but when we have no choice, we're ultimately grateful for the lifesaving measures the hospital makes available to us.

Although everyone is anxious about a hospital stay, people with diabetes have an added concern: giving up control of their diabetes management. At home, you decide the timing of your meals, take any insulin or pills your doctor has prescribed, and check your own blood sugar. In the hospital, much of this is taken out of your hands. The meal trays are delivered according to a system that works best for the entire hospital, the staff may use a blood glucose meter that differs from yours (or not use a meter at all), and your medicines may be changed, depending on the reason for your admission. If your admission was elective, or scheduled, there are ways to plan ahead so you can reduce your anxiety about putting your diabetes management in the hands of strangers. But even if you end up in the hospital unexpectedly, and there's little or no time to plan, having a general idea of what's likely to happen will help you feel less anxious.

A basic understanding

First, it helps to understand the fundamental difference between hospital, or acute, care and chronic care. Diabetes management at home is chronic care. You're not sick and don't need lifesaving treatment; instead you use your self-management skills to keep yourself healthy. When there's been a change in your body that is making you sick, however, or when you have surgery, your body's needs change. Intensive measures are called for; you require acute care. If you don't recognize the basic difference between hospital care and chronic care, you're bound to be upset and frustrated, because the first place you'll see the difference is in blood sugar goals that are higher than those you aim for at home. The primary reason for these higher goals is that the stresses of illness make your home goals difficult or impossible to achieve.

Your diabetes medicine may need to be changed when you're in the hospital. Surgery, medical procedures, and infections cause the body to secrete counterregulatory, or stress, hormones that raise blood sugar levels. High blood sugar interferes with both wound healing and the ability of white blood cells to fight infection. Thus, if you already inject insulin, you may need a change in your dose. If you usually take oral medicine, you may need short-term insulin therapy while you are in the hospital and perhaps for a few days after you are sent home. Once the levels of stress hormones return to normal, your doctor will most probably put you back on your usual medicines.

And keep in mind that if you are scheduled for surgery, the focus shifts from managing diabetes to healing. Your body needs the best environment it can get for healing, and the consensus is that this calls for a blood sugar goal of between 120 mg/dl and 180 mg/dl before, during, and after surgery. As you won't be in charge—in part because you won't feel up to it and in part because state health rules make the hospital responsible for all medicines a patient takes—you'll need someone to take over for you, such as your family doctor or endocrinologist. Team management

in diabetes is a common practice, so when you have surgery, not only your surgeon but also your medical doctor is part of the team.

Planning for an elective admission

If your admission is elective, rather than the unexpected result of an emergency or a serious illness, you'll have time to make some preparations.

Timing. If you're scheduled for an elective surgical procedure, for example, you'll be expected to report to the hospital at a certain time on the day it's to take place. Although some tests and procedures do not interrupt your eating schedule and require no changes in your diabetes care, for most procedures you will not be able to eat after midnight. Try to arrange it so that you will be scheduled early in the morning. A longer fast may raise your blood sugar, because your liver will release glycogen (stored sugar). People who live far from the hospital may prefer to be scheduled later. In that case, ask for specific guidelines about when to begin fasting.

Medication. You will need to ask your doctor how to adjust your medication the day before and the day of the procedure. This is the case both for procedures that require you to stay in the hospital and for procedures done on an outpatient basis. (See "Outpatient Surgery" on page 35.) If you take insulin, it is common practice to use one-half of your usual dose of longer-acting insulin (such as NPH or Lente) the morning of the procedure; if you take glargine (Lantus), you would take one-half of your usual dose at bedtime the night before the procedure. Although you won't be eating, this provides enough insulin to manage the effects of stress hormones. Because everyone has different insulin sensitivity, you will need guidance from your doctor about how much insulin to use on the day of or the night before the procedure. If you use an insulin pump, you will need to find out in advance if the hospital staff is familiar with pump therapy. Blood sugar control for most one-day surgeries or procedures can be managed without disconnecting from the pump. With major surgery or severe blood loss, insulin given via pump or injection is not absorbed well, and intravenous insulin is preferred.

If you take oral medicines known as thiazolidinediones or sulfonylureas, they are usually continued until the morning of the procedure. Thiazolidinediones include rosiglitazone (brand name Avandia) and pioglitazone (Actos). Sulfonylureas include glimepiride (Amaryl), glipizide (Glucotrol and Glucotrol XL), and glyburide (DiaBeta, Micronase, and Glynase PresTab). The sulfonylurea chlorpropamide (brand name Diabinese), however, has a very long action in the body, which means the pill you take on Monday is still working on Tuesday. For that reason, your doctor may advise you to stop chlorpropamide a few days prior to the procedure. Metformin (Glucophage) can have rare but serious side effects if your kidneys aren't working properly or if you become severely dehydrated. Depending on the procedure, you may be told to stop using metformin on the day of the procedure and not to start using it again until your kidney function has been reevaluated. Similarly, if you're going to have any x-ray or radiologic procedure using dye that contains iodine (such as an angiogram, CT scan, or intravenous cholangiogram), you'll be told to stop using metformin at the time of or prior to the procedure and for 48 hours afterward until your kidney function has been evaluated.

More to ask your doctor. In addition to getting full instructions about what medicines to take and when to take them, there are a number of other matters you might wish to discuss with your doctor. The doctor will probably tell you to call if you get a sore throat, a fever, or a cold before you're scheduled to go to the hospital for surgery; the surgery may have to be postponed so the infection won't complicate your recovery. Otherwise, you'll want to know how often you will see your own doctor while you're in the hospital and who will manage your diabetes care. You'll need information about whether you should bring your own medicines to the hospital. And you'll want to ask how long your hospital stay is expected to last, what sort of help you'll need at home afterward, and when you may return to work. Take along a list of these and any other questions you have when you go to see your doctor.

Last but not least. Before you leave for the hospital, make a list of the medicines you take, when you take them, and in what doses. Note also what your usual blood sugar range is. This list should become part of your record at the hospital, a reminder to those who are looking after you that this is your normal regimen.

Blood glucose monitoring

You make daily decisions based on blood glucose testing and have come to rely on it. You'd feel more secure if you could use your own meter in the hospital. In fact, you can. However, the hospital staff cannot use your meter results to make decisions about medication because of state health department rules. Blood glucose meters designed for hospital use may look like yours, but there are important differences. The hospital system has to conform to state standards, which require, among other things, that frequent control tests be done on hospital meters to assure that they are accurate. The hospital cannot accept responsibility for a meter that it does not test. So you may want to leave your own meter

OUTPATIENT SURGERY

An estimated 80% to 90% of all surgical procedures are performed in an outpatient setting. With outpatient surgery, most people go home the same day. If your recovery is slower than expected, however, you may have to stay overnight.

Depending on the procedure, you will need the following:

■ A ride to and from the hospital or outpatient center and some help when you get home
■ Guidelines for oral medicine or insulin adjustment before and after the procedure
■ Guidelines and instruction concerning your care after the procedure or surgery
■ Guidelines for expected blood-glucose goals immediately after the procedure and on the following days
■ Guidelines for when to monitor your blood glucose, what number is too high or too low, and when to call for dose adjustment
■ Instruction concerning the reason for a new medicine and what its possible side effects are

at home for the duration of your hospital stay. You may be allowed to use your own lancing device and lancets for the hospital blood tests, however.

Dealing with low blood sugar

Once you're in the hospital, it's quite possible you'll experience swings in blood glucose level. Although the staff will work very hard to prevent it, you could be sent for a test, get delayed, and miss a meal, resulting in low blood sugar. Be prepared to alert the nursing staff at the first symptom. Most hospitals have protocols for treating low blood sugar with glucose tablets and a snack, but you may encounter staff who insist on adding four packets of sugar to an 8-ounce cup of orange juice (a total of 46 grams of carbohydrate). As you know, overtreatment of low blood glucose only leads to high blood glucose later on and should be avoided. So remember, you can refuse to be overtreated and ask to see a supervisor.

Food issues

Humorous get-well cards make constant reference to miserable hospital food; it's a universal joke. Some hospitals have hired hotel-based chefs to add their skills to the mix, while hospital chefs strive to serve tasty, healthful food to hundreds of patients. Sometimes, when you don't feel well, nothing tastes good. If your family or friends choose to bring you food from home, they'll need to consult with the nurses and dietitians so that it is part of your meal plan. When you're feeling better, you might want to ask to see the dietitian for an updated meal plan or for guidance about food choices relating to the reason for your hospitalization. Perhaps you need to gain weight and want to know how to fit high-calorie foods such as cream soups or milk shakes into your diabetes meal plan.

Another food-related concern is what's in the intravenous drip (IV). When Frank was admitted to the hospital for abdominal surgery, he called home in a panic. "They're killing me here," he whispered. "I have diabetes and I'm getting an IV filled with dextrose! That's sugar, you know." Frank's daughter quickly called the nurses' station, only to be reassured. The nurse explained to Frank and his daughter that since he couldn't eat food yet, the best source of fuel for his body and healing was the intravenous dextrose. It wasn't a mistake. Quite the contrary: the amount of dextrose was being carefully calculated so that Frank's liver wouldn't release stored sugar and contribute to high blood sugar. Frank and his daughter felt better and also learned to ask questions. No one needs unnecessary anxiety.

The clear liquid diet can also be a worry if you don't understand why you're getting it. Regular Jell-O, apple juice, regular ginger ale, and Italian ices (not sugar-free) are all part of the clear liquid diet. A food is considered a clear liquid when it has no residue like that found in milk or orange juice. After surgery or any problem with your stomach or intestines, the first foods you are offered are clear liquids. Your body isn't ready to digest solid food yet, but you need calories as fuel for healing. You are not offered sugar-free foods because you need calories, and these clear liquids provide lots of calories in small portions. It is the same principle that applies to managing sick days at home.

Patient's rights

A copy of the Patient's Bill of Rights is given to every patient admitted to the hospital. One of your rights is to know the name and position of every member of the hospital staff who serves you. No one should begin to ask you questions about your health until you know that person's name and position. Another right is to be able to get the information you need to understand what's going on. Apart from anything else, this can help you make your hospital stay a safe one. If, for example, you're given something you don't think you should be getting, like Frank, or if you're not getting your medicine when you expect it, ask a question.

DEALING WITH THE EMERGENCY ROOM

Have you seen the television show *ER*? Although the stories are exaggerated to thrill the TV audience, the fast pace, quick thinking, and lifesaving measures are real. You may be admitted to the emergency room for diabetes-related problems such as severely low blood sugar levels or dehydration from continued vomiting. Or your problem may have nothing to do with your diabetes; you may have chest pain, for example, or injuries from a motor vehicle accident.

In the emergency room, everyone needs help NOW. Meals get delayed, snacks may be missed, and, unless it is the reason for your admission, diabetes management may be neglected. It's unlikely that anyone will have thought to bring along your medicines, meter, or snack foods. You will probably need to speak up to make sure your diabetes is not forgotten. Since you may be sitting in the waiting room for hours, it helps to have a friend or family member with you who can go get you a snack, call home for your supplies, and speak up for you if you don't feel able.

Keeping a list of medicines and a summary of your medical history in your wallet with your insurance cards will make it easier for the emergency room nurses to get you the help you need. And remember, some insurance companies require that you call them when you are admitted to an emergency room or within a certain number of hours or days—or they won't pay the bill. You can imagine how easily that step is forgotten when you are sick and upset!

Most of the time everything's as it should be, but occasionally you'll pick up on a problem. If you're not feeling well enough to do this for yourself, get a friend or relative to do it for you.

If you have a grievance, such as dissatisfaction with your care, a patient representative on the hospital's staff should help you handle it. This person can also help you communicate with your medical team, if you feel they're not answering your questions. The patient representative is your advocate and acts on behalf of patients and families in situations involving hospital administration and other departments and services. The patient representative also interprets the hospital's philosophy, policies, and services for you, your family, and visitors.

Going home

Hospital stays get shorter and shorter. Most people are anxious to get home, but before you are discharged, make sure that you are ready to leave, have adequate help at home, and are given proper discharge instructions. Ideally, it is best to have a friend or family member with you to hear the discharge instructions. The instructions should include not only information about any new medicines and your activity level but diabetes guidelines also. Make sure you know how often to check your blood sugar, the blood-glucose goal range after discharge, and your oral drug or insulin dose. You need to be aware of when to call for a change in dose, food, and eating guidelines, and when to schedule a follow-up appointment for review of your diabetes management as well as for a general medical or surgical follow-up. You should know to call your doctor if you have very wet or blood-soaked bandages, fever, persistent nausea or vomiting, moder-ate or large amounts of ketones in your urine, or a decrease in the amount of urine.

The extent of home health services available to you will depend on your needs and your insurance coverage. Every hospital has a discharge planning department, and a member of its staff will visit you and help you plan for going home. If you are new to insulin therapy, the staff member can arrange for a nurse to visit you in your home and continue the instruction you receive in the hospital. After discharge for a diabetes-related admission, it is helpful to see a diabetes educator for a review or attend a diabetes education program. Diabetes education provided when you are in the hospital is usually very limited, because it is hard to learn when you don't feel well, and the hospital stay can be very short.

We hope you won't need to be admitted to the hospital any time soon, but if you do, we hope this article allayed some concerns. Expectant mothers? Well, that's another article. ❏

GETTING THE MOST FROM HEALTH-CARE VISITS
by Teresa Pearson, M.S., R.N., C.D.E.

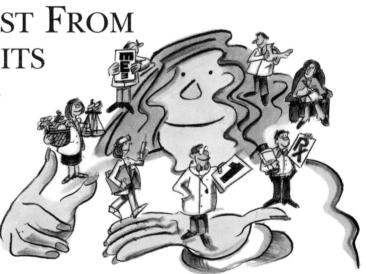

People with diabetes typically visit their health-care providers fairly frequently— at least four times a year if they follow current recommendations. Without good insurance coverage, the cost of these visits can add up. But even with good coverage, there is still a considerable cost in terms of time and effort. All too often, people feel as though they spend too long in the waiting room, not enough time in the examination room, and they still go home with their questions unanswered.

Clearly, this is an expensive way to waste your time. So how can you get more for your time and money? One of the keys to getting more from your health-care visits is to plan for them. Another is to stay informed about your diabetes and advances in diabetes treatment. Here are some tips to help you take care of yourself and take advantage of what your health-care providers have to offer.

Preparing for appointments

Your interactions with your health-care providers will vary depending on their specialty and your needs. Your initial visit to a given provider will likely be some-what different—possibly longer—from subsequent visits. Routine appointments are likely to cover different ground than those made because you're ill.

Whatever the case, you are more likely to get what you want from a visit if you know what you want when you walk in the office door. Take time to prepare for your visits by thinking about what you would like to ask or tell your health-care provider. Do you need help interpreting your blood glucose monitoring results? Are you concerned about a new symptom? Do you need help planning for an upcoming event such as a long trip? Remember that you're entitled to have an agenda for health-care visits.

Another way to get more out of appointments is to anticipate what information your provider is likely to want from you. Bring along any referral forms or records—such as your blood glucose log or food diary—that are relevant to the appointment. If you aren't sure what to bring with you, call the office and ask before your appointment.

Primary-care provider

When you meet with a primary-care provider (probably a medical doctor but possibly a nurse practitioner) for the first time, you will most likely be asked many questions about your health and be given a complete physical exam. You may also be asked to fill out a written health questionnaire. Be prepared to talk about (or write down information about) your personal and family health history, any recent illnesses, and any symptoms related to your diabetes. If you don't know whether a symptom is related to your diabetes, ask your provider.

Your primary-care provider will want to know what drugs and supplements, if any, you currently take, so bring a list of the names and doses of all the prescription medicines, over-the-counter products, vitamins and minerals, and other dietary supplements you take. You can also just put all your pill bottles in a bag and bring it with you. Your provider may also ask about your level of physical activity and your diet.

If you have recently been diagnosed with diabetes, your doctor's goal for your initial visit will be to get to know you and to set out a plan of care. If you already have a plan of care but are changing doctors for whatever reason, your doctor's goal for the initial visit will be to get to know you and to learn about your diabetes and how you care for it.

What are your goals? What concerns do you have about your health or your diabetes? What would you like to know about your doctor? To get the most out of these visits, write down your questions and concerns before the appointment. Try to prioritize your questions so that you ask the most pressing first.

At subsequent visits, your provider will evaluate how well your diabetes care plan is working, both by examining you physically and taking a history of how you've been doing since your previous visit. If you have started taking a new drug or dietary supplement since your last visit, bring it with you so your doctor can enter it in your medical record. Follow-up visits are your chance to describe what has worked and what has not worked for you in managing your diabetes.

If you consult with an endocrinologist or any other specialists, it is important to continue your relationship with your primary doctor as the coordinator of your health-care team. To make sure your doctors can communicate with one another about your care, be sure they have one another's names and contact infor-

mation. Ask them to forward notes to each other after they have seen you. If there is a difference of opinion between your team members, ask for clarification. Suggest that they consult with one another any time they or you feel it would enhance your care.

Diabetes nurse educator

A diabetes nurse educator can teach you about your diabetes and help you to learn the skills you need to manage it. Some of those skills include learning to inject insulin if you use insulin, learning to monitor your blood glucose and keep a log of your blood glucose levels, and learning to use your monitoring results as a guide to adjust food, activity, and medicines.

If you have just been diagnosed with diabetes, your nurse educator will want to get to know you and help you learn how to carry out the plan of care your doctor has recommended. He or she will review your health history and will most likely ask about your day-to-day routine. You may be asked questions about the type of work you do and your schedule. You may also be asked about your typical eating patterns and patterns of physical activity. This information will help your diabetes nurse educator help you develop a daily diabetes care regimen that will fit your lifestyle.

Your diabetes nurse educator can also direct you toward other sources of information that can help you manage your diabetes. While you may sometimes work one-on-one with your educator, you may also be advised to enroll in diabetes education classes, in which skills are taught in a group setting. Different people learn best in different ways, so ask your diabetes educator what options you have in your community or diabetes treatment setting, and think about which options might suit you best.

To get the most out of follow-up visits with your nurse educator, bring your blood glucose records, along with any notes you've kept about your eating patterns, physical activity, and medicines. Such notes can help you uncover the reasons behind blood glucose levels that are out of target range. Since stress can affect your blood glucose levels, it also helps to keep notes in your log regarding stressful events or sources of chronic stress. And be sure to note any illnesses or infections, including colds, the flu, and even periodontal disease, which can affect blood glucose control.

You may also come to appointments with certain goals, questions, or priorities. Maybe your monitoring is going fine but you'd like to find a less painful lancing device. Let your educator know what information or help you need to make your diabetes management tasks easier.

Dietitian

An individualized meal plan is key to your overall diabetes care plan, and a registered dietitian can help you develop one. At your initial visit, it is important to tell your dietitian what medicines you are using to control your diabetes and what kind of exercise or physical activity you currently do. You will want to bring your blood glucose records, so the dietitian can assess your current level of control. And of course, you will want to talk about food.

Your dietitian will most likely ask you to describe your eating habits and your food preferences. To prepare for the visit, it helps to keep a food diary in which you write down everything you eat for several days before the visit. This information, along with your blood glucose records, will help your dietitian guide you in designing a food plan that best suits you and your lifestyle and helps you manage your diabetes.

If you already have a meal plan, a visit to the dietitian provides the opportunity to discuss how well it is working and whether you would like (or need) to make changes. Bring a written copy of your meal plan with you to the appointment, along with any notes you've made about difficulties sticking with it. Remember, a meal plan only works if you can follow it.

Many people find it helpful to schedule at least a yearly visit with a dietitian—to keep their nutrition knowledge up to date, learn more about how food and eating habits can affect blood glucose levels, and to make sure their meal plan still fits their lifestyle and diabetes care regimen.

Other specialists

In addition to your primary-care provider, diabetes nurse educator, and dietitian, you may need to consult other specialists from time to time. Being prepared for these visits is important as well.

Eye doctor. At least once a year, you should have a dilated eye exam to check for signs of diabetic retinopathy. Remember to tell your eye doctor about your diabetes, how you control it, your current level of blood glucose control, any diabetes complications you have experienced, and any other medical conditions you may have, such as high blood pressure. Your eye doctor will also want to know about your family's health history, since many health problems have a hereditary component. You will likely also be asked about any changes in your health since your last visit. To make sure you remember all the details, write this information down beforehand and bring it with you.

Podiatrist. At some point, you may need to see a podiatrist. Some people with diabetes see a podiatrist on a regular basis to monitor the condition of their feet and have their toenails trimmed. Others see one only when they have a foot problem such as a wound, infection, or other foot complication.

Most likely, your podiatrist will want to know what kinds of shoes you wear and what kind of exercise you do, so come prepared with that information. If you have questions about the shoes you wear or any products you use on your feet, such as lotion, bring them with you to the appointment.

Behavioral health professional. If you are struggling with the emotional stresses of adapting to and living with diabetes, you may want to see a behavioral health professional. It's possible that this person will want to see a copy of your meal plan or blood glucose records, but that would be something you decide on together. The best advice one can give is to keep your appointments and show up on time. Beyond that, you and your behavioral health-care provider can decide together how to put your time together to good use.

Pharmacist. You will most likely see your pharmacist more often than any other health-care provider, and while you might not make an appointment to see a pharmacist, you may sometimes have questions for him or her about the medicines you take. If you do, bring the medicine with you to the pharmacy counter. That way, the pharmacist can see exactly what you're taking. (If you're on the phone with the pharmacy, have the medicine container in hand when you call.) And remember that the only way your pharmacist can warn you of possible drug interactions is if he or she knows about all the prescription drugs, over-the-counter products, and supplements you take.

Your pharmacist may also be able to answer questions about your blood glucose meter. Again, it helps to have the meter with you when you ask your questions, especially if they're about the functioning of the meter.

What to ask

To manage your diabetes as well as possible, you should know how and when to monitor your blood glucose at home. You and your doctor should have a mutually agreed upon target range for your blood glucose as well as a target HbA_{1c} test result. You should know how to respond to blood glucose levels that are out of target range.

In addition, you should know what medicines you have agreed to take, how and when to take them, and what precautions to keep in mind while using them. You should have a food plan and a physical activity plan that you understand how to follow. You should also know how to manage your diabetes when you've got a cold, the flu, or another illness.

If you have high blood pressure, you may also want to monitor your blood pressure at home, and getting accurate results with a blood pressure meter depends on knowing how to use it correctly. You should know when to schedule follow-up visits with members of your health-care team. And you should know when and how you will find out the results of any lab work or procedures that are done.

If there is anything on this list you don't know, use it as the beginnings of a list of questions to ask your health-care team. It's a good idea to write down both the questions you want to ask and the answers you receive. If the explanations are too technical, ask for clarification. Some people like to bring a family member or a friend with them to doctor visits to lend an extra set of ears or hands to take notes.

Sick-day plan

Because having diabetes can complicate even minor illness, and because even minor illness can affect blood glucose control, everyone with diabetes should have a sick-day plan. If you don't currently have one, ask your health-care team to help you develop one, then keep it in a handy location. Your sick-day plan should include the following information:
■ How and when to modify your usual diabetes medication plan
■ A schedule for monitoring your blood sugar
■ Instructions for testing for ketones
■ Instructions for taking your temperature
■ A list of over-the-counter drugs you can take when ill
■ Instructions on when to call the doctor
■ Phone numbers for your doctor, pharmacy, and friends you can call on for help

In general, people with diabetes are advised to take their usual doses of insulin or pills when they are sick, even if they have no appetite. This is because illness usually causes blood glucose to go up. However, it is also important to consume at least some carbohydrate and to drink plenty of fluids while you are sick. If you cannot eat, substitute regular soft drinks, juice, or other liquids or soft foods in place of your usual carbohydrates. Weigh yourself daily to determine if you are losing weight as a result of dehydration. Check your temperature every four hours to see if you are running a fever.

By having a sick-day plan and following it, you may be able to prevent your illness from becoming an emergency. If in doubt about what to do, call your doctor's office or your clinic's or health plan's nurse advice line. You should also call to report any changes in your condition, particularly if it worsens.

Dealing with emergencies

Not all emergencies can be prevented, so it's important to know what to do before an acute situation

RECOGNIZING GOOD DIABETES CARE

The American Diabetes Association (ADA) recommends that you visit your primary health-care provider every three months to monitor your health and diabetes control. By following the ADA Standards of Care, you and your provider can reduce your risk for the complications associated with diabetes. Here's what needs to be done and how often:
■ Blood pressure: every visit
■ Complete foot exam: every year
■ Dilated eye exam: at least once a year
■ Glycosylated hemoglobin (HbA_{1c}) test: every 3–6 months
■ Kidney function (microalbumin test): at least once a year
■ Lipid profile: every two years if most recent one normal; every year if most recent one not normal

In addition, talk with your primary-care provider about the following:
■ Quitting smoking—if you smoke—and options to help you quit
■ How you are managing your diabetes on a daily basis
■ Your blood glucose monitoring
■ Taking aspirin every day
■ Exercising regularly, preferably for 30 minutes most days of the week
■ Managing your weight
■ Seeing a diabetes nurse educator and a dietitian at least once a year
■ Seeing other specialists, such as a podiatrist or ophthalmologist, as needed

develops. Here are some basic rules of thumb when making a decision about who to call and when:
■ If you experience chest pain, difficulty breathing, profuse bleeding, or any other symptom that indicates a potentially life-threatening condition, call 911.
■ If you are unable to keep food down for more than six hours or if you are having severe diarrhea, particularly if you have lost more than 5 pounds in the past 24 hours, call your clinic's or health plan's nurse advice line (or your doctor's 24-hour line) for advice.

Some other reasons to call for advice include the following: your temperature remains over 101°F while using acetaminophen regularly, you have moderate to large amounts of ketones in your urine, or you feel unusually sleepy or can't think clearly. Ketones in your urine and feeling sleepy or mentally fuzzy can be signs of impending diabetic ketoacidosis, a life-threatening condition, and should be addressed immediately.

■ If you experience frequent, severe, or unexplained low blood glucose, blood glucose consistently above your target range, or a sudden change in your vision, call your primary-care provider right away. All of these can be signs of underlying problems and should be checked out without delay. Other symptoms that should be reported quickly to your health-care provider include having a sore that won't heal and having feelings of numbness or tingling in your hands or feet.

■ For less urgent questions about your medicines, less severe fluctuations in your blood glucose, and trouble with your food or exercise plan, call your health-care provider's office for an appointment during usual business hours.

If your life is truly in danger, your first priority is getting medical attention. You can worry about such things as insurance forms once your condition has stabilized. However, by wearing a medical ID bracelet or necklace, you make sure the people helping you know who you are and that you have diabetes.

If you plan to call your doctor's office or an advice hotline, having complete information available when you call will help the person you speak to decide how better to help you. Be prepared to describe the problem, when it began, and your symptoms. If you are experiencing nausea, vomiting, or diarrhea, indicate how long it has been going on. Describe any pain you are having (a dull ache or a sharp, stabbing pain) and where it is located. Report your blood glucose level and whether you have ketones in your urine, as well as your temperature, pulse, and breaths per minute. If you have ever had this problem before, describe what you did for it.

According to the American Society of Internal Medicine, 70% of a correct diagnosis relies on what you tell your doctor. The more complete your information, the easier it is for a nurse or doctor to advise you on managing the situation at home or getting to a medical facility to be seen.

Staying healthy

With all things considered, the best way to manage your diabetes and avoid problems is to stay healthy. Take care of your body as carefully as you would a prized possession. If you smoke, ask your health-care team for help with quitting. Get help developing a meal plan and exercise plan. Check your blood glucose regularly, write your numbers down, and learn how to use the information to adjust your food, physical activity, and medication. Check your feet daily for pressure sores, blisters, calluses, and other changes. Maintain good dental health and have a professional teeth cleaning at least twice a year. Make and keep regular appointments with your health-care team.

Most important, educate yourself. It will help you ask better questions and make better decisions about your care. ❑

WHO'S WHO ON YOUR TEAM?

by Martha Jo Dendinger, C.M.P.

It's often said that two heads are better than one. When it comes to diabetes management, sometimes three or four or five heads can be even better. Although the day-to-day management of your diabetes is largely up to you, controlling your diabetes is easiest when you have a team of professionals backing you up. Different members of your team can bring specialized knowledge to your diabetes care. One may be able to help you craft an effective meal plan, while another can keep tabs on your vision, and another can help you set up an appropriate exercise program.

Because the diabetes team often comprises health professionals from many different disciplines, you may feel a little unclear about what role each person plays in your overall health care. But getting to know the members of your team—or working with your doctor to assemble a team if you don't already have one—gives you the advantage of knowing who to turn to when you have a problem with your diabetes control.

Why a team?

Going to just one doctor seems to suffice for most people, so you may wonder why you need a whole team. Let's look at some of the reasons for making diabetes care a group effort.

Diabetes is a complex disease that affects the entire body, but some parts of it need special care and attention. The eyes, the kidneys, and the feet, for example, are especially susceptible to the effects of high blood sugar. Just as sports teams have specialists for different jobs—the quarterback, the running back, the kicker in football; the pitcher, the catcher, and outfielders in baseball—the diabetes management team requires specialists to attend to different parts of the body.

Your primary-care physician, although a key player on your team, cannot play all the positions, or fulfill all of your health-care needs. You will need an optometrist or ophthalmologist for eye exams and to help you with problems specific to the eyes. If kidney function is a concern, you may be referred to a nephrologist. A podiatrist can provide specialized foot care. And there are many other experts you may need to call upon to help with some aspect of your diabetes care.

Rest assured that not all of the specialists listed in this article are needed by everyone with diabetes all of the time. You may never need to consult some or many of these specialists. Which health-care professionals you need on your team depends upon your particular situation, including the degree of control you maintain and any complications you may have.

The basic players

The captain of your diabetes team is, of course, you. But there are a few "core" players who should be within arm's reach to help you with the diabetes fundamentals. They are the following:

Primary-care physician. Your primary-care physician, also known as a family practitioner, general practitioner, or internist, can provide much of your diabetes care. Many physicians who treat people with diabetes are endocrinologists, medical doctors who have additional training in the study of endocrine glands (including the pancreas) and their functions.

Some people get their primary care from a nurse practitioner, a licensed nurse with advanced training in a specialized area of nursing, such as women's health or pediatric medicine. Nurse practitioners may practice independently or in a doctor's office, and in most states they can write prescriptions.

Two other professionals you may meet in your doctor's office are the nurse and the physician assistant. Nurses perform many functions in the doctor's office such as taking blood pressure and drawing blood samples. Some also provide counseling on particular subjects such as diet and exercise, and many can help explain aspects of your treatment or help with communication with your physician.

Some nurses, often called diabetes nurse educators, have specialized training in diabetes treatment and education. They can help with many diabetes basics, including showing you how to monitor your blood glucose and how to inject insulin. Depending on the nurse's place of employment, such instruction might be offered on a one-on-one basis or in a group or classroom setting.

Physician assistants practice medicine under the supervision of a doctor, doing everything from conducting physical exams to assisting in surgery. In many states, they are authorized to prescribe drugs. Physi-

cian assistants usually have two years of undergraduate education followed by another two years of specialized medical education.

Dietitian. No matter what type of diabetes you have, a meal plan that is tasty, helps control your blood sugar, and fits into your lifestyle is the holy grail of diabetes management. A dietitian can provide basic nutrition education and design a meal plan customized to your needs. A registered dietitian has fulfilled certain requirements set by the credentialing agency of The American Dietetic Association. People with diabetes may wish to seek out a dietitian who is also a certified diabetes educator (see below) or who takes a special interest in diabetes meal planning. (Note that a "nutritionist" is not the same as a registered dietitian. If you are considering seeing someone who claims to be a nutritionist, ask about the person's training and credentials to make sure you are getting advice from a knowledgeable source.)

Dentist. Everyone's team should include a dentist. Tell your dentist, periodontist, orthodontist, or oral surgeon about your diabetes and how you treat it. With this information, your dental-care provider should be willing to set your appointment times to accommodate your insulin or meal schedule. This information may also suggest a need for more frequent exams or cleanings to maintain healthy teeth and gums and to help combat gingivitis, a disease of the gums to which people with diabetes are very susceptible.

Pharmacist. Also known as druggists, pharmacists fill prescriptions. They are also great resources for information on both prescription and nonprescription drugs, including side effects and potential interactions between drugs. In many states, pharmacists can also check blood pressure, administer immunizations, and provide screening for certain diseases. While you may see several doctors, experts suggest that you have only one pharmacist, who can keep track of all of your drugs and note any potential problems such as harmful drug interactions.

Certified diabetes educator. Some physicians, nurses, dietitians, pharmacists, and other health-care providers are certified diabetes educators (C.D.E.'s). To be certified as a diabetes educator, a health-care professional must have provided at least 2,000 hours of direct diabetes patient education and have passed a rigorous exam on diabetes education and treatment. It's a good strategy to ensure that at least one of your team members is a C.D.E.

Supporting players

Many people with diabetes have only a doctor and a pharmacist on their team, but there are times when a little extra help is called for. Just as a sports coach will turn to the bench for a specialist, in diabetes manage-

ALPHABET SOUP?

The field of health care is growing broader, and at the same time, more health-care professionals are concentrating on specific areas of expertise. Various certification boards have popped up to license them, resulting in an abundance of degrees and licenses. The abbreviations for many of these specialists can get a bit confusing. Here's a list of some of the more common abbreviations you might encounter.

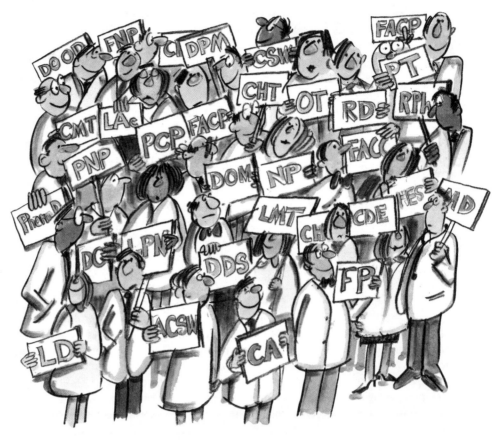

A.C.S.W. – accredited clinical social worker

A.P.R.N. – advanced practice registered nurse

A.R.N.P. – advanced registered nurse practitioner

B.S.N. – bachelor of science in nursing

C.A. – certified acupuncturist

C.D.E. – certified diabetes educator

C.H.E.S. – certified health education specialist

C.H.T. – certified hand therapist (a physical therapist who specializes in treatment of the hand)

C.M.T. – certified massage therapist

C.P.N.P. – certified pediatric nurse practitioner

C.P.T. – certified pump trainer

C.S.C.S. – certified strength and coordination specialist

D.C. – doctor of chiropractic

D.D.S. – doctor of dental surgery

D.M.D. – doctor of dental medicine (dentist)

D.O. – doctor of osteopathy

D.O.M. – doctor of Oriental medicine; usually an acupuncturist

D.P.M. – doctor of podiatric medicine

F.A.C.C. – Fellow of the American College of Cardiologists

F.A.C.P. – Fellow of the American College of Physicians

F.N.P. – family nurse practitioner

F.P. – family practitioner

L.Ac. – licensed acupuncturist

L.C.S.W. – licensed clinical social worker

L.D. – licensed dietitian

L.M.T. – licensed massage therapist

L.P.N. – licensed practical nurse

M.D. – doctor of medicine

M.S.N. – master of science in nursing

M.S.W. – master of social work; master of social welfare

N.P. – nurse practitioner

O.D. – doctor of optometry

O.T., O.T.R. – occupational therapist, occupational therapist-registered

P.A., P.A.-C. – physician's assistant, certified physician's assistant

P.C.P. – primary-care physician

Pharm.D. – doctor of pharmacy

Ph.D. – doctor of philosophy

P.N.P. – pediatric nurse practitioner

Psy.D. – doctor of psychology

P.T. – physical therapist

R.D. – registered dietitian

R.D.H. – registered dental hygienist

R.N. – registered nurse

R.N.C., R.N.,C. – registered nurse-certified

R.Ph. – registered pharmacist

R.P.T. – registered physical therapist

ment the same strategy can be useful: Your doctor may refer you to other professionals when your needs could best be met by someone else. For example, a neurologist, pain management specialist, or physical therapist may be able to offer the best treatment for painful neuropathy. A mental health professional or member of the clergy can help you cope with life changes and stresses brought on by diabetes and its management. Here are some of the more common specialists (in alphabetical order) you may want to have on your bench and how they can help you manage your diabetes.

Clergy. While the majority of your team members are focused on the physical aspects of your care, good treatment involves addressing spiritual needs also. Some religious leaders, in addition to offering spiritual guidance, are trained in counseling or other services and may be a good source for referrals.

Exercise specialist. Exercise is a crucial part of diabetes management, so it pays to plan it carefully and get help if you need it. Start by asking your doctor if your medical condition or fitness level makes some activities better choices than others. For more help, see what's available in your community. Many gyms and health clubs have personal trainers who can help you come up with an appropriate exercise routine. Your diabetes clinic may have an exercise physiologist on staff who can work with you to develop a program that will be both safe and healthful. Whoever you choose to work with, make sure that person is willing to learn about your diabetes and what it takes to control it during your chosen physical activity.

Massage therapist. Massage therapy can help reduce stress and improve circulation, both of which are pluses in diabetes management. Many types of massage can relieve muscle pain. So-called "therapeutic" massage is usually performed by a physical therapist with the intent of treating a specific ailment such as lower back pain. "Relaxation" massage is intended to soothe overall stress and tiredness.

Mental health professional. Caring for your psychological health is as important as caring for your physical health. Chronic illness and its treatment can bring on depression, anxiety, anger, and relationship problems. And these can seriously hinder your diabetes control, not to mention your enjoyment of life. To deal with your feelings and learn new ways to cope with life, you may wish to see a mental health professional. There are many types of mental health professionals with different qualifications. These include trained counselors, psychologists, and psychiatrists. Treatment usually entails group or individual therapy sessions. Psychiatrists, who are M.D.'s, may also prescribe drugs when appropriate. Counselors and psychologists are usually not medical doctors.

Nephrologist. A nephrologist is a medical doctor who specializes in the kidney. Your primary-care physician may refer you to a nephrologist if there are concerns about your kidney function. Kidney problems are a major complication of uncontrolled diabetes.

Neurologist. A neurologist is a medical doctor who specializes in the nervous system. You might see one for treatment for neuropathy, or nerve damage, caused by long-term or uncontrolled diabetes.

Occupational therapist. If diabetes complications have made movement or accomplishing everyday activities difficult for you, an occupational therapist can teach you ways to more easily do such tasks as cooking, cleaning, driving, and dressing, as well as checking your blood sugar and injecting insulin.

Ophthalmologist. The American Diabetes Association recommends that everyone with diabetes get a yearly dilated eye exam to check for diabetic retinopathy, a common diabetes complication. All ophthalmologists and some specially trained optometrists are qualified to perform dilated exams. Ophthalmologists have an M.D. degree and are authorized to diagnose and treat eye disease, perform surgery, and prescribe drugs. An ophthalmologist will also have an understanding of how medical conditions—such as diabetes and high blood pressure—can affect the eyes.

Optometrist. Some optometrists focus their practice on testing vision and prescribing corrective lenses. However, more and more are broadening their practice to diagnose and treat eye disease, and some are licensed to prescribe certain drugs.

Physical therapist. Injuries or neuropathy may require the assistance of a physical therapist, who can help you manage pain and improve mobility using exercise, heat, cold, or water therapy. Many physical therapists also help people with chronic illnesses or injuries design customized exercise plans.

Podiatrist. Podiatrists specialize in treatment of the feet and ankles, although they often diagnose conditions that affect the whole body, such as vascular disease, based on symptoms in the feet and legs. They can perform certain types of surgery and prescribe drugs. Your primary-care physician should examine your feet at every visit but may refer you to a podiatrist for specialized care.

Social worker. Also known as a case manager, a social worker can provide counseling for people with diabetes or other chronic illnesses. Social workers can also connect you with community resources and help you find practical solutions for life changes brought on by diabetes and its management, such as moving from home to an assisted-living center or changing jobs.

Support group. Many people with diabetes find the camaraderie of a support group very helpful. Being able to talk with other people with diabetes not only can help you feel less alone, but it can help you develop new perspectives on diabetes and new methods of dealing with day-to-day management challenges. A support group can also be beneficial for spouses and caregivers who might not have anyone else to confide in.

Recruiting your team

You probably already have a primary-care physician and a pharmacist on your team. If you're pleased with the services they provide, by all means stick with them. But know that other options are available to you if you're looking for a change. It's important to trust your doctor and to feel that he or she pays sufficient attention to your health needs. If you feel that you can't communicate with your doctor or that your doctor can't or won't give you the help you need, it may be time to look elsewhere. Most managed care plans require that your doctor be on a preapproved list, but you should be able to choose another doctor from that list.

Whenever you need special assistance with your diabetes management, start with your primary-care physician or endocrinologist—for two main reasons. First, many health-care plans require you to obtain written referrals from your primary-care physician before seeing a specialist, or they will not pay for the treatment. Most primary-care physicians have lists of specialists for referrals.

Another reason to start with your primary-care physician is that new members of the team should agree with the basic treatment plan and philosophy set by your doctor. This is very important: The primary-care physician, as coach for you and your team, must know about all the specialists you are seeing to make sure that their treatments and prescriptions do not conflict. Having open lines of communication and a good rapport among the members of your team can make it very effective. After all, to win the game you need not just a complete team but one that works together. ❏

ADDITIONAL RESOURCES

For more information on the specialties described in this article, or to find the name of a specialist in your area, contact the organizations listed below.

AMERICAN ACADEMY OF MEDICAL ACUPUNCTURE
(800) 521-2262
www.medicalacupuncture.org

AMERICAN ACADEMY OF NEUROLOGY
(651) 695-1940
www.aan.com

AMERICAN ACADEMY OF OPHTHALMOLOGY
(415) 561-8500
www.eyenet.org

AMERICAN ACADEMY OF OPTOMETRY
(301) 984-1441
www.aaopt.org

AMERICAN ACADEMY OF PHYSICIAN ASSISTANTS
(703) 836-2272
www.aapa.org

AMERICAN ASSOCIATION OF DIABETES EDUCATORS
(800) 338-3633
www.aadenet.org

AMERICAN DIABETES ASSOCIATION
(800) 232-3472
www.diabetes.org

THE AMERICAN DIETETIC ASSOCIATION
(800) 366-1655
www.eatright.org

AMERICAN MASSAGE THERAPY ASSOCIATION
(847) 864-0123
www.amtamassage.org

AMERICAN NURSES ASSOCIATION
(800) 274-4ANA (274-4262)
www.ana.org

AMERICAN OCCUPATIONAL THERAPY ASSOCIATION
(301) 652-2682
www.aota.org

AMERICAN PHYSICAL THERAPY ASSOCIATION
(800) 989-APTA (989-2782)
www.apta.org

AMERICAN PODIATRIC MEDICAL ASSOCIATION
(301) 571-9200
www.apma.org

AMERICAN PSYCHOLOGICAL ASSOCIATION
(800) 374-2721
www.apa.org

AMERICAN SOCIETY OF EXERCISE PHYSIOLOGISTS
(218) 723-6297
www.css.edu/asep

AMERICAN SOCIETY OF NEPHROLOGY
(202) 367-1190
www.asn-online.com

JUVENILE DIABETES RESEARCH FOUNDATION INTERNATIONAL
(800) JDF-CURE (533-2873)
www.jdf.org

NATIONAL ASSOCIATION OF SOCIAL WORKERS
(800) 638-8799
www.socialworkers.org

NATIONAL CERTIFICATION COMMISSION FOR ACUPUNCTURE AND ORIENTAL MEDICINE
(703) 548-9004
www.nccaom.org

DEALING WITH FEELINGS

DEALING WITH THE DIAGNOSIS
WHERE DO YOU GO FROM HERE?

by Kenneth Ruge, D.Min.

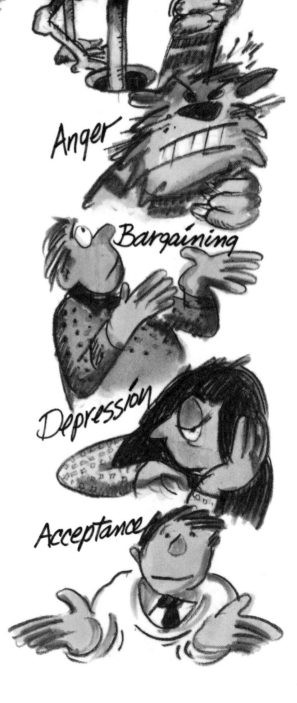

While taking a walk several months ago, I heard someone call my name and turned around to see a rather distinguished looking, bearded man who seemed completely unfamiliar to me.

"Ken, don't you recognize me? It's Paul!" he said. Sure enough, it was an acquaintance I had not seen in six years. He had grown a beard and looked like a different man, which explained my inability to recognize him at first. But as we chatted and walked together, I discovered that his neat new facial hair was not the only change in his life since we were last in touch. He told me he had finally quit an office job that he had disliked for 20 years and was actually making his living as a sculptor and art instructor at several schools in the area. In fact, a show of his work was coming up soon at one of them! He also told me that he was about to marry a woman he had met in one of his classes and become stepfather and step-grandfather to a wonderful new family. So he was to be a bachelor no more, on top of everything else, with age 60 approaching!

When I asked him how he had made so many changes so quickly, his answer took me completely off guard. "Well," he said, "five years ago I learned that I have diabetes, and..." He went on to describe how vibrant and wonderful his life had become, even thanking diabetes for sending a signal that, as he put it, "It was time to get my house in order."

Paul's story inevitably led me to think about another acquaintance, Sarah, a woman who has also had diabetes for several years. Unlike Paul, however, she has cut herself off from friends and family and resists following her diet and self-care regimen—even blaming God and her family for ending the productive, happy part of her life.

I began to wonder how two people of similar age and with essentially the same health concerns could react so differently. I began to see that either approach—viewing diabetes as a wake-up call or a curse—is a choice that each person decided to make. And it is a choice you can make, too. Armed with the right information and attitude, you can still make the most of your life despite diabetes, and you can even change your life for the better.

Shock and reorganization

Whether you've known for a while that you have diabetes or were recently diagnosed, you already know that this challenging condition requires you to rethink a lot of your life. How you engage in that process might be the key to whether you become a Paul or a Sarah as you restructure your life and move on. To explain this kind of learning experience, Virginia Satir, one of the pioneers of family therapy, created the Shock and Reorganization Model.

Shock occurs when you suddenly get new information, such as finding out you have diabetes, that conflicts with your sense of who you are. Life as you know it is suddenly disrupted by profound new issues that you have no choice but to deal with, whether or not you understand them at the time.

Reorganization follows, in response to the initial shock. You find a new way to put the pieces of your life back together, reorganizing your self-image, activities, and relationships.

I see these steps at work in the life of a friend who recently learned he has diabetes. It was indeed a shock. The news ushered in a period of profound personal adjustment, which was made more difficult by the fact that his life seemed to be in perfect order before the diagnosis. Steve is a successful stockbroker who is happily married and has two wonderful young children. Suddenly, he feels his health has been taken away from him. Steve acts like someone grieving the loss of a loved one. He is sometimes difficult to live with at home. He says he feels exhausted—not so much because of his diabetes, but because of the stress of adjusting to change. Yet even in these tough days, he's beginning to put his life back together in a thoughtful, constructive way. As Steve learns to deal with changes in his physical health, his attitude is turning back toward more positive thoughts. His wife and friends know that he's going to adjust and that he'll be all right.

But will Steve merely cope with diabetes, or will he reach some better, transformed life, as my friend Paul did? Perhaps the answer to that question lies in the writings of Dr. Elisabeth Kübler-Ross, a psychiatrist and authority and counselor on issues related to death.

Stages of change

According to Dr. Kübler-Ross, when people confront a significant loss or major life change such as the onset of a chronic illness, the loss of a loved one, the loss of a job, or a divorce, they adjust to the change in a series of predictable stages. Regardless of the source of distress, most people go through the stages of denial, anger, bargaining, and depression before reaching the final stage of acceptance.

Denial. This is the first, ostrich-like response. When someone first learns that he has diabetes, for example, he is likely to react by sticking his head in the sand and saying, "This is not happening! This can't be happening to me! This is not who I am!" When confronted with any life-altering news that doesn't fit a person's sense of who he is, this is a natural first response.

Anger. In this second stage, the person begins to wonder, "Why me? This is unfair! What did I do to deserve this? Why is my health being affected?" He may even become angry at God (who serves as a handy scapegoat for unwanted life changes), or he may blame his spouse, friends, or family members for his new problems.

Bargaining. In this stage, people begin to consider making changes. The newly diagnosed person with diabetes may have thoughts such as, "If I don't eat Snickers bars for the next six months, then everything will be fine and I'll be back to normal. And I'll walk every day, too. OK, is that a deal?" Of course, watching your diet and maintaining an exercise program will help blood sugar control, but you know that diabetes will not go away. Even though such thoughts usually do not result in changes that improve the situation, bargaining allows people to grapple with how they are going to change their lives. Yet it isn't the ultimate answer, since people cannot erase changes in their lives.

Depression. As people start to accept the permanence of these changes, they usually get the blues. They lose hope, lack energy, experience trouble sleeping, or see a drop in libido. At this point, many people also report that they're just going through the motions of daily life. "The horizon seemed a kind of bleak gray," one woman recalls, "and I thought it would stay that way forever." Such depression saps peoples' sense of hope and sense of the future. But after they have gone to this dark place, the gloom lifts and they can move on.

Acceptance. A new day dawns somewhat gradually. People begin to accept the new changes and they envision a future—a new life that takes diabetes into consideration. They can see new possibilities and new

Dealing With Feelings

options for themselves. With the support of family and friends, advice and guidance from health-care professionals, and some healthy reevaluation, they can move ahead with a restored sense of hope.

How these stages help

Knowing about these stages of change is helpful. It provides a framework for people to understand their feelings and lets them know that others have had similar experiences.

Knowing about these stages also lessens the chances of getting stalled in one stage and not moving on. It's easy and seductive, for instance, to get stuck denying one's diabetes by not taking medicines, not exercising, and not monitoring your blood sugar. It's equally tempting to get stuck in depression and self-pity, casting yourself as a victim of a capricious God, your genetic makeup, or your past habits. Denying your feelings of anger or depression is another way you can get stuck moving through the stages. But if you realize where you are in the process, you stand a better chance of breaking out, moving on, and finding new meaning and rewards.

If you're going through such a process (or if you're supporting someone who is), it may help to know that people usually work through the five stages several times over and not always one after the other. In fact, most people spiral back and forth through the stages, gravitating slowly toward acceptance. One day they're working on acceptance issues, then the next day they're bargaining, angry, or depressed. It takes time and patience and inner courage to accept your feelings as you move this process along.

From acceptance to mastery

Once a person with diabetes reaches acceptance, he can view diabetes not as a loss, but as an opportunity to reorient his life and priorities. That's clearly what Paul did. He incorporated all his changes and restructured his life magnificently.

When people reach acceptance, they often say they now occupy a new kind of landscape—a place that's different from where they lived before all the changes took place. Often, they start to review the past.

When you have reached this stage of the change process, you too may find yourself considering how you've lived your life up to this time. What's been important to you? What would you have done differently? You're really starting a new chapter! Another characteristic of this stage is that time may become more precious to you. We're not immortal. And our choices may be limited. But these thoughts aren't necessarily limiting or morose. In fact, they may be an invitation to take risks and redirect our lives to where we really want to be.

SUGGESTED READING

To read more about personal growth and development in the face of adversity, look for these books in your local bookstore or library:

WHERE DO I GO FROM HERE
An Inspirational Guide to Making Authentic Life and Career Choices
Kenneth Ruge
McGraw-Hill
New York, 1998
This book by the author of this article offers readings and exercises for people engaged in self-discovery and personal redirection using a practical, spiritual vantage point.

THE WHEEL OF LIFE
A Memoir of Living and Dying
Elisabeth Kübler-Ross
Scribners
New York, 1997
This biographical book leads the reader through life lessons that can be learned by confronting and passing through life's great challenges.

GIFT OF THE RED BIRD
A Spiritual Encounter
Paula D'Arcy
Crossroad Publishing Company
New York, 1996
Ms. D'Arcy lost her husband and young child in an accident. This inspiring book tells of spiritual insights she gained while taking a wilderness retreat in search of healing and answers.

SEVEN HABITS OF HIGHLY EFFECTIVE PEOPLE
Stephen R. Covey
Fireside Books
New York, 1989
Mr. Covey offers seven suggestions to help individuals overcome personal chaos or crisis. These tips highlight lifestyle changes for a more effective and fulfilling life.

SOUL MAPPING
An Imaginative Way to Self-Discovery
Nina H. Frost, Kenneth C. Ruge, and Richard W. Shoup
Marlowe
New York, 2000
The authors, through wide-ranging questions and exercises, help you understand more clearly who you were, who you are, and who you most want to be.

As that new horizon becomes brighter and better defined, many of us can focus on what is truly important to us. An exercise developed by Stephen Covey (author of several books, including *Seven Habits of Highly Effective People*) can help you achieve that level of insight. In this exercise, imagine yourself sitting in the back pew at your own funeral service. No one can see you as you listen to eulogies about you delivered by four different people. The first eulogy is given by a colleague, who talks about what you were like at work. The second speaker is a friend, who talks about you as a member of your social circle. The third is a relative, who describes your home and family life. The fourth is a member of your religious community, who recalls you in that context. Listen closely as you sit in your imaginary pew. What would those four people say, honestly, about you? Is that the kind of eulogy you would like to hear? If not, what are you going to do about it?

Certain questions will arise in your mind as you go through this exercise. What qualities would you like to be remembered for? What is most important in your life? What are your values? What do you stand for? Are you living your life according to those values and beliefs? These questions offer an opportunity to orient yourself toward a more authentic you.

Creating a spiritual tie

As you set your life back on center and start moving ahead, you might also want to bring another level of self-discovery into the process. You might say, "OK, I'm in a new place. My health is back in my control. I'm sorting out my values. But are these new life changes also a spiritual opportunity for me?"

They probably are. In the words of author Paula D'Arcy, "God is in the detours." She means that any cataclysmic life change offers an opportunity to ask the spiritual questions, "What am I supposed to be

doing with my life?" and "What does God intend for me?"

I recall my own father working out those issues. Dad faced hurdles and losses like the rest of us, but he still somehow managed to reorient his life toward a more spiritual plane. For one thing, he had diabetes back in the days before many of the medical advances that are available today. For another, he lost his wife at a relatively early age. I recall that he went through stages of loss similar to those I describe above—certainly through anger and depression. Yet through it all, he defined a new role for himself as a teacher and spokesperson in a 12-step recovery program. Helping other people became a very meaningful opportunity for him to put his diabetes in perspective and to get his life back in order after my mother's death. Despite the difficult challenges, he used them to open doors to new ways of thinking that were both meaningful and personally authentic.

Finding your path

So, where are you supposed to go as you begin this new chapter in your life? It may mean drawing closer to family and friends. It may mean discovering and following your passion—whether it's a long-deferred dream or some new interest. It may mean taking a new role as you encourage acts of healing and reconciliation among your family members and friends. Or it may mean an increased devotion to spirituality or health or nature. Life is an open book. You can write your own story.

As you navigate your unique journey, try to remember that your path may not be exactly what it at first seems—a hard road, blocked by high obstacles and tough challenges. It is really an opportunity for you to redesign your life in a fuller and more authentic way. As you walk this new walk, I wish you good luck, good friends, and Godspeed. ❑

GETTING UP
WHEN YOU'RE DOWN

by William H. Polonsky, Ph.D., C.D.E.

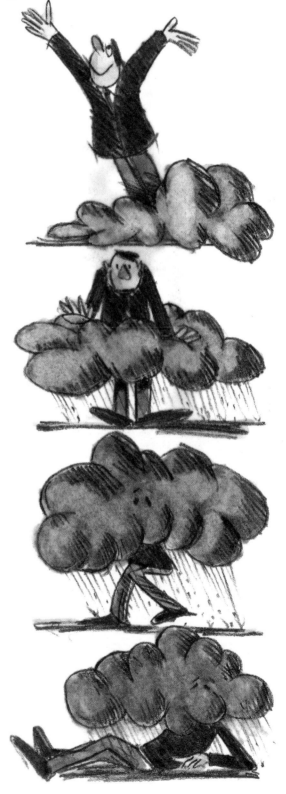

We all have times when we feel overwhelmed and stressed. Now and then, a sense of gloom and sadness may cast a pall over our whole day. Luckily, for most of us, such feelings come and go and rarely reach a deep level of despair. For some, however, such feelings are a constant companion that can lead to significant problems in family relationships, jobs, and quality of life. This type of depression, called *major depression,* can be a very serious and sometimes life-threatening problem. To make matters worse, when this form of depression is combined with diabetes, a very nasty interaction frequently happens: Depression can make it much more difficult to manage diabetes and, in turn, diabetes can make it more difficult to recognize and treat depression.

The good news is that depression is not a shameful weakness or an incurable curse. Rather, this problem, which is born of a complex interplay of biology and life experience, is a thoroughly treatable illness. If you feel those blues are playing longer than normal, ask for help; chances are that with treatment, the depression will lift and you can get back to feeling like your old self.

A common experience

For 40 years, Duane had been a relatively happy and successful engineer with a large Midwest corporation. When he retired last year at 65, he expected a time of delicious relaxation and happiness. Instead, he spent most of his days aimlessly working on household tasks he cared little about (and which he never did get around to finishing) and arguing with his wife more and more (and often about the silliest things).

All this left him feeling increasingly grumpy. Over time, he found it harder and harder to get a good night's sleep; he often woke up early in the morning and couldn't fall back to sleep. He felt lonely, worried, and tired all the time, found it difficult to concentrate on anything, and was slowly losing interest in most of the things that had previously given him pleasure. With little to do, he was feeling increasingly worthless and even began to have recurrent thoughts about his own death.

Duane had developed diabetes in his early 50's and had never found it very difficult to manage, until recently. Since his retirement, he became increasingly fond of chips, crackers, and cookies, especially late at night. His blood sugar level climbed to well above 200 mg/dl, he was gaining weight, and his doctor told him that it was probably time to begin insulin. Duane knew that he had to make some major changes in his life, but he didn't know where to start or where to find the motivation to begin.

Though Duane didn't know it, he was suffering from a major depressive disorder. He had most of the major characteristics that are used to diagnose the illness, including changes in feelings (such as a sad mood and the loss of pleasure), negative thoughts (such as feelings of worthlessness and recurrent thoughts of death), and changes in behavior (with resulting insomnia, chronic fatigue, and weight gain).

Like Duane, many people suffer in silence. Either no one recognizes that something is wrong or the depressed person never asks for help. As a result, the burden of depression may continue for years and years. Duane's story also illustrates the fact that depression is not about being "crazy" or having a "weak mind." And it is much more than just feeling sad. Depression is a coherent group of mental and physical symptoms that can afflict any of us, regardless of how bright, stable, or successful we have been in our lives.

Depression is not a rare event. Among the general population, 5% to 8% of people will experience a major depressive disorder at some time in their lives. However, among those people who have diabetes, the rate is at least doubled. Approximately 15% to 20% of people with diabetes will experience major depression. When we add in the milder forms of this illness, it is obvious that a very large number of people with diabetes are likely to encounter depression at least once in their lives. And it is especially important to worry about depression if you have diabetes, since depression can sap your motivation and make it even harder to deal with diabetes self-care tasks.

The roots of depression

What causes depression? In most cases, it is caused by a confusing combination of factors. We know that biology can play an important role, ranging from the broad influence of heredity to other biological changes such as neurotransmitter levels in the brain and hormone levels in the body. The social environment can also be important; job and family stresses, the loss of a loved one, and feelings of loneliness can all contribute to depression. In addition, our thinking styles are very significant. For example, depression is more likely to occur in those people who characteristically see themselves as powerless or out of control in their own lives. Researchers at the University of Pennsylvania have found that this particular style of thinking, known as "pessimistic explanatory style," is a strong predictor for the development of depression.

Diabetes can also contribute to depression. When blood sugar levels are chronically high, for example, you may feel more down and lethargic. Most people do not know that chronically elevated blood sugar levels can lead to significant biological changes in mood, including such feelings as depression and increased fatigue. Indeed, sometimes these changes occur so gradually that you hardly notice that you are feeling different. In many of these cases, regaining good control of blood sugars may cause a dramatic improvement in depression.

Biology aside, the ongoing struggle of coping with diabetes may also lead to depression. Feeling that you are constantly failing with your diabetes regimen, or that you are all alone in your struggle to manage diabetes, or feeling hopeless in the face of long-term complications can lead to a sense of "diabetes burnout" and eventually depression.

One of the reasons people with diabetes may be more likely to develop depressive disorders is because of the tricky ways in which these two problems can interact. As in Duane's case, depression can lead to a loss of motivation and poorer diabetes self-care, which can lead to chronically high blood sugar levels followed by greater fatigue and lethargy, which can then worsen your mood. In other words, depression can interfere with diabetes management, and that can in turn exert a negative impact on depression, leading to a difficult downward spiral that can prove quite hard to reverse.

Symptoms of depression

How can you tell if you are depressed? Surprisingly, it is not as easy as you might think. Many people experience just the physical symptoms of depression (such as insomnia and appetite changes) without ever really noticing any *feelings* of depression. To make matters worse, in people with diabetes, studies show that depression is recognized and treated in less than one-third of those who are suffering. If you suspect that you may be living with depression, consider the following symptoms:

■ Do you feel depressed, tearful, or empty most of the time?

■ Have you experienced changes in your sleep pattern such as difficulty falling asleep, staying asleep, or sleeping more than usual?

■ Have you experienced changes in your appetite such as eating much more or much less than usual, resulting in a significant change in your weight over a relatively brief period of time?

■ Do you frequently feel so anxious that you can't sit still?

■ Have you lost interest or pleasure in most of your common activities?

■ Have you noticed that it is more difficult to concentrate on tasks?

■ Do you feel worthless or excessively guilty about the past most of the time?

■ Do you frequently think about your death or have thoughts about suicide?

If you have been feeling down for more than two weeks and you recognize two or three of these symptoms or more, you should take some action as soon as possible. Odds are good that you may be suffering from depression. The good news is that, in many cases, *depression is curable.* There is no need for suffering to continue when brief and effective treatments are available.

Seeking treatment

What action should you take? Most important, begin by talking to your doctor. He or she can help you determine what is causing these symptoms, uncover any physical factors that may underlie the depression (such as thyroid disorders or certain prescription drugs), and help you to develop a plan for treatment.

To overcome depression, you and your doctor should consider these major strategies:

Psychotherapy. A series of large-scale studies sponsored by the National Institute of Mental Health have shown that structured psychotherapy with a mental health professional can help to overcome depression. In particular, a psychotherapy approach that includes *cognitive–behavioral strategies* seems to be one of the most effective. These studies have shown that over half of those patients who receive such treatment recover from their depression quickly, usually within three months. In this type of brief, action-oriented counseling, the psychotherapist and patient team up to figure out how the patient's thoughts, feelings, and actions may be maintaining the depressive disorder and then develop specific methods for making necessary changes.

In Duane's case, for example, his psychotherapist helped him to realize that his depression had primarily resulted from his retirement, which had led him to the incorrect belief that he was no longer needed and that his life no longer had value. By challenging these negative thoughts and by encouraging small behavioral changes (Duane began volunteering at a local museum), a cascade of changes soon followed: Duane's self-esteem began to lift, his sleep patterns improved, he felt renewed energy, and he developed a closer relationship with his wife.

Psychotherapy approaches such as these are designed to help people cope more effectively with stressful life circumstances and, thus, may also be beneficial in preventing the recurrence of depression. Oddly enough, many people with major depression avoid psychotherapy, because they believe that it is just for those who are "weak." On the contrary, people who use psychotherapy are actually quite brave; after all, they are willing to risk confrontation with their personal fears and vulnerabilities.

FOR MORE INFORMATION

More information about depression, referrals, and support can be obtained by calling or writing to these organizations or by visiting their Web sites:

NATIONAL INSTITUTE OF MENTAL HEALTH
(301) 443-4513
www.nimh.nih.gov

NATIONAL DEPRESSIVE AND MANIC-DEPRESSIVE ASSOCIATION
730 N. Franklin Street
Suite 501
Chicago, IL 60610-7204
(312) 642-0049, (800) 826-3632
www.ndmda.org

NATIONAL MENTAL HEALTH ASSOCIATION
1021 Prince Street
Alexandria, VA 22314-2971
(703) 684-7722, (800) 969-NMHA (969-6642)
www.nmha.org

To read more about depression, check out these books at your local library or bookstore:

FEELING GOOD
The New Mood Therapy
David D. Burns
Avon Books
New York, 1999

PSYCHING OUT DIABETES
A Positive Approach to Your Negative Emotions
Richard H. Rubin, June Biermann, and
Barbara Toohey
Lowell House
Los Angeles, 1999

DIABETES BURNOUT
What to Do When You Can't Take It Anymore
William Polonsky
American Diabetes Association
Alexandria, Virginia, 1999

LEARNED OPTIMISM
Martin F. P. Seligman
Simon & Schuster
New York, 1998

Antidepressant drugs. Three major classes of antidepressant drugs are currently used, and all have been proven to alleviate depression: Tricyclic antidepressants (the most well-known is amitryptiline, or Elavil); selective serotonin reuptake inhibitors (or SSRI's, which include fluoxetine, or Prozac); and monoamine oxidase (MAO) inhibitors. MAO inhibitors are used the least often of the three classes because they require a special diet.

Like psychotherapy, over half of the people who take antidepressant medicine recover quickly from their depression. However, despite their proven helpfulness, antidepressant drugs have developed a bad reputation over the years and still lead to people being or feeling stigmatized. The truth is that antidepressants are not addictive and they are not "happy pills." In most cases, they can help people to feel more like their old selves and, in combination with psychotherapy, help them to more effectively confront the very real and difficult beliefs, feelings, and situations that need to be resolved.

Antidepressants alone are probably the best choice for those who cannot talk about their problems as well as those who don't have the time or money available for psychotherapy. Also, for people who are very depressed, antidepressants can be used to help them improve enough to become receptive to psychotherapy.

Exercise. While reaching out for professional intervention is the most important thing you can do, there are steps you can take on your own that can support the process of overcoming depression. Indeed, given that feelings of powerlessness are so closely linked to depression, taking *any* positive action is likely to be a valuable step.

So take action to become physically active, especially if you tend to be a sedentary soul. A brief walk around the neighborhood each morning is a good way to clear your head and reduce stress (not to mention all the other benefits of physical exercise on diabetes and general health). And there is good scientific evidence that regular physical activity may generate important biological changes that may aid in reducing depression. These may include direct changes in the levels of the same neurotransmitters that are influenced by antidepressant drugs. So you don't even have to enjoy it immediately; just walk each day for one week and then decide for yourself if your mood has improved and if it was worth doing.

Confidants. One of the toughest things about major depression is the overpowering sense of isolation you may feel. Even when surrounded by a loving family, it is easy to feel very alone. You may feel that no one does (or can) understand what you are going through. Take a risk and reach out to make real contact with one person, asking him or her to listen to you and talk with you, without trying to solve your problems. Having a confidant can have a very significant impact on overcoming depression.

If having a confidant is not possible, put your thoughts and feelings to paper. Specifically, start a journal or write a letter to someone you trust. In a series of innovative research studies, Dr. James Pennebaker and his colleagues have shown that the simple act of writing down your thoughts and feelings can have a major influence on mood. Even if you never share your journal or mail your letter, you can begin an important process that can help you overcome your depression.

Avoid alcohol abuse. Unfortunately, the most common (and most foolish) treatment for depression is the liberal use of alcohol (or recreational drugs). While excessive use of booze can be a temporary escape that takes you away from depression and dulls the pain for a short while, it actually serves over time to *worsen* depression. For one thing, excessive alcohol use interferes with the body's ability to enter a state of deep, restful sleep. Frequent drinking binges lead you to become increasingly deprived of restorative sleep, resulting in more and more fatigue as the days pass.

Excessive alcohol use also serves to further isolate you from people who might offer support and activities that might make you feel better. Alcohol abuse can interfere with your work and your relationships, and eat away at your self-esteem. If you are suffering from depression and drinking excessively, you are pouring gasoline on a fire. At this stage, seeking outside help is imperative.

Improve your glycemic control. As noted earlier, chronically elevated blood sugar can lead to chronic fatigue and other mood changes that can exacerbate depression. By bringing blood sugar levels back into a lower range, many people find that their moods brighten and their energy levels climb. For example, early in the course of Duane's psychotherapy, Duane was convinced to follow his doctor's advice to begin insulin. Within the week, his mood and energy improved, which motivated him to pursue the initial behavioral changes he and his therapist planned. So to overcome depression, talk with your doctor about taking more aggressive action to improve your diabetes management, especially if your blood glucose levels are chronically elevated.

Rays of hope

If you are experiencing major depression, please know that you are not alone and that there is no need to give up hope. Depression is remarkably common in people with diabetes, partly because of the unfortunate interaction between diabetes and depression. The good news is that depression is absolutely treatable. By talking with your doctor, you can set up an effective treatment plan that may involve psychotherapy, antidepressant medicines, and a host of personal behavior changes. Why put it off? ❏

DEALING WITH "DIABETES OVERWHELMUS"

by Richard R. Rubin, Ph.D., C.D.E.

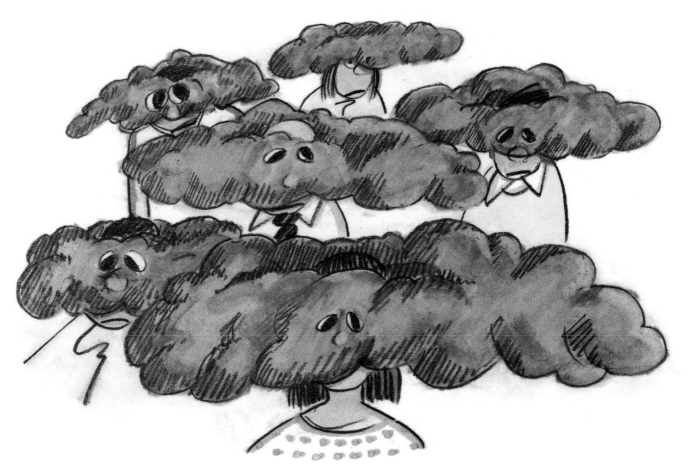

Janice sat stuck in an extra-long backup on the highway after a stressful day at work. The traffic jam gave her plenty of time to think about what she had to do when she got home. First, she should check her blood sugar level, and with all the stress she was feeling, it was sure to be high. In fact, it had been high most of the time recently.

Janice hated having high blood sugar. It made her feel rotten: tired, worried, and guilty all at once. You might think that feeling bad would motivate her to do something about her blood sugar control. But instead, it seemed to drain all the energy she might have put toward getting back on track. Over the past couple of weeks, she had been checking her blood sugar less frequently and telling herself she didn't need to because it was sure to be high. She knew her rationale for not checking didn't make sense, but still...

Even though she wasn't monitoring her blood sugar regularly, Janice knew it was high because she was frequently running to the bathroom to urinate. In addition, she had pretty much given up on her walking program. She knew she had hit bottom when she sat in front of the television one night and ate an entire pint of ice cream after the rest of her family had gone to sleep.

Janice's work had become more demanding in the past couple of months, but not enough to explain how badly things were going. "I used to do a decent job with my diabetes," Janice said to herself. Then, sitting there on the highway, gridlocked 50 yards from her exit, she yelled, "What's wrong with me?"

I'd say Janice is suffering from a condition I call *diabetes overwhelmus*. At the moment, she is simply overwhelmed by the demands of diabetes. That's not to say these are the only demands she is dealing with. Stress at work, at home, and in other important parts of her life are also contributing to her burden. But the demands of diabetes seem to be playing a big part in her distress. That's why I think Janice may be suffering from a bout of diabetes overwhelmus.

A common problem

Diabetes overwhelmus is very common, and it's common for one simple reason: Diabetes is a very demanding disease. It's there all the time, 24 hours a day, 365 days a year, and it never goes away. The things you need to do to care for it—such as lance your fingers several times a day to check your blood sugar level—are no fun. Most people don't enjoy having to exercise regularly and eat carefully, either. Perhaps most frustrating of all is that even when you do all the things you are supposed to do, there is no guarantee that your blood sugar will stay where you want it or even be predictable. And to top off the burden, there are the unpleasant physical effects of high and low blood sugar levels.

Given the responsibilities and stresses that come with having diabetes, it's no surprise that many people suffer from at least occasional bouts of diabetes overwhelmus. In fact, the real surprise may be that for most people, these bouts are only occasional. I'd like to tell you what I've learned about ways to protect yourself from diabetes overwhelmus and to get back on your feet if you are feeling overwhelmed.

Preventing diabetes overwhelmus

Avoiding feeling overwhelmed by your diabetes is very important, and Janice is a perfect illustration of why. Until recently, she was feeling good, her stress levels were under control, and she wasn't feeling overwhelmed. That gave her the motivation and energy she needed to take care of her diabetes. As a result of her attentive self-care, Janice's blood sugar levels were usually close to normal, she felt good physically, and she felt in control of her diabetes. However, when her stress level began to mount, feeling overwhelmed made it harder to care for her diabetes. As she stopped performing parts of her regular diabetes self-care routine, her blood sugar levels rose, she felt worse physically, and she felt more and more overwhelmed.

What you need to do to keep diabetes overwhelmus from your door is probably unique to you. That's because everyone's life is a little different and everyone's diabetes is a little different. I've learned over the years that the source of diabetes overwhelmus is often a very specific issue, what I call a "sticking point." A sticking point is like a piece of grit in the gears: It isn't very big, but it can cause a lot of trouble. Clearing your sticking point is often the key to resolving diabetes overwhelmus.

The first step is to identify your sticking point. Even if you aren't currently feeling overwhelmed, you may want to try to identify your sticking point: It could help protect you from becoming overwhelmed. Think about what's hardest for you right now about living with diabetes. If the first answer that comes to mind is "everything," you probably are feeling overwhelmed. However, if your first answer is something like "my diet" or "testing my blood," you are close to identifying the problem.

Whatever your first response, try to be more specific. You'll know you have identified a real sticking point when you can picture yourself in the situation. For example, "I can't stop snacking between dinner and bedtime," is a specific sticking point, as is "I can't get myself to check my blood sugar at work before I eat my lunch." I can picture each of these situations perfectly.

One of the great things about sticking points is that once you identify one, you can almost always find a way to clear it. So taking the time to identify your current sticking point is a big first step toward dealing with diabetes overwhelmus. You are working like a football referee, digging through the pile of players to find the one who has possession of the ball.

Once you have identified a sticking point, you can use your experience to clear it. Here's how: Think about a time when you didn't feel so stuck dealing with the issue you have identified. It doesn't matter if this has rarely been true, or if it has been a long time since it was true. Try to recall even one time when you weren't struggling as hard as you are now. What was different then?

When I asked one man this question, he realized that the only times he didn't snack nonstop between dinner and bedtime (his sticking point) were those evenings when his young granddaughter came to visit. He started spending more time with her, babysitting a couple of nights a week (to the delight of his son and his daughter-in-law, who appreciated the time off). The evenings he didn't babysit, he called his granddaughter on the phone. The result: The man cut out the extra snacking altogether three to four evenings a week, and he cut back a lot most other nights. Was it a miracle? If so, it's a miracle you can make happen in your own life.

In addition to identifying your sticking points and finding ways to clear them, there are other ways to protect yourself from developing diabetes overwhelmus or to banish it if it has you down. I've found that people who are feeling overwhelmed almost always lack one or more of three things: information, skills, or support. Naturally, your need for each of these may vary from time to time, even from day to day. If you start taking a new medicine to lower your blood sugar, for example, you might need information to be sure you are taking it as prescribed and you know what its potential benefits and side effects are. If you just got a new blood sugar meter, you want to be confident you have the skills to use it. And if you are having a bad diabetes day or a longer stretch of diabetes difficulty, you might need some extra support.

Here are some good sources of information and support and some good ways to build your diabetes self-care skills:

Sources of information

When it comes to your diabetes, you are the expert. You know yourself and your life better than anyone else possibly could, and once you have a little experience with diabetes, you know what management tools and techniques work best for you. After all, you make the vast majority of the decisions that affect your blood sugar control and your health. Every time you eat carefully, exercise, check your blood sugar, take your medicine, or call your health-care provider, you are making a decision. And every time you don't do one of these things, you are making a decision as well. To figure out why you are not sticking to your self-care plan and what you can do about it, use the process of identifying sticking points and solutions.

Your health-care provider is another good source of information and an especially important one if you have just been diagnosed with diabetes. He or she should be an expert in the clinical management of diabetes, just as you are (or will soon become) the expert in your own diabetes. The two of you are a team, and to be a really good team, you have to work together, each member contributing expertise. Both of you need to do your part. If your diabetes team is running smoothly, you are blessed. If it isn't, be sure you are doing your part, then think about what you can do to get more from your health-care provider. When working on this problem, it often helps to talk to other people with diabetes about their experiences.

Books, magazines, and the Internet are also sources of information about diabetes, including the emotional side of diabetes. I've written some books with other people that you might want to look at, including *The Johns Hopkins Guide to Diabetes,* which I wrote with an endocrinologist, Christopher Saudek, and a diabetes nurse educator, Cynthia Shump. I also wrote *Psyching Out Diabetes* with June Biermann and Barbara Toohey, and a book for the parents of children with diabetes, *Sweet Kids,* with Betty Page Brackenridge. Another book I recommend if you are struggling with the emotional side of diabetes is *Diabetes Burnout,* by William Polonsky. Magazines, including *Diabetes Self-Management, Diabetes Forecast,* and *Diabetes Interview* and newsletters like the *Diabetes Wellness Letter,* for which I write a monthly column, are also good information resources. The World Wide Web is also full of fascinating facts about diabetes and diabetes management.

The American Diabetes Association (ADA) publishes a variety of pamphlets (many of them free) and books in addition to their membership magazine. The Association also sponsors educational programs and has a Web site (www.diabetes.org) with lots of diabetes information. Join the ADA and make use of its services to stay up to date.

Building skills

As important as information is for controlling diabetes overwhelmus, it is only part of the puzzle. Having the skills you need to put that information into action is even more important. That's where the rubber meets the road. The best way to sharpen your diabetes self-management skills is to get some training. And the best place to get trained is a diabetes self-management education program that has been recognized by the ADA. You can find out about ADA-recognized programs in your area by calling your local ADA affiliate

FOR FURTHER READING

These books may help prevent diabetes overwhelmus by providing basic information about diabetes and its care as well as tips on coping emotionally.

THE JOHNS HOPKINS GUIDE TO DIABETES
For Today and Tomorrow
Christopher Saudek, Richard R. Rubin, and Cynthia Shump
The Johns Hopkins University Press
Baltimore, Maryland, 1997

AMERICAN DIABETES ASSOCIATION
COMPLETE GUIDE TO DIABETES,
2ND EDITION
Bantam Books
New York, 2000

PSYCHING OUT DIABETES
Richard R. Rubin, June Biermann, and Barbara Toohey
Lowell House
Los Angeles, 1999

SWEET KIDS
How to Balance Diabetes Control and Good Nutrition With Family Peace
Betty Page Brackenridge and Richard R. Rubin
American Diabetes Association
Alexandria, Virginia, 1996

DIABETES BURNOUT
What to Do When You Can't Take It Anymore
William H. Polonsky
American Diabetes Association
Alexandria, Virginia, 1999

(look in the phone book for the number). If there are no such programs close to you, you might try another program, but be sure it emphasizes hands-on training and not simply lecturing.

Sources of support

Just as you are a good source of information about your diabetes, you are also one of your best sources of support. You know what makes you feel truly good—and what sort of quick fixes you later regret. Does walking the dog improve your mood? Does sitting quietly in your backyard make you feel calmer and more in control? How about calling a friend for a chat? Buying a new magazine? Whatever works for you, find a way to do it more often. It will feel great, and it will remind you that you can take really good care of yourself.

Your family and friends can be important sources of support as well. Your diabetes affects everyone who loves you and cares for you, and the way these people deal with your diabetes can have a powerful effect on the way you manage it. That's why it's important to do all you can to maximize the help and minimize the hassle you get from other people. Let other people know how much you care about them, and be as clear as you can be about the things they can do to help make your life with diabetes a little easier. Sometimes you may need practical help, such as having a prescription picked up at the pharmacy. Other times you may need someone to listen to you vent about whatever diabetes-related problem is bugging you at the moment.

Support groups, whether sponsored by the ADA, a local hospital, or a diabetes Web site, can also be good sources of support. If you are looking for this kind of help, you might have to search a bit to find a group that's right for you. When you find the right one, you'll be glad you invested the time and energy.

The support you get from family, friends, and other sources can go a long way toward banishing diabetes overwhelmus, because this kind of support helps relieve stress, and it builds your faith in other people and in yourself. My son has had diabetes for 21 years, since he was 7. When he was about 12, I said I wished his diabetes would go away. I'll never forget his response: "I don't. It's not that I like diabetes; in fact I hate it. But because of diabetes I can take care of myself better than any other kid I know. I wouldn't give that up for anything." I know there are days my son feels otherwise, but his bouts with diabetes overwhelmus are rare, and they generally pass quickly. May the same be true for you. ❏

WHEN YOU NEED SOMEONE TO TALK TO
HOW TO CHOOSE A THERAPIST
by Robert Taibbi, L.C.S.W.

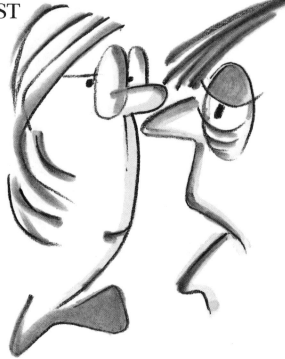

Ed has not been feeling like himself lately. Ever since the new contract started at work he has been constantly worried about deadlines. Not only has his mind been running a thousand miles an hour, but he has been tense and irritable with his staff. At home he has had little energy or desire to do anything, and he has had trouble sleeping. His wife is worried about how quiet and withdrawn he has become.

It has been almost two years since Martha's 30-year-old son, Mike, moved back home after he and his wife separated. At first Martha enjoyed having him around, but lately his comings and goings late at night and his not helping out around the house or paying the bills have started to irritate her. Last night they had a long argument but, as usual, little was resolved. She doesn't necessarily want him to move out, but she certainly doesn't want things to continue the way they are.

A human problem

It's what makes us all too human, perhaps, the way problems—in ourselves, with our work, in our relationships—have a way of spilling out across our lives, filling us with anxiety, anger, and frustration. Not only do problems make it hard for you to enjoy what you have and difficult for you to think about anything else, they create stress, and stress can undermine your diabetes management.

Under emotional strain your concentration can easily be disrupted, making it more difficult for you to pay attention to glucose monitoring, meal planning, and all the things you know you need to do to stay healthy. Physically, stress can trigger hormones that release glucose. While this can provide energy for handling an anxiety-producing situation, it can also raise your blood sugar and wreak havoc on your diabetes regimen.

Fortunately, most of our problems have a way of resolving. Sometimes we're able to take active steps to solve the problem. For example, Ed may find a way to bring in some extra workers to help meet deadlines and reduce his pressure. Other times, time itself or circumstances outside our control change the situation. In Martha's case, Mike may find a new job out-of-state or go back to his wife, effectively removing the source of Martha's concern.

But sometimes problems linger. Sometimes, in spite of our best efforts, we don't know what to do about problems, or what we try doesn't work. We feel physically drained or knotted up. Those crummy feelings stay cooped up inside. They keep pulling us down. It's times like these that talking to a therapist may be just what we need.

What therapy is

Hold on. Before you start picturing some bearded guy in a white coat who talks with a German accent and spends a couple of years and your son's college tuition asking you how you felt about your mother when you were five years old, realize that this isn't what therapy is all about.

It also isn't about someone finding out that you really are crazy and locking you up in a hospital, or reading your mind and uncovering some deep dark secret you've never revealed to anyone. Nor is therapy a personality makeover that removes all your inhibitions or gives you too many.

Instead, therapy is a place to talk about your problems, ideas, and feelings with someone who won't make you feel guilty or ashamed and who doesn't claim to already know what is best for you. Therapy is a place where someone will listen to you, hear you out, and, best of all, help you to hear yourself.

Therapy is also a process, one that involves sorting out and discovering what your problems really are and exploring options for resolving your problems. It won't make your life stress-free, but it can help you develop the skills to determine what you need and to convey your needs to others.

Ed, for example, may come to realize that it's not his job but rather long-standing problems at home that are making him irritable and depressed.

Martha may discover that her conversations with Mike go nowhere because she is still talking and reacting to him as though he were 10 years old.

How long therapy takes varies. As with other forms of medical care, insurance companies have in the past few years pushed for less long-term, more short-term work. While 8 to 12 therapy sessions is now a common length of treatment, your therapy could take longer if you are trying to tackle a number of problems at one time, or if your problems have been going on for a long time.

What's more, it takes time for the therapist to get to know you and understand the problems you see. And it takes time for you to feel comfortable with your therapist and to try out new behaviors and perspectives and integrate them into your life. A therapist should, generally speaking, be able to give you an idea of how long the process may be expected to take within the first few sessions.

The many faces of therapy

Okay, so maybe therapy could be helpful. But how do you decide who to see?

You have a number of choices. Although there are many different types of therapists, the main therapeutic professions are psychiatry, psychology, social work, counseling, and psychiatric nursing.

Psychiatrists are medical doctors who are specifically trained in psychiatry. While many of them stick strictly to talking, problem-solving therapy, because they are physicians they are also licensed to dispense medication—for depression or anxiety, for example—and they can admit patients to the hospital.

Psychologists are not medical doctors, but instead they usually have a doctorate degree in psychology. Part of their expertise includes psychological testing—including personality tests and educational tests—which is often a useful way of gathering information.

Social workers, counselors, and psychiatric nurses usually have master's degrees in their respective fields, with specialized training in therapy. They cannot write prescriptions for medicine nor do they do testing, but they often blend family, educational, or medical perspectives into their work.

While the therapy field may seem divided by different professions, in actuality what each type of professional does on a day-to-day level is more similar than different. A therapist who is a social worker, for example, may do the very same type of therapy as a psychologist.

What does tend to make one therapist's everyday work different from another's is the therapist's theoretical orientation to therapy itself. While there are a multitude of therapeutic approaches—from the original Freudian analysis to New Age body–mind techniques—the primary schools of thought are *psychodynamic, cognitive–behavioral,* and *systemic.*

Psychodynamic. For psychodynamic therapists, problems stem from the past, particularly from one's relationship with one's parents and from old hurts that color how one sees oneself and others in the present. These therapists believe that by unraveling the past and its pains and by seeing it how it was rather than how it seemed, a person can stop repeating the same mistakes over and over again and become free to feel and act differently in the present.

Cognitive–behavioral. For cognitive–behavioral therapists, the problem and solution are in the present, not in the past. Specifically, they believe that much of how you feel about a situation comes from how you think about it. The way we talk to ourselves and exaggerate and distort what is happening—telling ourselves, for example, that the hard time we're having now proves that we're failures and will never do better in the future—can make us feel depressed or nervous. By being aware of these distorted thoughts and changing them, as well as deliberately trying out new behaviors, problems can be seen more realistically and can be solved.

Systemic. Whereas psychodynamic and cognitive–behavioral therapy focuses on what has happened or is happening to the individual, systemic therapy looks at what happens between people in their relationships. Rather than unraveling an individual's past or thoughts, a systemic therapist tries to unravel the unhealthy patterns that a couple or a family create and are locked into. While these patterns are often learned—a husband, for example, may get angry and blow up at his wife just like his father blew up at his mother—the focus is on becoming aware of what sets off these negative cycles and stopping them before they create bad feelings or become emotionally destructive.

Because problems are seen as originating from relationships, the therapy usually involves inviting family members or friends into the therapy process so the therapist can see how people interact and then help to change the patterns replicated right there in the room.

Making a choice. With all these choices how do you choose? One practical starting point, of course, is to find out what your insurance company will cover. Some companies will only reimburse certain types of therapists or those from an approved provider list.

Beyond that, you should consider your own preferences in terms of orientation: Do you think your problems are tied to your past? To your relationships? To your thoughts? Do you feel like you need to understand where this all started? Do you need help trying out new behaviors? Or do you think it would useful to have a forum to talk things out with your spouse or mother or whoever? .

While many therapists combine a number of approaches in their work—behavioral exercises, for example, with some exploration of the past—working with a therapist who thinks the way you do can help you feel more comfortable and will make the process more effective and efficient.

In the room

So what really happens once you sit down across from the therapist?

The traditional therapy session runs about 50 minutes, and it may take a session or two for the therapist to hear about the problems you're worried about and to get the background information he or she needs. Again, depending on his or her orientation and background, the therapist may ask you to fill out a questionnaire, give some medical or family history, or bring in some of your family members.

Ed's therapist, for example, may ask him to keep a log of when he gets most frustrated on the job. The therapist may compare his reaction to his boss with past reactions to his father, or may suggest that Ed see his family doctor for some antidepressant medicine.

Martha's therapist may suggest that she bring Mike to the next session so they can talk about Martha's concerns. Or she may help Martha role-play (that is, act out) a conversation with Mike to explore how she could talk to Mike without his getting angry. Exactly what happens will depend largely on the therapist's orientation.

Regardless of a therapist's orientation, everything you say in therapy will be confidential. Your therapist cannot tell anyone about anything you said unless he or she has your permission. The only exceptions are cases where there is suspicion of physical or sexual abuse, or fear that your life or someone else's life is in danger. Your therapist should explain his or her policy on confidentiality to you in the first session.

After the first few sessions, you should have a good idea of just what the therapist thinks the problem is and what the goals of therapy might be. For Ed, the goal might be to reduce his stress by doing more things with his family. For Martha, it might be to figure out why she feels guilty about confronting Mike.

While individual therapy sessions will have their ups and downs (not every session will produce a life-changing revelation), they should generally build on each other. In addition they should include time for checking on progress or problems during the week, for continuing to discuss a particular topic (for example, a past divorce), as well as for suggestions for the following week. Even if you do not see any dramatic changes, you should find yourself feeling somewhat better—a bit less anxious, less worried, and clearer about what needs to be done—within a few sessions.

Getting started

If you think talk therapy might help you sort out some of the problems in your life, here are some guidelines to get you started:

Check with your doctor. Not all bad feelings are emotional. Sometimes there are medical reasons for the way you are feeling. Depression, for example, can be a side effect of some medications, and anxiety can be a symptom of a physical ailment. Seeing your doctor and ruling out medical issues first will help the therapist get on track more quickly.

Get referrals. Your doctor may be able to give you the names of some therapists. Check as well with friends who may have been in therapy. Your workplace may have an employee assistance program that can refer you to qualified therapists in your area. If you don't have insurance, your local mental health association can refer you to mental health centers and private therapists in your area who set fees based on your income and expenses.

Think about your own expectations. Before you talk to a therapist, think about what you're looking for in terms of orientation, personality, and your preference for a man or woman. Consider what you see to be the most productive direction and focus of the therapy. And decide what your limits are in terms of fees. Not only will you be taking a more active role in your treatment, you'll be more likely to find what you want.

Do a phone interview. Once you've come up with a list of names and expectations, make some calls. Ask about the therapist's qualifications, experience with your problem, and orientation. Take note of how comfortable you feel talking to him or her on the phone and how well he or she listens. If the therapist suggests you come in for an initial consultation, clarify whether there is a charge. Bring your list of questions with you. But don't feel committed to start therapy with anyone if you would rather shop around.

You can change your mind. If after a couple of sessions you feel like it isn't working out the way you had hoped, if you still feel uncomfortable, or if you feel like you are being strong-armed into talking about things you absolutely don't want to talk about, bring it up directly with your therapist. Don't feel, however, that you're obligated to stay, or that this is in some way good for you. Therapy is a service, and you always have the right to change your mind.

Just as it's important to turn to your doctor for help in managing your diabetes, it's important to seek help when life problems become overwhelming or simply more than you can handle on your own. A therapist may be just the person to give you that help. ❑

OPENING NEW DOORS
BROADENING YOUR SELF-IMAGE
by Robert Taibbi, L.C.S.W.

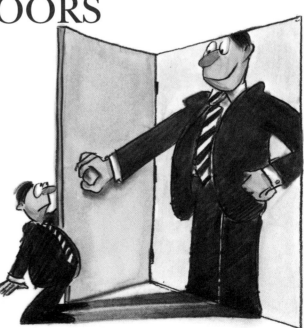

Sam will be the first to admit that he's a couch potato. While his older brother was the lean and mean star athlete in school, Sam was the nerd, the unathletic klutz, the last to get picked for any team. Now that he's an adult, Sam would much rather spend his time surfing the Web or tinkering with the software on his computer than going for a walk or a bike ride. He's read enough to know that regular exercise would improve his health in many ways, including making it easier to control his blood sugar. "But," he says, "I'm no good at sports. I would look ridiculous attempting to jog in the park or pump iron at the gym." Sam can even imagine the other guys snickering—the way his brother used to—were he to don a sweat suit and do anything resembling exercise.

Give Ellen a computer manual or even a page full of small print and her eyes start to glaze over. While she's good at working with her hands—sewing quilts and making many of her own clothes—school was always a struggle. Ellen thinks of herself as slow, and anything that sounds unfamiliar or technical can quickly overwhelm her. While she diligently reads food labels at the grocery store, the way her dietitian suggested, she gets confused trying to balance calories with carbohydrates, fat, saturated fat, cholesterol, fiber, and calcium—and the advice to eat three to five fruits and vegetables every day. "It's too much to keep in mind all at once!" she tells herself. And instead of trying to puzzle it all out, Ellen often resorts to eating the sample menus her dietitian wrote out (even though she's getting tired of them) so that she doesn't have to do any calculations.

Unlike Ellen, Tom does fine with information; it's people he has a hard time with, especially if they are in positions of authority or importance. His weekly meetings with his supervisor at work are exercises in anxiety, it's hard for him to have more than a two-sentence conversation with the minister at church, and he's never the guy to complain to a store manager about poor service.

Tom's shyness also affects his interactions with his doctor. Since being diagnosed with diabetes, Tom has read a lot about it and has come to a fairly sophisticated understanding of the condition. He feels that his current diabetes-care plan doesn't optimally control his blood sugar, and he's concerned about how this will affect his health down the line. But he just can't bring himself to speak with his doctor about it. He always gets too nervous at his appointments and never manages to broach the subject. Tom would also like to join a diabetes support group, but he can't bear the thought of talking in front of so many strangers at once.

Sam, Ellen, and Tom are all motivated to take care of their diabetes, but each one of them is having trouble with a certain aspect of his or her care. And in each case, the problem clearly originates with the person's self-image.

What is self-image?

We all believe we have a pretty good idea about what we're like: attractive, plain, disorganized, smart, emotional, cautious, fun-loving, etc. We also believe we know what others are like: strong, weak, dependable, loving, intimidating, sneaky, honest, manipulative. Based on these impressions, or images, of ourselves and others, we make choices, construct relationships,

and form the patterns and routines that make up the bulk of our lives.

It's good that we do. Without a sense of who we are, we'd feel adrift, anxious, fraught with the prospect of having to redefine ourselves each day. By using our self-image as a sort of psychological anchor, we're able to hold ourselves steady in the face of all that's new, confusing, and potentially overwhelming in the world that is around us.

But sometimes, holding steady holds us back. Clinging firmly to our beliefs about ourselves can keep us from noticing how out-of-date or distorted our images of ourselves may be. It can prevent us from appreciating positive qualities we already possess and make it difficult for us to see that we're capable of changing aspects of ourselves that we wish were different.

Sam, for example, may never play in the pros. But it's the lingering mental image of himself as an overweight, nerdy eight-year-old that keeps him from finding out that with a steady dose of moderate exercise, he could not only transform his body, but also his longstanding, but inaccurate, view of himself.

Similarly, while Ellen may learn slowly, she's certainly capable of learning, in spite of what she's come to believe. With some patience and effort, she could not only better understand her meal plan, but in the process, come to realize that her assumptions about herself aren't 100% true.

And while Tom may struggle with social situations now, he can, by learning and practicing some basic social skills, come to handle them more easily. His view of himself as a shy person, however, undermines his confidence.

Only by questioning and going beyond our familiar assumptions can we create an image of ourselves that more fully represents who we are.

Once upon a time

It's easier to talk about changing than to actually do it, of course. The ways we think of ourselves and our world are well-entrenched. Developmental psychologists now tell us that it is in the first three years of life that we form the template upon which we view ourselves and the larger world. Infants who are well cared for and who feel content and secure with their parents come to feel that the world is safe, that people are trustworthy, and that they themselves are loveable. Infants who are neglected or mistreated not only feel anxious, angry, and afraid, but also learn on the most basic level that the world can be hurtful, that people are not dependable, and that they need to take care of themselves, be careful, and not make too many demands. Most of us fall somewhere in the middle, leaving these early years with a mix of positive and negative feelings and a handful of core beliefs about

Dealing With Feelings

ourselves, other people, and ways of getting our needs met.

As we grow into school age, these initial impressions and assumptions are whittled and honed by family life and our experiences in the increasingly larger world. Early on, for example, Sam may have tried to follow in the footsteps of his athletic brother, but soon realized that he was physically no match. Discovering that he could get more of his parents' attention by being precocious and good with gadgets, he learned to put his energy there, and left sports behind.

Ellen may have been placed in the slow reading group at school and may have found that her parents not only didn't get upset about the mediocre grades she brought home, but they seemed, in fact, to expect them. It was only when her grandmother introduced her to quilting that Ellen found something that caught her enthusiasm and earned her the recognition from adults that she needed.

Similarly, Tom, already frightened by overbearing parents, could easily have carried those same feelings over to school, where he was uncomfortable and cautious around his stern teachers. Never feeling safe enough to speak his mind, Tom's way of holding back and holding in gradually became, as the years passed, both his style of relating to others, and the way he looked at himself and his social skills.

Throughout our teenage years and beyond, our self-image consolidates and becomes more fixed, and we begin to gather around us people who support our view of ourselves. In high school, Sam hung out with other computer enthusiasts who thought like him. Ellen joined a quilting group, where her handiwork was appreciated and she didn't feel dumb. Tom eventually married a woman who finds his shyness attractive, is outgoing herself, and is willing to speak up when he can't. By our late teens, the self-image we began creating at birth has become the foundation upon which we build our life and lifestyle.

By and large, this system works. When we stick with our self-image, our world stays intact, and we know who we are. But this stability comes at a price. If we adhere too rigidly to our self-image, we can lose the flexibility we need to accommodate to the changes that occur over time. Our old self-image, created in a time long gone, may no longer be appropriate for our needs and can constrain our potential.

The courage to change

Most of us could use an "upgrade" of our self-image, particularly when we sense that our needs aren't being met. But how to do it? Here are some ways to get started:

Make a list. Take a minute and write down your basic assumptions about yourself and others. How would you describe yourself to someone? What is your strongest personality trait, your greatest weakness, your greatest talent? What is your basic view of others? How trustworthy, dependable, or caring are they? What are your core beliefs about the purpose of life, the way the world works? Be as honest with yourself as possible.

Evaluate. Now go over your list, looking for what may no longer apply. Is it really true, for example, that you're impulsive or foolhardy, as you once thought? Or have you changed over the years, becoming more deliberate or cautious when situations require it? Is income or job title still your measure of success? Or have some other criteria, such as relationships or your satisfaction with your work, become more important? Do you still believe that people need to pull themselves up by their own bootstraps? Or have life experiences made you think that seeking help from others is sometimes the better way to go?

If Sam were to mull through his list, he might decide that it's finally time to stop comparing himself to his brother and thinking of exercise as the stuff of star athletes. If he actually looks at the guys jogging in the park, he'll see that a lot of them resemble him more than they do his brother. He may acknowledge that it would be more productive (and healthful) to find some type of moderate physical activity that he enjoys and can do regularly.

Even though Ellen may never really enjoy "bookish things," she can learn to be more patient with herself and to resist the urge to give up before she tries. She may be surprised at just how helpful reading and studying new information can be.

And there's no reason for Tom to keep feeling like a nervous 10-year-old, assuming that others will criticize him if he says what he thinks or asks for what he needs.

Take a careful look at your beliefs about yourself and how they affect your life. Are there beliefs that are holding you back, preventing you from achieving your life goals or from being the person you want to be? Are there parts of who you are that you would like to change? Do not assume that your persona is set in stone: There are no limits to what you can become.

Make a plan. Once you've nailed down the specific aspect of your self-image that you want to change, come up with a plan. Think small. Think slow. Sam can't expect to run 5 miles by next week, but he can take a walk around the block after dinner. Ellen may not understand the whole meal-planning booklet the first time she reads it, but if she goes over it a few times, she will probably learn something. At the very least, she'll be able to formulate some questions to ask her dietitian. Tom may not be able to turn the tables on his supervisor at their next meeting, but he can make a contract with himself to attend at least one support group meeting.

Remember that your self-image was formed from your life experiences, so it will take new life experiences to change it. By taking small steps and doing things that feel a bit awkward at first, you will become more comfortable with the whole notion of taking risks, and your confidence and ability to take bigger ones will increase. Slowly, but truly, your self-image will expand.

Expect resistance and setbacks. Just because you're making progress doesn't mean that parts of you won't be kicking and screaming along the way. Expect excuses to pop up: You're too tired to exercise, you're too rushed to remember to bring a good snack to work, you're wasting your time, you're really not that smart or that organized. Why bother attempting to change anything when you're bound to fail, the way you always do?

What you're hearing, no doubt, are replays of the real messages you probably heard while growing up. It takes time to shut off those old, discouraging, critical messages and replace them with encouraging, positive messages.

RAISING CONFIDENT KIDS

The best time to start developing a positive self-image is in childhood. By helping children create a positive foundation in themselves, we give our kids the tools they need to face challenges and continue to grow throughout their lives. Here are some tips for helping children get off to a good start:

Don't say don't. When our kids get frustrated or irritated, want to quit doing their homework or taking their insulin, or get tired of watching their diet all the time, it's easy for us parents to start lecturing: "Don't get so discouraged." "Don't be a quitter." "You need to change your attitude." While our intentions may be good, our children tune in to how we sound rather than to what we say. Instead of feeling encouraged, they feel scolded.

Over time, such messages become internalized. That's to say, our children repeat those messages in their heads, scolding and criticizing themselves when they feel frustrated or fed up, make a mistake, or don't do as well as they'd like to. More often than not, such self-talk endures into adulthood.

So instead of trying to verbally whip our children into shape, it's better to take the time to listen, to empathize with their feelings ("It sounds like you are feeling really frustrated today"), and to help them figure out what they can do in order to solve the problem.

Accentuate the positive. Stating the positive is always better than pointing out the negative. Children need to feel supported. They need to know from those close to them what they do well, what they seem to enjoy most, and where their uniqueness and creativity lie. Again, over time, these positive statements are transformed into inner words of encouragement.

Encourage risk taking. No, you don't want to encourage your kids to hang off the water tower or play chicken with cars. But do try nudging your children to say hello when they feel socially awkward, encouraging them to try a new class even though they know nothing about the subject, or persuading them to go out for a sport even though they may wind up spending a lot of time on the bench. Especially for children dealing with the challenges of ongoing physical conditions like diabetes, learning at an early age to tackle what's difficult helps them feel less different and helps them develop the strong self-confidence and resiliency they need to handle the many obstacles of adult life.

Resist using your child as a report card for yourself. It's tempting to measure our own abilities as parents by the outcome of our children. If they're successful, we're successful; if they fail in some way, it somehow reflects on us. Thinking this way pushes us to control, shape, and make children what we need them to be. We try to use them to make up for our own inadequacies, missed dreams, and uncompleted tasks. And in doing so, we wind up creating the seeds of the problems we're hoping our children will avoid.

Instead of outcome, think process. Think of your job as a parent as providing the environment, the love, the guidance, and the support your child needs to grow in his or her own way and to discover just who he or she really is. Rather than always looking ahead, trying to orchestrate some distant goal that you feel is important, measure the success of your parenting by your ability to appreciate the moment, the present, the quality of the time spent together here and now.

Be a good role model. If you're able to admit to and learn from your mistakes, take risks, and expand your own boundaries over the course of your life, you offer your child a model for how it can be done. The best gift you can give to your child is the best you.

Staying positive can be tough, because change is almost never smooth or steady. Sam may be gung-ho about exercise for the first two weeks, then feel too sore or have made too little progress and want to quit. Ellen may carefully read some nutrition pamphlets, not grasp the concepts presented at all, and really feel like she's stupid. Tom's experience at the first support group meeting may go a hundred times better than he expected, but at the second he may find himself wanting to run out the door when the room gets quiet for more than a few minutes, or people ask him to say something about himself.

Getting off to a slow start, taking "two steps forward, one step back," is to be expected, and keeping that in mind is the best antidote. If you believe that ups and downs are a normal part of the change process, you won't be surprised by the downs, and you will know that in spite of them, you're still changing and moving forward.

Get support. In addition to giving yourself positive messages and support, it helps to have the support of others. Let those close to you know what you're trying to do, and let them know how they can help. Tom, for example, may ask his wife for pointers on introducing himself to the support group members and chatting during the coffee break. Ellen may want to have her sister (who enjoyed school) look over her nutrition information with her, or she may want to schedule some extra sessions with her dietitian. Sam may take out a trial membership at the local health club and sign up for group exercise sessions instead of doing push-ups alone in his basement.

Persevere. Who you are now is a culmination of all that has passed. You've put years into becoming the person you are, so you can't expect changes, even small ones, to happen overnight. You're not only learning to move against your own habits and instincts, you're literally etching new thought pathways in your brain. With continued practice, these new pathways will replace the old ones, and new habits will replace the old, worn-out ones. By changing what you do, you change who and how you are. Just give yourself time. ❏

TALKING WITH YOUR DOCTOR
PROBLEMS AND SOLUTIONS

by Martha M. Funnell, M.S., R.N., C.D.E.

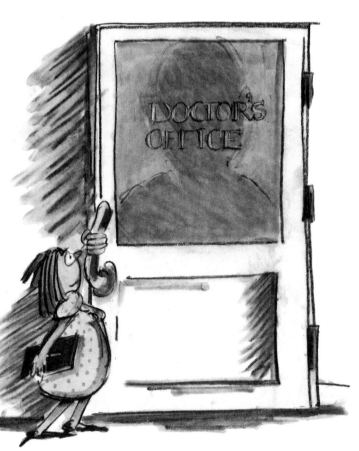

How do you feel before you go to your doctor appointments? Are you looking forward to talking over any problems or concerns that you have? Do you have questions that you know will be answered? Or are you anxious and worried that your doctor will "scold" you for not losing weight or doing the other things that he or she recommended at your last visit? Do you tend to forget to bring your monitoring records? Or do you keep two sets of books—one with your real blood sugar numbers and one with more desirable numbers to show your doctor?

If you ever dread doctor visits, you may think you'd dread them less if you were able to follow your doctor's advice more closely. But the way you feel about doctor visits probably has less to do with what you've done to take care of your diabetes than with your relationship with your doctor. If you and your doctor work closely together, then visits become opportunities for discussion and problem-solving, whether or not you have been able to lose weight, exercise more, stop smoking, or keep your blood sugar within a certain range. If you do not have this type of relationship with your doctor, it's easy to feel intimidated, ashamed, or frustrated at your appointments.

Becoming equal partners

In the traditional doctor–patient relationship, the doctor tells the patient what to do to take care of himself, perhaps writes a prescription, and then the patient goes home and follows (or attempts to follow) the doctor's orders. The doctor is largely responsible for the outcome of the treatment. This type of relationship works well for acute illnesses such as strep throat or the flu, where getting better is a matter of taking medicine and resting for a set amount of time. It doesn't work so well for chronic diseases like diabetes.

Many people use this traditional model when they establish a relationship with their diabetes doctor. They expect that the doctor will be responsible for their care and for the outcome of the treatment plan. But diabetes care is primarily given by the person who has it, not by the doctor. And many of the "doctor's orders" are for changes in the way one lives one's life. For most people, however, it isn't possible to change eating and exercise patterns just because someone tells them they should.

Having diabetes means that you and your doctor need a different kind of relationship, where you combine what you know about yourself, diabetes, your lifestyle, and your values with what your doctor knows about diabetes to create a plan that will work for you. It also means accepting responsibility for much of your own daily decisions, care, and outcomes.

If you currently have a more traditional relationship with your doctor and you are satisfied with it, there's no need to change it. However, some people with diabetes feel frustrated by their relationships with their doctors. They feel they are not getting the care they need. And this frustration can affect how they choose to or are able to take care of themselves.

Resolving frustrations

By examining and perhaps changing the way you communicate and interact with your doctor, many of the concerns you have regarding the care you receive from your doctor can be resolved. However, changing a relationship is easier said than done. You and your doctor are accustomed to your traditional roles. And for most people, including health professionals, stepping outside the way they usually behave represents a major change. However, because the way you are able to care for your diabetes can have such a large impact on the quality of your life, you may decide it is worth the effort. Here are some suggestions to help you deal with some common frustrations.

"My doctor tells me what I 'should be' doing, but I'm not sure I agree."

Imagine that you and a friend were building a garage. If your goal was to have everything done precisely and your friend's goal was to finish as quickly as possible, you would probably have a hard time working together until you came to some agreement. The same is true in managing diabetes. If your doctor's goal is for you to lose 50 pounds, and your goal is to lose 10 pounds, you will probably have different opinions of your progress and success until you come to some understanding.

You may never have thought about your goals for diabetes, but you do have them. To determine what your goals are, think about the answers to these questions:
- What would I like my blood sugar to be most of the time?
- What would I like to weigh?
- How often do I want to exercise?
- How often am I able or willing to test my blood sugar?
- How hard am I able or willing to work to reach these goals?

It is important to tell your doctor what your goals are and what you are willing and able to do. Ask your doctor his or her opinion of your goals and about different options for reaching your goals. Having a discussion about goals will help to shift the focus from what you are or aren't doing now, to what you plan to do in the future.

"My doctor is in too big of a hurry."

Doctors are in a hurry these days. They have a lot of pressure to see more patients in less time. Unfortunately, this can make you feel rushed or feel that you are not important. Because speedier visits are a reality, however, it's up to you to do everything you can to get what you need in a shorter period of time. For example, you can take off your shoes and socks when you arrive in the examination room so your doctor can examine your feet more efficiently. You can bring your blood sugar records in a readable format. And you can prepare yourself for your visit so you know what you want to accomplish.

If you're truly not getting what you need, tell your doctor that you feel rushed and that you have more to discuss. If you still don't feel you get enough time, you may want to consider changing doctors. Many people worry about hurting their doctor's feelings by going to a different doctor. It may help to remember that you are paying for your doctor's services. If you're not getting the service you need, you certainly have the right to speak up.

"My doctor expects too much of me and scolds me if I don't do what he or she wants."

Bringing in your blood sugar records for the doctor to see can feel a lot like taking your report card home to your parents. That's because the traditional doctor–patient relationship is very much like a parent–child relationship. But you are an adult now, dealing with a chronic illness. Blood sugar records aren't just for your doctor: They give you the information you need to take care of yourself every day. Your relationship with your doctor needs to recognize your role as an equal partner and decision maker. To establish an equal relationship, tell your doctor what your goals are and what you are willing and able to do to work toward these goals.

Part of taking responsibility for your part of the relationship is being honest on your blood sugar records and about other health behaviors such as diet, exercise, and smoking. Tell your doctor what you honestly believe you can do and what will help you to reach your goals. If you feel intimidated, practice what you want to say to your doctor at home before your appointment. One way you might respond to scolding is to say, "I am trying as best I can. It would help me to hear a positive suggestion about how I can do this better."

"I can't understand what my doctor is talking about."

Doctors often use medical terms that most people don't understand. If your doctor does this, say you don't understand and ask for an explanation in lay terms. Repeat back what you think the doctor said. It may help to make a statement such as, "I want to be sure I understand. Is what you're saying...?"

"I don't get my questions answered."

Your doctor should take the time to answer your questions, but you may be able to get some of the information you need from other sources. Lots of general information about diabetes is available in books, from various diabetes organizations, through support groups, and on the Internet. One benefit of printed materials is that you can read through them at your own pace and reread them as many times as you need. Of course, you will probably have questions about your own care that cannot be answered by a book or a pamphlet.

To get answers from your doctor about your own care, write down your questions before you go to your appointment. Tell your doctor at the start of the visit that you have questions. If your questions aren't answered or you don't understand, ask for clarification or for a referral to a diabetes educator or dietitian.

"My doctor isn't a diabetes 'expert.' Is that a problem?"

Many people with diabetes are cared for very well by physicians who are not endocrinologists or diabetologists. Family doctors, general practitioners, internists, nurse practitioners, and others often treat diabetes. The important thing is to have a health-care provider who is knowledgeable and interested in diabetes and with whom you can establish a good working relationship. No matter what type of provider you see, it is in your own best interest to be well-informed. If you read

STAYING INFORMED

For more information about diabetes, as well as referrals to professionals or resources in your area, call the following organizations or visit their Web sites:

American Diabetes Association
(800) DIABETES (342-2383)
www.diabetes.org

American Association of Diabetes Educators
(800) TEAM-UP-4 (832-6874)
www.aadenet.org

The American Dietetic Association
(800) 877-1600
www.eatright.org

National Diabetes Information Clearinghouse
(800) 860-8747
www.niddk.nih.gov/health/diabetes/ndcc.htm

about new therapies in the newspaper or see something on television, bring the information to your appointment and ask your doctor if it would work for you.

"My doctor is always referring me to other people such as nurses, dietitians, ophthalmologists, and podiatrists."

Part of diabetes care includes education, screening, and sometimes care for diabetic complications. Most physicians can't provide all of these services on their own. Referrals to specialists are therefore in your best interest. In fact, you may have a bigger problem if you are not referred to any other providers. If that's the case, ask your physician if you should be. For example you might say, "I read that people with diabetes need their eyes examined once a year by an eye-care specialist. Could you refer me to one?"

Change for the better

Change in any relationship takes time and persistence. Since you may see your doctor only once or twice a year, you may doubt that change in this relationship is possible or worth the effort. It's true that much of the work is up to you: You will need to spend time thinking about your goals, writing down questions, and keeping careful records of your blood glucose levels. And in spite of your best efforts, you may not get all the results you want in one appointment or even two. But keep trying. The relationship you have with your doctor strongly affects how well you are able to care for yourself, and how well you care for yourself affects both your short-term and long-term health and your quality of life. Putting in the extra effort to make your doctor–patient relationship a partnership is indeed worth the effort. ❑

SURVIVING DIABETES AS A COUPLE

by Kenneth Ruge, D.Min.

T il diabetes do you part? No way! A spouse's diabetes needn't destroy your marriage. It's a challenge, to be sure, but like other tests of your marriage relationship, diabetes can offer a chance to connect with your husband or wife on a more profound spiritual level and perhaps even deepen your relationship.

Getting the news

The phone rings just as Paul gets back to his office from lunch, the very minute he was expecting Phyllis to check in after her visit to the doctor. He answers on the first ring.

"Hi, honey," he says, "What did the doctor say?"

"Well, we've got some things to think about and some changes to make," Phyllis replies with a breezy cheer that tells Paul she's really worried. "The doctor says I have diabetes."

Phyllis goes on to talk about blood sugar levels, the pills she needs to pick up at the pharmacy, and losing weight, but Paul can't quite focus on her words. His mind is racing. He and Phyllis end the conversation in their usual way by talking about what's for dinner and saying, "Love you, honey." But a big, hollow space hovers behind the words today, a space that's rapidly filling up with fears and doubts.

Paul hangs up the phone, but he's not thinking about the information Phyllis gave him. It was too much to absorb in one dose. Instead, his mind drifts onto some words he spoke 24 years ago, the day he and Phyllis were married: "...for richer or poorer, in

sickness and in health...." Paul finds some strength in those words but not an immediate end to his fears. He spoke those words with her, took that vow. He'll support Phyllis, of course. He always has. But how will diabetes change their lives? How sick will his wife become? Paul also wonders about himself. Will he be able to learn what he must about the disease?

"Do I have what it takes to do what I have to do?" Paul asks aloud. Then, distracted, he turns toward his work.

Marriage vows

Though Paul is worrying, he's actually taken a positive step by recalling the vows taken in his marriage ceremony. Those vows represent a reassuring commitment to stand together during rough times, even if an illness comes along. The variety of situations presented in the words "for richer or poorer, in sickness and in health" also reminds Paul that he and his wife have already faced challenges: other illnesses and certainly the "poorer" days of their early years. If they overcame those challenges, perhaps they are up to the test of confronting this new disease.

In his own way, Paul is already starting to put his new situation in context. Diabetes will not end his marriage. The disease will be just one theme in the ongoing story of their years together and in the story of how well they are living their lives.

My colleague Arthur Caliandro, minister of Marble Collegiate Church in New York City, believes that when we come to the pearly gates, we're asked two questions. The first is, "What have you done with what you've been given?" And the second is, "How have you loved?"

Those are good questions to keep in mind when a marriage faces the challenge of diabetes. If you and your spouse are "given" diabetes, what will you do with it? Will you love well, or poorly? Those are not simple questions. Even when you've made a firm resolve to support your spouse and manage the disease in a mature, problem-solving way, you'll encounter roadblocks along the way. A complex disease inevitably invites depression, resentment, and guilt into even the healthiest relationships. Yet with flexibility, intelligence, and a firm resolve, you can find ways to keep your marriage not just stable, but growthful and loving too.

Start with open communication

Open communication between you and your spouse is the foundation that lets you adjust to new challenges and still remain close. This style of communicating hinges on your ability to express a supportive, positive outlook that lets your partner know you are going to hang in there with him or her. But there's also a harder part: having the courage to talk about shadowy issues such as doubt, guilt, and anger.

The fact is, those darker issues need to be aired. When you talk about the negatives, you bring them to the conscious level in your relationship and reduce their power. If you hide them, they can only exert damage. I have seen marriages where husband and wife conceal their fears. In these couples, the husband and wife often start avoiding each other and may eventually become emotionally estranged. (In Alcoholics Anonymous, there's a saying that goes, "You're as sick as your secrets." That's strong stuff, but it does reflect the fact that secrets can make resentments more powerful.)

When confronting a husband's or wife's diabetes, it is only natural to feel angry and resentful. Harboring those feelings is nothing to feel guilty about. After all, your spouse "brought" illness into your life together. From his or her side of the equation, your spouse is equally prone to experiencing anger, fear, and guilt. This is especially likely if he or she has avoided exercise, become overweight, or overindulged in junk food or alcohol. In such cases, normal fears can be compounded by thoughts such as, "I brought this problem on myself. I created it, so why do I deserve to get better now?"

You and your spouse may have already established ways to talk openly about such fears and frustrations. If not, diabetes may actually represent an opportunity to start now, lifting your relationship to a higher plane. It may even afford you a new way to contribute to your marriage and grow closer.

If you have children, make the effort to communicate with them openly, too. With young children, especially, it is important to provide an understandable context for the disease by making a statement like, "Dad's diabetes is something we'll have to watch, but he will have a good, long life if we all pitch in." Without that kind of information, young children have no way of knowing just how ill a parent is. They may start to harbor unrealistic fears.

Define a healthy, caring role

A woman named Mary became her husband's primary care-giver for his diabetes. She read up on the topic, bought the right foods, visited dietitians, and made sure that her husband monitored his diet and blood glucose levels and took his medicine. After all, her husband was a busy man and he needed help! Yet, Mary was surprised at her husband's response to her efforts. He seemed withdrawn at times, even angry. And from her side of the relationship, Mary had another problem. She was beginning to resent her role, even though she had taken it upon herself.

Taking on the role of care-giver may seem like a positive, giving step to take. In many cases, it is. But it can also be taken too far. You need to support your partner, but you also need to allow him or her the independence to take responsibility for self-care, as an adult.

That outlook—assuming that both partners will behave responsibly when faced with a problem, as adults—is essential to keeping a marriage strong. Even in situations where one partner eventually becomes quite ill and dependent, it is important to allow that partner the responsibility for self-care for as long as possible.

Above all, avoid the temptation to move into a custodial relationship prematurely. By a custodial relationship, I mean a relationship where you act like the parent and your spouse acts like the child. In this relationship, you pester your spouse by continually asking, "Did you take your pill?" or "Did you take your shot?" If you assume that role when it is not needed, you run the risk of destabilizing your marriage. You can even create a "marital time bomb," a slow, ticking resentment in your spouse that will later explode.

It is healthier to find ways to support the changes your spouse has to make without taking over. If your partner must start to lose weight, exercise, and monitor foods, the ideal way to support those changes is to take part in them yourself. That is, start paying attention to your own diet, and start an exercise program, too.

Another vital step is for you and your spouse to utilize separate support networks. While you need to rely on each other, each of you should claim time to spend alone with close friends with whom you can openly discuss your hopes, fears, angers, and frustrations. You may even find it healthy to learn to complain about your new role, without self-blame or guilt. If you don't have a place to communicate your frustrations, you run the danger of developing a toxic relationship, in which you build up resentments against your partner. You may even be creating another "time bomb" that will cause *you* to explode.

If you lack the friends to support you, seek out a support group or the counseling of a therapist or a minister. Such "outside-the-marriage" support also has the potential to take on added importance if, later down the line, your spouse becomes quite ill. In that eventuality, you may well need a healthy, external forum to voice reluctance, anger, and ambivalence without expressing those feelings directly to your spouse.

Establish boundaries

At the same time you are reaching out to people for support, you may need to set up boundaries to keep other people from intruding into your marriage relationship. In effect, you may need to erect some defensive shields around you and your spouse. In many large, close families, there are relatives who will eagerly intrude to assume a caretaking function when they hear about a health problem. It can take a bit of "spine" to set ground rules that let these would-be helpers know that you and your spouse have a primary loyalty to each other and to your marriage. You appreciate the good will, but you are making the care decisions as a couple, yourselves.

Like allowing your spouse to administer self-care, demanding respect for your marriage is an adult thing you can do to protect your marriage and your spouse.

Chase away blame and shame

In the years after his wife developed diabetes, Jerry felt increasingly resentful. Half of his kitchen was taken up with foods and medicines that he found intrusive in his home. He found his wife's need to give herself injections disquieting, even disturbing. Their sex life had died away. When he thought about his wife, he could only think about what her disease was doing to their lives. Although he never used the word "blame," it was eroding their marriage. Jerry still loved his wife, so he was haunted by shame over his selfish feelings. He hid them. Things were on a downward cycle, and the only relief available to him came from avoiding the issue and, ultimately, avoiding his wife too.

When illness enters a relationship, blame and shame often follow close behind. The ill person blames himself or herself for having the health problem. The well person often experiences shame over

past actions that contributed to the problem. For example, the well person might think, "I never helped my husband lose weight, even though I've known for years that he needed to. Now I've made him sick."

Many people find it hard to deal personally with blame or to discuss it openly with a spouse. Even if they have the courage to air the problem, they don't really believe that their spouse has the ability to help them get past it. After all, the husband or wife is inside the family system, which can make it hard to be objective. This is one reason why counselors, ministers, or doctors outside your circle of intimacy may be required to help break the blame/shame cycle and get a troubled relationship back on track.

Another way to keep blame from infecting your marriage is to actively practice forgiveness by letting go of hurts or anger about things that happened in the past. Rather than storing up resentments, you can "let the pressure out" so you don't harbor grudges or guilt from the past. You might start out by testing your own ability to ask for forgiveness and to apologize. Just introducing that kind of language into your relationship can open new areas of communication about forgiveness.

To move on, you may even need to cultivate a kind of amnesia about some past hurts, rather than storing up every little transgression. It may be best to purposely forget thoughts like, "Last Thanksgiving you cooked a giant meal, even though you knew I was dieting" or "John always wanted to exercise, but I always poked fun at him and refused to join him." With some conscious effort, you can learn to stop blaming yourself for the things done or left undone. A marriage should have that kind of ecology: a process that disposes of negative emotions. Often, starting that process is as simple as making a decision to let the negatives go.

Keep love alive

How can you help love thrive in the face of a disease like diabetes? One very good approach can be found in *The Good Marriage*, a book by Judith Wallerstein and Sandra Blakeslee. Their advice? Cultivate a double vision in your marriage, in which you maintain an idealized, romantic vision of your marriage alongside the more mundane one. On the everyday side, you know the person you're married to, warts and all, problems and illnesses. On the idealized side, you hold to a romantic vision of your relationship, a vision of your spouse that embodies an idealized quality of loving sweetness. In her studies of marriages, Wallerstein has found that people who hold those two visions at the same time are more successful in maintaining healthy, long-lasting relationships.

You might also try adding a level of shared spiritual value beneath the day-to-day routines of living

Dealing With Feelings

together. You might tell yourself, "We've taken those marriage vows, we're on a path together, growing and learning from each other every day in a divine presence." Adding that spiritual level of support can be a very important tool in keeping disease and other problems from derailing a relationship. In fact, one study conducted by David Olson at the University of Minnesota determined that shared spiritual values represented the greatest factor in whether or not a marriage lasted beyond 11 years.

Yet another way to keep diabetes from becoming the defining characteristic of your relationship is to actively seek a larger perspective on the problem. The employees of Apple Computer coined the phrase, "Perspective is worth 20 IQ points." One way to gain that perspective is to "reframe" the illness, or learn to view it in a different way. One Tibetan Buddhist teacher writes, "There are no problems, there is only how we look at things." He's telling us that if we can view problems as opportunities for spiritual growth, we can find a healthy alternative way to live. While it would be unnatural to relish life's serious problems, you can learn to integrate them as part of the process of life and living well together.

Strive to avoid the trap of seeing your marriage in the context of diabetes. By keeping a larger perspective, you can find ways to view diabetes the other way around: within the context of a rich, rewarding married life.

Keep your sex life alive

If diabetes-related problems arise around sexual abilities, it is very important to not just give up and deny your need for sexual closeness. As the sneaker ads say, it may be necessary to make a commitment to "just do it" and then to find a way, seeking medical help for the problem if needed. There are ways to be coached and counseled to help you maintain a satisfying sexual relationship despite physical problems. A close physical relationship with your spouse is something that you are entitled to. Don't simply give up.

Finding spiritual courage

Sheila found herself feeling terribly alone when, after years of successful self-care and maintenance, her husband began to experience problems with his vision and circulation. She faced the bleak fear that he would soon develop serious complications from diabetes. Where would she find the courage to cope with them?

Courage is not some rare characteristic of mythic heroes. It is simply the ability to do what needs to be done in the face of adversity. It is a quality that you and I have, though we may not discover it until we find it

A MORE PERFECT UNION

If you would like to read more about keeping your marriage strong and growing, here are three books you may enjoy:

WHY MARRIAGES SUCCEED OR FAIL...
And How *You* Can Make Yours Last
John Gottman
Fireside Books
New York, 1995

WELL BEING
A Personal Plan for Exploring and Enriching the Seven Dimensions of Life: Mind, Body, Spirit, Love, Work, Play, and Earth
Howard J. Clinebell, Jr.
HarperCollins
San Francisco, 1992

THE GOOD MARRIAGE
How & Why Love Lasts
Judith S. Wallerstein and Sandra Blakeslee
Warner Books
New York, 1996

necessary to love sacrificially, that is, to do what is in the best interest of ourselves and our families.

You *can* find courage. One starting point is to become involved, if possible, in the healthy spiritual community of a church, synagogue, mosque, or other place of worship. The setting you choose should afford you a place to be vulnerable and to feel a sense of healing and community. If both you and your spouse are part of it, all the better. If your spouse is unable or uninterested, you might consider seeking out such a community yourself.

Another way to find courage is to learn to value every day you have together. In my practice as a psychoanalyst, I counsel one client with a terminal disease. This wonderful man really knows that he only has a certain amount of time left. He's often in Paris on business, where he stays in a hotel room that overlooks the Eiffel Tower. He told me that each morning when he's there, he opens the doors to his balcony, looks out, takes a deep breath, and says, "This is the day the Lord has made. Let us rejoice and be glad in it." There's one more day to get into, one more day to revel in the present, to live fully. What a gift!

If this man has learned to see the beauty and promise of each day, you can, too. Learn to value your time together with your husband or wife. It is a gift so precious, diabetes cannot take it away. ❑

BLOOD GLUCOSE CONTROL

DO YOU KNOW YOUR A$_{1C}$'s?

by David E. Goldstein, M.D.

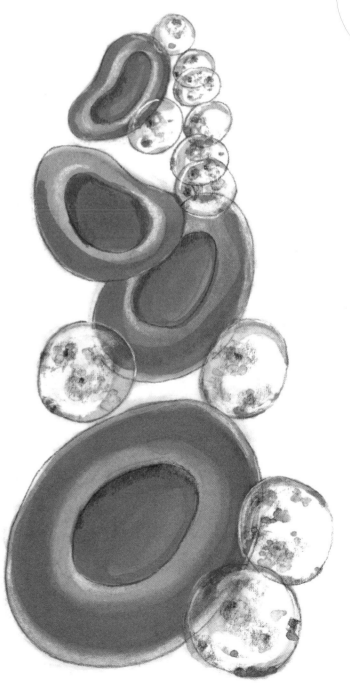

You probably already know that our tissues are fed by the blood that courses through our veins. A protein in those blood cells, called hemoglobin, acts like a tiny waiter, carrying oxygen to nourish our cells from our brains down to our toes. But hemoglobin doesn't just specialize in oxygen. It can also carry glucose molecules. This discovery, which occurred in the 1950's, led to the development of a remarkable test that has improved the management of diabetes.

The test is known by such names as the glycosylated hemoglobin test, glycated hemoglobin test, and glycohemoglobin test. Using a single drop of blood, obtained at any time of day, without regard to the blood glucose level at the time of testing, it gives an indication of a person's average blood glucose level over the preceding three to four months. A few variations of this test exist; each one focuses on a slightly different portion of the hemoglobin molecule. You may have already heard of the most commonly used version: the glycosylated hemoglobin A$_{1c}$, or HbA$_{1c}$, test—often called simply the A$_{1c}$ test. If you have diabetes, you need to know how the test works and how it can help your diabetes care.

How the test works

Fortunately, oxygen's bond to hemoglobin is a loose one that allows oxygen to be released in the tissues where it is needed. The tie between hemoglobin and glucose is quite different, however. Once glucose attaches to a hemoglobin molecule, it binds very tightly for the life of the red blood cell carrying that hemoglobin molecule—about three to four months. During each red blood cell's life span, as blood glucose levels rise, so does the likelihood that the hemoglobin in that red blood cell will trap glucose molecules. Not surprisingly, therefore, the amount of glycosylated hemoglobin in the blood sample—the sample's "A$_{1c}$ level"—is an accurate measure of a person's average blood glucose level over time.

For people who do not have diabetes, the average blood glucose level is about 100 mg/dl; this corresponds to an A_{1c} level of about 5%. In other words, in a person who does not have diabetes, one in every 20 hemoglobin molecules has a glucose molecule attached to it. In people with diabetes, A_{1c} levels are usually elevated, but how high depends on the average blood glucose level during the past four months. On average, people with diabetes have an A_{1c} level of approximately 10%. That's twice the level in people without diabetes. However, the A_{1c} level can be 20% or more if the diabetes has been poorly controlled.

Although the existence of glycosylated hemoglobin has been known since the late 1950's, the relationship between glycosylated hemoglobin and blood glucose was not fully understood until the mid-1970's when a clinical test was first developed. In the late 1980's, the American Diabetes Association recommended A_{1c} testing as part of routine diabetes care. Thus, this test is relatively new, and some people with diabetes and their health-care providers still do not know about it.

Why measure A_{1c}?

For many years, scientists debated whether the long-term complications that can develop in people with diabetes—problems with the eyes, kidneys, nerves, and blood vessels—are related to how high the blood glucose level is over time. In essence, the debate was as follows: Does blood glucose control matter? You might think that such a simple question would be easy to answer. However, scientists could not find a way to accurately measure a person's blood glucose control over the many years necessary to watch for the development of complications.

This changed in the late 1970's when the A_{1c} test became available. With this new test, it was finally possible to answer the question of whether blood glucose control is related to diabetic complications. Since that time, several studies have shown conclusively that in people who have diabetes, the risks for developing complications and for showing progression of previously diagnosed complications are directly related to blood glucose control.

The most important of these studies was the Diabetes Control and Complications Trial, or DCCT, which was completed in 1993. Almost 1500 people with Type 1 diabetes participated in the study for up to nine years. The study volunteers were divided into two treatment groups: intensive and conventional. To measure blood glucose control over the course of the study, participants had regular A_{1c} tests. In the intensive treatment group, study volunteers worked hard to keep their blood glucose levels as close to the normal range as possible. They did this by testing often and adjusting their treatment accordingly, so that their A_{1c}

came out close to normal. In the conventional treatment group, study volunteers took good care of their diabetes but did not strive for any specific blood glucose or A_{1c} levels; the primary treatment goal was to prevent symptoms due to either high or low blood glucose levels.

The study was terminated after nine years (it was supposed to last 10 years) because the study participants in the conventional treatment group had developed or shown progression of many more eye, kidney, and peripheral nerve complications than study volunteers in the intensive treatment group. The only difference between the two treatment groups that could explain the striking differences in outcome was their blood glucose control. In the intensive therapy group, participants had an average A_{1c} of 7%, which indicated an average blood sugar level of about 150 mg/dl. The people in the conventional therapy group had A_{1c} levels of about 9%, or an average of about 230 mg/dl.

Regardless of which treatment group the study volunteers were in, their risks of developing and/or showing progression of complications were directly linked to how high their A_{1c} levels were during the study. In summary, the DCCT proved that blood glucose control matters, and A_{1c} is the best way to measure overall blood glucose control.

Using the A_{1c} test

Now that you know what A_{1c} is and why it is important to measure, let's cover some practical issues.

1. How often should I have this test performed? Most experts agree that everyone who has diabetes should have an A_{1c} test at least twice a year. People who take insulin should have the test more often: about three to four times a year. You and your doctor can best decide exactly how often you should have the test. Some people with diabetes find it very useful to have their level checked monthly to confirm that their blood glucose control is consistent with the results of their daily blood glucose self-monitoring. For other people, especially those whose diabetes is very stable, it may be fine to have the test about twice a year just to keep tabs on their progress.

Most current A_{1c} testing methods require only a tiny drop of blood. The blood is obtained simply by pricking a finger, just as you would do for a self-test with a blood glucose monitor. In fact, for most A_{1c} testing methods, it actually takes less blood than for home blood glucose testing.

2. How do I interpret the A_{1c} test results? This can be tricky. A national standardization program for the United States was started in 1996, but some laboratories still do not take part in it, which means they may produce different test numbers for the same blood sample. (For more information about the standardization initiative—known as the National Glycohemoglobin Standardization Program, or NGSP—visit its Web site at www.missouri.edu/~diabetes/ngsp.html.)

You should ask your doctor what the nondiabetic range is for the test you take. Typically, the nondiabetic range is about 4% to 6%. Then discuss with your doctor what your A_{1c} goal should be. In general, the American Diabetes Association recommends that the goal be below 7%, assuming use of a standardized test "traceable to the DCCT reference method." Goals, however, should be individualized and should take into account a number of factors. For example, if you take insulin and are subject to frequent hypoglycemia without warning signs, the A_{1c} goal might be somewhat higher than for a person who does not have hypoglycemic unawareness. On the other hand, if you don't use insulin or oral hypoglycemic drugs, you can (and should) aim for an A_{1c} level in or very near the nondiabetic range, since you don't have to worry about hypoglycemia.

Age may be an important factor, too. In young children with Type 1 diabetes, recurrent hypoglycemia may affect intellectual development. Thus, A_{1c} goals may need to be slightly higher than for older patients. Similarly, for elderly patients, risks for heart attacks and strokes may be increased with hypoglycemia. In these patients, A_{1c} goals may need to be adjusted upward slightly for safety. Regardless, we should remember that in the DCCT, A_{1c} levels about 1% above the upper limit of normal for the test were associated with much better outcomes than A_{1c} levels about 2% higher. Thus, if your A_{1c} level is 11% or 12%, and the nondiabetic range for your laboratory is only up to 6%, you need to take immediate action.

It is also important to note that in the DCCT very few study volunteers were able to maintain their A_{1c} levels in the nondiabetic range. Thus, for a person with Type 1 diabetes, aiming for A_{1c} levels in the non-diabetic range may not be a realistic goal or even a safe one, given the risks of hypoglycemia. (The DCCT also showed that the closer the A_{1c} level is to the nondiabetic group, the greater the risks for serious hypoglycemia.)

3. Is the A_{1c} test result ever wrong? Like all laboratory tests, the A_{1c} test has its limits. Even the best laboratories mix up samples once in a while. If the test result does not "fit" with your home blood glucose testing results or with previous A_{1c} test results, ask to have it repeated. Depending on how the laboratory measures A_{1c} (there are many different ways to measure it), some drugs may interfere with the test result, giving a falsely high or low report. Some red blood cell abnormalities—including inherited problems such as sickle cell disease and thalassemia, and acquired problems such as immune damage to red blood cells from reac-

tions to certain drugs and chemicals—can also affect the test result. All types of anemias will falsely lower the test result. Fortunately, these types of problems are not common. Regardless, if you or your doctor believe the A_{1c} test result does not make sense, ask to have the test repeated, perhaps by a different laboratory or by using a different method in the same laboratory (most large reference laboratories have these services available).

4. How are changes in blood sugar control reflected in the A_{1c} test? Although the A_{1c} test averages all the blood glucose ups and downs over the previous three to four months, it is not a simple average of all these blood glucose levels. It is a *weighted average*. The A_{1c} test result is affected much more by recent blood glucose levels than by older ones.

Thus, a big improvement in blood glucose control during the month before the test will make the results look as if overall blood glucose control during the past four months was better than it actually was. Conversely, higher blood glucose levels for several weeks just before obtaining the test will suggest that blood glucose levels were quite a bit higher during the past four months than they actually were.

These peculiarities of A_{1c} are an important reason why infrequent A_{1c} testing may provide misleading information about a person's actual long-term blood glucose control. This also means that a big improvement (or worsening) in blood glucose levels can be detected by a change in the A_{1c} test result fairly quickly—within a month or so. Therefore, it is not necessary to wait four months to document the change.

The fact that the test is a weighted average can be a bit confusing. You may find five different experts giving five different answers to the question of how far back the A_{1c} test measures. The simplest answer is about four months, but probably the most accurate answer is that the test best reflects the average blood glucose during the past two to four months, particularly if there have been quite a few ups and downs in blood glucose levels.

5. What if my doctor does not want to order this test for me? You may need to educate your doctor. Bring in this article or point your doctor to the American Diabetes Association's "Clinical Practice Recommendations" that are published yearly in the medical journal *Diabetes Care*. Once you start using the A_{1c} test, in no time at all you and your doctor will find that this test has become an old friend.

In summary, management of diabetes has taken a giant leap forward since the development of the A_{1c} test. Not only has the test finally allowed scientists to show that blood glucose control counts, it also offers people with diabetes objective information on how well they are doing in their efforts to stay healthy. ❏

THE LOWDOWN ON LANCETS AND LANCING DEVICES

by Virginia Peragallo-Dittko, R.N., M.A., C.D.E.

Years ago, a man told me that he had stopped checking his blood sugar because "the lancelot hurt a lot." I immediately imagined Sir Lancelot with a sword and grimaced. We laughed at the play on words, and I learned two important lessons. First, it is worth the time and effort to find a product that minimizes the discomfort of a fingerstick. Second, learning to manage diabetes includes learning new words that may sound foreign. Let's start this article on lancets and lancing devices by defining some words.

Lancet. This is a pointed piece of surgical steel encased in plastic. The point is used to stick your finger to get a blood sample.

Lancing device. The lancing device pushes the lancet into your skin and then retracts it; its action is controlled by a spring. It controls the depth of penetration of the lancet—and allows the user to change that depth—through one of several mechanisms.

Drawing blood. This term has nothing to do with pencils, paper, or artistic talents. Instead, it describes what happens when you stick your finger with a lancet: that is, you cause your finger to bleed, or you draw blood.

Lancing devices

When you purchase a blood glucose meter, a lancing device is usually included with the meter. Some products give you the option of changing the depth of penetration by changing the plastic cap (sometimes called a platform) at the end of the device. Many products have a feature that allows you to dial in the penetration depth. Generally, children and adults with sensitive fingers prefer a shallower puncture; adults with callused fingers may need a deeper puncture to get an adequate blood sample.

The lancing device packaged with your meter may not be the best one for you. It makes sense to try it, but if you can't get enough blood or it hurts too much, there are plenty of other devices to try.

After a while, the spring in a lancing device weakens, and it gets harder to draw blood. You have a few options. You can purchase a new lancing device and use this as an opportunity to try a new product. You can call your diabetes educator, who may have a free sample to give you. Or, if your device came with your meter, the meter manufacturer may replace it at no charge.

Franz, a professional musician, felt managed by his diabetes because he had frequent and severe swings in his blood glucose. He couldn't check his blood glucose because he played the violin and wouldn't risk injury to his fingers. But now, Franz and anyone else who is reluctant or unable to stick his fingers have another option: lancing devices, such as the Microlet Vaculance, designed for obtaining capillary blood from body sites other than the fingertips. Potential sites include the fleshy side of the palm between wrist and little finger, the underside of the forearm, the abdomen, and the outer thigh. Such devices may be particularly useful for anyone with hand injuries and for women who have had mastectomies. After a mastectomy, women are advised not to draw blood from the hand on the side of the body from which a breast was removed. Injury or infection of the arm or hand on that side increases a woman's risk of developing *lymphedema,* or swelling of the arm. Meters that have been approved to measure blood from alternate sites such as the forearm are packaged with their own lancing devices that help bring the blood to the surface of the skin.

Some people choose not to use a lancing device; they just stick their finger with a lancet. The trouble with this courageous technique is that you can't control the depth of penetration: You may have to stick yourself more than once to get enough blood, or you may stick yourself too deeply and bleed more than necessary.

If you choose to use a lancet without a lancing device, you may want to try one of the single-use, safety lancets. They combine a lancet and spring in one unit. Because they are designed for use in hospitals and can be used only once, they are more expensive than other models.

Lancets

Choosing the right lancet is as important as using the right lancing device. One way in which lancets differ is in the *gauge,* or width of the metal point that sticks your finger. The higher the gauge, the smaller the hole in your finger. So a 30-gauge lancet makes a smaller hole than a 23-gauge lancet. Many people find that a 30-gauge lancet hurts less, but everyone's sensitivity is different.

A potential drawback to using a higher-gauge lancet is that you may not get enough blood when you do a fingerstick. If you're having trouble getting an adequate drop of blood, the gauge of the lancet is something to consider. You may get a larger drop of blood from a lower-gauge lancet (one with a larger point) and avoid doing repeated fingersticks just to get one blood sugar result.

Most lancets fit into any lancing device, but there are exceptions. The Softclix device can only be used with Softclix lancets. Long-body lancets are only compatible with certain lancing devices, such as the Autolet II.

Controlling costs

In any discussion of diabetes products, cost is an issue. Many people reuse lancets a few times to save money. (Reuse is not advised for children.) The main concern about reusing lancets is infection. Your best defense against infection is to wash your hands well before lancing your finger. Do not use alcohol on your finger, since alcohol dries out your skin and may alter your blood glucose reading. However, if you have soiled hands, don't have access to running water, and must use alcohol to clean your finger for a blood glucose check, make sure the alcohol is completely dry before lancing your finger.

Another concern about reusing lancets is that the point gets duller each time you use it. When this happens, sticking your finger hurts more and draws blood less efficiently. Using alcohol on a lancet can have a similar dulling effect, because alcohol removes the protective coating on the metal. For that reason, don't use alcohol on your lancets. Between uses, simply store the lancet in the lancing device without attempting to clean it.

Some insurance companies contract with one lancet manufacturer and provide only one product through their medical supplier. If that product is not the best lancet for you, you could pay out of pocket for the lancet of your choice, or you could contact the diabetes case manager at your insurance company. Sometimes a company will allow you to purchase lancets locally and submit the receipt for reimbursement.

Laser lancing device

Someday, we'll make the transition from conventional blood glucose monitoring to noninvasive technology, and the laser lancing device is the beginning of that transition.

The Lasette Plus laser lancing device produces a laser beam that draws blood from your fingertip by vaporizing water molecules in the skin tissue. Rather than tearing the skin like a conventional lancet, the Lasette Plus actually removes a tiny bit of skin, so you feel a slight sensation of pressure. The width of the hole is equivalent to that produced by a 28-gauge lancet.

GETTING ENOUGH BLOOD

For many people, the hardest part of blood glucose monitoring is getting an adequate blood sample. Here are some tips to improve your chances of getting enough on the first try.

■ Wash your hands in warm water, rubbing them together vigorously to increase blood circulation to your fingertips.

■ Hang the hand to be pricked at your side for 30 seconds so the blood can pool in your hand. (You will see the veins in your hand distend and fill with blood.)

■ Shake the hand to be pricked as though you were shaking down a thermometer.

■ After you puncture your finger, gently milk it (from the bottom knuckle to the fingertip) as though you were squeezing toothpaste from the bottom of the tube. Milking the whole finger works better and is preferred over just squeezing the fingertip.

■ Try using a different lancet or lancing device.

■ Switch to a meter that requires less blood.

■ The shaded areas in the illustration below are the best spots for a fingerstick. Aim for the sides of the fingers, between the tip of the finger and the last knuckle. Avoid pricking the very tip of the finger, the middle of the pad, and the back of the finger. These areas have more nerve endings, so you may feel more pain.

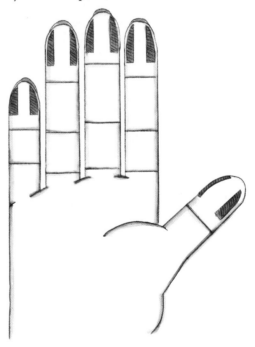

The Lasette Plus costs $995 for home use, including a trial pack of disposable cartridges for 240 blood samples. Each additional cartridge costs approximately $30. The Lasette Plus requires proper maintenance and instruction. It has 16 different power settings and a rechargeable battery.

Tips and techniques

Whatever method or device you use to draw blood, your goals are the same: to get a drop of blood large enough to do an accurate blood glucose check with the least amount of pain. To minimize discomfort, it helps to prick the side of your finger. The sides have a good blood supply and fewer nerve endings than fingertips. Be sure to prick the meaty sides of your fingers—not too close to the cuticle, but not directly on the center pad of the fingertip. To get an adequate blood sample, press the lancing device firmly against your finger. Some people choose to use the same fingers repeatedly and build up a callus; others rotate fingers. Both groups say their method hurts less.

You may read about using earlobes as an alternate site for drawing blood. It's not impossible, but earlobes bleed a lot, and you have to be very coordinated to get the blood onto a test strip. Drawing blood from the toes is never advised because of concerns about infection and decreased blood flow to the feet.

If you find that your fingers bruise from fingersticks, it may be because the lancet is penetrating too deeply. Using a lancing device with dial-in depth settings may be part of the answer.

You also need to allow your blood to clot following the fingerstick. A helpful technique is to put the blood sample on the strip, then firmly hold a tissue to the puncture site while you are waiting for the blood sugar result. If you take the drug warfarin (brand name Coumadin) or other types of anticoagulant or antiplatelet drugs, you will need to firmly hold the puncture site for at least 30 seconds.

Children may not be willing to sit still long enough after a fingerstick to allow the bleeding to fully stop. In the grand scheme of things, this is not critical. But if you can make clotting the blood part of the habit for blood glucose monitoring, it will help prevent bruises and black marks on your child's fingers.

If you work outdoors or find that the skin on your fingers cracks, you may want to try one of the skin creams specially formulated for fingers. Some skin cream makers offer free samples so you can try it before you buy it.

Doing regular fingersticks is no fun for anyone, but finding the right combination of lancets and lancing device can make the procedure less painful. If you're not happy with the products you currently use, we encourage you to consult your diabetes educator and to shop around. Surely there's a combination out there that's right for you. For information on lancing techniques, see page 77. ❑

HOW ACCURATE IS YOUR METER?

by Virginia Peragallo-Dittko, R.N., M.A., C.D.E.

Since they came on the market in the late 1970's, home blood glucose meters have revolutionized diabetes care. With a meter, you can measure your blood glucose level at any time, and within seconds, you can decide whether to eat some food, how much to eat, or how much insulin to take. Self-monitoring also allows you to find patterns in your blood glucose levels and evaluate how well your food choices, exercise, and medicines are controlling your diabetes. But the more you rely on your blood glucose meter, the more you may find yourself asking the question "How accurate are the results?"

There is no simple way to answer the question, so fasten your seat belts: We're about to enter the technical world of the clinical laboratory.

What is accuracy?

The dictionary definition of accuracy is "freedom from mistake or error." Most of us take that to mean that a meter that is accurate will be dead-on: If it reads 100 mg/dl, our blood glucose level should be exactly 100 mg/dl.

But blood glucose meters for home use are not that accurate. The American Diabetes Association recommends to meter manufacturers that the performance goal for their products should be a total error of less than 10% at blood glucose levels of 30 mg/dl to 400 mg/dl, 100% of the time. In that case, a blood glucose reading of 68 mg/dl on your meter could actually range from 61 mg/dl to 75 mg/dl, and your meter would be considered accurate. Why that range is considered good enough and what you can do to reduce the error as much as possible is covered later in this article.

Another part of the dictionary definition of accuracy is "degree of conformity of a measure to a standard or a true value." For blood glucose meters, the laboratory is the standard against which they are judged. But anyone who has compared their meter readings with their lab results knows that the two are often different. To understand why they are different and how they can be compared in spite of the difference, it helps to know a little about the heart and circulatory system.

The cardiovascular system is an elaborate transportation network that carries blood throughout the body so that nutrients can be delivered to cells and waste products can be escorted away. The heart pumps the blood, pushing it through large muscular tubes called arteries. Large arteries connect to smaller ones, which in turn connect to capillaries, tiny tubes that run throughout the body. Capillaries lead into veins, which carry the blood back to the heart, completing the circle.

As blood circulates, exchanges take place between the blood in the capillaries and the body cells. Glucose and oxygen leave the capillary blood to supply the cells, and waste products enter the blood from the cells. The capillaries deliver this blood to the veins, which carry it back to the heart and lungs to pick up more oxygen and begin the cycle again.

By the time blood reaches the veins, some of the glucose in it has been transferred to other tissues, so the blood flowing through the veins has less glucose than the blood flowing through the capillaries. However, the difference between the two varies depending on when you last ate. After a fast of eight or more hours, the difference between the level of glucose in capillary blood and in venous blood is very small. After a meal, the difference can be quite large, as blood glucose levels rise and the rate of glucose transfer into the tissues accelerates. The circulatory system after a meal is like a city bus at rush hour: The overall number of passengers is higher, and the rate at which they enter and leave the bus is higher.

Since meters use samples of blood from capillaries and labs use blood from veins, a certain amount of difference is expected in the results, even if the samples are taken at the same time. Both measurements may be accurate, but each shows what is happening in your body at a different point in the transportation system. As stated earlier, however, the difference should be small if you have fasted for at least eight hours before the tests.

But even if you have fasted, the results may not be the same. That's because some meters measure the glucose level of whole blood, while laboratories measure the glucose level of *plasma,* the fluid part of blood.

Whole blood is composed of plasma (sometimes called *serum*) and three formed elements: red blood cells, white blood cells, and platelets. The glucose content of red blood cells is about 20% less than the glucose content of plasma, due to the density of the red blood cells. If the plasma glucose level is 100 mg/dl, then the concentration of glucose in the red blood cells would be about 80 mg/dl. Since whole blood consists of approximately equal portions of plasma and red blood cells, a mixture of the two would yield a glucose value of 90 mg/dl. So if you measure your blood glucose with a meter that gives whole blood readings and compare it with the laboratory result, your meter will read about 11% to 15% *lower* than the lab.

Most meters use a drop of whole blood on a test strip. But some meters read the plasma glucose level or have been programmed to calculate the plasma glucose level and give it on the readout. (See "Which Meter Reads Which?" on page 80.) A meter that gives plasma glucose levels will have results that are closer to the lab's. For tips on comparing your meter's blood glucose readings to the ones that you get from your doctor, see "Comparing Your Meter With the Lab" on page 82.

Since a meter that gives whole blood values and a meter that gives plasma values will have different results for the same blood sample, the American Diabetes Association recently revised its suggested blood sugar goals to take the two systems into account. The updated goals are as follows: When using a meter that gives whole blood glucose levels, the target goal before a meal is between 80 mg/dl and 120 mg/dl. When using a meter that gives plasma glucose, the target goal before a meal is between 90 mg/dl and 130 mg/dl. These goals may not be achievable by everyone. Your doctor can help you establish individualized blood glucose goals.

What is precision?

When evaluating a blood glucose meter, it's important to consider not just the accuracy of the product, but also the *precision.* To be considered precise, a given meter must be able to consistently produce the same results. Before a new product is released, manufacturers usually test a meter's precision by conducting an experiment in which the same blood sample is analyzed a minimum of 20 times. That way, they can determine how much the results may vary.

A meter can be precisely wrong, meaning that you repeatedly get the same reading, but it is wrong. To understand this idea better, think of throwing darts at

WHICH METER READS WHICH?

Some meters report whole blood glucose levels and others are calibrated to report plasma glucose levels. (Either way, the technique is the same: the user places a drop of blood, usually from a fingerstick, on a strip.) Plasma glucose readings are roughly 10% to 15% higher than whole blood readings, so it's important to know which your meter gives. Here's a list of which meter gives which:

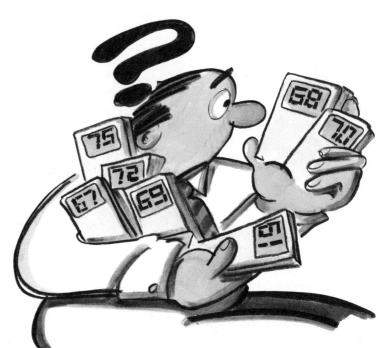

Whole blood

Accu-Chek Instant (Roche Diagnostics)

Accu-Chek Simplicity (Roche Diagnostics)

Duet Glucose Control Monitor (LXN Corporation)

ExacTech (MediSense)

ExacTech RSG (MediSense)

One Touch Basic (LifeScan)

One Touch Profile (LifeScan)

Prestige (Home Diagnostics)

Plasma calibrated

Accu-Chek Active (Roche Diagnostics)

Accu-Chek Advantage* (Roche Diagnostics)

Accu-Chek Compact (Roche Diagnostics)

Accu-Chek Complete* (Roche Diagnostics)

Accu-Chek Voicemate* (Roche Diagnostics)

AtLast Blood Glucose System (Amira Medical)

FastTake (LifeScan)

FreeStyle (TheraSense)

Glucometer DEX (Bayer Corporation)

Glucometer Elite (Bayer Corporation)

Glucometer Elite XL (Bayer Corporation)

Glucometer Encore (Bayer Corporation)

In Charge Diabetes System (LXN Corporation)

MediSense 2 Card† (MediSense)

MediSense 2 Pen† (MediSense)

One Touch Ultra (LifeScan)

Precision Xtra (MediSense)

Precision QID (MediSense)

Precision QID Pen (MediSense)

Sof-Tact (MediSense)

SureStep (LifeScan)

Whole blood or plasma

The following products can be programmed to report either plasma or whole blood glucose levels:

Assure (Chronimed)

Checkmate Plus (QuestStar Medical)

Prestige IQ (Home Diagnostics)

Prestige LX (Home Diagnostics)

Select GT (Chronimed)

Supreme II (Chronimed)

* These products can be used with either Advantage strips or Comfort Curve strips. Accu-Chek now makes both Advantage and Comfort Curve strips to give plasma blood glucose levels. But older Advantage strips (those with lot numbers beginning with 4 or below) give whole blood readings.

† The MediSense 2 Card and MediSense 2 Pen are no longer on the market. However, people who have these meters can use them with Precision QID strips, which give plasma glucose levels.

a dartboard. If you consistently hit the same area of an outer ring, your results are precise. But because you did not hit the bull's-eye, they are inaccurate.

While a meter can be precise but not accurate, it can't be accurate without being precise. If it's accurate, meaning that the result is the same when measured against a reference method (the laboratory), it will be reproducible, or precise.

How the user affects meter accuracy

The user of a meter plays a critical role in securing accurate results. You will have false results, despite the accuracy and precision of your meter, if you have an inadequate blood sample, a soiled meter, an uncalibrated meter, or defective strips.

Inadequate blood sample. Despite advances in technology with some meters, some things never change. Even with strips that require only a tiny amount of blood, it's still possible to provide a blood sample that's too small, and the meter will give a false result. Some meters have a feature that signals the user when the blood sample isn't big enough. But this feature creates a false sense of security because users assume that if they don't get the signal, they've given an adequate sample. Don't be fooled! The meter will only signal you about a blood sample it can't process; any other sample—even an inadequate one—will go through, but the results may not be accurate, although some newer meters on the market have been designed to not provide a reading if the blood sample is inadequate.

The instruction booklet packaged with your meter should include a picture of an adequate blood sample. Anything less will give you false results. If you can't find the instruction booklet, call the toll-free number on the back of your meter and the manufacturer will send you another copy.

Another way to be sure of your technique is to demonstrate how you use your meter to a diabetes educator at every opportunity, especially if you've been using the meter for a long time. The more comfortable we get using a machine, the more careless we become. (Think about how you drive your car. Remember when you began to drive and you *always* signaled before changing lanes?)

Soiled meter. Some of the meters on the market still need to be cleaned, and not cleaning them can lead to inaccurate results. Meters measure blood glucose in one of two ways: using *color reflectance* or using *sensor technology*. With reflectance meters, the glucose in a drop of blood reacts with an enzyme in the strip, changing the color of the strip. The meter reads the

darkness of the strip and gives a numeric readout of the blood glucose value. On these meters, the window that allows the meter to read the strip may need to be cleaned. If it's dirty, you'll get a false high reading. Check your user's manual for instructions on how and how often to clean your meter.

Meters that use sensor technology measure small electrical currents produced by the chemical interaction between the glucose in the blood and the chemicals on the reagent strip. These meters usually don't require cleaning since blood does not come in contact with the meter.

Lack of calibration. Almost every meter needs to be calibrated. That's the meter's way of letting itself know which factory-coded batch of strips you are using. If your meter doesn't have automatic calibration, you'll need to push a button or insert a calibrator (code strip) when you open a new package of strips. Directions for calibration should come with both your meter and each package of strips.

Mail-order companies typically send a large shipment of packaged strips that share the same calibration code number. But even if the calibration code is the same, laboratory specialists advise you to recalibrate each time you open a box or vial of strips. Not only does it help with accuracy, it keeps you in the habit of checking the code. Forgetting to change the calibration code is a common error that leads to false results.

Heat or cold. Extremes of heat and cold also affect the accuracy of the readings. Many meters have a temperature warning indicator that alerts the user when the air temperature is above or below the operating range of the strips. If your meter does not have this feature, you might want to check the owner's manual so you know when to be concerned.

Defective strips. Strips should be stored in the vial or foil wrapping they come in, according to the manufacturer's guidelines. Not doing so could lead to false results. You also need to be aware of your strips' expiration date. That's the date after which the manufacturer will no longer stand behind the accuracy of the strips.

Cindy and her doctor were surprised when her recent glycosylated hemoglobin (HbA_{1c}) result was in her goal range, because her blood glucose log showed readings that were consistently high. (The HbA_{1c} test indicates a person's level of blood glucose control over the past two to three months.) Her doctor suggested that Cindy repeat the HbA_{1c} test and check with her diabetes educator about the blood glucose readings. During the troubleshooting process, they realized she had been using expired strips. Cindy's uncle had given her his unused strips when he changed to a different meter, and she never checked the expiration date.

Be alert to extremes of heat, cold, or humidity in the storage of your strips. You can control how the strips are stored in your home, but you can't control how they're stored in transit. If your shipment of strips sat baking in the back of a delivery truck on the way to your house, they could be defective.

You can make sure that your strips are still good by using *control solution* on the first strip of a new box. Every meter is compatible with a control solution, but not all meters can use the same one. A bottle of control solution may come packaged with your meter when you buy it, or you may have to call the meter manufacturer to get a bottle. Because it expires with time, you need to get a fresh bottle every three months. Many health insurance plans cover control solution.

Use the control solution on a strip and check it in the meter as if it were a drop of blood. The acceptable range of results for the control solution is printed on the vial or package of strips or on an insert in the control solution package. If the acceptable range for the control solution is 83 mg/dl to 140 mg/dl, and the reading is 106 mg/dl, you know that the meter and strips are working properly. If the results are out of range, call the manufacturer's toll-free customer service number.

Some people mistakenly believe that the acceptable range printed on the package of strips or on the control solution bottle is also the acceptable range for their own blood sugar level. This is not necessarily the case. Your blood sugar goals should be discussed with your health-care provider.

Why aren't the meters 100% accurate?

Even if you work to perfect your technique, there is a certain amount of error that is inescapable. Although it can be hard to accept, a little bit of error is part of every type of test. Standards are set to determine what type and amount of error is unavoidable and what type and amount is unacceptable. When it comes to blood glucose monitoring, the type and amount of error that would be *clinically relevant* is unacceptable. A clinically relevant error is one that would affect your treatment decisions. For example, it would be unacceptable if your blood glucose readings were so far off that you thought your blood sugar was in range when it was really quite low. In this case, you wouldn't know to treat for hypoglycemia.

Many meters do not achieve the ADA goal of less than 10% error at blood glucose levels from 30 mg/dl to 400 mg/dl, 100% of the time. That may be in part

COMPARING YOUR METER WITH THE LAB

The best way to determine whether your readings are accurate is to test them against the results you get from the laboratory. The advanced equipment there allows technicians to make exact measurements. If your self-monitoring results match the ones you get from the lab, you'll know they're accurate. If not, consult your diabetes educator, who can help you figure out what's the problem. Here are some tips for making the comparison:

■ Compare your meter against a blood glucose test performed in a laboratory. Don't bother comparing against another meter; neither system is considered a laboratory standard.

■ Compare a *fasting* blood glucose level only. After-meal readings will differ between capillary blood (as measured on your meter) and venous blood (as measured in the lab).

■ Remember that a meter that gives whole blood glucose levels will have a reading 11% to 15% lower than the lab.

■ To compare meter and lab results, the two tests must be done at the same time. Perform a fingerstick check just prior to having blood drawn from your arm. (Doing the fingerstick after the blood is drawn from your arm is impractical since you have to hold the gauze to your arm after the venipuncture). Doing a fingerstick at home either before or after the venipuncture allows too much time between the readings for a valid comparison.

■ The venous blood that was collected into a tube must be spun by a centrifuge machine to separate the red blood cells from the plasma within 30 minutes after the time the blood sample was taken. If it is not, the glucose in the blood will begin to break down, and the results will not accurately reflect the blood glucose levels at the time the sample was collected. Although you have no control over when the specimen is centrifuged, you can ask the lab technician about the time frame.

■ Comparing meter to lab involves a fingerstick and a venipuncture. If the lab technician offers to place a drop of blood from the venipuncture needle on your meter strip, don't accept the offer. Some strips are designed for capillary blood only and will give false results if venous blood is used.

because the Food and Drug Administration (FDA) does not require meters to meet ADA goals for market approval. The ADA goals are voluntary goals; the FDA standards are less stringent. The good news is that studies show that clinical errors due to inaccurate blood glucose self-monitoring are uncommon. This is reassuring, but we still need to challenge blood glucose meter manufacturers to meet or exceed the ADA performance goal.

Decision making

If you use your meter correctly, the meter readings are as accurate as we can expect from a pocket-sized, portable meter designed for home use. The meter readings are much more accurate than the urine-testing results used years ago or the blood glucose monitoring method of visually matching a strip to a color chart.

The key issue is how the readings affect your decision making. Let's say that you plan to use blood glucose monitoring results to evaluate the effect on your blood glucose of eating two cups of pasta. It doesn't matter whether the result is 250 mg/dl or somewhere between 225 mg/dl to 275 mg/dl. The result is out of range, and two cups of pasta is too much for you within your current diabetes-care regimen. Or let's say you have symptoms of hypoglycemia and your blood glucose is 72 mg/dl (which could really be anywhere from 65 mg/dl to 79 mg/dl). You would still have to treat the symptoms, even if the meter reading doesn't match the textbook definition of hypoglycemia.

Still, anything less than a true value is frustrating when you're working hard to keep your blood glucose within range. Many people walk the line between in-range readings and low readings and use the numbers to fine-tune their insulin dose and meal plan. For them, it is hard to accept that a blood glucose reading of 180 mg/dl might actually be 162 mg/dl to 198 mg/dl. In choosing a bedtime snack, someone taking insulin might decide to eat 20 grams of carbohydrate at 162 mg/dl, 15 grams at 180 mg/dl, and 10 grams at 198 mg/dl. Fortunately, there are some things that you can do to create an environment for less variable readings:

Use only one meter. Your results will be most consistent if you use the same meter all the time. But since it isn't always practical to use the same meter, at least use the same model and strips. Don't use different kinds of meters; choose one model and stick with it.

Because your meter and strips are precise, using the same meter exclusively will yield consistent readings. If the true blood glucose level is 180 mg/dl and your meter reads 162 mg/dl, your meter will always read in the 160 mg/dl range for levels around 180 mg/dl. Over time, you will learn how to react to the readings. When Oscar says that he starts to feel symptoms of hypoglycemia when his blood glucose is less than 90 mg/dl, he means 90 mg/dl *on his meter.*

If you've accumulated a collection of different meters, choose one, and donate the others to your local diabetes program. Of course, any testing is better than none, even if you can't stick to just one meter. Since Shondell always checks her blood glucose before she drives, she bought a meter that has features making it easier to check and get results in a few seconds. She doesn't use that model at home because her insurance company won't pay for the strips. Although her readings are not the most consistent, she is much safer when driving than if she didn't check.

Look for patterns. Remember that the overall pattern of your blood glucose readings, not individual readings, is used to prescribe medicines or evaluate goals. Most people who monitor their blood glucose can describe their blood glucose patterns in general terms. For example, you might be able to say, "My readings are higher in the morning but lower as the day goes on" or "The readings always go up at night." This is the type of information your doctor uses to choose your drugs or plan your insulin routine. As far as your health-care team is concerned, it doesn't matter if your readings aren't 100% accurate because they still show your blood glucose patterns.

Have your HbA$_{1c}$ checked. Use your glycosylated hemoglobin (HbA$_{1c}$) to evaluate the big picture. If your HbA$_{1c}$ is elevated, your treatment plan will need to be revised. If your recorded readings don't reflect the HbA$_{1c}$ results, you'll need to find the reason for the discrepancy. It usually has nothing to do with the meter. It may indicate that you are not checking your blood glucose when it is elevated. (Many people check only their fasting blood glucose and miss the elevated readings after meals.)

A shared burden

There's a lot to consider when discussing the accuracy of blood glucose readings. To secure accurate readings, half of the burden falls on you and half on the manufacturer. It can be frustrating to realize that blood glucose readings aren't always correct. But the bottom line is that it is possible to secure readings that are accurate enough to guide your self-management decisions. ❏

TREATING TYPE 2 DIABETES WITH DIET AND EXERCISE

by Barbara N. Campaigne, Ph.D., and
Carol Younkin, R.N., M.Ed., C.D.E., C.H.E.S.

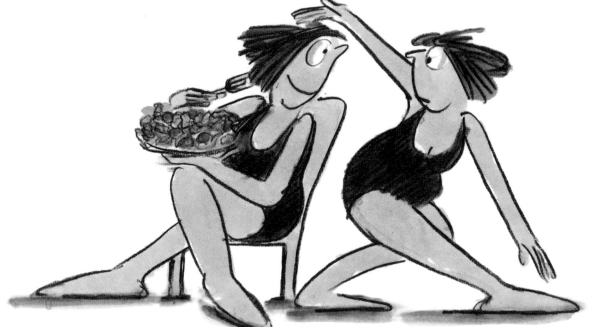

If you have Type 2 diabetes, you've no doubt been told to "watch your diet and get plenty of exercise." Diet and exercise are cornerstones of any diabetes control regimen. In fact, Type 2 diabetes can sometimes be managed with diet and exercise alone. Yet few people with Type 2 diabetes receive useful advice on how to change their diet and exercise habits.

Your diabetes meal plan is not just about "going on a diet." While your meal plan may be designed to help you lose weight, it is also designed to keep your blood sugar level stable. Following a meal plan that distributes carbohydrates evenly throughout the day helps prevent periods of high blood glucose. And a diet that is low in fat and includes lots of fruits and vegetables can help bring down high blood pressure—a common problem in Type 2 diabetes.

Exercise is important for managing diabetes because it lowers blood glucose, both by burning glucose for energy and by increasing the cells' ability to take glucose from the blood. Exercise can also help lower blood pressure. And it can diminish your appetite and boost your mood, making it easier to stick to your diabetes-care plan.

Together, diet and exercise can help you lose weight and keep it off, and weight loss also makes insulin more effective. Even a modest weight loss of 8 to 10 pounds can help control blood glucose levels and blood pressure levels.

To determine whether you are a good candidate for controlling your diabetes with diet and exercise alone, talk to your doctor. Because each person's body, lifestyle, and diabetes are different, each person's nutrition needs are different. No single eating plan is effective for everyone. Likewise, each person's ability and willingness to exercise is different, so each person needs an individualized physical activity plan. For these reasons, this article covers only general advice on diet and exercise therapy. You and your diabetes-care team can work out a specific plan for you.

When diet and exercise aren't enough

Diet and exercise alone may not work for everyone. Nor will they work all the time, so it's important that you don't judge yourself by whether you use diabetes medicines. Some people feel that they are failures when they cannot control their blood sugar with diet and exercise. But the United Kingdom Prospective Diabetes Study (UKPDS), a major study of people with Type 2 diabetes, established a better measure of success. Results of the UKPDS show that keeping your blood glucose level close to the normal range by any means necessary can prevent or delay complications. It did not find any additional benefit to managing blood sugar with diet and exercise alone. So to avoid complications, there may be times when you want to complement your diet and exercise plan with insulin or pills.

When first diagnosed with diabetes, some people have extremely high blood sugar levels. This can result in *glucotoxicity,* an effect caused by a buildup of glucose in the body, which impairs the insulin-producing beta cells in the pancreas and slows the release of insulin into the bloodstream. If you have just been diagnosed with Type 2 diabetes, you may need pills or insulin to lower high blood glucose levels. Once the levels come down, you may be able to stop the drugs on your doctor's recommendation.

Even if you have been successfully managing your diabetes with diet and exercise, there may be times when your body cannot supply enough insulin or may have trouble responding to its own insulin. This may happen when you are ill, under stress, or have an infection. It is not unusual for a person who is ill to require insulin or glucose-lowering pills temporarily to better manage blood sugar during the illness. Weight gain, which reduces the cells' ability to use insulin, or pregnancy may also make pills or insulin necessary.

Another reason you may need to add pills or insulin to your regimen is that Type 2 diabetes is progressive. With time, your pancreas becomes less able to produce enough insulin to keep your blood glucose in the normal range and your cells become more resistant to insulin—particularly, for women, at menopause. So eventually you may need the extra help of diabetes pills or insulin to manage your diabetes.

First steps first

So just how do you manage your diabetes with diet and exercise? Let's take a look at the first steps: education and blood glucose self-monitoring. In general, people who know more about diabetes and how it affects their bodies manage their diabetes more effectively, so it's worth your while to learn as much as you can. There are many ways to learn about diabetes. An important first step is to meet with a certified diabetes educator (C.D.E.) to learn the skills you need to carry out your diabetes management plan. A C.D.E. is a health-care professional who has received special training in diabetes treatment and education. Ask your doctor to recommend a diabetes educator, or, to find one near you, call the American Association of Diabetes Educators at (800) 832-6874 or use the referral service on the Association's Web site, www.aadenet.org.

Another way to learn about diabetes is to attend diabetes classes. Many hospitals, diabetes clinics, and community centers hold them, generally for no or low cost. For more information about diabetes education programs in your area, call your local chapter of the American Diabetes Association (ADA) or the national office, at (800) DIABETES (342-2383), or visit the ADA Web site at www.diabetes.org.

Blood glucose self-monitoring is key to managing diabetes, because it tells you whether your blood glucose is in the target range. For meters that give results for whole blood, the ADA recommends a target blood glucose range of 80 mg/dl to 120 mg/dl before meals. The target range after meals is 100 mg/dl to 180 mg/dl, and at bedtime it is 100 mg/dl to 140 mg/dl. For meters that give plasma readings, the ADA recommends a target range of 90 mg/dl to 130 mg/dl before meals, 110 mg/dl to 200 mg/dl after meals, and 110 mg/dl to 150 mg/dl at bedtime. Your personal goals may differ from these recommendations. Talk to your doctor about the blood glucose goals that are right for you.

Blood glucose self-monitoring also lets you know how certain foods or activities affect your blood sugar, and it allows you to make immediate decisions and adjustments to your diet and exercise plan. If your blood glucose level is slightly high, for example, you may decide to exercise for a bit longer than usual to bring it down or to eat something for your next meal that will not raise it much.

You should check your blood glucose frequently at first, until you have found the diet and exercise regimen that keeps your blood sugar in target range. The times to check your blood glucose are before eating, two hours after eating, before exercising, 15 minutes after exercising, and at bedtime, although you don't need to check at all of these times every day. (Your health insurance company may not cover adequate supplies for frequent checking, but having your doctor write a prescription for a certain amount of supplies may help get some of them covered.) Once you've established a pattern and settled on a diet and exercise plan, you may be able to cut back on blood glucose monitoring. However, if you get a result that is unusually high or low, or if you alter your treatment plan, resume more frequent testing.

Having a glycosylated hemoglobin (HbA$_{1c}$) test every three to six months allows you to double-check how well your plan is working. (The HbA$_{1c}$ test indicates your average level of blood sugar control over the preceding two to three months.) As long as your HbA$_{1c}$ result is below 7%, you don't need to add pills or insulin. However, if it is over 8%, your management plan is not adequately controlling your blood glucose and should be changed.

MEAL-PLANNING RESOURCES

Planning meals and counting carbohydrates is easier when you have the recipes and nutrition information you need at your fingertips. The books listed below offer just that. You can order *Quick & Easy Meals and Menus* exclusively from Diabetes Self-Management Books by calling (800) 366-3303 or by logging on to the Web site www.DiabetesSelfManagement.com. The others in the list and several other books in the series called *Month of Meals* can be ordered from the American Diabetes Association by calling (800) 232-6733 or logging on to http://store.diabetes.org.

THE DIABETES CARBOHYDRATE AND FAT GRAM GUIDE
Lea Ann Holzmeister
The American Dietetic Association and the American Diabetes Association, 2000

DIABETES MEAL PLANNING MADE EASY
Hope Warshaw
American Diabetes Association
Alexandria, Virginia, 2000

MONTH OF MEALS
Ethnic Delights
American Diabetes Association
Alexandria, Virginia, 1998

MONTH OF MEALS
Vegetarian Pleasures
American Diabetes Association
Alexandria, Virginia, 1998

QUICK & EASY MEALS AND MENUS
Marjorie Hollands and Margaret Howard
Diabetes Self-Management Books
New York, New York, 1997

If you do not require pills or insulin to manage your diabetes, it does not mean that your diabetes is "mild" or "borderline." You either have diabetes or you don't. And don't be fooled into thinking that your diabetes is cured because you have been able to stop taking insulin or diabetes pills. You still have diabetes; it is just well controlled, and your body is able to use its own insulin.

Diet

No one diet plan works for everybody; your diet needs to be tailored to you. A registered dietitian (R.D.) is the best person to help you with this. Together you can develop a meal plan that takes into account your blood glucose, blood pressure, and weight goals, your lifestyle, and your food preferences. Health conditions that are commonly related to Type 2 diabetes, such as high cholesterol and high blood pressure, may also be managed with diet, and your dietitian should consider these as you develop an eating plan.

To stay healthy, your body needs a balanced diet that provides adequate nutrients and a minimum of six to eight glasses of water or other nonalcoholic liquids a day—and more than that on days you exercise. The three types of nutrients from which your body receives energy are carbohydrate, protein, and fat. All three are important. Current American Diabetes Association (ADA) guidelines recommend that no more than 30% of most people's total daily calories come from fat (less than 10% from saturated fat), 10% to 20% from protein, and the rest from carbohydrate. (The recommendations vary slightly for people whose LDL cholesterol level is high.)

Carbohydrate is the source of energy that most affects your blood sugar levels. Eating a lot of carbohydrate at one time will cause your blood glucose to rise. But most of your energy comes from carbohydrates; your body needs them, so don't try to avoid them. Instead, eat a little bit at a time. When you divide your total calories from carbohydrates into five or six snacks or small meals per day, you may eat as little as 200 calories from carbohydrates each time. Combining each serving of carbohydrate with protein and fat, which have a smaller effect on blood glucose, may slow the digestion and absorption of the carbohydrate, thus lessening the rise in blood glucose caused by the meal. Your dietitian can help you devise a meal plan of small, frequent meals that evenly distribute the carbohydrate, protein, and fat you eat over the day.

When choosing which kinds of carbohydrate-containing foods to include in your meals, remember that while all carbohydrates raise blood glucose, some make better choices. Because foods such as whole grains, fruits, and vegetables contain more vitamins, minerals, and fiber, consider picking them over simple sugars, such as table sugar and honey, and processed carbohydrates, such as white flour.

Check your blood glucose about two hours after meals. High blood sugar levels at that time are harmful and are a sign either that your body is not using its own insulin or that it does not have enough. Many scientists believe that high blood sugar levels after meals are responsible for the complications of diabetes. (For more information about high blood glucose after meals, see the article "High Blood Sugar After Meals" on page 92.) Unless your HbA_{1c} is less than 7%, you should not hesitate to take pills or insulin if recommended by your doctor. Do whatever it takes to keep your blood sugar levels as near to normal as possible after meals and possibly prevent complications.

Physical activity

Adding more physical activity to your life yields immediate results. Because your body burns glucose during exercise, your blood sugar levels will begin to drop soon after beginning a session of increased physical activity. With this in mind, you may want to consider exercising about two hours after a larger meal, when your blood sugar may be higher.

Exercise also lowers blood sugar by decreasing insulin resistance, a common problem in Type 2 diabetes in which cells do not respond properly to insulin. Insulin resistance reduces the amount of glucose that cells can absorb from the bloodstream for energy, even when plenty of insulin is available. An exercise session lowers insulin resistance for about a day, so it is important to be active every day to maintain this benefit. (For more tips on exercise, see the article "Getting Started and Staying Motivated" on page 234.)

If you have never done regular exercise, you should check with your doctor and get an OK before beginning a program. According to the recommendations of the ADA and the American College of Sports Medicine (ACSM), people who have diabetes and are over 35 should have an exercise test before beginning an exercise program. Anyone who has had Type 2 diabetes for 10 years or longer or who has eye, kidney, or nerve problems associated with diabetes should also be tested, as should anyone with peripheral vascular disease or any risk factors for heart disease other than diabetes.

Once you've gotten your doctor's OK to participate in regular physical activity, you may want to work with a certified instructor to develop an exercise program. Certified instructors who have knowledge of diabetes management, such as an ACSM exercise specialist, are the most helpful. To locate an ACSM-certified specialist or instructor, or for additional information on exercise, contact the American College of Sports Medicine at (317) 637-9200; the organization's Web site, www.acsm.org, also offers useful information.

The U.S. Surgeon General's Report on Physical Activity and Health, the ACSM, and the U.S. Centers for Disease Control and Prevention recommend that everyone accumulate at least 30 minutes of moderate physical activity on most days of the week. If you are not currently active, you may need to gradually work up to 30 minutes of moderate activity a day. The best types of activities are those that use the large muscle groups and that last from 20 minutes to an hour or more. These activities include walking, jogging, hik-

MODERATE PHYSICAL ACTIVITY

Here are some examples of moderate-intensity physical activity. The items at the top of the list are less vigorous than the ones at the bottom. Even if you're not up to the length of time listed, keep in mind that any amount of activity can improve your health.

Washing and waxing a car (45–60 minutes)

Washing windows or floors (45–60 minutes)

Playing volleyball (45 minutes)

Playing touch football (30–45 minutes)

Gardening (30–45 minutes)

Wheeling self in wheelchair (30–40 minutes)

Walking (1¾ miles in 35 minutes)

Shooting baskets (30 minutes)

Bicycling (5 miles in 30 minutes)

Social dancing, fast (30 minutes)

Pushing a stroller (1½ miles in 30 minutes)

Raking leaves (30 minutes)

Walking (2 miles in 30 minutes)

Doing water aerobics (30 minutes)

Swimming laps (20 minutes)

Playing wheelchair basketball (20 minutes)

Playing basketball (15–20 minutes)

Bicycling (4 miles in 15 minutes)

Jumping rope (15 minutes)

Running (1½ miles in 15 minutes)

Shoveling snow (15 minutes)

Stair-walking (15 minutes)

Modified from the U.S. Surgeon General's Report on Physical Activity and Health 1996

ing, skating, rowing, cycling, swimming, dancing, and cross-country skiing. (For more examples of moderate activity, see "Moderate Physical Activity" on this page.) In general, activities that are less intense should be done for more time. But any activity will help control your weight and your blood sugar levels.

To prevent injury, it's important to start each exercise session with a warm-up. Begin your aerobic activity at a low intensity to gradually get your muscles warmed up and your heart pumping, then stretch lightly without bouncing. The warm-up should last about 10 minutes.

After exercise, allow for a cool-down period. Gradually slow the pace at the end of your activity. Then stretch your muscles for another 5 to 10 minutes—as when warming up—to allow your body to relax and your heart rate to return gradually to a resting pace.

To keep track of the effect exercise has on your blood sugar, check it right before exercise and about 15 minutes after you stop exercising and notice the difference. If your blood glucose is higher than 300 mg/dl before exercise, you may not have enough insulin available to transport glucose into the cells. Not only does this mean that your cells won't get the energy they need to perform the activity, it means your blood glucose level will go even higher as your liver automatically responds to physical exertion by releasing more glucose into the bloodstream. To find out whether an exercise session will raise or lower your blood glucose, take a brief, slow walk, then check your blood glucose again. As long as light activity lowers your blood glucose, you can proceed with your regular activity.

Exercising too hard for your current level of fitness can also cause a rise in blood sugar after exercise. Slow your pace the next time you exercise, and make sure enough insulin is available by checking your blood glucose before you start.

A person with Type 2 diabetes who does not take diabetes pills or insulin is at no greater risk of hypoglycemia than someone who does not have diabetes. Although your body may show signs of low blood sugar—such as dizziness, rapid heartbeat, cold sweats, blurry vision, headache, or irritability—it normally responds by releasing stored glucose into your bloodstream to bring your blood sugar back up naturally. Still, if your blood sugar is below 100 mg/dl before exercise, eat or drink at least 15 grams of carbohydrate for every 30 minutes of planned exercise. Then wait 15 minutes. Test, and if your blood sugar level is over 100 mg/dl, start exercising. If you experience any symptoms of low blood sugar during exercise, stop and check your level. If it is below 70 mg/dl, eat or drink 15 grams of carbohydrate, then check it again after 15 minutes.

Putting the pieces together

No matter how you manage your diabetes, sticking to your self-care plan is easier when you get the moral and practical support you need from the people around you. You also need support from your diabetes-care team. Regularly scheduled visits with your doctor are necessary to perform recommended checks to make sure that your diabetes is in control and that you have not developed complications. Just as important are periodic visits with your dietitian, who can help you modify your meal plan if you're tired of it or if it's no longer meeting your needs. Your diabetes educator can make sure your self-monitoring technique is up to par and answer questions that arise about controlling your blood sugar. And all of these health-care professionals can provide new information to keep your knowledge of diabetes up to date. ❏

NEW OPTIONS FOR TREATING TYPE 2 DIABETES

by Diane M. Karl, M.D., and Matthew C. Riddle, M.D.

Drug treatment of Type 2 diabetes used to mean either sulfonylurea pills or insulin injections—one or the other. The approach was straightforward: If your diabetes did not respond to a sulfonylurea, you stopped the pills and started taking insulin. Once you started insulin, it was pretty certain you would continue to take it for life. And using insulin and pills together was considered a strange idea. Times have changed. Much as ice cream isn't just vanilla or chocolate anymore, treatments for Type 2 diabetes have multiplied, and combinations of them are routine. Let's look at some of the possibilities.

Stepping up

One of the forces leading us to rethink our tactics for treating Type 2 diabetes is the rapid appearance of several new kinds of drugs, each of them effective for some people and in some situations. These include, besides new sulfonylureas and new insulins, metformin (brand name Glucophage; generic versions were approved for marketing in the United States in 2002), acarbose (Precose), miglitol (Glyset), pioglitazone (Actos), and rosiglitazone (Avandia). Two new oral treatments are repaglinide (Prandin) and nateglinide (Starlix), which resemble the sulfonylureas but have some distinctive features. (For brief descriptions of how the new drugs work, see "Diabetes Pills" on page 90.)

Since all these classes of drugs work in different ways, we can add two (or even more) together to get better results. We also know that the ability of the pancreas to keep up with the body's insulin needs decreases as we get older, so a person with Type 2 diabetes is likely to find it more difficult to control blood sugar over time. Combining oral pills often allows good control of blood glucose to continue and delays the need for insulin injections. A very common combination is a single daily dose of one of the new sulfonylureas, glimepiride (Amaryl) or extended-release glipizide (Glucotrol XL), which stimulate the pancreas to produce more insulin, plus two or three doses of metformin, which reduces blood glucose levels and also helps control food intake and weight.

In many people with Type 2 diabetes insulin will still eventually be needed (that's why Type 2 diabetes is less likely to be called non-insulin-dependent diabetes these days—it's too confusing). To save money and make treatment easier, there is now much interest in finding a safe and effective way of starting insulin outside of a hospital setting. Adding an insulin injection or injections to pills is one such way. This approach has several advantages. The old way consisted of stopping the pills and learning how to handle insulin vials, draw up and inject insulin, increase blood glucose testing, and adjust to the risk of low blood sugar—all at the same time. When oral pills and insulin are overlapped, there's less of a need to learn everything at once. Blood glucose levels will not soar (as they can when the pills are stopped cold) however slowly the doses of insulin are increased, because the oral pills haven't stopped working entirely. They just aren't quite enough to maintain good blood glucose control by themselves any longer. Low doses of insulin, usually in a single injection, are all that's needed to restore control. Adding insulin while continuing oral medicines may be called "step-up" therapy.

Stepping down

There is the possibility of "step-down" therapy as well. In the past, before the new oral medicines became available, many people were started on insulin as soon as treatment with a sulfonylurea alone had failed. Many of them now have quite good control with one or, more often, two injections of insulin. Most of these people will have had diabetes for less than 10 or 15 years. If one or more oral pills are added back to the regimen, even better blood glucose control may be possible, and some people may be able to decrease the number of injections they take to just one. A few may be able to stop insulin entirely while maintaining good blood glucose levels with combinations of oral pills. Of course, since Type 2 diabetes is almost always a gradually progressive condition, it's likely that insulin will become necessary again for most, but they may welcome even a temporary holiday from injections, a "step-down" from insulin to oral pills.

Stepping across

Finally, let's consider the situation of people with Type 2 diabetes who have been taking insulin for some time but are still unable to keep blood sugar levels where they want them. Often their difficulty lies in the fact that injecting insulin corrects only one of the two causes of high blood glucose in Type 2 diabetes, namely, insulin deficiency and insulin resistance. All people with Type 2 diabetes have insulin deficiency. That is, they are less able to make more insulin when the body's needs are greater than someone who has not inherited the tendency to diabetes. But besides this, their muscle and fat tissues may respond less well to insulin than other people's tissues do, reducing their uptake of glucose. Such people are said to have "insulin resistance, " and they often need very large amounts of injected insulin to get blood glucose levels down. Even 150 or 200 units daily may not be enough for some, and large doses like this may increase the tendency to gain weight or have low blood sugar. Adding oral pills to the regimen can help some of these people a lot. Combination therapy may "rescue" them from unsuccessful control with insulin alone. Three medicines sometimes used for this purpose are metformin, pioglitazone, and rosiglitazone. Metformin, as noted before, reduces blood glucose levels and helps control food intake and weight. Pioglitazone and rosiglitazone work directly on muscle and fat to improve the effects of insulin. (Troglitazone [Rezulin], a drug related to pioglitazone and rosiglitazone, was also often used for this purpose but was withdrawn from the market in March 2000 after it was linked to dozens of cases of liver failure, many of them fatal.)

So combination therapy can delay the need to use insulin, make starting insulin easier, permit stopping insulin for a while, and restore good control when insulin alone is ineffective. Before getting to the specifics of how to do this, however, we need to look at two other key issues: our blood glucose targets and the role of lifestyle changes in reaching them.

Benefits of good control

Study after study shows us the importance of blood glucose control in preventing diabetic complications in people with both Type 1 and Type 2 diabetes. The American Diabetes Association (ADA) suggests a goal for morning blood glucose levels of under 120 mg/dl and a goal for glycosylated hemoglobin A_{1c}, or HbA_{1c}, of under 7%. HbA_{1c} is a measure of average blood glucose over time, and the ADA advises that if it goes over 8%, a significant change in treatment should be made. We agree. An elevated HbA_{1c} value should be the signal that tells us to move to the next level of treatment, in a continuous stepwise fashion. We can use this important test to help us know when we need to step up treatment and when we are successful in stepping down.

It's worth remembering that lifestyle changes, specifically significant weight loss and increased physical activity, increase the body's sensitivity to insulin. This increased sensitivity results in a need for less diabetes medicine of any kind—the ability to move down a step. Diabetes in a person who has been taking insulin can then sometimes be controlled without insulin. Not everyone is able to make and maintain big changes in eating and exercise habits, but those who do can see dramatic benefits.

DIABETES PILLS

NONSULFONYLUREAS

GENERIC NAME	BRAND NAME	HOW IT WORKS
Acarbose	Precose	Delays digestion of carbohydrate and glucose absorption; taken before meals to prevent high blood glucose levels after meals.
Metformin	Glucophage	Decreases production of glucose from the liver.
Metformin, extended release	Glucophage XR	Decreases production of glucose from the liver.
Miglitol	Glyset	Delays digestion of carbohydrate and glucose absorption; taken before meals to prevent high blood glucose levels after meals.
Nateglinide	Starlix	Stimulates release of insulin from pancreas; taken with or before meals to prevent high blood glucose levels after meals.
Pioglitazone	Actos	Increases muscle and fat cell sensitivity to insulin, reducing insulin resistance.
Repaglinide	Prandin	Stimulates release of insulin from pancreas; taken with or before meals to prevent high blood glucose levels after meals.
Rosiglitazone	Avandia	Increases muscle and fat cell sensitivity to insulin, reducing insulin resistance.

SULFONYLUREAS

GENERIC NAME	BRAND NAME	HOW IT WORKS
Glimepiride	Amaryl	Stimulates release of insulin from pancreas.
Glipizide	Glucotrol	Stimulates release of insulin from pancreas.
Glipizide, extended release	Glucotrol XL	Stimulates release of insulin from pancreas.
Glyburide	DiaBeta, Glynase, PresTab, Micronase	Stimulates release of insulin from pancreas.

COMBINATION

GENERIC NAME	BRAND NAME	HOW IT WORKS
Metformin plus glyburide	Glucovance	Decreases production of glucose from the liver plus stimulates release of insulin from pancreas.

Also, when a very high blood glucose level is treated successfully, *glucotoxicity* reverses. Glucotoxicity occurs when high blood glucose levels both impair the ability of the pancreas to produce insulin and make insulin resistance worse. When glucotoxicity is reversed through successful treatment, it may then be possible to step down in treatment.

How combination therapy works

With all this in mind, let's look at a few examples of how people with Type 2 diabetes might experience our present combination treatment options.

Helen is in her 60's. She learned she has Type 2 diabetes when she was 50 years old, a typical age for diagnosis. She was given a lifestyle program and at first did very well in keeping her fasting blood sugar levels under 120 mg/dl. About a year later, however, she noticed that the levels were creeping up, and her HbA_{1c} rose above 7%. Her doctor started her on metformin, and her diabetes remained under control again for around four years. When her HbA_{1c} increased to 8% despite renewed efforts at weight loss, a sulfonylurea was added. This, too, worked well for a time. When Helen reached 60 years of age, however, her blood glucose was again over target levels. Her doctor felt it was time for insulin. He decided to continue both of her oral pills at slightly reduced doses while adding insulin once a day, in the evening. He sent Helen to a diabetes nurse educator, who taught her how to inject insulin. The insulin dose was increased slowly until her morning blood glucose level was below 120 mg/dl on her home meter. Her oral medicines continued to work, keeping her blood glucose in a good range for the rest of the day. By the time Helen needs to take two or more injections of insulin to keep her diabetes under good control, she will be very comfortable with how to take her insulin, and the transition will be easier. Helen's story illustrates how step-up therapy usually works.

Frank's experience is somewhat different. His diabetes was discovered when he was 46 years old and went to see his doctor because of extreme thirst and excessive urination. His blood glucose level was 500 mg/dl at the time, and he was hospitalized and started on two injections of insulin a day. He remained in good control of his blood sugar levels on his insulin injections, with an HbA_{1c} of 6.2%, although he did get low blood glucose once or twice a week. He is 5′11″ tall and weighed 240 pounds when he learned he had diabetes. At age 52, by which time he weighed 250 pounds, he asked his doctor if he still needed insulin. His doctor did the following to find out. First, he started Frank on metformin while reducing the insulin dose slightly. When Frank's blood glucose remained in a good range, his doctor increased his metformin and stopped his morning insulin dose. Then, when glucose control remained good, he stopped the evening insulin, but Frank's morning blood glucose jumped up to around 200 mg/dl. A sulfonylurea was added, and good control was restored. Frank was able to step down from insulin therapy because he'd had diabetes for a relatively short time, and also because he probably had glucotoxicity at the time of diagnosis, which was increasing his level of insulin resistance. The best way for Frank to prolong the time before he needs to start using insulin again is to lose weight and begin that exercise program he's been thinking about.

A third patient, Louise, is 58 years old and has had diabetes for 18 years. She started using insulin five years ago after pills no longer controlled her blood glucose. Her insulin dose was gradually increased to 160 units a day, given in three injections. Despite these large doses, her HbA_{1c} was 9.6%, well above the recommended target. Louise, who is 5′4″ tall, has always had problems with her weight, and her sense of failure at being unable to control her diabetes has made trying to diet even harder—185 pounds at the time of diagnosis, she later weighed in at 215. Her weight problem and the fact that large doses of insulin weren't controlling her blood glucose are both signs of insulin resistance, making Louise a good candidate for pioglitazone or rosiglitazone, both of which decrease insulin resistance by making muscle and fat cells more sensitive to insulin. Her doctor kept her on insulin but added pioglitazone to her regimen. He also reminded her to check her blood glucose regularly to watch for a glucose-lowering effect. After two weeks, she started to see blood glucose levels in the 150 mg/dl to 200 mg/dl range, and by four weeks she had some readings of 120 mg/dl. Her doctor then increased her pioglitazone dose and began reducing her insulin gradually. Six months later, Louise had an HbA_{1c} value of 7.1%, and her insulin dose had been reduced to 100 units a day given in two injections. Louise has stepped down in insulin dose and number of injections, but more important, she has significantly improved her blood glucose control.

We think combination therapy for Type 2 diabetes is here to stay. Indeed, a combination of two often used drugs, metformin and glyburide, in a single pill (Glucovance) was introduced in the United States in 2000. How combination therapy applies to you, or to any individual person, depends on several factors: the way diabetes has developed in your body, how long you've had it, your lifestyle, and the treatments you're now using. Ask your physician how the new drugs might be helpful for you now or in the future. Let's take advantage of all these new choices. ❏

HIGH BLOOD SUGAR AFTER MEALS
WHY IT MATTERS

by Robert S. Dinsmoor

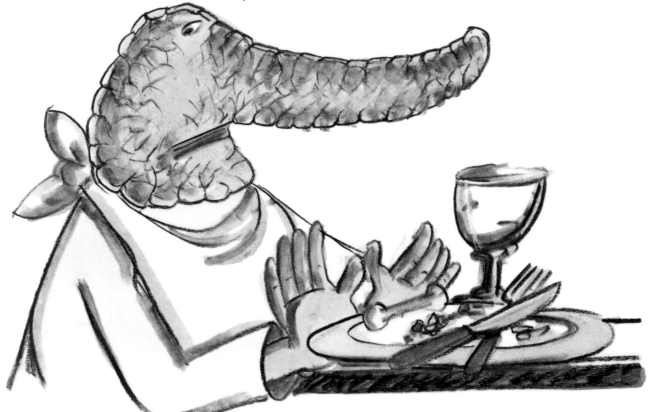

You have Type 2 diabetes and you think you're doing everything right: You eat a balanced diet, you take your medicines when you're supposed to, and you check your blood glucose level dutifully before every meal just like your doctor advised, and it's always under 150 mg/dl. But then you get your hemoglobin A_{1c} (HbA_{1c}) tested, and it's soaring—over 9%. (A desirable HbA_{1c} test result is less than 7%, and anything over 8% is cause for concern.) What's happening? The culprit may be *postprandial hyperglycemia,* or high blood glucose levels following meals.

Postprandial, or after-meal, hyperglycemia can occur even when fasting blood glucose levels—the ones you check before eating—are relatively normal. It can disrupt overall diabetes control (as indicated by a high HbA_{1c} result), and it may significantly increase your risk of heart disease and other diabetic complications. But you can do something about it.

A common problem

To understand why postprandial hyperglycemia is especially common in people with Type 2 diabetes, it helps to understand how the pancreas normally manufactures and secretes insulin, and how that process changes during the early stages of diabetes.

In people who don't have diabetes, the pancreas continually alters its insulin output in response to changes in blood glucose levels. The pancreas secretes a small, steady flow of insulin all the time to allow any glucose in the blood to be used for energy. When a person eats a meal or snack and more glucose enters the bloodstream, the pancreas senses this and secretes more insulin.

Insulin secretion in response to meals occurs in two distinct phases: In the first 10 minutes after glucose enters the bloodstream, there is an early burst of insulin release, the so-called *first-phase* insulin secretion. This is followed by the *second-phase* insulin secretion, a sustained release of insulin that may last for several hours. Researchers believe that the first-phase insulin secretion contains insulin the pancreas has already manufactured and stored in the periphery of the beta cells, the site of insulin formation. They believe the second-phase secretion releases newly formed insulin that the pancreas has just manufactured in response to the blood glucose rise.

Diabetes researchers believe one of the early changes that occurs in the body as Type 2 diabetes develops is loss of the first-phase insulin secretion following a meal. This means that not enough insulin enters the bloodstream as quickly as it is needed, resulting in high blood glucose levels after meals. In some cases, the pancreas compensates by secreting more insulin in the second phase, which can lead to high levels of insulin in the bloodstream. (Eventually, as diabetes progresses, second-phase insulin secretion is reduced, leading to hyperglycemia before meals as well as after.)

Even though postprandial hyperglycemia is common in people with Type 2 diabetes, it often goes undetected, according to Mark Feinglos, M.D., Professor of Medicine at Duke University Medical Center in Durham, North Carolina. Most likely, this oversight is due to the way blood glucose control is typically assessed in people with Type 2 diabetes. Most official guidelines recommend two ways of measuring blood glucose. The first is the HbA_{1c} test, a lab test that indicates a person's average blood glucose control over the preceding two to three months. The other is the fasting, or *prandial*, blood glucose level you check on your meter before meals.

Doctors are beginning to realize, however, that these two tests don't give the whole picture. "Everyone's looking at what blood sugar is doing when it's at the lowest, but nobody looks at the response to a meal," Dr. Feinglos says. "There are some individuals in whom fasting or premeal blood glucose levels look fine, and then you look at their hemoglobin A_{1c} and it's not fine. And then you measure the postprandial blood glucose level and you realize there's a significant problem that no one has been looking at."

Uncovering the problem

It has long been established that high blood glucose levels can increase the risk of microvascular (small-vessel) diabetic complications—diabetic retinopathy, nephropathy, and neuropathy—in people with either Type 1 or Type 2 diabetes. Furthermore, chronic high blood glucose in people with Type 2 diabetes is known to be a risk factor for macrovascular (large-vessel) complications of diabetes such as atherosclerosis, which can lead to heart disease, stroke, and peripheral

vascular disease (narrowing of blood vessels in the legs or arms). Researchers are now starting to put together the specific connection between postprandial hyperglycemia and diabetic complications. Here is some of the evidence:

■ After meals, people with Type 2 diabetes typically experience, along with high blood glucose levels, an increase in blood lipids—especially very-low-density lipoproteins (VLDL's). While a brief rise in lipid levels has no significant effect, VLDL levels that stay high are thought to greatly increase the risk of heart disease.

■ A number of large studies that have involved people with and without diabetes, such as the Paris Prospective Study and the Honolulu Heart Study, have shown that the higher a person's after-meal blood glucose levels, the greater his or her risk of heart disease, heart attack, and early death.

■ Studies of people with Type 2 diabetes have shown that, statistically, after-meal blood sugar levels are a better predictor of heart disease than are fasting blood glucose levels. So someone with high blood sugar levels after meals may be prone to heart disease even if he or she has normal levels before meals.

■ At least one study has shown that in people with Type 2 diabetes, postprandial blood glucose levels are also more closely tied to heart disease risk than are HbA_{1c} test results. This means that someone with a relatively normal or only slightly elevated HbA_{1c} result—but high blood glucose after meals—would be more likely to develop heart disease.

■ The Kumamoto Study, a Japanese study that evaluated the effects of blood glucose control on microvascular complications in people with Type 2 diabetes, showed that postprandial hyperglycemia (blood glucose levels above 180 mg/dl) raised the risk of diabetic retinopathy and diabetic nephropathy.

Treating postprandial hyperglycemia

Traditional therapies for Type 2 diabetes, including diet, sulfonylurea drugs, and insulin, can keep overall blood glucose levels from spiraling out of control, but they don't do a good job of targeting postprandial hyperglycemia in particular. While dietary modifications such as eating smaller meals and increasing fiber intake can slow carbohydrate absorption and contribute to lower blood glucose levels after meals, they often are not enough to adequately control after-meal hyperglycemia.

Neither Regular insulin nor sulfonylureas (which stimulate the pancreas to secrete insulin) really come close to mimicking the first-phase burst of insulin after meals. Molecules of Regular insulin tend to clump together and are slow to break apart in the body. As a result, Regular insulin must be injected 30 to 60 minutes before meals. It peaks too slowly to completely manage the blood glucose elevations following meals, and it stays in the bloodstream longer than is necessary. The effects of sulfonylureas also last well beyond the meal, setting the stage for low blood sugar after all the glucose from the meal has been absorbed.

Several newer drugs do a better job of controlling postprandial hyperglycemia. Let's look at some of the newer options:

Alpha-glucosidase inhibitors. A class of drugs called *alpha-glucosidase inhibitors,* or "starch blockers," block the action of enzymes that break down carbohydrates in the small intestine, thus slowing the absorption of carbohydrate into the bloodstream. This doesn't prevent glucose from entering the bloodstream altogether, but it "flattens out" the blood sugar peak following meals. One alpha-glucosidase inhibitor, acarbose (brand name Precose), has been available for a number of years, and another one, called miglitol (Glyset), became available on the U.S. market in February 1999.

Because of the way acarbose and miglitol work—slowing the digestion of carbohydrates in the small intestine—both often cause bloating, diarrhea, and flatulence. These side effects can be minimized by starting with a small dose and slowly working up to the most effective dose. With both drugs, the unpleasant gastrointestinal effects should diminish with time.

Meglitinides. Drugs in the class called *meglitinides* lower blood sugar by stimulating insulin secretion by the pancreas, but they are different from sulfonylureas, and they work much faster. Currently, two drugs in this class are available in the United States: repaglinide (Prandin), approved by the Food and Drug Administration (FDA) in April 1998, and nateglinide (Starlix), approved by the FDA in December 2000. Although they do not mimic the first-phase insulin response

DIABETES DRUGS

Each class of diabetes drugs works differently, and some are better than others at controlling high blood sugar after meals. Among those that target after-meal blood glucose are drugs in the alpha-glucosidase inhibitor class, rapid-acting insulins, and the meglitinides. If your after-meal blood glucose levels tend to be high, talk to your doctor about whether any of these drugs might help you. Controlling postprandial hyperglycemia depends on finding the diet and drug or combination of drugs that works best for you.

DRUG CLASS	EXAMPLES	HOW IT WORKS
Alpha-glucosidase inhibitors	acarbose (Precose) miglitol (Glyset)	Slows carbohydrate digestion and glucose absorption into the bloodstream by blocking the action of digestive enzymes in the small intestine.
Biguanides	metformin (Glucophage)	Decreases production of glucose from the liver.
Insulin	aspart (Novolog) lispro (Humalog) Regular	Carries glucose into cells to be used for energy or stored as fat.
Meglitinides	nateglinide (Starlix) repaglinide (Prandin)	Stimulates the pancreas to release a quick burst of insulin.
Sulfonylureas	chlorpropamide (Diabenese) glimepiride (Amaryl) glipizide (Glucotrol, Glucotrol XL) glyburide (DiaBeta, Glynase, Micronase)	Stimulates an extended release of insulin by the pancreas.
Thiazolidinediones	pioglitazone (Actos) rosiglitazone (Avandia)	Increases muscle and fat cell sensitivity to insulin, reducing insulin resistance.

exactly, these meglitinides significantly raise insulin levels following meals and lower fasting blood sugar levels, blood sugar levels after meals, and HbA_{1c} levels. Nateglinide works even faster than repaglinide.

Rapid-acting insulin. Until recently, the only insulin used to handle mealtime blood glucose elevations was Regular insulin. However, in August 1996, an even faster-acting insulin, called lispro (Humalog), became available. Unlike Regular insulin, lispro has been chemically modified and dissociates quickly, thus entering the bloodstream and acting sooner. Lispro should be injected within 15 minutes before or immediately after a meal. Because it works more rapidly than Regular, it handles mealtime blood glucose elevations better than Regular. And because it disappears from the system more quickly, it is unlikely to cause hypoglycemia between meals. Another rapid-acting insulin, insulin aspart (Novolog), received FDA approval in June 2000.

Drug combinations. Doctors have traditionally avoided combining insulin and sulfonylureas out of concern that the two together could dramatically and unpredictably raise the levels of insulin in the bloodstream, leading to sudden, severe hypoglycemia. Now there are a number of other drugs that work by different mechanisms, including metformin (Glucophage), rosiglitazone (Avandia), and pioglitazone (Actos). In many instances, they can be combined safely with insulin or with other pills. This has expanded the range of possibilities for combining insulins and oral drugs to create drug regimens that come closer to mimicking natural insulin secretion by the pancreas.

Treatment pays off

Treating postprandial hyperglycemia appears to have far-reaching, positive effects. Dr. Feinglos and his colleagues at Duke University Medical Center looked at the effects of adding mealtime insulin lispro to sulfonylureas in people with Type 2 diabetes whose blood glucose did not stay in target range with sulfonylureas alone. (The study was published in the October 1997 issue of *Diabetes Care*, a journal for medical professionals.) As one might expect, adding insulin lispro lowered their blood glucose levels after meals, and it also lowered their average HbA_{1c} levels. What the researchers didn't expect was that it also lowered their fasting glucose levels. No one knows why treating postprandial hyperglycemia improved fasting blood glucose levels in this study, but Dr. Feinglos speculates that it may have subtly improved insulin secretion or somehow increased the body's sensitivity to insulin. Therapy with insulin lispro also lowered the participants' triglyceride levels and total cholesterol levels and raised their "good" HDL cholesterol levels— changes that would be expected to lower their risk of cardiovascular disease.

An after-dinner hint

If you have been getting unexplained high HbA_{1c} test results despite fasting blood sugar levels in your target range, it may be a good idea to test your blood sugar two hours after meals. If it is high (say, over 160 mg/dl), postprandial hyperglycemia may be the root of your problem, and you should discuss these results with your physician. In addition to indicating that a change in drug regimen may be in order, checking after meals can tell you how different meals (for example, pasta versus hamburgers) affect your blood sugar. Knowing this can guide you in setting carbohydrate consumption goals for each meal so that your diet and drug regimen can work together to help you meet your blood glucose goals. ❏

INSULIN AND INJECTION DEVICES

INJECTING INSULIN 101

by Eve Gehling, M.Ed., R.D., C.D.E.

Does the thought of getting a shot—any kind of shot—sound scary to you? Sometimes flu, tetanus, or novocaine shots can hurt or leave you feeling sore afterward. It's no surprise that the mere sound of the word "needle" or "shot" can make some children and adults cringe.

But what about insulin shots? Do they really compare to tetanus or flu shots? Should the thought of taking shots scare someone with diabetes away from starting insulin therapy? Not at all; insulin shots don't have to be scary or painful.

Injecting insulin can be quite easy if you use the right supplies and develop the right technique. In fact, after learning to inject insulin, people often remark that their fear of taking a shot was worse than the actual shot; poking a finger for a blood glucose check often hurts more. Insulin shots hurt less than other types of shots in part because insulin doesn't need to be injected into a muscle or vein like other drugs; it should be injected into the fatty tissue right beneath the skin. In addition, the needles used for insulin shots are very short and very thin. They even have a silicone coating on them so they slip into the skin easier.

Of course, even insulin shots can be painful or difficult to take if you don't know how to use your equipment correctly. Whether you're new at taking shots or a seasoned veteran, it's a good idea to review your injecting technique from time to time. Without good technique, not only can shots be uncomfortable, but it can also be difficult to attain good diabetes control.

Start with the right supplies

When you start using insulin, your health-care provider should advise you on what supplies to get and how to use them. He or she should also keep you informed of new products you may find helpful. Here are some of the supplies you'll need:

Insulin. Your doctor will tell you what type of insulin to get, how much to take, and when to take it. It's important to get and use the exact type of insulin your doctor prescribes because insulin can vary in strength and speed.

In the United States, insulin is made from pork or is synthesized to be identical to human insulin. Its strength is measured by its concentration. The most common strength is 100 units of insulin per milliliter; it is known as U-100 insulin. On occasion, people who need to take very large or tiny doses of insulin may be advised to use other strengths (such as U-500 or U-10).

Insulin comes in four different speeds: rapid-acting, short-acting, intermediate-acting, and long-acting. The faster-acting insulins begin lowering blood glucose more quickly after injection than the slower-acting insulins, and they continue working for a shorter amount of time. Some insulins last for only two hours, while others can last for an entire day.

Syringes. When choosing a syringe, there are four things to consider: which insulin concentration it's designed for, its capacity, the needle gauge (or thickness), and the needle length. Always choose a syringe that's designed for the insulin strength that you use. For example, if you use U-100 insulin, use U-100 syringes; otherwise, you will inject the wrong amount of insulin. Common syringe capacities are $\frac{3}{10}$-cubic centimeter (cc), $\frac{1}{2}$-cc, and 1-cc. The small, $\frac{3}{10}$-cc syringe is designed for people who take less than 30 units of insulin per dose. The $\frac{1}{2}$-cc syringe works best for doses of 25 to 50 units, and the larger, 1-cc syringe holds doses up to 100 units of insulin. Choose the smallest syringe barrel that can hold the total insulin dose you need to take. This will make reading the unit increments on the syringe barrel easier.

Needle gauges range between 27 and 31. The higher the gauge, the thinner the needle. Pick a needle gauge that feels most comfortable for you. Needles also come in different lengths, such as $\frac{5}{16}$ inch and $\frac{1}{2}$ inch. Some insulin pen needles are as short as $\frac{1}{3}$ inch. The needles are short to help prevent insulin injections from going in too deeply. Ask your doctor which length needle he or she recommends for you.

Cleansers. To minimize the risk of infection, you'll need to make sure your hands and the site where you will inject the insulin are clean before taking your shot. For this, you'll need soap and water for your hands and rubbing alcohol and cotton balls (or alcohol swabs) for your injection site.

Other tools. For people who don't want to use a syringe, there are a number of alternative insulin-injecting devices. People who need to take insulin at work, school, or when traveling may want to use an insulin pen. Each pen is about the size of a Magic Marker, contains a small cartridge of insulin, and uses a disposable needle. Pens are available in different types and styles and are easy to carry in a purse or pocket. (For a description of pens sold in the United States, see "Insulin Pens" on page 102.)

Another way to take insulin without a syringe is to use an insulin pump. About the size of a pager, a pump delivers a continuous supply of insulin through a small tube and a needle, which is usually inserted into a person's abdomen. Pumps work well for people who take multiple doses of insulin each day.

Yet another option is a spray injector, which uses high pressure to "spray" insulin in a fine stream through a person's skin without a needle.

Preparing an injection

Although alternatives exist, injecting with a syringe is a fundamental skill in insulin management. Even people who use an insulin pump, insulin pens, or a spray injector may occasionally need to inject with a syringe. Knowing how to use a syringe carefully and consistently can prevent costly mistakes such as incorrect doses, damaged needles, and wasted insulin. Here's how it's done:

■ Gather your supplies.

■ Wash and dry your hands using soap and water.

■ Inspect your insulin. Check its appearance and its expiration date. Rapid-acting insulins (lispro [Humalog] and aspart [Novolog]) and short-acting insulin (Regular) should be clear and colorless like water. All longer-acting insulins (NPH, Lente, Ultralente, and glargine [Lantus]) should have a cloudy, milky, or marbled look. If your insulin is past its expiration date, has clumps or crystals in it, or looks discolored, frosted, or thick, do not use it. Get a new bottle.

■ Clean the top of the insulin bottle with an alcohol swab. If you're using a new bottle of insulin, remove the protective cap from the bottle. Do not remove the rubber stopper or metal band under the cap. The rubber stopper keeps the insulin bottle sealed between uses.

■ Mix the insulin. If you use a longer-acting insulin, gently roll the bottle between your hands or tip the bottle at least 10 times. Rolling the bottle between your hands also warms the insulin, which can make the injection more comfortable. Never shake a bottle vigorously, because shaking can make bubbles in the insulin.

■ Prepare your syringe. Remove the cap from the needle carefully so that it does not get damaged or dirty by touching something. Pull the plunger to draw air into the syringe. The amount of air you draw in should equal the amount of insulin you need to take.

■ Inject air into the bottle. Insert the needle through the rubber stopper on the insulin bottle. Push the syringe plunger to inject all of the air into the bottle.

■ Draw up the insulin. Turn the bottle upside down (with the syringe still inserted) holding it with one hand. Make sure the tip of the needle is well covered by insulin inside the bottle. If it's not, switch to a new bottle. With your other hand, slowly pull back on the plunger to draw the correct dose of insulin into the syringe.

■ Look for air bubbles in the syringe. Without removing the needle from the bottle or changing the position of the syringe or bottle (they should still be upside down and vertical), hold the syringe at eye level. If you see any air bubbles, tap the side of the barrel a few times with your finger to allow the bubbles to float to the top of the syringe. Gently push the plunger to inject the air bubbles back into the insulin bottle. Pull back again on the plunger to redraw your dose of insulin. Repeat this step as needed if you see more bubbles in the syringe.

■ Remove the needle from the bottle.

■ Double-check your dose by looking to see that the end of the plunger is in line with the mark for your dose. The syringe is now loaded and ready to use.

Preparing a mixed injection

If your doctor recommends you take two different insulins at the same time, you may have to take two separate shots, or you may be able to mix the insulins in the same syringe so you only have to take one shot. Consult your doctor and the insulin vial insert before mixing, because not all insulins can be mixed. If you mix two different insulins in one syringe, always draw up the fast-acting insulin first and the slow-acting one second. If the bottle of fast-acting insulin, such as Regular, were to get contaminated with slow-acting insulin, such as NPH, the insulin might not work as quickly as it usually does.

The first several steps for preparing a mixed injection are similar to those for preparing a single dose:

■ Gather your supplies.

■ Wash your hands.

■ Clean the tops of the insulin bottles.

■ Mix the longer-acting insulin.

■ Prepare your syringe.

■ Inject air into the bottle of longer-acting (cloudy) insulin. Holding the syringe in one hand, pull back on the plunger to draw air into the syringe equal to the amount of longer-acting insulin, in units, you need to take. Hold the longer-acting insulin bottle upright and insert the syringe needle downward through the rubber stopper on the bottle. Push the syringe plunger to inject all the air into the bottle.

■ Remove the syringe from the bottle without drawing up any insulin.

■ Inject air into the bottle of fast-acting insulin. Draw air into the syringe again, this time in an amount equal to the dose of fast-acting insulin you need to take, in units. Insert the syringe needle through the rubber stopper on the fast-acting insulin bottle. Push the syringe plunger forward to inject all the air into the bottle.

■ Draw up your fast-acting insulin first. Turn the bottle (with the syringe inserted) upside down, holding it with one hand. Make sure the tip of the needle is covered by insulin inside the bottle. With your other hand, slowly pull back on the plunger to draw up your fast-acting insulin dose.

■ Look for air bubbles in the syringe. Hold the syringe, which should still be in the bottle, straight up at eye level. If you see any air bubbles, tap the side of the barrel so that the bubbles can float up to the top of the syringe. Gently push the plunger to move the bubbles back into the insulin bottle. Then, redraw your correct insulin dose by pulling back on the plunger again.

■ Remove the needle from the bottle.

■ Draw up your longer-acting insulin second. Insert the needle into the longer-acting insulin bottle. Turn the bottle and syringe upside down. Jiggle the bottle gently to allow any air bubbles in the insulin to rise to the top of the bottle. Make sure the tip of the needle is in insulin. Pull back on the syringe plunger until the amount of insulin in the syringe is equal to the sum of the fast-acting and long-acting insulin doses.

■ Remove the needle from the bottle and double-check your dose. The syringe is now loaded and ready to use.

Preparing an insulin pen

Some insulin pens have removable insulin cartridges; others are prefilled with insulin and are disposable. It's important to read the instructions that come with your pen to learn how to dial in your dose and use its other features. To get you started, though, here are some basic steps to follow when using a pen:

■ Gather your supplies.

■ Wash your hands.

■ Prepare your pen. Remove the pen cap. Check the insulin to verify that it's the type your doctor prescribed, that it hasn't expired, and that it's not discolored, frosted, or lumpy. If the insulin looks wrong, do not use it. Use a new insulin cartridge or a new disposable pen.

■ Attach a needle to your pen. Follow the directions that come with your pen for attaching a needle. Leaving the needles attached between shots is not recommended because it can allow air to come into the needle or insulin to leak out.

■ Mix the insulin well. Roll the insulin pen between the palms of your hands or tip it back and forth at least 20 times to mix the insulin.

■ Prime your pen. To ensure your pen is working, do a trial "air shot" before injecting insulin into yourself. Dial the pen to deliver two or three units of insulin. Hold the pen like a pencil, with the needle pointing up. Tap the barrel of the pen to let any air bubbles in the insulin cartridge float to the top of the cartridge. Push down firmly on the pen's injector button to "shoot" insulin into the air. If the pen is working, you should see a couple of drops of insulin come out of the needle. If nothing comes out, try doing another air shot. If insulin still doesn't come out of the needle, your pen may be low on insulin, or the needle may not be connected properly. Refer to the directions that come with your pen for troubleshooting tips.

■ Set your dose. Dial the pen to deliver the amount of insulin you need to take. You should hear clicking as you turn the dial. Your pen is now loaded and ready to use.

Injecting insulin

Once your syringe or insulin pen is loaded, you're ready to inject the insulin. Here's how:

■ Choose an injection site. The most common sites to inject are in the abdomen, upper arms, thighs, and buttocks. Don't pick a site that is near a mole or scar or that is within two inches of your navel.

■ Make sure the site is clean. If the skin where you'll be injecting insulin is dirty, clean the area with soap and water or an alcohol swab. Let it dry.

■ Gently pinch up a fold of skin surrounding the site you've selected. Hold it firmly with one hand.

■ Insert the needle. Holding the syringe or pen like a pencil, insert the syringe or insulin pen needle straight into the pinched-up skin, that is, at a 90° angle. (A 90° angle is the standard recommendation, but some thin adults or children may find it helpful to inject at a 45° angle.) Make sure the needle gets all the way into the fatty tissue below the skin, but not so deep that it hits the muscle below.

■ Inject the insulin. Push the syringe plunger all the way in with a slow steady motion or firmly press the insulin pen injection button. The injection should take a couple of seconds, unless you take a very small dose. Let go of the skin.

■ Remove the needle. Pull the needle straight out. You may gently press on the injection site with your finger for a couple seconds. Do not rub or massage

A PICTURE IS WORTH...

Learning to inject insulin is easier when you can watch it being done. In lieu of a live demonstration, a few of the steps are illustrated below. It can also be helpful to have a diabetes educator observe your injection technique periodically.

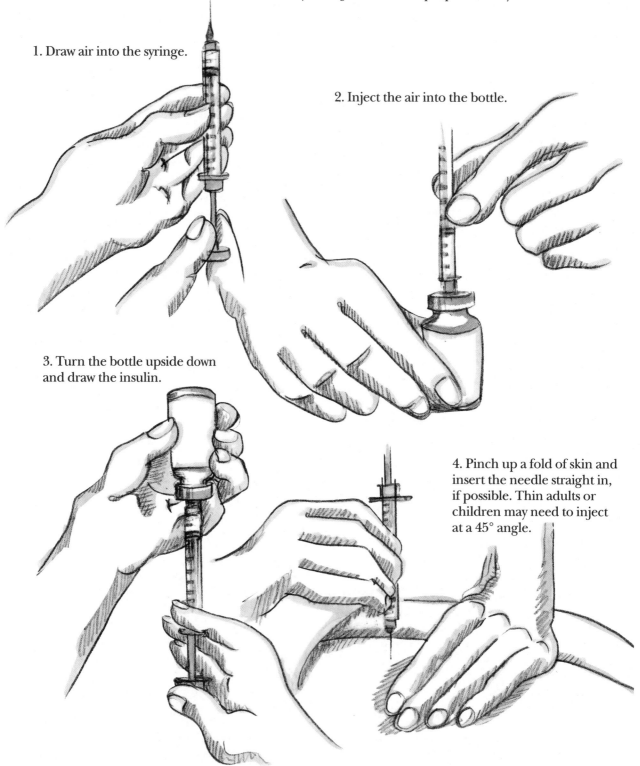

1. Draw air into the syringe.

2. Inject the air into the bottle.

3. Turn the bottle upside down and draw the insulin.

4. Pinch up a fold of skin and insert the needle straight in, if possible. Thin adults or children may need to inject at a 45° angle.

the skin where the insulin is injected; it can affect how fast the insulin is absorbed and acts within the body.

Site rotation

While it may be tempting to inject into the same spot all of the time, doing so can cause the skin to become thick and hard (a condition called hypertrophy) or pitted and dented (a condition called lipoatrophy). When skin tissue becomes damaged in these ways, insulin injected at these sites may not be absorbed consistently by the body, and that can make it harder for you to control your blood glucose levels.

To keep skin healthy, it's important to establish a pattern for picking different sites within an injection area, such as the abdomen. For example, you might mentally divide your injection area into a grid of columns and rows. Move across or down the grid, picking new injection sites that are at least a finger's width away from where you last injected.

Sharps disposal

The last step to injecting insulin is to properly dispose of any used needles and syringes. Besides being the tidy thing to do, it prevents needle-stick injuries.

Don't throw syringes into garbage cans where someone else could accidentally get poked. Instead, put your used syringes in a puncture-resistant container with a tight-fitting lid. You can purchase storage containers from a drugstore or create your own using a plastic laundry soap or bleach bottle. Before throwing the bottle out, fasten the lid securely with strong tape and write "do not recycle" on the bottle. Some counties require all used syringes, needles, and lancets to be destroyed. Be sure to check with your local waste authority to learn what rules apply where you live.

When you travel, you may want to take further steps to reduce the chance of someone else reusing your syringes or incurring a needle-stick injury. To stop someone else from reusing a syringe, you can remove the plunger from the syringe and bend or break it in half. If you see a sharps-receptacle discreetly hanging on a wall in a public or hotel restroom, use it to dispose of your supplies. Otherwise, consider taking your used syringes and needles home where you know you can safely dispose of them. To store small numbers of used syringes, use an empty, plastic 20-ounce soda or water bottle. Empty 35-millimeter film canisters work great to store used needles and lancets.

If there's any chance that someone could get accidentally stuck by your needles, use a needle-clipping device that snips off and stores used needles. Your drugstore should sell one. Don't try to cut the needle off with scissors; doing so can cause a needle to go flying off or fall and get lost.

Frequently asked questions

As you encounter new situations and become more familiar with injecting, you may have more questions about how to do it. Even people who've been injecting insulin for years sometimes have questions. Some of the most common questions are answered below. If you have a question that is not answered here, ask your diabetes educator, who can help you review your injection technique periodically.

Is it safe to reuse syringes?
Disposable syringes are designed to be used once so they remain sterile, straight, and sharp. However some people prefer to reuse their syringes. While this may make financial sense, it can make injections progressively less comfortable. With each use, the needles become duller, and the tip becomes slightly bent.

If you reuse syringes, discuss it with your health-care provider to make sure you know how to do it safely. After each use, carefully recap the needle, and don't reuse the syringe if the needle gets bent or comes into contact with an unclean surface. Don't clean the needle with alcohol between uses; doing so can remove the silicone coating that helps it slide easily into the skin.

Is it OK to fill syringes ahead of time?
In some instances, yes. If you have trouble seeing or are unable to draw up your own insulin, your doctor may advise you to have someone else—a family member or home health nurse—help you prefill your syringes. However, because some insulins mix together better than others, ask your doctor if it's OK to mix your insulin ahead of time. Buying premixed insulin is also an option.

Prefilled syringes should be kept refrigerated with the needles pointing up until they're needed. This reduces the chance of any crystals forming inside the needle, which could plug it up. Discuss with your doctor or diabetes educator how long it's safe to store prefilled syringes, so you prepare only as many as you need for any given time. Before injecting a prefilled syringe, gently turn the syringe back and forth in your hand to remix and warm up the insulin.

How do people inject insulin when dining out?
When dining out or traveling away from home, you may sometimes need to inject insulin in a public place. If your companions know about your diabetes, you may feel comfortable giving yourself an injection in the abdomen or thigh at a restaurant table. To do so, lift up the bottom of your shirt or sweater or raise the hem of your shorts or dress to expose your injection site. Some people inject through a single, thin layer of clothing, and studies have found that this practice does not increase the risk of infection. If you inject quickly, the people around you will most likely

be too busy to notice what you're doing. If you feel more comfortable injecting in private, look for a restroom or quiet place nearby you can go to.

What should I do if clear fluid or blood leaks out of my injection site?

Clear fluid or blood leaking out of an injection site after you remove the needle is not something to get alarmed about. The clear fluid is insulin, and when it leaks out, it's often because the needle wasn't inserted all the way into the skin or because it was removed too quickly. To solve this, count to five before removing the needle from your skin after an injection. If you use an insulin pen or take large doses of insulin, you may want to count to 10 to give the insulin a little longer to disperse under the skin. If some leaks out, put a finger over the injection site and apply gentle pressure for five to eight seconds to stop the leak. If quite a bit of insulin leaks out, check your blood glucose level a few hours later to see if you got enough insulin to control your diabetes.

INSULIN PENS

Many people prefer insulin pens over syringes because of their ease of use and penlike appearance. Pens come in two types: disposable (or prefilled) and nondisposable. Disposable pens, as the name suggests, come already filled with a set amount of insulin; once you have used up the insulin, you throw the pen away. With a nondisposable pen, you generally replace the insulin cartridge when it is empty. Both types of pens require a pen needle, which is screwed onto the tip of the pen before injection. Pen needles come in various lengths and thicknesses.

The following is a list of insulin pens currently for sale in the United States.

AUTOPEN
OWEN MUMFORD, INC.
(800) 421-6936
Autopen AN 3000: Nondisposable. Delivers up to 32 units of insulin in 2-unit increments.
Autopen AN 3100: Nondisposable. Delivers up to 16 units of insulin in 1-unit increments.
Autopen AN 3800: Nondisposable. Delivers up to 42 units of insulin in 2-unit increments.
Autopen AN 3810: Nondisposable. Delivers up to 21 units of insulin in 1-unit increments.

Both the AN 3000 and the AN 3100 can accept any Eli Lilly or Novo Nordisk 150-unit insulin cartridge. The AN 3800 and the AN 3810 accept 300-unit cartridges.

B-D PENS
BECTON, DICKINSON AND COMPANY
(800) 237-4554
B-D Pen: Nondisposable. Delivers up to 30 units of insulin in 1-unit increments.
B-D Pen Mini: Nondisposable. Delivers up to 15 units in ½-unit increments.

Both pens can accept Eli Lilly or Novo Nordisk 150-unit cartridges.

DISETRONIC PEN
DISETRONIC MEDICAL SYSTEMS
(800) 280-7801
Disetronic Pen: Delivers up to 80 units of insulin in 1-unit increments. Has a refillable cartridge that holds 315 units of any type of insulin.

ELI LILLY PENS
ELI LILLY AND COMPANY
(800) 545-5979
All Eli Lilly pens are prefilled with 300 units of insulin, delivered in 1-unit increments. There are four varieties:
Humalog Pen: Contains lispro insulin.
Humalog Mix 75/25 Pen: Contains 25% lispro and 75% longer-acting insulin.
Humulin 70/30 Pen: Contains 70/30 insulin.
Humulin N Pen: Contains NPH insulin.

Eli Lilly also makes cartridges for use with nondisposable pens that are produced by other companies. These cartridges have a capacity of 150 units and contain either lispro, Regular, NPH, or 70/30 insulin.

NOVO NORDISK PENS
NOVO NORDISK PHARMACEUTICALS
(800) 727-6500
NovoPen 1.5: Delivers up to 40 units in 1-unit increments.
NovoPen 3: Delivers from 2 to 70 units in 1-unit increments.
Novolin Prefilled Pen: Can deliver up to 58 units in 2-unit increments. Available filled with Regular, NPH, or 70/30 insulin.

Novo Nordisk also manufactures cartridges for use with nondisposable pens. They come with Regular, NPH, or 70/30 insulin in 150-unit and 300-unit sizes.

If a drop or two of blood leaks out of an injection site, don't worry. You probably just hit a tiny blood vessel beneath the skin. However, if this happens frequently, ask your diabetes health educator to review your injection technique.

Sometimes when I inject insulin I feel a burning sensation. What can I do to minimize this?

Burning or pain when you inject could be caused by a number of things, including the following:

■ A skin cleanser. If you use alcohol to clean your injection site and you inject your insulin before the alcohol dries completely, the shot could sting a little bit.

■ Cold insulin. If you're using refrigerated insulin, let it warm up to room temperature before using it. If you can't wait, gently roll the syringe or bottle between your hands to warm the insulin up (and mix it at the same time) before injecting it.

■ Reused needles that have dull or bent tips. This can be avoided by using a new needle each time you take insulin.

■ Injecting technique. If you inject the needle too slowly or move the needle around under the skin after it's inserted, it can cause the injection site to feel sore or bruised.

■ Tense muscles. To relax the muscles in the area you'll be injecting, take several deep breaths while you concentrate on relaxing, and exhale as you insert the needle.

I'm scared of needles. Is there any other way I can take insulin?

There are a number of ways to inject insulin using special tools or devices. You may want to try an automatic injector, which is available at most drugstores. It hides the entire syringe from view. All you have to do to inject your insulin is hold the device next to your skin and push a button, which inserts the needle effortlessly into your skin. You could also try an insulin spray injector, which doesn't use any needles. In the future, more options will exist.

If I accidentally inject an air bubble or two when I take my insulin shot, will it harm me?

Although injecting a bubble or two of air isn't dangerous, it does mean that you won't be getting your full dose of insulin. This could cause your blood glucose levels to run high later in the day. If this happens often, it can make controlling your diabetes difficult.

My eyesight isn't the best. What can I do to see the lines on a syringe better?

There are a number of ways to make injecting insulin easier for people with low vision:

■ First, make sure there is good lighting where you take your injections. If the lighting is dim, it will be hard to read the syringe.

■ If you're having difficulty seeing the numbers on the syringe, try using a syringe magnifier.

■ To see how much insulin you've drawn more easily, try using a syringe that has a different colored plunger than the lines on the syringe barrel.

■ If the aforementioned measures aren't enough, try using a preset dose gauge that can help you measure the space between the end of the syringe barrel and the plunger.

■ Try using a variable-dose insulin measurement tool or an insulin pen. They indicate units with clicks that are either felt or heard.

■ If you can't tell which insulin bottle is which, identify different bottles using textured tape, a rubber band, or some other marker.

For more information about insulin management tools that can help people with impaired vision, ask your diabetes educator.

It's hard for me to hold a syringe steady because I have arthritis. What can I do to make injecting insulin easier?

If you have difficulty drawing up insulin or holding a syringe steady, you may want to try an automatic injector or insulin pen. Another idea would be to experiment using needle guides and insulin bottle stabilizers that help you hold the bottle correctly and withdraw a specific preset insulin dose. If you're drawing up insulin into a syringe, hold the syringe against a straight wall to make reading the syringe numbers easier at eye level.

Staying sharp

If you follow these steps to injecting insulin, you'll quickly find that with practice, it can be pretty easy. But don't rush through it once you've become comfortable with the procedure. It's too easy to make a mistake. Perform each step carefully every time you inject. To ensure that you maintain good technique, review these steps periodically with a diabetes educator. ❑

ALL ABOUT LISPRO
A New Kid on the Block
by Susan L. Barlow, R.D., C.D.E.

W hen it went on sale in August 1996, lispro (brand name Humalog) was the first new insulin product introduced to the diabetes marketplace in more than a decade. It was also the first in a whole new category of insulins, the analogs. And it initiated an entirely new class of insulins, known as rapid-acting insulins.

By 1998, sales of lispro comprised about one-third of the total short-acting and rapid-acting insulin market. Now that lispro is being used by hundreds of thousands of people with diabetes, it is timely to explore how it affects management of the condition.

Lispro is a human insulin analog (which is where the name Humalog comes from). That is, lispro has the same functions as human insulin without having exactly the same chemical structure. The objective behind its development was to find an insulin that would start lowering blood glucose levels faster than Regular human insulin, reach peak effectiveness sooner, and stay in the body for a shorter time, in other words, an insulin that would more closely simulate the body's own response to a meal. Lispro is almost identical to the human insulin produced within the body. The difference is that the order of two amino acids is reversed on one of the two protein chains that make up insulin, from proline and lysine to lysine and proline (giving rise to the generic name, lispro). It is this reversal that makes lispro act faster than other insulins.

Let's spend some time examining how insulin produced naturally by the body works, how lispro mimics this, and what advantages lispro might offer to a person with diabetes.

About insulin

Insulin's primary function is to regulate blood sugar, or blood glucose, levels so that they're neither too high nor too low. Insulin stimulates muscles and other tissues to transport glucose and amino acids into cells, promoting growth and preventing protein breakdown. In the liver, insulin promotes the uptake and storage of glucose and inhibits new glucose formation. It also helps convert excess glucose into fat.

In people who do not have diabetes, the insulin-producing cells in the pancreas release small amounts of insulin throughout the day, a process known as *basal secretion*. This low level of insulin secretion balances the sugar that the liver makes during periods of fasting (overnight and between meals), thus helping to maintain normal blood sugar levels.

In people with diabetes who inject insulin, longer-acting insulins, such as Lente, NPH, or Ultralente, serve as basal insulins. They are not ideal, though, since most tend to have an extended peak action time and duration, which can cause problems with delayed low blood sugar due to individual variation in absorption. In short, the longer-acting the insulin, the less predictable its action time from person to person and from injection to injection in the same person. The table "Insulin Action Times" on page 106 shows the different types of insulins, their approximate onset (how long it takes until they start lowering blood glucose), peaks (the time during which they are most effective), and duration of action (total time during which they lower blood glucose).

When food is eaten, blood glucose levels rise. In people who do not have diabetes, the pancreas acts to control the rising levels by quickly releasing an appropriate amount of insulin (called a *bolus* of insulin). Once the food has been completely absorbed, the insulin secretion returns to the lower, basal rate. In people with diabetes, blood glucose levels after meals have been controlled primarily with Regular insulin. Unfortunately, its effects are delayed for 30 to 60 minutes or so after an injection, because the drug must be absorbed through tissue under the skin and into the bloodstream to work. This means Regular insulin must be taken 30 to 45 minutes before a meal or snack so it will be peaking at the same time as blood glucose levels are peaking. Another drawback is that Regular insulin stays in the bloodstream for several hours. So there is still a tapering amount of Regular insulin at work in the body after the food has been digested and absorbed.

Ideally, insulin therapy should closely mimic the normal basal and food-stimulated (bolus) release of insulin. Enter...lispro—at least for the latter. Lispro starts working more quickly than Regular insulin and does not keep on lowering blood glucose for as long. Its effects more closely resemble those of insulin naturally secreted from the pancreas in response to food.

Benefits of lispro

So what implications does lispro have for the person with diabetes currently using Regular insulin? There are several, including increased lifestyle flexibility, mealtime convenience, lower blood glucose levels after meals, fewer episodes of low blood glucose during the night, and a more consistent and predictable insulin response. Let's examine each one of these in a little more detail.

There is no doubt that lispro increases the potential for lifestyle flexibility. Studies have shown increased satisfaction with insulin treatment among people using lispro. The ability to "dose and eat" allows more spontaneity. It is easier to deal with delays in restaurant service, flight delays and changes in airports, and erratic schedules. Lispro grants the flexibility of skipping meals, too: If a meal is skipped, the dose of lispro is simply skipped until food is eaten. (Of course, this only works if lispro is combined with an appropriate type and dose of a basal insulin). Because it does not stay in the bloodstream for a long time, lispro also decreases the potential for delayed low blood glucose levels, an unwelcome surprise for any person with diabetes.

Mealtime convenience is a high priority for people with diabetes. When instructed on the use of Regular insulin, most people with diabetes are taught by their diabetes educator to inject 30 to 45 minutes prior to a meal. There are several problems with this. If you are in a crowded restaurant and your reservation or service is delayed, your blood glucose can drop too low before food arrives. For children and toddlers who may be picky eaters, an injection of insulin can lead to a severe case of low blood glucose if their appetites or attitudes don't match the amount of insulin that has been injected.

According to a survey done by the International Diabetes Center in Minneapolis, more than 40% of those surveyed who'd had diabetes for one year to 55 years did not comply with the 30- to 45-minute time delay recommended between Regular insulin administration and food consumption. In studies conducted by Eli Lilly and Company, lispro's developer, the statis-

tics were even worse. The company found that nearly 70% of people timed their dose of Regular insulin incorrectly, taking their injection less than 20 minutes before a meal. With lispro, the timing issue is virtually eliminated.

Given the action times of Regular insulin, shortening the interval between injection and meal consumption will affect a person's blood glucose response (and, thus, blood glucose control) after a meal. In clinical trials involving people with Type 2 diabetes, 722 participants taking Regular insulin had an average blood glucose level of 250 mg/dl two hours after a meal. The American Diabetes Association's target range for blood glucose levels two hours after a meal is between 100 mg/dl and 180 mg/dl. In another study, the blood glucose levels of people with Type 2 diabetes using lispro were 30% lower one hour after a test meal, and 53% lower two hours after, compared with Regular insulin therapy. In a third study, people with Type 1 diabetes who used lispro had an average blood glucose level of about 120 mg/dl two hours after eating a carbohydrate-rich meal, compared to 180 mg/dl with Regular insulin.

Perhaps one of the scariest and most dangerous aspects of diabetes management, no matter what your age or therapy, is the threat of low blood glucose during the night, while you're sleeping. In a study by Lilly with over 1,000 participants, people with Type 1 diabetes treated with lispro before dinner had fewer episodes of low blood glucose between midnight and 6:00 AM when compared to those treated with Regular human insulin. The study demonstrated a 30-day rate of low blood sugar that was statistically significantly less in the lispro-treated group.

What about predictability and consistency of response? As the action times table shows, the longer-acting the insulin, the more extended the time range, or time–action curve, of onset, peak, and duration. It has long been established that the more extended the time–action curve of an insulin, the less predictable the response. This means that the ability to predict when the insulin might peak is lessened, which can lead to unexpected highs and lows in blood glucose. Another problem with traditional insulin such as Regular is that the larger the dose, the longer the time–action curve. This elongation of the insulin action, based on dose only, makes this short-acting insulin behave more like NPH or Lente. Lispro, however, whatever the dose, responds within the same time range. Thus, predictability is greater, making diabetes management less of an art and more of a science.

You may be wondering about the overall effect of lispro on such things as weight and long-term glucose control (as measured by glycosylated hemoglobin A_{1c}, or HbA_{1c}). Analysis of combined data from several studies in people with Type 1 or Type 2 diabetes showed no statistical difference in weight gain between those treated with lispro and those treated with Regular human insulin. The reduced need for snacks in people using lispro as their mealtime insulin may contribute to less weight gain, since they may not be treating low blood sugar as frequently. As for HbA_{1c}, long-term blood glucose control (over a period of one year) tended to be only slightly better in people using lispro (and it was not considered statistically significant).

Remember that HbA_{1c} levels are contingent on control of both premeal as well as postmeal blood glucose levels. Lispro is designed to affect blood glucose control after meals and, thus, is only one component in overall therapy, along with an appropriate basal insulin, proper nutrition, and self-monitoring of blood glucose. (If you use an insulin pump, of course, you won't use the longer-acting insulins, only Regular or a rapid-acting insulin like lispro.)

Is it right for you?

So, now that you know the features and benefits of lispro, how do you know if it is right for you? There are several questions to ask yourself, in consultation with your health-care provider or diabetes educator.
1. Are you currently using Regular insulin?
2. Do you have an unpredictable schedule or a busy lifestyle?
3. Do you eat out often?
4. Do you want greater convenience and flexibility when it comes to managing your diabetes at mealtimes?
5. Are you interested in upgrading your therapy or are you already on an intensive treatment regimen (multiple daily injections or insulin pump therapy)?
6. Do you experience variability in your insulin action depending on where you inject (site) and how much you inject (dose administered)?
7. Do you have gastroparesis (a condition of delayed stomach emptying which is one of the long-term complications of diabetes)?
8. Are you a picky eater or do you have an erratic eating schedule?
9. Are you able to consistently wait 30 to 45 minutes after injecting Regular before eating?
10. Are your after-meal blood glucose readings in the range of 100 mg/dl to 180 mg/dl?
11. Have you been free of low blood sugar episodes since your last visit to your health-care provider?

If you answered "yes" to Questions 1 through 8, but "no" to Questions 9 through 11, you might be a candidate for lispro. Discuss the potential application of a rapid-acting insulin like lispro in your treatment regimen with your health-care professional.

Obviously, lispro may not be for everyone. If your diabetes is already well controlled, there may be no reason to change therapy. And lispro is not a panacea

INSULIN ACTION TIMES

Different types of insulin take different amounts of time to begin working, to reach peak effectiveness, and to leave the body. Only approximate ranges are given here; in practice, action speeds will vary from person to person.

Insulin type	Onset (hours)	Peak (hours)	Duration (hours)
REGULAR	½–1	2½–5	4–12
NPH	1–3	4–12	up to 24
LENTE	2–4	7–15	up to 24
50% NPH 50% REGULAR	½–1	2–12	12–18+
70% NPH 30% REGULAR	½–1	2–12	up to 24
ULTRALENTE	4–10	6–16	24+
GLARGINE	1–2	virtually none	24
LISPRO	up to ¼	½–1½	up to 5
ASPART	up to ¼	½–1½	up to 5

for diabetes control. Unless you use a pump, it is strictly a mealtime insulin and still needs to be combined with an appropriate type and dose of a basal insulin. Those who are unwilling to take more injections per day also may not benefit from a switch to lispro. People who like to graze all day or eat several smaller meals would have to take more injections, so this type of eater may not be the ideal candidate for lispro either.

Why would a person with diabetes elect to use lispro? The convenience and flexibility it offers for mealtimes, contributing to a more spontaneous lifestyle, is probably the reason most people switch. Improved control of blood glucose, not in the form of long-term control as measured by HbA_{1c}, but in the reduction of daily episodes of low blood glucose and high blood glucose, is another major advantage of lispro over Regular human insulin. Then there are many people with diabetes who are simply eager to upgrade their therapy and try new technologies and advances for improved diabetes management. Finally, diabetes is a progressive disease that warrants options in treatments to keep blood glucose controlled.

Lifestyle changes (a new job, a move, pregnancy, illness, and so on) also require alternative therapies so that an adaptive plan can be developed to meet your new schedule needs.

Making the switch

Once you have made the decision to switch to lispro, there are some rules of thumb that can be followed to make the transition smooth and easy. See "Practical Tips for Switching to Lispro" on this page. It is important to continue self-monitoring of blood glucose, and even to increase the frequency, when you initiate a change in your therapy, such as switching to a new insulin.

Other immediate concerns that come to mind include storage, mixing with other insulins, and special precautions. As with any insulin, lispro is best stored in the refrigerator, where there is very little loss of potency. At room temperature, all insulins lose 1½% of potency per month. However, insulin is best injected and absorbed when administered at room temperature. So keep the current bottle at room temperature and use it within a month, and store extra

PRACTICAL TIPS FOR SWITCHING TO LISPRO

■ If blood glucose levels are running high before meals or between meals, substitute lispro (Humalog) for Regular insulin unit for unit. Do not switch to lispro if only your fasting blood glucose (the level upon awakening) is high.

■ If blood glucose levels are normal while using Regular, decrease the lispro dose by 20% when switching since lispro works more efficiently.

■ If you develop low blood sugar between meals with Regular, decrease the lispro dose by up to 50%.

■ If you are switching from Regular to lispro for your suppertime insulin, your bedtime NPH may need to be increased because you are losing some of the nighttime coverage that Regular provides. You will no longer need to eat a bedtime snack. If you do eat a snack, you will need to cover it with an injection of lispro.

■ If you want more freedom around the timing of lunch and your food choices at lunch, use lispro at lunch and decrease your morning NPH by up to 50%.

■ If you have gastroparesis (delayed stomach emptying), injecting lispro after eating, when blood glucose starts to rise, may help. Check with your diabetes caregiver.

■ If you currently take Regular with meals, changing to lispro will mean you need to add a background insulin (NPH, Lente, or Ultralente) during the day, or, alternatively, you will need to add 1 to 2 units of Regular to your lispro dose.

■ When you begin using lispro, check your blood glucose level two hours after meals for the first several days. A two-hour goal of 140 mg/dl to 160 mg/dl is a safe range. To mimic a nondiabetic glucose pattern, the blood glucose level two hours after a meal should be within 20 mg/dl to 40 mg/dl of the level before the meal. Many people comment on how much better they feel after meals when using lispro. In particular, they notice they no longer feel hungry between meals, an effect that can be caused by late-working Regular.

■ Parents of toddlers or children who have picky appetites or are slow eaters should administer lispro *after* the child eats.

■ Teens who experience high blood glucose levels because of growth hormones and puberty may not need to reduce their overall insulin dose when switching from Regular to lispro. Switching unit for unit works well.

bottles in the refrigerator. Do not expose insulin to temperatures above 85°F or below 40°F because it begins to degrade at these temperatures.

Like Regular human insulin, lispro can be mixed with basal insulins such as NPH, Lente, or Ultralente. Always draw up the lispro first ("clear before cloudy"). The injection must be given immediately after drawing up the insulin. Remember again that lispro is primarily used as a mealtime insulin that needs to be balanced with an appropriate type and dose of a basal insulin.

Because lispro acts more quickly than other insulins and clears from the bloodstream faster, special precautions revolve around the prevention of blood glucose levels that are too low or too high. If a person injects lispro and waits longer than 15 minutes to eat, the potential for low blood glucose is extremely high. Unless injected lispro is balanced with an appropriate background, or basal, insulin for fasting periods (between meals and overnight), the potential for high blood glucose is also very high. A switch to lispro insulin requires intensive education from your doctor or diabetes educator to prevent an increase, rather than the expected decrease, in the number of times that blood glucose levels are too low or too high.

Looking ahead

The future of insulin analogs is bright. A second rapid-acting insulin, aspart (Novolog), was approved by the U.S. Food and Drug Administration in 2000; its action profile is similar to that of lispro. The agency the same year also approved an analog long-acting insulin, called glargine (Lantus), which works in an essentially peakless manner and lasts for some 24 hours. A number of other analogs are in various stages of research.

I hope this article has stimulated you to consider at least discussion with your health-care provider on the benefits of rapid-acting insulin, such as lispro. Such an insulin is like the perfect dinner guest: It arrives on time for dinner, and it doesn't stay beyond its welcome! ❑

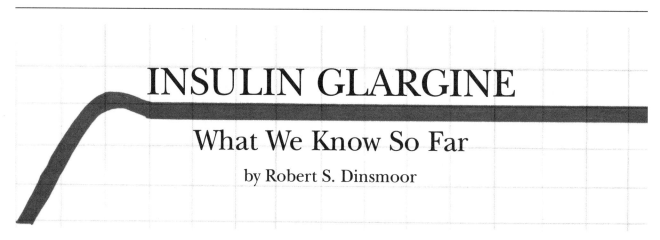

INSULIN GLARGINE

What We Know So Far

by Robert S. Dinsmoor

Insulin glargine (brand name Lantus), the newly available long-acting insulin preparation, may well turn out to improve diabetes treatment significantly. It enters the bloodstream gradually and predictably and has a "peakless" activity profile, all of which could make it an ideal long-acting insulin. But do these properties actually translate into better blood sugar control in the real world? Here's what the best available evidence shows—and what we don't yet know.

Room for improvement

Why do we need a better long-acting insulin anyway? What's wrong with the other products on the market? To understand the shortcomings of these products, it helps to understand how insulin regimens are designed.

In a person who doesn't have diabetes, the pancreas continually secretes a stream of insulin, called the *basal insulin* secretion, to enable the body to use the glucose that is in the bloodstream even during fasting and between meals. When the person eats a meal, the pancreas secretes extra insulin to help the body use the glucose from the carbohydrate that was ingested.

In a person with Type 1 diabetes, whose pancreas has lost the ability to make and secrete insulin, insulin regimens are designed to mimic this pancreatic insulin secretion as closely as possible. Often, a short-acting insulin (Regular insulin) or a rapid-acting insulin analog (lispro, brand name Humalog; aspart, brand name NovoLog) is injected to take care of the postmeal glucose rise. A longer-acting (or basal) insulin, such as NPH, Lente, or Ultralente, is given to meet the body's basal insulin needs.

Some people with Type 2 diabetes also take insulin. When diet, exercise, and oral agents fail to adequately control a person's blood sugar level, a doctor may add a basal insulin to the treatment plan. If the condition progresses and most of the ability to secrete insulin is lost, multiple daily injections, with shorter-acting mealtime insulin injections as well as basal insulin, may become necessary, much as in a person with Type 1 diabetes.

NPH. NPH, which stands for neutral protamine Hagedorn, is currently the most commonly used basal insulin preparation. The insulin is bound to a protein called protamine, which makes it less soluble in the body and extends its duration of action.

According to Novo Nordisk, the company's NPH (Novolin N) begins to work about 1½ hours after injection. It "peaks" (has its strongest effect) about 4 to 12 hours after injection, and its effects can last up to 24 hours. Lilly's Humulin N has its peak around 3½–9½ hours after injection and can last 13½–24 hours. NPH's pronounced peak and the fact that its effects may not last a full 24 hours can make blood glucose levels more difficult to control.

The sometimes wide ranges given by manufacturers for insulin activity profiles reflect that each person's unique body chemistry, as well as circumstances at the time of and after an insulin injection, can affect how insulin acts in the body. For example, dose size, injection site, and physical activity level can all affect the activity of insulin.

Figuring out when to take NPH can be tricky. If NPH is given before dinner, its effects may wear off during the night, causing high blood sugar in the morning. Giving it at bedtime, on the other hand, may set the stage for either nighttime hypoglycemia (low blood sugar) or high morning blood sugar. A 10 PM injection, for instance, would reach its peak around 4 AM, when a person is likely to be asleep, and possibly cause hypoglycemia. Decreasing this dose could lead to insulin deficiency between 5 AM and 8 AM, when the body is most resistant to insulin's effects, causing high morning blood sugar.

Lente and Ultralente. Both Lente and Ultralente are crystallized suspensions of insulin with zinc added to prolong their effects. Lente insulin has a slightly longer activity profile than NPH—Novolin L reportedly lasts up to 22 hours or so, while Humulin L may last 21–26 hours—although both Lente and NPH are extremely variable in their effects. Like NPH, Lente has a pronounced peak (at 7–15 hours for Novolin L and 7–14 hours for Humulin L) and its effects are extremely variable.

Ultralente is the longest-acting insulin preparation on the market, with effects lasting up to 23–36 hours for Humulin U. Despite this long duration of action, which can be highly beneficial, it acts much like NPH and Lente, with a distinct peak somewhere between 8 hours and 16 hours after injection. The absorption rate of Ultralente is also extremely variable.

The goods on insulin glargine

Like lispro and aspart, insulin glargine is an insulin analog or "designer insulin." Insulin analogs are artificially produced forms of insulin in which the insulin molecule has been altered to produce a more desirable effect. Whereas lispro and aspart are designed to work more quickly than Regular, glargine is designed to work longer than NPH or Lente.

Glargine is synthesized from harmless *E. coli* bacteria that have been modified with recombinant DNA technology. In the glargine molecule, the amino acid *asparagine* has been replaced by *glycine* at one position, and two *arginine* molecules have been added to another position. These changes make glargine less soluble at the body's natural pH (acidity level). Once injected into the skin, glargine forms a precipitate, which is absorbed very slowly and evenly into the bloodstream. The U.S. Food and Drug Administration (FDA) approved glargine for marketing in April 2000; its manufacturer, Aventis Pharmaceuticals, announced its widespread availability in May 2001.

For many years, researchers have been studying how glargine behaves in the body. The research shows that glargine is indeed absorbed very slowly into the bloodstream (its effects lasting 24 hours) with little variability and with no peak activity level. In theory, these properties could make it an ideal long-acting insulin product, improving blood glucose control while, at the same time, lowering the risk of hypoglycemia. In practice, however, not enough clinical studies have been done yet to say whether it is, in fact, an ideal basal insulin.

What the research shows

Even before insulin glargine was approved, researchers began testing its effects on blood glucose control both in people with Type 1 diabetes and in people with Type 2. Specifically, these studies have been comparing the effects of glargine with those of NPH, since NPH is the most commonly used basal insulin. In these studies, people were randomly assigned to receive either one or two injections of NPH or one injection of glargine as part of their regimen. The researchers then compared blood glucose control and the frequency of hypoglycemia in the two groups. The results of several of these clinical trials have appeared in the journal *Diabetes Care*.

Julio Rosenstock, M.D., and colleagues at the Dallas Diabetes and Endocrine Center in Dallas, Texas, studied the effects of glargine in 256 people with Type 1 diabetes who had previously been on multiple-daily-injection regimens using NPH. They were randomly assigned either to receive glargine in place of NPH or to stay with their previous NPH regimen for four weeks. People in the glargine group turned out to have somewhat lower fasting plasma glucose levels than the NPH group, leading the researchers to conclude that glargine was "more effective in lowering fasting plasma glucose levels than NPH in patients with Type 1 diabetes."

Robert Ratner, M.D., of the MedStar Clinical Research Center in Washington, D.C., along with colleagues in other locations, studied the use of glargine in 534 people with Type 1 diabetes who had previously followed multiple-daily-injection regimens using NPH and Regular insulin. Roughly half of them were randomly assigned to follow a regimen of glargine at bedtime plus Regular before meals; the other half were assigned to receive their previous regimen of once- or twice-daily NPH plus mealtime Regular. Both groups were followed for up to 28 weeks. The study showed that the group that switched to glargine had lower fasting plasma glucose levels as well as fewer episodes of hypoglycemia.

Philip Raskin, M.D., of the University of Texas Southwestern Medical Center in Dallas, and colleagues in the United States and Canada studied glargine in people previously treated with once- or twice-daily NPH plus insulin lispro. Roughly half were randomly assigned to receive glargine in place of NPH; the other half continued to receive their previous insulin regimen for 16 weeks. Of those in the glargine group, 29.6% reached their target fasting blood glucose level of 119 mg/dl, whereas only 16.8% of the NPH group reached these target levels. However, there were no differences in their glycosylated hemoglobin (HbA_{1c}) levels, which indicate long-term blood glucose control, and there were no differences between the two groups in their rates of hypoglycemia. The researchers concluded that glargine was "at least as effective" at controlling blood sugar as once- or twice-daily NPH.

So far, at least two clinical trials of glargine have been carried out in people with Type 2 diabetes. Hannele Yki-Jarvinen, M.D., at the University of Helsinki in Helsinki, Finland, and colleagues at the Hoescht Marion Roussel Deutschland Clinical Development in Frankfurt, Germany, studied the effects of glargine in 426 people with Type 2 diabetes who had previously been unable to control their blood glucose using diabetes pills. They were randomly assigned to receive either bedtime NPH or bedtime glargine in addition to their previous regimen of pills, and they were followed for one year. The glargine group had lower blood glucose levels after dinner than the NPH group, as well as less nocturnal hypoglycemia. According to the researchers, "These data support use of insulin glargine instead of NPH in insulin combination regimens in Type 2 diabetes."

Dr. Rosenstock at the Dallas Diabetes and Endocrine Center and colleagues across the United States studied glargine in 518 people with Type 2 diabetes who had been receiving NPH insulin with or without mealtime Regular insulin. Half of them were randomly assigned to receive either glargine once daily or NPH once or twice daily. Those who had previously been taking Regular as part of their regimen continued to do so. Both groups were followed for 28 weeks. Once-daily bedtime glargine was shown to be as effective as once- or twice-daily NPH at improving and maintaining blood glucose control. Furthermore, the glargine group had a lower risk of nighttime hypoglycemia and less weight gain than the NPH group.

Research indicates that glargine is at least as safe as NPH, with similar rates of "adverse events." As with all insulins, the most common adverse event with glargine is hypoglycemia. In one study, the use of glargine was associated with worsening of diabetic retinopathy. However, none of the other studies has found such an association, and researchers believe it to be a statistical fluke. Nonetheless, there is an ongoing clinical trial with glargine looking specifically at this issue.

In an editorial in the May 2000 issue of *Diabetes Care,* John Buse, M.D., Ph.D., at the Diabetes Care Center at the University of North Carolina in Durham observed that in his practice, the most dramatic positive results with glargine have been in people who had been unable to control their blood glucose levels adequately without high rates of hypoglycemia, despite trying every combination of available insulin formulations. He also speculated that using glargine in combination with a rapid-acting insulin such as lispro could eventually be the "poor man's pump," offering an effective, more convenient, and less expensive alternative to insulin pumps. In people with Type 2 diabetes, he says, it may turn out to be suitable for those with moderate insulin deficiency and as a basal insulin for those with more complete insulin deficiency.

Taken together, this research suggests that glargine has some benefit over NPH insulin, at least in certain situations. Yet not all doctors and researchers completely agree on how to use this information. Some are eagerly embracing this new product while others are more cautious and insist that more studies are needed to confirm these beneficial effects and rule out adverse effects.

Is insulin glargine for you

The first rule of thumb when considering changes to your insulin regimen should be, "If it isn't broken, don't fix it." In other words, if you're able to control your blood sugar level with your current diabetes treatment plan, why change it?

Aventis Pharmaceuticals, the manufacturer of Lantus, suggests that Lantus may be most useful in the following situations:

■ If your blood sugar is too high despite the best efforts to control it with diet, exercise, and oral agents.
■ If you're currently using an intermediate-acting insulin (such as NPH) once a day and want 24-hour basal coverage.
■ If you would rather take one injection of glargine rather than two injections of NPH.

If you're interested in glargine, speak with your doctor, and if you do switch to glargine, plan on working closely with him or her during the transition. Since the effects of switching insulin formulations can be unpredictable, it is important to know what to do in the event of very high blood sugar or hypoglycemia. Be prepared, too, to check your blood glucose levels more frequently for at least a week after making the switch, particularly at bedtime and in the middle of the night, to find out exactly what effect glargine is having. Make sure you and your doctor establish guidelines for contacting your health-care team should problems arise

Words to the wise

There are some minor drawbacks and risks associated with the use of insulin glargine, as well as some precautions to keep in mind when using it. They are the following:

■ It should not be diluted or mixed with any other insulin or solution, because it may physically react with them, altering its activity profile in an unpredictable way.
■ Pregnant women should not use glargine because of potential safety issues.
■ As with any drug or insulin, people who develop allergic symptoms to glargine should not use it.
■ Glargine is associated with temporary pain at the injection site, which is probably a result of glargine's acidity.

The introduction of glargine could wind up being a real boon to diabetes treatment, but until the necessary studies are conducted, doctor and patient alike should approach this new product with caution and common sense. ❏

AN INSIDER'S LOOK AT INSULIN PUMP THERAPY

by Gary Scheiner, M.S., C.D.E.

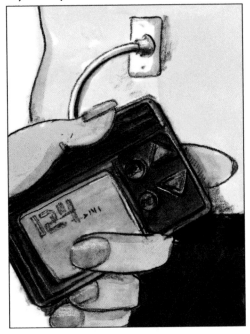

It's days like today that make me glad I went on an insulin pump. It's Saturday, and despite having two little rugrats at home, I was able to sleep until 9:30 (miracles do happen). Today was the day to clean out the basement—something I've been promising my wife I'll do for, oh, about a year. After testing my blood sugar (it was 131 mg/dl), I lowered the basal rate on my pump and decided to skip breakfast and get right to work.

By 1 o'clock, I was covered with dust and little specks of drywall, but the basement was in pretty good shape. I disconnected from my pump temporarily and hit the shower. By the time I was able to grab a bite to eat around 2 o'clock, my blood sugar was 82. I hit a few buttons to deliver a small dose of insulin, just enough to cover the carbohydrate in a leftover turkey sandwich and some stuffing. As I ate, I pondered that age-old question: Why does turkey get worse with age, but stuffing get better?

At 3 o'clock, we took the kids to the latest computer-generated, animated movie. Having grown up on a steady diet of the classics (Bugs Bunny and Scooby Doo), I'm not big on today's kids' movies. But the popcorn—that's another story: I live for movie theater popcorn. And not the little kiddie-size cup! Daddy gets the jumbo size, complete with the free refill, perfect to take home for tomorrow's football games. I figured that the jumbo bag had about 80 grams of carbohydrate, so I took my bolus of insulin and raised my basal rate to cover the delayed blood sugar rise caused by the fat in the "butter" topping.

After the movie, my blood sugar was 202 (perhaps I underestimated the amount of carbohydrate in the popcorn), so I touched it up with a 2-unit bolus. We picked up the babysitter and then met up with some friends for a few friendly games of bowling (guys vs. gals), followed by a late dinner. I think the popcorn shifted my center of gravity a little bit, because my game deteriorated big-time, and the ladies got to choose the restaurant. No all-you-can-eat buffet tonight.

The hostess at the "café" told us there would be a 30-minute wait for a table, so I tried the old "I'm diabetic and I'll die if I don't eat right away" bit, but it didn't work. Seems the hostess recognized my insulin pump, and she knows from a friend who wears one that I don't have to eat according to a schedule. Oh, well. Despite looking pretty stupid, I had a really good time. And my blood sugar at bedtime was a tidy 128.

So, let's see. If I was still on insulin injections, I probably would not have been able to sleep late without getting high blood sugar from delaying my morning shot; I couldn't skip breakfast without going low; work through the morning without going low again; eat a big bag of popcorn one hour after lunch without going very high; bowl through dinnertime without going low; delay dinner without going low; or go to bed with a decent reading because the fat from the popcorn would have shot my blood sugar up.

Today, tens of thousands of Americans wear insulin pumps. While that may seem like a lot, consider that there are nearly one million people with Type 1 diabetes in the United States and millions more with Type 2 diabetes who take insulin. Still, the number of pumpers is increasing by more than 20% each year as pumping gains wide acceptance in the medical community and insurance industry. Pump users rarely discontinue the pump to go back to injections. In fact, the major reason more people have not gone on insulin pumps is a simple lack of knowledge of what pump therapy has to offer.

How does a pump work?

The insulin pump is as close a substitute as we have to a healthy, working pancreas. It mimics the pancreas by releasing small amounts of short- or fast-acting insulin (such as Regular or lispro) every few minutes. This is called a *basal rate* of insulin. The basal rate is designed to keep the blood sugar level steady between meals and during sleep. When food is eaten, the pump is programmed (at the touch of a button) to deliver a larger quantity of insulin right away to cover the carbohydrate in the meal. This is called a *bolus* of insulin. The bolus can also be adjusted based on the blood sugar level and amount of planned physical activity.

With a pump, you get the right amount of insulin at the right time: large amounts when you eat, and small amounts between meals and while you're sleeping. This system cannot be duplicated with multiple injections of insulin because intermediate- and long-acting insulins (NPH, Lente, and Ultralente) typically provide an uneven flow of insulin, not the steady, continuous flow that the body needs. Because the pump's basal rate holds the blood sugar steady between meals, you can vary your schedule as much as you like in terms of meals, activities, and sleep. In other words, you can live a more normal life.

The pump itself is a beeper-size device that contains a cartridge filled with short- or fast-acting insulin. The pump's onboard computer runs a motor that pushes insulin from the cartridge through a tube and into your body. The motor is powered by a battery, which generally must be changed every six to 12 weeks.

To get the insulin under your skin, an *infusion set* is worn. Most infusion sets feature a small, flexible, plastic tube that is inserted just under the skin with a needle that is immediately removed. The infusion set is usually worn on the abdomen, buttocks, or hip and is taped securely in place. A new infusion set is inserted every two to four days. Today's pumps are equipped with multiple safety features that ensure against accidental insulin delivery.

Who should consider a pump?

Insulin pumps are ideally suited for people whose pancreas produces little or no insulin, including anyone with Type 1 diabetes and those with Type 2 diabetes who have been shown to produce little of their own insulin through a lab test called a C-peptide test. And unless your last name is Trump, you will need to have adequate insurance to use an insulin pump. Pumps cost around $5,000, and the supplies that go with them cost $1,000 to $2,000 a year. Luckily, most medical insurance now covers at least part of the cost of an insulin pump and supplies.

There are also certain skills that are needed to use a pump successfully. While programming the pump is simple for most people, an ability to press a few buttons with confidence is needed. Changing the infusion set is easy enough to be performed by a child, but it does require a certain amount of dexterity and the ability to follow directions. Pump users should be prepared to test their blood sugar levels several times every day and learn how to count carbohydrates so that insulin boluses can be matched to food intake. It is also very important to keep good written records of blood sugar readings, insulin doses, grams of carbohydrate eaten, and physical activities.

Pump pros and cons

Before making the jump to or from a pump, it is only fair to take a look at both the pluses and minuses.

Based on my 10 years' experience on shots, five years on the pump, and feedback from hundreds of other pump users, here are some of the main benefits of pump therapy:

More desirable blood sugar levels. Reductions in HbA_{1c} are common in those whose test results are often high on shots. (The HbA_{1c} test, a blood test that should be done two to four times a year, is an indicator of blood sugar control over the preceding two to three months.) There are also fewer "high to low" and "low to high" swings.

Fewer episodes of low blood sugar. By using only short- or fast-acting insulin, there is no intermediate- or long-acting insulin peaking when you're not eating (although the new long-acting insulin glargine is said to be essentially peakless). This makes pump therapy a good choice for those with frequent lows or an inability to detect low blood sugar (hypoglycemia unawareness).

A more flexible lifestyle. Raise your hand if you can eat, sleep, and exercise at the same times every day. For those of you with your hands down, the pump lets you choose your own schedule.

Precise dosing. With a pump, you can dose within tenths of a unit. This is ideal for people who are sensitive to very small insulin doses, such as children and lean adults.

Convenience. There is no need to draw up syringes every time you need insulin; just reach to your side and press a few buttons.

No shots. Multiple daily insulin injections can be uncomfortable and cause skin problems. The pump's infusion set is changed two to three times a week.

Easy adjustments. Basal rate changes permit good blood sugar control during periods of growth, illness, seasonal sports, menstruation, and fasting.

Weight control. With a pump, snacks are not required between meals to prevent hypoglycemia. You will have flexibility with meals when setting your nutrition goals.

Novelty. Just as cool graphics and sounds help motivate some people to use exercise equipment, the high-tech aspect of the pump can add a dimension of excitement and fun to one's diabetes care.

There are also drawbacks to pump use, including the following:

A learning curve. Don't expect good control right away. It usually takes a few months to get the basal and bolus doses regulated and to adjust to using the pump.

Inconvenience. Wearing the pump around the clock, even during sleep, can become awkward once in a while.

Technical difficulties. As a mechanical device, pumps are prone to occasional infusion set clogs, battery failures, computer glitches, and damage due to typical wear and tear.

Skin problems. Skin can become irritated from infusion set adhesive, and infections can occur if infusion sets are worn too long or are inserted improperly.

Risk of ketosis. The absence of long-acting insulin with pump use can present a problem if insulin delivery is interrupted for more than a few hours. Very high blood sugar can occur, and ketones, a sign that your body is burning fat for fuel rather than glucose, may appear in the bloodstream and urine. Ketones can be detected at home with a urine test and corrected by drinking lots of water and taking insulin with a syringe.

Infusion set changes. Every couple of days, the pump user must change the infusion set. This procedure, which generally takes between three and 10 minutes, involves numerous steps and can be momentarily painful or traumatic for the novice pump user.

Living with a pump

I am often asked, "Is it easy to live with your pump?" to which my response is always, "It's a lot easier than living with my kids."

The pump should not force anyone to change his routine or avoid his favorite activities. In fact, it will probably free you up to take part in a wider range of activities with minimal interference from your diabetes.

Many infusion sets feature a "quick disconnect" mechanism that allows the user to temporarily unhook the pump and tubing for situations such as bathing, contact sports, and intimacy. All pumps are either waterproof or have a waterproof case, so the pump can be worn in or around the water if you choose. The pump itself has a secure clip and is usually worn on a belt or waistband or in a pocket. A variety of cases and fashion accessories make the pump easy to wear in just about any situation.

When you sleep, you continue to need a basal flow of insulin, so the pump must be worn through the night. This does not usually present any problems, because the pump can be clipped to sleepwear, kept in a pocket, put under a pillow, or simply placed next to you in the bed. The pump's tubing is long, strong, and taped in place very securely, so nothing is likely to pull out or disconnect while you sleep.

If looks are a concern, consider that insulin pumps have the look and size of a beeper and are very easily concealed. If you're still worried about your personal appearance, don't forget that Miss America 1999, Nicole Johnson, wore an insulin pump throughout the pageant!

Ingredients for success

Let's face facts. Just about anyone who has insulin-dependent diabetes and a decent insurance policy can

INSULIN PUMP MANUFACTURERS AND DISTRIBUTORS

Contact the following companies for more information about the insulin pumps they manufacture or distribute and for more information about pumping in general.

ANIMAS CORPORATION
(manufacturer of the R-1000 Insulin Pump)
590 Lancaster Avenue
Frazer, PA 19355
(877) YES-PUMP (937-7867)
www.animascorp.com

DISETRONIC MEDICAL SYSTEMS, INC.
(manufacturer of the H-Tron Plus Insulin Pump)
5151 Program Avenue
St. Paul, MN 55112-1014
(800) 280-7801
www.disetronic.com
www.disetronic-usa.com

INSULIN INFUSION SPECIALTIES
(the largest independent distributor of insulin pumps in the United States, carrying all pumps and diabetes product lines)
2601 N. Hullen Street, Suite 200
Metairie, LA 70002
(800) 838-PUMP (838-7867)
www.insulininfusion.com

MINIMED, INC.
(manufacturer of the 508 Insulin Pump)
18000 Devonshire Street
Northridge, CA 91325-1219
(800) MINIMED 646-4633
www.minimed.com

go on an insulin pump. But to succeed with a pump takes preparation and follow-through.

I would never discourage a person from going on a pump because of problems with blood sugar control. Difficulty keeping blood sugar within target range is often caused by using intermediate- and long-acting insulins and a failure to match insulin precisely to the body's needs. The criteria that I consider the most important for those seeking an insulin pump are the following:

■ Motivation and interest in going on a pump.

■ A true state of insulin dependence, meaning either Type 1 diabetes or Type 2 with little or no insulin production.

■ Adequate resources to afford the pump and supplies, either through insurance coverage or cash reserves.

■ The ability to handle basic button-pushing and infusion set change procedures. (This can be done by a parent or guardian if the user is very young or physically or mentally challenged.)

Certain skills are essential to make a successful transition to the pump. Ideally, these should be taught and mastered prior to starting on the pump:

■ Carbohydrate counting, using grams rather than exchanges or choices.

■ Blood glucose monitoring before meals and at bedtime (four times a day as a minimum).

■ Full record-keeping of blood sugar readings, insulin doses, carbohydrate intake, and physical activities.

■ Self-adjustment of insulin doses, based on blood sugar levels, carbohydrate intake, and physical activity.

■ The basic principles of pump therapy, including basic pump operation, infusion set function, basal rates, and boluses.

Successful pump use will also require adequate follow-up and fine-tuning once the pump is initiated. This should include the following:

■ Periodic basal rate testing, which involves fasting for an 8–10 hour interval and testing blood sugar to see if it is holding steady. If blood sugar levels are rising or falling, the basal rate should be adjusted and the test repeated until readings are steady.

■ Fine-tuning of bolus formulas, based on record-keeping.

■ Prompt troubleshooting and prevention of emergencies such as diabetic ketoacidosis, a condition characterized by very high blood glucose, dehydration, and ketones in the bloodstream and urine.

■ Use of advanced pump features such as extended boluses and temporary basal rates.

The next step

The decision to use an insulin pump is an important one to you and your family, so discuss it with them and with your doctor. If your doctor is not familiar with insulin pumps or simply dismisses them as a waste of time, consider asking your doctor for the name of a diabetes specialist who may be more knowledgeable on the subject. Ideally, it is best to work with a doctor who invites your input and has a team of diabetes educators who can assist you with your pre-pump education and post-pump blood sugar management.

To learn more about pump therapy, contact one of the insulin pump manufacturers or distributors listed on this page. Find out if there are insulin pump support groups in your area. Support group meetings offer an excellent forum for meeting other pumpers and finding out about their personal experiences since starting pump therapy. ❏

GETTING THE MOST OUT OF INSULIN THERAPY

by Priscilla Hollander, M.D., Ph.D.

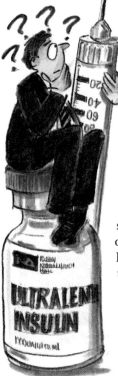

It has been almost ten years since the publication of the landmark Diabetes Control and Complications Trial (DCCT). This study was the first to show that the development of complications in Type 1 diabetes is related to blood glucose levels. Further studies, such as the Kumamoto study done in Japan and the United Kingdom Prospective Diabetes Study, have demonstrated a similar link in Type 2 diabetes. The DCCT and the Kumamoto study also showed that aggressive therapy aimed at obtaining the best possible blood glucose levels is the key to optimal treatment for people with diabetes. For people who use insulin, aggressive, or intensified, therapy is defined as taking multiple injections of insulin or using an insulin pump.

This has led to individual improvement for many people, but it is clear that there are many more who could benefit. The intensified approach to a diabetes regimen is not right for everyone, but for most people who require insulin, for both Type 1 and Type 2 diabetes, it offers great promise. This article explains the key elements of an intensified insulin program, with the emphasis on how to best use insulin.

Keys to tight control

For an intensified insulin program to work, a number of key considerations must be taken into account and a number of key components need to be in place.
Target glucose goals. The first step is to set your target glucose and glycosylated hemoglobin (HbA_{1c}) goals. The HbA_{1c} test is used to measure average blood glucose control over an extended period. Goals should be set in conjunction with your doctor and health-care team. Ideal control has been defined as daily blood glucose levels in the normal (nondiabetic) range and an HbA_{1c} below 6.0%. However, studies like the DCCT show that for those who can reach and maintain an HbA_{1c} of 7.0%, the risk of complications is decreased dramatically. The lesson here is that any improvement in HbA_{1c} can be helpful.

Individualized goals. If an individual is prone to episodes of hypoglycemia, or blood glucose levels that are too low, glucose goals may be set higher than they would be otherwise. However, for some people, low blood sugar may result from an insulin regimen that does not match food intake and exercise. By getting a better balance, they may be able to decrease the number of low blood sugar episodes and actually lower their HbA_{1c}. For those whose blood glucose levels tend to be high, setting intermediate blood glucose goals may be best. Once these goals are reached, they can be set lower.

Frequent self-monitoring. To obtain the best control, blood glucose monitoring three to four times a day is needed, usually before meals and in the evening. If a new regimen is being started, even more frequent testing, such as following meals and during the night, may be helpful to fine-tune your insulin dosages.

The key to using blood glucose results is to record them in a way that gives adequate information. Keeping a written record book allows evaluation of the overall pattern of blood glucose levels. Using the memory function on most blood glucose meters can be helpful, depending on the programs in the meter. Some meters have a small screen and a computer program that allows visual access to a readout similar to a record book. However, if the meter allows you to see only the result of your last blood glucose check or an overall average, you won't be able to follow patterns or see trends.

Using correct technique when checking your blood glucose level is important for accurate results; check your technique every so often by demonstrating it to your doctor or diabetes educator.

Glycosylated hemoglobin tests. The glycosylated hemoglobin, or HbA_{1c}, test is a long-term index of blood glucose control that gives the average percent of glucose in the blood over the preceding 8 to 12 weeks. An HbA_{1c} test should be done every three to four months to help assess and confirm overall blood glucose control. The test result should be consistent with blood glucose levels obtained on your meter. If it is not, your technique may need improvement, or more testing, such as after meals, may be needed to evaluate your insulin regimen.

Meal plan. For most people, the greatest barrier to blood glucose control is the right meal plan. In the

TABLE 1: INSULIN ACTION TIMES

Different types of insulin have different action times—that is, they take different amounts of time to begin working, to reach peak effectiveness, and to leave the body. Only approximate ranges are given here; in practice, action speeds will vary from person to person.

INSULIN	TYPE	ONSET (HOURS)	PEAK (HOURS)	DURATION (HOURS)
Human	Regular	½–1	2½–5	4–12
	NPH	1–3	4–12	up to 24
	Lente	2–4	7–15	up to 24
	Ultralente	4–10	6–16	24+
Analog	Lispro	up to ¼	½–1½	up to 5
	Aspart	up to ¼	½–1½	up to 5
	Glargine	1–2	Virtually none	24

DCCT, people with the best blood glucose control were those who did the best job of balancing food and insulin. Methods such as the exchange system and especially carbohydrate counting allow people to match rapid- and short-acting insulins to varying food intake. The current approach to diet is to individualize and pursue flexibility. Food can be added or subtracted and the insulin dose adjusted accordingly. Everybody with diabetes should see a registered dietitian for help with developing an appropriate meal plan.

Sometimes people on intensified regimens gain weight. This gain comes from three sources and can be avoided. First, when blood glucose levels are high, up to 800 calories a day in excess glucose may be lost in the urine. When the insulin regimen is improved, the goal is to eliminate excess glucose. With the right balance of food and insulin, the body will utilize all the food that is eaten. But if you continue to eat at the same level as before, you will gain weight.

A second way to gain weight is to eat extra food, thinking that because you are increasing your insulin to cover it, there is no problem. But if you take in more calories than you use, your weight will increase.

A third way to gain weight is to overtreat episodes of low blood sugar, using more quick-acting carbohydrate than necessary to correct the low blood sugar.

Physical activity and exercise. Generally, regular physical activity and planned exercise lower blood glucose. For people on conventional fixed insulin regimens, sporadic or variable exercise often leads to low blood sugar. With intensification, the ability to adjust your insulin dose to balance your anticipated physical activity can help you fit in exercise and still maintain excellent blood glucose control.

Team approach to treatment. Routine appointments with your doctor are important for monitoring your blood glucose control and for assessing and treating complications. Other key members of the diabetes-care team are the nurse educator and dietitian. Both of these individuals play essential roles in helping people achieve the self-management skills needed to successfully implement an intensified regimen.

Self-management skills. Knowledge about the various aspects of diabetes is necessary for self-management of diabetes on a day-to-day basis. To make an intensified regimen work, the person with diabetes must be in charge. He or she needs to be able to make decisions about diet, to make insulin dose adjustments, and to understand how to avoid and treat low blood sugar. Education is fundamental to gaining these skills.

Choosing the right insulin regimen. This may be the most important component of setting up an intensified insulin regimen. Ideally, an insulin regimen that mimics perfectly the function of normal beta cells, the insulin-producing cells of the pancreas, could be developed for each person. However, as most people with diabetes know, this is not always an easy task.

How insulin works

To understand what is needed for a successful insulin regimen, you have to understand how insulin works in a person who does not have diabetes. If diabetes is not present, blood insulin levels are low until food is eaten. Eating serves as a stimulus to the beta cells, and insulin output is sharply increased for 60 to 90 minutes. Just enough insulin is released to metabolize the amount of food eaten, and no more. Thus, neither low blood sugar nor high blood sugar results.

An important player in the glucose story is the liver. It is literally a storehouse of glucose. If the blood glucose level is too high, the liver will siphon off the extra glucose for storage. If blood glucose starts to

TABLE 2: Common Regimens Using NPH Plus Regular, Lispro, or Aspart Insulin

Here are five examples of the ways in which NPH can be combined with Regular, lispro, or aspart insulin. These are among the most commonly used regimens in the United States. Which regimen works best depends on the individual's needs.

MORNING	NOON	EVENING	BEDTIME
NPH plus Regular, lispro, or aspart	no injection	NPH plus Regular, lispro, or aspart	no injection
NPH plus Regular, lispro, or aspart	no injection	Regular, lispro, or aspart	NPH
NPH plus Regular, lispro, or aspart	Regular, lispro, or aspart	NPH plus Regular, lispro, or aspart	no injection
NPH plus Regular, lispro, or aspart	Regular, lispro, or aspart	Regular, lispro, or aspart	NPH
Regular, lispro, or aspart	Regular, lispro, or aspart	Regular, lispro, or aspart	NPH

fall, as it does between meals or if a person fasts, the liver will release glucose into the blood. Interestingly, the signal to the liver is not glucose itself but the level of insulin in the blood. If the insulin level is high, as after a meal, the liver will absorb glucose. If the insulin level is low, as between meals, the liver will release glucose.

An insulin regimen must provide two important kinds of insulin: basal insulin and bolus insulin.

■ *Basal insulin* is the background insulin present throughout a 24-hour period to provide a level of insulin between meals and overnight sufficient to suppress glucose release by the liver.

■ *Bolus insulin* is insulin given before meals to cover the food eaten during the meal and to prevent blood glucose elevation following the meal.

Insulin types

The various types of insulin provide the building blocks for making up an insulin regimen. There exist several classes of insulin: rapid-acting insulins (lispro and aspart), short-acting insulins (Regular), intermediate-acting insulins (NPH and Lente), and long-acting insulins (Ultralente and glargine). Almost all insulins now available are human insulins or specially designed analog insulins that differ in time of action or other characteristics. Currently, lispro (brand name Humalog), aspart (Novolog), and glargine (Lantus) are the only analog insulins approved by the U.S. Food and Drug Administration.

Approximate action times for several insulin types are listed in Table 1 on page 116. Action times include onset, or how long it takes for insulin to begin acting; peak time, or the time during which insulin is most effective; and duration, or how long insulin continues

to act. For a given insulin, these figures may differ slightly from person to person.

The short- and rapid-acting insulins (Regular, lispro, and aspart) are used as bolus insulins. Regular insulin must be taken approximately 30 to 45 minutes before a meal, while lispro or aspart can be taken at the start of a meal. Results of blood testing one hour after a meal and just before the next meal can be used to help determine the appropriate premeal dose of such insulins.

NPH or Lente insulin can be used to provide basal levels. Both of them take longer to peak than Regular, lispro, or aspart, and they may be able to cover a meal such as lunch. To be effective, they usually need to be given twice a day.

Ultralente insulin and the newest analog, insulin glargine, have longer durations and give lower levels of basal or background insulin than the intermediate-acting insulins. This may make them better as once-a-day background insulins than the intermediate insulins. Ultralente has a slight peak, but insulin glargine is essentially peakless.

Insulin regimens

In selecting or redoing your insulin regimen, the underlying principle is to use the simplest regimen that allows fulfillment of your goals. This may be one of numerous multiple-injection regimens or it may be a regimen based on using the insulin pump.

Multiple injections. It is possible with the insulins available today to be quite creative in a multiple-injection regimen. A total of 39 different regimens were used in the DCCT, and at that time lispro, aspart, and glargine were not available.

There are a number of regimens that are commonly used and make good sense. Common NPH reg-

TABLE 3: Common Regimens Using Ultralente Plus Regular, Lispro, or Aspart Insulin

Here are four examples of the ways in which Ultralente can be combined with either Regular or lispro insulin (and in one case, NPH). Which regimen works best depends on the individual's needs.

MORNING	NOON	EVENING	BEDTIME
Regular, lispro, or aspart	Regular, lispro, or aspart	Regular, lispro, or aspart	Ultralente
Regular, lispro, or aspart	Regular, lispro, or aspart	Ultralente plus Regular, lispro, or aspart	no injection
Ultralente plus Regular, lispro, or aspart	Regular, lispro, or aspart	Ultralente plus Regular, lispro, or aspart	no injection
Ultralente plus Regular, lispro, or aspart	Regular, lispro, or aspart	Regular, lispro, or aspart	NPH

TABLE 4: Common Regimens Using Glargine Plus a Short- or Rapid-Acting Insulin

Here are three examples of the ways in which glargine can be combined with short- or rapid-acting insulin. Whether Regular, lispro, or aspart is used depends on individual choice and need.

MORNING	NOON	EVENING	BEDTIME
Regular, lispro, or aspart	Regular, lispro, or aspart	Regular, lispro, or aspart	Glargine
Glargine plus Regular, lispro, or aspart	Regular, lispro, or aspart	Regular, lispro, or aspart	no injection
Glargine plus Regular, lispro, or aspart	Regular, lispro, or aspart	Regular, lispro, or aspart	Glargine

imens using Regular, lispro, or aspart as a bolus insulin are listed in Table 2 on page 117. The first regimen, NPH and bolus insulin twice a day, has the advantage of simplicity. The disadvantages are that nighttime low blood sugar can occur, and the noon meal is not always well covered. The second regimen in the table moves the evening NPH dose to bedtime, thus helping to avoid nighttime low blood sugar, and provides better control over the fasting blood glucose.

Regimen three adds a noon dose of short- or rapid-acting insulin to the basic two-injection regimen. This gives better control of the noon meal, but it may not control overnight glucose as well as regimen two. The fourth regimen involves four injections and addresses all the problems, including lunch and overnight glucose control. The fifth option is also a four-injection regimen but does not include a morning dose of NPH. This regimen works for people whose bedtime NPH carries them through 24 hours.

For some individuals, NPH, even in small amounts, appears to provide too high a background insulin. A shift to Ultralente or glargine as a background insulin may be the right step for them (see Table 3 on this page for examples of regimens with Ultralente). These background insulins used in conjunction with

bolus insulin, as in the first through third regimens in Table 3, may be a good choice for individuals with variable routines. The biggest problem with Ultralente and glargine regimens is that for some people these regimens are not sufficient to suppress glucose production by the liver overnight. Another approach to erratic and high fasting-blood-glucose levels is shown in regimen four: Ultralente (or glargine) in the morning and NPH at bedtime. This allows low basal levels during the day and a higher level during the night.

For many people with diabetes, and especially those who are prone to hypoglycemia, glargine may be a better choice as a background insulin than NPH or Ultralente. Glargine in combination either with a rapid-acting insulin such as aspart or lispro or with Regular insulin given at each meal can mimic the action of a normally functioning pancreas (see Table 4 on this page). If you use glargine, remember that it cannot be mixed with another insulin in the same syringe but must always be given separately. Although glargine is usually given once a day prior to bedtime, usually 9 PM to 10 PM, it may actually work better for some people when given in the morning instead.

The insulin pump. This device is about the size of a beeper and contains a syringe, reservoirs for insulin, a

TABLE 5: Sᴀᴍᴘʟᴇ Bᴀsɪᴄ Iɴsᴜʟɪɴ Rᴇɢɪᴍᴇɴ

In a basic insulin regimen, the same amount and type of insulin is injected at the same time every day. Blood glucose goals are achieved by maintaining consistency in diet (both the amount of food eaten and the times at which it is eaten) and exercise (both the timing and amount of activity). In the example below, such measures kept blood glucose levels close to the target goal range—60 mg/dl to 120 mg/dl.

	MORNING		NOON		EVENING		BEDTIME	
Day	Blood Glucose (mg/dl)	Insulin (units)	Blood Glucose (mg/dl)	Insulin (units)	Blood Glucose (mg/dl)	Insulin (units)	Blood Glucose (mg/dl)	Insulin (units)
1	101	5 Regular 8 NPH	98	none	113	7 Regular	83	21 NPH
2	119	5 Regular 8 NPH	109	none	94	7 Regular	125	21 NPH
3	69	5 Regular 8 NPH	74	none	120	7 Regular	105	21 NPH

TABLE 6: Sᴀᴍᴘʟᴇ Aᴄᴛɪᴠᴇ Iɴsᴜʟɪɴ Rᴇɢɪᴍᴇɴ

In an active insulin regimen, insulin can be added or subtracted in response to blood glucose levels or in anticipation of more or less food or activity than usual. Adjusting your insulin accurately requires working out an insulin supplementation scale with your doctor. In this example, insulin additions or subtractions are in parentheses.

	MORNING		NOON		EVENING		BEDTIME	
Day	Blood Glucose (mg/dl)	Insulin (units)	Blood Glucose (mg/dl)	Insulin (units)	Blood Glucose (mg/dl)	Insulin (units)	Blood Glucose (mg/dl)	Insulin (units)
1	167	5 Regular 8 NPH (+1 Regular)	105	none	59	7 Regular (−1 Regular)	97	21 NPH
2	100	5 Regular 8 NPH	126	none	184	7 Regular (+2 Regular)	132	21 NPH
3	97	5 Regular 8 NPH	84	(+2 Regular)*	103	7 Regular	123	21 NPH

* Indicates units of Regular taken for a change in food intake.

TABLE 7: Sᴇʟꜰ-Mᴏɴɪᴛᴏʀɪɴɢ Rᴇᴄᴏʀᴅs

Keeping good records of your blood glucose levels and insulin injections is key to developing a basic insulin regimen. The example below shows what type of insulin was injected and when, as well as the blood glucose level at the time of injection. This person's target goal range was 60 mg/dl to 120 mg/dl. The high levels at noon indicate that an adjustment is needed.

	MORNING		NOON		EVENING		BEDTIME	
Day	Blood Glucose (mg/dl)	Insulin (units)	Blood Glucose (mg/dl)	Insulin (units)	Blood Glucose (mg/dl)	Insulin (units)	Blood Glucose (mg/dl)	Insulin (units)
1	99	6 Regular 10 NPH	146	none	117	3 Regular 7 NPH	132	none
2	101	6 Regular 10 NPH	183	none	106	3 Regular 7 NPH	113	none
3	87	6 Regular 10 NPH	157	none	98	3 Regular 7 NPH	79	none

small micropump, and a microchip. Insulin is pumped through a length of thin, flexible tubing connected to a needle inserted in the abdomen. The pump is usually worn on a belt, and the tubing and needle are changed every two to three days.

Pumps can be programmed to deliver a constant low rate of rapid- or short-acting insulin as background insulin, and can be set to change the infusion rate automatically; usual rates may vary anywhere from 0.5 to 2.0 units of insulin per hour. A bolus dose of insulin can be delivered by pushing a button on the pump before you eat. Insulin pumps can be very effective for individuals whose erratic or poor absorption of intermediate- or long-acting insulin makes it difficult to set up a predictable background insulin.

Special considerations

One major challenge in choosing the right insulin regimen is to find one that prevents a high fasting blood glucose. There are several reasons why a blood glucose level may be high. One is that background insulin is too low to control glucose output by the liver overnight. Another is the rebound effect, in which too much background insulin early in the night results in a low blood glucose level around 1 AM to 4 AM, causing the liver to release a surge of glucose. The third possible reason is the "dawn effect." Blood glucose may stay level through the first part of the night but start to rise around 3 AM to 4 AM. The rise is caused by the release of hormones such as adrenaline and cortisol. Part of your body's mechanism for waking you up, they also depress insulin levels, thus activating glucose release from the liver. Determining which problem is causing elevated blood glucose levels in the morning may require a series of blood glucose checks at around 3 AM.

Setting up an insulin regimen

How much insulin do I need? Which regimen should I use to have better control or more flexibility? When you are making these decisions, considerations such as your weight, your daily schedule, how physically active you are, your food preferences, and the time of your meals all play a role. You can use your present insulin regimen as a starting point.

In a basic insulin regimen, blood glucose goals are achieved by maintaining consistency in diet, exercise, and basal and bolus insulin. Insulin supplementation—in which insulin is added or subtracted on the basis of blood glucose levels, anticipated food consumption, or physical activity—is not needed or used. This basic regimen is adequate for some people (see Table 5 on page 119), but others need greater flexibility. In fact, most people need an active insulin regimen. The active regimen uses the basic regimen as a foundation, but it allows the user to add or delete doses of short-acting

insulin to bring the next blood glucose value into target range (see Table 6 on page 119).

The first step when considering intensification is to establish or reestablish your basic insulin regimen. The key to evaluating and changing the basic regimen is *pattern control*. In general, the principles of using pattern control to adjust insulin include first establishing blood glucose goals and then looking for a glucose pattern. Patterns can help identify which insulin and dose is responsible for what, and what changes might need to be made. Table 7 on page 119 provides a simple example of blood glucose patterns. In this example, the person's blood glucose levels before lunch consistently exceed the target blood glucose goals of 60 mg/dl to 120 mg/dl. Therefore, the morning Regular insulin should be increased. Table 7 shows a basic insulin regimen using NPH and Regular insulins, but the principles are the same for regimens that use Ultralente and glargine as background insulins and lispro or aspart as rapid-acting insulins.

Begin by collecting your data. For four to seven days, continue your routine activities, trying to be consistent in activity and food. Test your blood glucose four times a day. With your data in hand, see if you can identify any patterns. If a change seems called for, the dose can be adjusted in small increments of 1 to 2 units. The effect of the adjustment should be observed for two to three days before further changes are made.

The second important part of your insulin regimen is supplementation. Supplements can be used to control day-to-day variations. The goal of any addition or subtraction of fast-acting insulin is to bring the next scheduled blood glucose value into target range. You can anticipate by adding insulin for extra food or compensate by adding insulin for a high blood glucose level. Insulin may be subtracted when extra activity is anticipated. All those following an active regimen would have a set of supplemental doses tied to blood glucose levels and based on their own goals. Supplement scales can be simple or complex. Addition or subtraction of insulin for food can be based on carbohydrate counting or experience. Many people have developed set supplements for particular foods such as pizza. If supplements are consistently needed at a certain time of day, this means that the basic insulin dose is not adequate and should be adjusted.

Intensification of your diabetes regimen may seem complex and may take some up-front effort, but the rewards of achieving success can be great. Improvement in blood glucose control is obviously a major goal, but many people find increased lifestyle flexibility and an improved feeling of well-being almost as important. If you feel that changes are needed in your current regimen, talk to your doctor and health-care team about working with them to establish a new program. ❏

DRUGS AND DIETARY SUPPLEMENTS

AN ASPIRIN A DAY
NEW RECOMMENDATIONS

by Daniel L. Lorber, M.D.

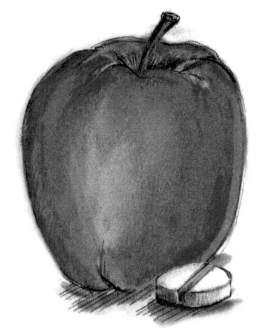

Heart disease continues to be the single most common killer of people with Type 2 diabetes, far surpassing any other chronic complication of diabetes as a cause of death. People with diabetes are two to four times more likely to die from heart disease than people without diabetes.

Diabetes alone raises a person's risk of heart disease. A sedentary lifestyle and poor physical condition compound that risk. Many people with Type 2 diabetes also have characteristics of the insulin-resistance syndrome ("Syndrome X"), including abnormal blood lipids (cholesterol and triglycerides), obesity, high blood pressure, and insulin resistance. When combined with the effects of chronic high blood sugar, these factors significantly raise the risk of developing blood clots and thickening of the lining of blood vessels—factors that further increase the risk of heart attack and stroke.

But the good news is that having diabetes doesn't mean you can't lower your risk. One of the newest weapons we have today to reduce the risk of heart attack and stroke is one of the oldest medicines available: aspirin.

For years, experts have recommended an aspirin a day to prevent the occurrence of a second stroke or heart attack. Whether that general recommendation applied to people with diabetes was unclear—until recently. In November 1997, the American Diabetes Association issued the recommendation that aspirin therapy be used by people with diabetes at high risk for heart disease to prevent not just a second but also a first heart attack or stroke.

What follows is a review of aspirin's role in preventing heart disease and a summary of the American Diabetes Association's recommendation.

How aspirin works

In people with diabetes, *platelets* (cell fragments that normally play a role in blood clotting after injury) are "stickier" and clump more easily than in people without diabetes. When blood sugar levels run high, platelets clump together and stick to each other and to blood vessel walls even more easily. Once platelets begin sticking together and to other cells, they begin to produce *thromboxane,* a hormone-like substance that promotes yet more clumping and eventually leads to a blood clot. Platelet clumping constricts blood vessels, making it difficult for oxygen-rich blood to flow to the heart, brain, and other organs throughout the body. When blood clots get stuck in blood vessels, a heart attack or stroke may result. Aspirin reduces the risk of heart attack and stroke by inhibiting the production of thromboxane.

Clinical studies support the use of aspirin to prevent a first or second heart attack in people with or without diabetes who are at risk for heart disease. The U.S. Physicians' Health Study, for example, found a

44% reduction in the risk of a first heart attack in men taking low-dose aspirin (325 milligrams every other day) after a five-year period. In 1994, the Antiplatelet Trialists' Collaboration conducted a massive review of studies that used aspirin and other antiplatelet therapy in people who had preexisting heart disease. The review found that in people at high risk for heart disease, aspirin in doses of 75 to 325 mg/day (milligrams per day) offered significant protection against heart attack, stroke, and death. However, the review also pointed out that there is not enough evidence to advise people at low risk for heart disease to take aspirin on a daily basis for preventive measures.

The largest study of aspirin therapy in people with diabetes is the Early Treatment Diabetic Retinopathy Study. It involved more than 3700 men and women with Type 1 or Type 2 diabetes, half of whom had preexisting heart disease. Results of the first five years of the study revealed a 28% decrease in heart attack risk as a result of daily aspirin treatment. Thus, it showed that aspirin is effective for the prevention of a first or second heart attack in people with diabetes. Similar results were found in the Antiplatelet Trialists' review and the U.S. Physicians' Health Study when data pertaining only to people with diabetes was examined.

Aspirin safety

In developing its recommendations, the American Diabetes Association noted the most common side effects of aspirin therapy and included precautions for safe use. The major risks of aspirin therapy are stomach irritation and bleeding. However, these side effects are rare when low doses of buffered aspirin (75 to 325 milligrams once a day) are used. The coating on buffered aspirin helps it to pass through the stomach undigested so that it can be absorbed in the intestine.

Some studies have also found a slight increase in hemorrhagic stroke (stroke resulting from bleeding from an artery supplying blood to the brain) in people on aspirin therapy. But their risk was not found to be significantly higher than that of people not taking aspirin.

Dosage

Currently, doctors generally recommend low-dose aspirin therapy in the form of one adult aspirin (325 milligrams) or one "baby aspirin" (81 milligrams) every day for protection against heart attack and stroke in people with risk factors for heart disease such as high blood pressure or abnormal lipid levels.

According to the Antiplatelet Trialists' review, most studies of aspirin and antiplatelet therapy found that low doses (75–81 mg/day) are as effective as, and pos-

ARE YOU AT RISK?

Diabetes is only one of the many factors that can increase your risk of developing heart disease. Some other factors that raise your risk include the following:

- Family history of heart disease
- Cigarette smoking
- High blood pressure
- Obesity (more than 20% above desirable weight)
- Albuminuria or proteinuria (protein in the urine)
- Total cholesterol greater than 200 mg/dl
- LDL cholesterol greater than 100 mg/dl
- HDL cholesterol less than 45 mg/dl in men and 55 mg/dl in women
- Triglycerides greater than 150 mg/dl

sibly are more effective than, large doses (up to 1500 mg/day) of aspirin. Doses of up to 325 mg/day have been shown to effectively reduce heart disease risk in people with conditions that involve the rapid production of new platelets, including diabetic vascular disease. Therefore, the American Diabetes Association recommends that buffered aspirin be used, in doses of 81–325 mg/day.

Summary of recommendations

Here is a summary of the American Diabetes Association's recommendations on low-dose aspirin therapy as of 2002:

1. Low-dose aspirin therapy should be used to prevent a second heart attack in men and women with diabetes who have large-vessel disease. Evidence of large-vessel disease includes a history of heart attack, chest pain, vascular bypass surgery or angioplasty, stroke, or peripheral vascular disease (narrowing of blood vessels in the arms or legs).

2. Aspirin therapy should also be considered to help prevent a first heart attack or stroke in all high-risk men and women with diabetes. (See "Are You At Risk?" on this page for a list of factors that place a person at high risk of heart disease.)

3. While aspirin therapy may be an effective prevention strategy for people at high risk for heart attack and stroke, it may not be right for everyone. It is not recommended for anyone under 21 or for people under age 30 with no cardiac risk factors. People with any of the following medical conditions may also be poor candidates for aspirin therapy:

- Allergy to aspirin
- Bleeding tendency
- Undergoing anticoagulant therapy
- Recent bleeding in the digestive tract
- Clinically active liver disease

It is possible that aspirin therapy may reduce the beneficial effects of so-called ACE inhibitor drugs in people with established heart disease; the American Diabetes Association suggests that alternatives to aspirin be considered for such people.

A new tool

You may already be taking measures to reduce your risk of heart disease, such as controlling your blood pressure and managing your blood lipids. Now, you may be able to add aspirin therapy to your efforts. Check with your doctor to see if it's right for you. Heart risk reduction can become as much a part of your daily routine as watching your diet, injecting insulin, and taking diabetes medicines. ❑

METFORMIN
How It Works
by Charles A. Reasner, M.D.

The diabetes drug metformin was big news when it came on the United States market in 1995. Although it had been available in Europe for 30 years and Canada for 20, it was the first drug in a class called *biguanides* to be sold in the United States since 1977. That entire class of drugs was pulled off the market at that time because of complications arising from some of them. But in view of three decades of safe and effective use abroad, in 1994, the U.S. Food and Drug Administration (FDA) was ready to reconsider and allow at least one biguanide, metformin, on the market, under the brand name Glucophage. The number of prescriptions for metformin skyrocketed almost immediately upon its market debut, and in its first five years some 5 million people were treated with it. In 2002 the FDA authorized the marketing of generic versions of the drug.

Unlike older diabetes drugs—namely, sulfonylureas and insulin—metformin does not increase the amount of insulin circulating in the blood. Rather, it lowers blood glucose by enabling the body to better use its own insulin. Since 1995, advances by researchers in their understanding of what causes Type 2 diabetes, combined with the results of recent clinical trials, have clarified the best ways to use metformin in treating Type 2 diabetes.

The main reason to use metformin is to lower blood sugar levels. Maintaining lower blood sugar levels significantly reduces the risk of developing *microvascular* (small blood vessel) complications. Microvascular complications include retinopathy (eye disease), nephropathy (kidney disease), and neuropathy (nerve disease).

In addition to lowering blood sugar levels, metformin has beneficial effects on blood lipids (triglycerides and cholesterol) and body weight. Elevated triglycerides and cholesterol and excess body weight (all of which are common among people with Type 2 diabetes) increase the risk for *macrovascular* disease, or diseases of the large blood vessels. An example of macrovascular disease is *atherosclerosis,* or narrowing of the arteries, which is known to raise the risk of heart attack and stroke. Metformin's effects on blood lipids and body weight may be as important as its ability to control blood sugar in preventing the complications associated with Type 2 diabetes.

This article takes a look at some studies that have demonstrated the wide-ranging benefits of metformin; it also discusses the use of metformin in combination with other diabetes drugs.

About Type 2 diabetes

Type 2 diabetes is characterized by two primary problems: insulin resistance and insufficient insulin secretion. Insulin resistance, which occurs first, leads to reduced uptake of glucose by muscle and fat cells and increased production of glucose by the liver. Normally, insulin signals the body's tissues to allow glucose to enter the cells. In a person with insulin resistance, this signal does not work well, and for a given amount of insulin, less glucose enters the cell.

Initially, individuals with Type 2 diabetes compensate for their insulin resistance by making two to three times more insulin than people who don't have diabetes. As the condition progresses, however, the insulin-producing cells in the pancreas, called the beta cells, get burned out by the high demand for insulin and produce progressively less insulin. This lack of insulin secretion causes blood sugar levels to rise. Eventually, the pancreas may make so little insulin that the person must inject insulin.

Insulin resistance can cause more trouble than just high blood sugar levels. People with insulin resistance are likely to have other conditions that are often referred to as components of the "insulin-resistance syndrome," or "Syndrome X." These conditions include obesity, high blood pressure, high triglyceride and cholesterol levels (but low levels of HDL cholesterol, the "good" cholesterol), and high levels of insulin in the blood (called *hyperinsulinemia*).

Each component of the insulin-resistance syndrome is a significant risk factor for heart attack and stroke. Since the cause of death in 70% of people with Type 2 diabetes is some form of heart or blood vessel disease, treatment of Type 2 diabetes must address these cardiovascular risk factors.

Microvascular complications

Numerous studies in recent years have shown that maintaining blood sugar levels as close to normal as possible reduces the incidence of microvascular (small blood vessel) complications associated with diabetes, which include retinopathy, nephropathy, and neuropathy. The Diabetes Control and Complications Trial examined the risk of developing microvascular complications in two groups of people with Type 1 diabetes. It found that persons with a glycosylated hemoglobin (HbA_{1c}) test result greater than 7% (indicating an average blood glucose level of about 140 mg/dl) had a dramatically increased risk of developing eye disease, kidney disease, or nerve disease. The HbA_{1c} test gives an estimate of a person's average blood sugar level over the past three months.

The importance of blood glucose control in preventing microvascular complications in people with Type 2 diabetes was shown in the United Kingdom Prospective Diabetes Study (UKPDS). In this study, 4,209 people newly diagnosed with Type 2 diabetes were initially treated with diet alone, with drugs that increased the concentration of insulin in the blood (either injected insulin or sulfonylureas), or with metformin. Metformin was given to overweight participants only.

The study began to enroll people in 1977, and participants were monitored for an average of 11 years. Those people initially treated with insulin or sulfonylureas had similar reductions in blood sugar levels and were able to maintain a 0.9% lower HbA_{1c} concentration than people initially treated with diet alone. The participants initially treated with diet alone maintained an average blood sugar level of approximately 175 mg/dl, while those treated initially with insulin or sulfonylureas had average blood glucose levels of 140 mg/dl. This modest reduction in blood sugar was associated with a 25% reduction in microvascular complications. In fact, 21% fewer people developed eye disease, 33% fewer people showed evidence of kidney damage, and 40% fewer people developed nerve problems. These results reinforce the need for aggressively lowering blood sugar levels in people with Type 2 diabetes.

Macrovascular disease

About 50% of people with Type 2 diabetes already have significant atherosclerosis, a form of macrovascular disease, at the time their diabetes is diagnosed. Atherosclerosis is a disease characterized by the buildup of plaques in the inner lining of the arteries. Such buildup narrows the opening through which blood flows and can lead to angina (chest pain), heart attack, and stroke. Given the very serious nature of atherosclerosis, it is imperative that treatment of people with Type 2 diabetes include measures to prevent and treat this problem. The use of metformin has been shown to reduce the risks associated with atherosclerosis.

In the UKPDS, metformin was shown to lower the risk of heart attacks and strokes when given as initial therapy to people who were overweight and had Type 2 diabetes. Here's what happened: About 1,700 overweight individuals newly diagnosed with Type 2 diabetes were randomly assigned to one of three treatment groups. Group 1 received initial dietary therapy. Group 2 was initially treated with either a sulfonylurea or insulin to address a lack of insulin secretion. Group 3 was started on metformin to address insulin resistance.

During the 11-year follow-up, participants treated with insulin or sulfonylureas or metformin maintained HbA_{1c} concentrations of 0.5% to 1% lower than participants treated with diet alone. Compared with the group treated with diet alone, those in the group that took metformin had a 29% reduction in microvascular (small blood vessel) complications. People initially treated with sulfonylureas or insulin had a 16% reduction in microvascular complications. (The difference in reduction between these groups was not considered statistically significant by researchers.) However, those individuals who were initially treated with metformin also showed a dramatic reduction in macrovascular complications, as compared with the diet-treatment group.

The surprising reductions in heart attacks, stroke, and diabetes-related and all-cause mortality seen with metformin therapy in the UKPDS confirm the benefits of a diabetes drug that addresses the cardiovascular risk factors associated with Type 2 diabetes as well as lowering blood sugar levels. Because of its beneficial effects on all components of the insulin-resistance syndrome, metformin is an ideal first drug for people with Type 2 diabetes.

Metformin's effects on blood glucose

Metformin lowers blood glucose in a couple of ways. It works mainly by preventing the liver from overproducing glucose. To understand how this works, it helps to know that not all of the glucose in your blood comes from the food you eat. Between meals and during the night, the liver can make glucose to meet the body's energy needs. In Type 2 diabetes, however, too much glucose is produced, resulting in high blood sugar levels. Metformin puts the brakes on this overproduction of glucose. It also reduces the amount of fat and cholesterol produced by the liver.

Metformin also lowers blood glucose by countering insulin resistance in the muscle and fat cells. That is, it makes muscle and fat cells more sensitive to insulin and better able to take in glucose after a person eats. Rather than circulating in the bloodstream after a meal, glucose can be used by muscles as a source of energy or converted into fat, or stored energy.

A large study designed to test the ability of metformin to lower blood glucose involved 451 people with Type 2 diabetes. For all of the participants, neither diet alone nor diet combined with a sulfonylurea had previously provided adequate blood sugar control. One group received a placebo (a pill that has no drug in it). The other group received metformin in a variety of doses: 500 milligrams (mg) a day, 500 mg twice a day, 500 mg three times a day, 1,000 mg twice a day, or 2,500 mg (1,000 mg with breakfast, 500 mg with lunch, and 1,000 mg with dinner).

At the end of 14 weeks, the group treated with metformin saw reductions in fasting blood sugar (the level before breakfast) and HbA_{1c} concentrations compared to the group receiving a placebo. When compared to placebo, metformin reduced mean fasting blood glucose by 19 mg/dl at the dose of 500 milligrams per day and by up to 78 mg/dl at the 2,000-milligrams-per-day dose. HbA_{1c} concentrations were similarly lowered: from 0.8% at the lowest dose to 2.0% at the 2,000-milligrams-per-day dose.

While the average daily dose of metformin prescribed by doctors in the United States was less than 1,400 milligrams per day, this clinical study showed that increasing the dose of metformin to 2,000 milligrams per day would benefit most people.

Effects on lipids

Metformin has consistently been shown to lower blood levels of triglycerides and cholesterol (collectively called blood lipids). Studies suggest that larger doses of metformin lower blood lipid levels more than smaller doses. In a study comparing the effects of 1,500 milligrams per day with 3,000 milligrams per day, the higher dosage led to a statistically significant decrease in triglyceride and cholesterol levels relative to placebo.

The lipid-lowering effect of metformin at dosages up to 3,000 milligrams per day suggests that higher doses of metformin may have a beneficial effect on cardiovascular risk factors, even when adequate blood sugar levels have been achieved with lower doses. For example, when metformin was given for 29 weeks at a dose of 2,500 milligrams per day, total cholesterol levels were reduced by 5%, while LDL-cholesterol ("bad cholesterol") levels were reduced by about 8% and triglycerides were decreased by a maximum of 16%. The effect of metformin on blood lipids is seen even in people who don't have diabetes, and it does not depend on changes in blood sugar levels or body weight.

Effects on body weight

Unlike other drugs used to treat diabetes—including sulfonylureas, meglitinides, and insulin—metformin is not associated with weight gain. In the UKPDS, after nine years of follow-up, body weight increased by 11 pounds in people treated with sulfonylureas and by over 15 pounds in people treated with insulin. In contrast, people treated with metformin or diet gained only slightly more than 2 pounds. Metformin has been shown to produce weight loss in both obese and nonobese people with Type 2 diabetes. Most of this weight loss appears to result from loss of fat tissue. Clinical studies have demonstrated that this weight reduction can be sustained for at least one year.

It has been suggested that metformin promotes satiety, or a feeling of fullness after eating, thus decreasing food consumption and producing weight loss. In a study that compared a daily dose of metformin of 1,700 milligrams to a daily dose of 850 milligrams, people receiving 1,700 milligrams per day achieved a maximum weight loss of approximately 17 pounds more than people taking a placebo. It should also be noted that when used together with sulfonylureas or insulin, metformin moderates the weight gain associated with these drugs.

Side effects

The most common side effects of metformin therapy are nausea and diarrhea, which occur in approximately 25% of people who take metformin. However, these side effects usually go away over time, and they may be minimized by starting with a low dose (one or two 500-milligram pills per day) and increasing the dose slowly. In addition, metformin should always be taken with meals. Larger doses of the drug do not appear to raise the incidence or the severity of side effects. In a large study in which daily doses of metformin were increased from 1,000 to 2,500 milligrams, there was no increase in the incidence of side effects when larger doses were given.

The most serious side effect associated with metformin is *lactic acidosis*, which is caused by a buildup of lactic acid in the blood. People with advanced kidney disease are at great risk of developing this complication and should not be treated with metformin. In fact, doctors should test kidney function in all patients before starting metformin therapy, as well as periodically after starting the drug and after a person has been exposed to any procedure that could cause kidney damage, such as surgery or use of a contrast dye.

Liver disease, congestive heart failure, and alcohol abuse (either chronic excessive drinking or "binge" drinking) all raise the risk of developing lactic acidosis, so people with any of these conditions should not use metformin. Since dehydration can also raise the risk of lactic acidosis, persons taking metformin should discuss with their doctor what to do during periods of illness or other special situations that might lead to dehydration.

Symptoms of lactic acidosis include feeling very weak or tired or having unusual muscle pain or unusual stomach discomfort. If you experience these symptoms while taking metformin, call your doctor. He or she will want to do a blood test to see if you have developed lactic acidosis.

In some people metformin may reduce the body's absorption of vitamin B_{12}, raising the risk of B_{12} deficiency, which can lead to nerve damage and other problems. Individuals who show signs of subnormal levels of the nutrient may be advised to take B_{12} supplements. There is some evidence suggesting that B_{12} deficiency attributable to metformin may also be reversible by taking calcium supplements.

Drug combinations

Early in the course of Type 2 diabetes, most people are able to achieve near-normal blood sugar levels by using one diabetes drug along with exercising and following a diet. Over time, however, a person's pancreas makes less and less insulin, making blood sugar control more difficult. Usually, combining diabetes drugs that work in different ways brings blood sugar levels back down to the desired range.

Drugs that increase insulin release. Sulfonylureas and meglitinides increase insulin production by the pancreas and can be used with metformin if metformin alone does not lower blood sugar levels enough. Studies have shown that the addition of either drug lowers blood glucose more than metformin alone.

In a study that enrolled 632 people, the blood-glucose-lowering effects of metformin and the sulfonylurea glyburide (brand names DiaBeta, Glynase, and Micronase) were shown to be additive. When metformin was combined with glyburide in 213 people, HbA_{1c} results dropped from 8.8% to 7.1% at week 29 of the study, total cholesterol levels fell from 216 mg/dl to 206 mg/dl, and triglyceride levels were lowered from 216 mg/dl to 194 mg/dl. By comparison, mean HbA_{1c} measurements and total cholesterol and triglyceride levels all rose in the study participants who continued therapy with glyburide alone.

Similar results were seen in another study, which enrolled 83 people who had an HbA_{1c} concentration greater than 7.1% when taking metformin alone. In this study, participants either switched to the meglitinide drug repaglinide, continued taking metformin, or took both oral pills. A synergistic effect—meaning the total effect was greater than the sum of the individual effects—was seen with the metformin-repaglinide combination.

In 2000 the FDA approved for marketing a combination of metformin and glyburide in one pill, with the brand name Glucovance.

Insulin. In many people with Type 2 diabetes, the beta cells in the pancreas eventually cease producing insulin. When this happens, the person must begin injecting insulin. However, even when a person with Type 2 diabetes requires insulin, there is good reason to continue taking one or more oral pills along with insulin. That's because injected insulin only addresses the problem of a lack of insulin secretion. It does not address the problem of insulin resistance. And unless that problem is addressed, a person with Type 2 diabetes is likely to require very large doses of insulin to keep blood glucose levels in the desired range. In fact, it is not uncommon for a person with Type 2 diabetes to require two or three times as much insulin as a typical person with Type 1 diabetes. Large doses of insulin stimulate the appetite, usually causing a person to overeat and gain weight.

A study done in 1993 involving 14 people with Type 2 diabetes demonstrates how large doses of insulin can affect body weight. After one month in the study, the 14 people required an average of 86 units of insulin per day to maintain blood glucose control. At the end of the six-month study, they required an average of 100 units of insulin per day to control their blood sugar levels. During these six months, the participants gained on average about 18 pounds in spite of monthly visits with a dietitian. The increase in body weight was directly related to the increase in the dose of insulin. As insulin doses increase and body weight goes up, a vicious circle is created, in which weight gain increases insulin resistance, which necessitates the use of more insulin, which causes yet more weight gain, and so on.

There are at least two good reasons to combine metformin with insulin in people with Type 2 diabetes who require insulin therapy: For one thing, the combination of metformin and insulin allows a person to achieve better blood glucose control, which lowers the risk of microvascular complications. For another, a reduction in risk factors associated with insulin resistance—excess body weight, high levels of LDL cholesterol, high levels of insulin in the blood, and high blood glucose—should result in a reduction in macrovascular complications. A number of studies have demonstrated the benefits of using metformin and insulin together.

A study published in 1998 in the journal *Diabetes* examined the effects of adding metformin to insulin in 43 people with Type 2 diabetes for whom approximately 100 units of insulin per day did not bring blood sugar levels into the desired range. Half of the people began taking metformin in addition to the insulin, and the other half took a placebo pill. Over the next six months, the dose of insulin was adjusted in both groups to try to achieve normal blood sugar levels. At the end of the six months, those treated with the combination of insulin and metformin required a mean of 33 fewer units of insulin per day than the placebo-insulin group, and their HbA_{1c} concentration was 1% lower. (In the UKPDS, a reduction in HbA_{1c} concentration of this magnitude resulted in a 25% reduction in microvascular complications.)

Factors associated with insulin resistance also can be improved by combining insulin with metformin. In a study of 51 people with Type 2 diabetes who were on an average daily dose of 126 units of insulin, the addition of metformin enabled them to lower the dose of insulin by 27 units per day and to obtain a 0.7% reduction in HbA_{1c} concentrations. In addition, people who took metformin lost 3 pounds and lowered their LDL (bad) cholesterol by 21 mg/dl.

After reviewing the two studies outlined above, the FDA gave its approval for the combined use of metformin and insulin.

More uses for metformin

There's no doubt metformin can be a big help to people who have Type 2 diabetes. But could it also help people who don't have it? In an ongoing study called the Diabetes Prevention Program, researchers are investigating whether metformin might be able to prevent or delay the onset of Type 2 diabetes in people at risk of developing it. They are also investigating whether metformin can slow down the progression of atherosclerosis in these same people. Other studies have shown that because metformin lowers insulin resistance, it is effective in treating such insulin-resistant conditions as polycystic ovary syndrome in women.

If you do not currently take metformin and this article has piqued your interest, we suggest you talk to your doctor about it. Besides the regular form of the drug, commonly taken two or three times a day, an extended release version is available (brand name Glucophage XR). Metformin is not for everyone, but for those who can take it, it can do a lot of good. ❏

OVER-THE-COUNTER DRUGS
WHAT'S SAFE TO TAKE?
by Kim Begany, R.Ph., Pharm.D.

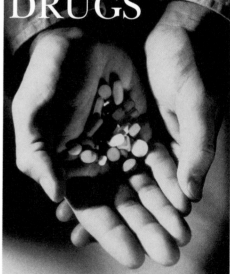

I t's Saturday afternoon and you begin coughing, develop a headache, or have a bout of diarrhea. You head down to the local pharmacy and face an aisle with hundreds of medicines. Which one is safe for you? You may already look for products that are sugar-free and alcohol-free, but are there other products you should avoid? Which ingredients in over-the-counter medicines might raise or lower your blood sugar? Are there any that might jeopardize your health or diabetes control in some other way?

This article takes a look at some of the most commonly used over-the-counter drugs and their effects and side effects, particularly those that might affect diabetes control. It lists many brand-name products and their active ingredients. (In some cases, generic products are also available with the same active ingredients.) However, because drug companies are constantly changing the ingredients in their products, it is important to read labels closely. For the same reason, it is impossible to provide an accurate list of sugar-free and alcohol-free products. If you are ever in doubt as to whether a product is safe for you to take, do not hesitate to ask your pharmacist or another health-care provider.

Pain relievers

Over-the-counter pain relievers are very effective in relieving mild pain and fever. There are many products to chose from, including acetaminophen, aspirin, ibuprofen, ketoprofen, and naproxen, as well as combinations of some of these.

While occasional use of nonprescription pain relievers, when taken as recommended on the package label, has little or no effect on blood sugar levels, there are some precautions to keep in mind. Aspirin, ibuprofen, ketoprofen, and naproxen can upset the stomach, and prolonged use of ibuprofen, ketoprofen, or naproxen, especially at high doses, can adversely affect the kidneys. Acetaminophen is rarely associated with stomach problems, but it can be toxic to the liver or kidneys if taken in doses larger than what's recommended on the package. High doses of aspirin (5 to 6 grams per day) can lower blood sugar levels.

If you require constant relief from pain for more than a few days, call your physician for advice on what to take. Oral pain relievers include the following:
- Acetaminophen (Tylenol)
- Acetaminophen, aspirin, and caffeine (Excedrin)
- Aspirin (Ascriptin, Bayer, Bufferin, Ecotrin)
- Ibuprofen (Advil, Motrin IB, Nuprin)
- Ketoprofen (Orudis KT)
- Naproxen (Aleve)

Even though external pain relievers, generally applied as ointments or creams to the skin, are often intended to relieve muscle aches, they may actually cause muscle pain or aggravate pain associated with neuropathy. Avoid products containing salicylic acid because they can irritate the skin and cause burning. Products containing capsaicin may be the most effective over-the-counter items for relieving painful neuropathy. But capsaicin may cause stinging, burning, or itching, and it may take three to four weeks to achieve optimal pain relief from a capsaicin cream.

External pain relievers include the following:
- Capsaicin (ArthriCare, Zostrix)
- Menthol (Absorbine, Flexall 454, Mineral Ice)
- Menthol and methyl salicylate (BenGay, Icy-Hot)
- Trolamine salicylate (Aspercreme, Myoflex, Sportscreme)

Upper respiratory symptoms

For the symptoms that commonly accompany the common cold, the flu, and some allergic reactions—runny nose, sneezing, sore throat, cough, muscle and joint aches, and fever—there is at least one product to address each, and more likely there are several. Many cold, flu, and allergy products contain active ingredients to relieve several or all of these symptoms at once. Typical remedies for upper respiratory symptoms include antihistamines, decongestants, cough relievers, expectorants, and pain relievers, and combinations of these ingredients.

Antihistamines (such as brompheniramine, chlorpheniramine, clemastine, diphenhydramine, doxylamine, and triprolidine) are found in most allergy, cold, and cough products. They dry the nose and eyes and relieve sneezing. All over-the-counter antihistamines cause drowsiness. Clemastine tends to cause the least amount of sedation. Be aware that these agents can cause impotence and loss of libido. If used sparingly, however, no adverse effects should be expected to occur.

A decongestant (such as phenylephrine or pseudoephedrine) is also found in most allergy, sinus, cold, cough, and flu products. Decongestants are used to relieve congestion in the nose and sinuses. Decongestants, generally speaking, may increase blood sugar. Topical products (nasal sprays), however, have less effect on blood sugar.

Dextromethorphan, a cough reliever, or antitussive, is found in many products. An expectorant, guaifenesin, is used to loosen phlegm in the throat and chest to make coughs more productive.

Most pharmaceutical companies make three to five versions of their product, each containing different ingredients or combinations of ingredients. For example, there's Robitussin (containing only an expectorant), Robitussin DM (containing an expectorant and a cough reliever), Robitussin PE (containing an expectorant and a decongestant), and Robitussin CF (containing an expectorant, a decongestant, and a cough reliever). This can be confusing, but it allows you to find a product that treats your specific symptoms and doesn't contain ingredients you don't need. That way, you avoid side effects from ingredients that are not giving you any relief. To avoid taking too much of any one ingredient, don't mix medicines without asking your pharmacist or other health-care provider first.

Products sold mainly for allergy relief include the following:
- Chlorpheniramine (Chlor-Trimeton)
- Diphenhydramine (Benadryl)
- Clemastine (Tavist Allergy)

Products intended to relieve one or more symptoms of colds, coughs, and the flu include the following:
- Antihistamine (Benadryl)
- Decongestant (Sudafed)
- Antihistamine and decongestant (Tavist-D, Dimetapp)
- Antihistamine, decongestant, and pain reliever (Motrin Cold and Flu)
- Antihistamine, decongestant, pain reliever, expectorant, and antitussive (Thera-Flu, Nyquil)

Nasal decongestant sprays and drops include the following:
- Oxymetazoline (Afrin, Dristan 12-Hour Nasal Spray, Vicks Sinex 12-Hour)
- Phenylephrine (Afrin Allergy, Dristan Nasal Spray, Neo-Synephrine, Vicks Sinex Ultra Fine Mist)
- Saline (Ocean)

Another option for relief of symptoms caused by the common cold or flu is a topical ointment such as Vicks VapoRub (containing camphor, menthol, and eucalyptus oil). These products, which are rubbed on the chest and throat, can relieve congestion and coughing with no bothersome side effects.

In addition to watching for the effects of over-the-counter cold and flu drugs on blood sugar, remember that infection itself tends to raise sugar levels. Close monitoring of blood sugar levels is necessary during a cold or flu.

Motion sickness products

Antihistamines are the primary nonprescription medicines used to prevent and control motion sickness. They can cause dry mouth, dry eyes, drowsiness, and urinary retention, as well as impotence or loss of libido. However, the occasional use of these products for motion sickness should have no long-term ill effects. Motion sickness products include the following:
- Dimenhydrinate (Dramamine)
- Meclizine (Bonine, Dramamine Less Drowsy Formula)

Sleep aids

Approximately one-third of all Americans suffer from insomnia, and many take over-the-counter products to help them nod off. However, if you have chronic sleep problems, see your doctor. An antihistamine is the active ingredient found in nonprescription sleep aids. As mentioned earlier, antihistamines can cause dry mouth, dry eyes, drowsiness the next day, and urinary retention. Impotence and loss of libido can occur if large doses are taken. Nonprescription sleep aids include the following:
- Diphenhydramine (Nytol, Sominex, Tylenol PM)
- Doxylamine (Unisom)

Stimulant products

Caffeine is the only stimulant approved by the U.S. Food and Drug Administration for nonprescription use. Moderate use is safe, but large doses can raise blood sugar levels.
- Caffeine (NoDoz, Vivarin)

Oral discomfort and oral hygiene

An occasional cold sore or canker sore can be effectively treated with an over-the-counter ointment. Persistent cold sores may need to be treated with a prescription medicine. Since products for treating cold sores, canker sores, and other types of mouth and tooth discomfort cause no adverse effects on blood sugar, they are safe for people with diabetes. Such products include the following:
- Benzocaine (Anbesol, Orajel, Zilactin-B)
- Camphor and phenol (Campho-Phenique)
- Dyclonine and allantoin (Tanac Medicated Gel)
- Docosanol (Abreva)
- Tannic acid (Zilactin)
- Tetracaine hydrochloride (Viractin)

Vaginal yeast infections

Nonprescription vaginal antifungal products are effective for treating most vaginal yeast infections, but not all vaginal infections are yeast infections. Self-treatment is most appropriate for women who have previously had a vaginal yeast infection diagnosed by a physician and who treated it with an over-the-counter product. It is also most appropriate for women who have no more than three vaginal infections per year and who have had none in the previous two months.

If you have never had a vaginal yeast infection diagnosed, have had more than three within the past 12 months, or have had one within the past two months, see your doctor before using an over-the-counter product. Frequent vaginal yeast infections can be a sign of high blood sugar or other serious medical problems; a physician should be consulted.

Over-the-counter antifungal products are available as suppositories, vaginal tablets, and creams. They include the following:
- Butoconazole (Femstat, Mycelex-3)
- Clotrimazole (Gyne-Lotrimin, Mycelex-7)
- Miconazole (Monistat 3, Monistat 7)

Premenstrual discomfort

Some women find relief from fluid retention, weight gain, bloating, and breast soreness associated with the menstrual cycle with over-the-counter products such as the following:

- Ibuprofen (Advil, Motrin, Nuprin)
- Pamabrom (Aqua-Ban, Diurex)
- Pamabrom and acetaminophen (Diurex PMS)
- Pamabrom, acetaminophen, and pyrilamine (Midol PMS, Pamprin Multi-Symptom, Premsyn PMS)

Gastrointestinal upset

Gastrointestinal complaints are common and can have any number of causes. Stress is a frequent cause of stomach and bowel upsets. Most problems are time-limited, and symptoms can be eased by home remedies or over-the-counter products. However, if you frequently experience gastrointestinal problems or your pain is severe, notify your physician. Frequent gastrointestinal symptoms can be a sign of diabetic gastroparesis, or slowed stomach emptying, which is best treated with advice and help from your health-care team.

Heartburn. Relief from heartburn, indigestion, or reflux can be attained with a stomach acid neutralizer or an acid blocker, which reduces production of stomach acid. Acid neutralizers (also called antacids) contain aluminum, calcium, magnesium, or sodium bicarbonate. Use of antacids containing magnesium can cause diarrhea. Use of products containing calcium or aluminum may cause constipation.

Recently, some prescription acid blockers were made available without a prescription. These products are stronger and more effective than antacids if heartburn or indigestion occurs frequently. These must be taken at least an hour before a meal.

Antacids on the market include the following:
- Aluminum hydroxide (Amphogel)
- Aluminum hydroxide and magnesium (Gaviscon, Maalox, Mylanta)
- Calcium carbonate (Tums)
- Calcium carbonate and magnesium (Rolaids, Mylanta Supreme)
- Magnesium hydroxide (Milk of Magnesia)
- Magaldrate (Riopan)
- Sodium bicarbonate, aspirin, and citric acid (Alka-Seltzer Original)

Over-the-counter acid blockers include the following:
- Cimetidine (Tagamet HB 200)
- Famotidine (Mylanta AR, Pepcid AC)
- Nizatidine (Axid AR)
- Ranitidine (Zantac 75)

Constipation. Causes of constipation are numerous, and while nonprescription laxatives are effective, they should be used with care. So-called bulk-forming laxatives can be used safely on a regular basis, but other types can actually interfere with normal bowel function if used too frequently. If constipation is a chronic problem, talk to your doctor about other possible treatments.

Laxatives are classified according to their mechanism of action. The different categories are bulk-forming, emollients, lubricants, saline, and stimulants. Try a bulk-forming laxative first. Don't ignore the urge to have a bowel movement. If necessary, try a stool softener. Bulk-forming laxatives include the following:
- Calcium polycarbophil (FiberCon)
- Methylcellulose (Citrucel)
- Psyllium (Fiberall, Metamucil)

The following products are stool softeners:
- Docusate calcium (Surfak)
- Docusate sodium (Colace, Correctol Stool Softener)

Other laxative products include the following:
- Bisacodyl (Correctol, Dulcolax, Fleets)
- Glycerin (Fleets glycerin suppositories)
- Mineral oil (Fleets Mineral Oil)
- Senna (Senokot)

Diarrhea. A common cause of diarrhea is a viral infection of the digestive tract. Diarrhea can also be caused by many medicines, particularly antibiotics. Over-the-counter antidiarrheals are effective at slowing the diarrhea, but they do not treat the underlying cause and may not be advisable in all cases. Antidiarrheals on the market include the following:
- Attapulgite (Diasorb, Kaopectate)
- Bismuth subsalicylate (Pepto-Bismol)
- Loperamide (Imodium AD)

Flatulence. Everyone produces gas, but some people produce an excessive amount that can be accompanied by pains and cramps. Avoiding foods that can produce flatus (such as beans, cabbage, onions, high-fiber foods, and dairy products if you have lactose intolerance) may be the most effective way to decrease flatulence. The gas caused as a side effect by prescription diabetes pills usually diminishes over time, as the body adjusts to the drug.

Pills or liquids that can be mixed with gas-producing foods are often very effective at reducing symptoms when food is the cause. Lactase enzyme is effective for many people who are lactose intolerant but would like to consume some dairy products. Alpha-galactosidase (Beano) can be added to beans and other foods to reduce the amount of gas produced. Simethicone is an alternative, but it must be used after symptoms occur. For relief from gas, try the following products:
- Alpha-galactosidase enzyme (Beano)
- Lactase enzyme (Dairy Ease, Lactaid)
- Simethicone (Gas-X, Mylanta Gas Relief, Phazyme)
- Simethicone, calcium carbonate, and magnesium hydroxide (DiGel)

Skin-care products

Keeping skin clean and moisturized is important for everyone and particularly for people with diabetes, who may be more susceptible to infection if blood sugar levels are high. Using a moisturizer prevents drying and cracking of the skin, which can let in infection. Minor cuts and scratches should be cleaned with soap and water. A mild first-aid cream or ointment can then be applied.

The active ingredients in dry skin products include the following:
- Glycerin
- Mineral oil
- Petrolatum

First-aid and mild wound-care products include the following:
- Polymixin B sulfate and neomycin (Neosporin)
- Polymixin B sulfate, bacitracin, and neomycin (Mycitracin, Neosporin Ointment)
- Povidone-iodine (Betadine)

Persons with diabetes can safely self-treat mild burns, sunburns, acne, and poison ivy, poison oak, or poison sumac with over-the-counter products. Remember, though, that all burns should initially be treated with cool water (not ice) to stop the burn process. If a condition worsens or shows signs of infection, contact your physician.

Products to ease burns and sunburns include the following:
- Benzocaine and methanol (Dermoplast)
- Benzocaine and benzethonium chloride (Lanacane)
- Lidocaine (Solarcaine)

Over-the-counter acne products include the following:
- Benzoyl peroxide (Benoxyl, Neutrogena Acne, Oxy Balance Cream, Oxy Balance 10)
- Salicylic acid (Aveeno Acne Treatment Bar, Clearasil, Noxzema, Oxy Balance Pads, Stridex Acne Pads)
- Sulfur (Fostril)

A variety of products exist that can tame itches caused by poison ivy, poison oak, poison sumac, insect bites, and in some cases eczema and similar problems. Among them are the following:
- Bentoquatam (Ivy Block)
- Calamine and diphenhydramine (Ivarest)
- Calamine and zinc oxide (Calamine)
- Diphenhydramine and zinc acetate (Benadryl Itch Stopping Cream)
- Hydrocortisone (Cortaid, Cortizone, Lanacort)
- Pramoxine and calamine (Caladryl)
- Pramoxine, camphor, and calamine (Aveeno Anti-itch)

Foot-care products

Good foot care is vital for people with diabetes. Numbness in the feet because of neuropathy may cause a person not to feel a hangnail, cut, or infection. Reduced blood circulation to the feet may impair the body's ability to heal small wounds on its own.

Probably the best thing you can do for your feet is to wear shoes that fit. It's also a good idea to inspect your feet daily for cracks, blisters, and abrasions. If you should detect any sign of infection, such as redness, warmth, swelling, or pus, you should see your doctor immediately.

The removal of corns, calluses, or warts should only be done under the supervision of a physician. Avoid over-the-counter callus, corn, and wart removers such as the following:
- Salicylic acid (Compound W, Clear Away, DuoFilm, DuoPlant)

Self-treatment of athlete's foot is generally safe for a person with diabetes. However, if the infection persists, consult your physician: An underlying infection may be hindering the healing process. The following products can be used to treat athlete's foot:
- Clotrimazole (Lotrimin AF)
- Miconazole (Micatin)
- Terbinafine (Lamisil Cream)
- Tolnaftate (Tinactin)

Weight-control products

Weight control is an important part of diabetes management. It is achieved most effectively by following a nutritious diet, exercising regularly, and modifying behaviors that lead to overeating or being sedentary. Over-the-counter weight-loss products, however, have generally had unimpressive results. Also, the only over-the-counter products available in the United States in recent years contained phenylpropanolamine (PPA), a decongestant that was also used in some cold preparations, which can elevate blood sugar and blood pressure. In late 2000, after researchers linked PPA with an increased risk of stroke, particularly among young women, the Food and Drug Administration requested that manufacturers withdraw products containing PPA from the market.

Smoking-cessation products

In addition to all its other health consequences, smoking increases a person's risk of developing diabetic complications. It decreases blood flow to the feet, raising the risk of developing foot ulcers; decreases blood flow to the penis, raising the risk of impotence; and dramatically raises the risk of stroke. Smoking cessation products can be very effective if you want to quit smoking. Many people find it helpful or even necessary to participate in a structured stop-smoking program, as well. Patches and chewing gum available over the counter to assist individuals in their efforts include the following:

■ Nicotine patches (Nicoderm CQ, Nicotrol)
■ Nicotine gum (Nicorette)

Taking care with OTC drugs

Diabetes isn't the only condition that can affect over-the-counter drug choices. Pregnant women should always consult their doctor about what's safe to take. People with chronic health problems such as glaucoma or liver or kidney disorders should do likewise. And elderly people, particularly those who use one or more prescription drugs, should discuss safe choices with their doctor.

When giving over-the-counter drugs to children, read the dosing instructions on the label. Many drugs only give dose information for children age two or older. However, some fever and pain medicines will soon bear labels listing safe doses for ages down to six months. If in doubt, call the doctor. Any parent of a child with diabetes should work out a written, sick-day care plan with the child's health-care team that specifies which drugs are safe to take at what doses during times of illness. Periodically review your child's plan with the health-care team as your child grows.

Even though over-the-counter drugs can be purchased by anyone, they have real effects and need to be treated with care and respect. Most are intended for occasional symptom relief or a short-term cure, not chronic use. If a label suggests an appropriate amount of time (days or weeks) to use the product, take that advice seriously. If you still have symptoms after that time, see your doctor for proper diagnosis and treatment. ❏

VITAMIN AND MINERAL SUPPLEMENTS
Do You Need One?

by Linnea Hagberg, R.D.

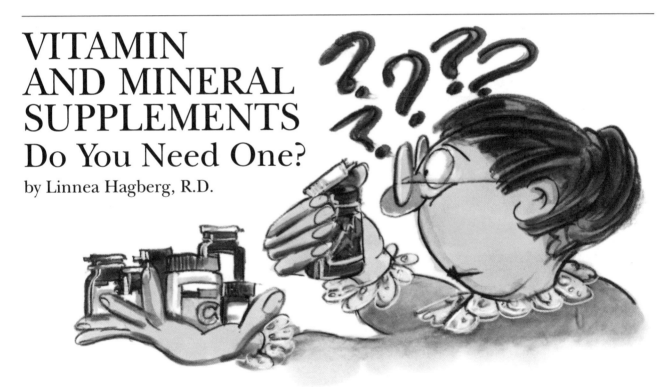

At the beginning of the 20th century, many vitamins had not yet been discovered. A few generations later, vitamin and mineral supplements had become a multi-billion-dollar industry. Navigating through the morass of media reports, advertising and label claims, and advice from coworkers, friends, and even near-strangers regarding supplements can be a tricky business, made more so by the nearly bewildering number and variety of products available. It can be difficult to distinguish between products that are essentially a modern version of snake oil and products with real health benefits, particularly when they are sold side by side.

It's clear that vitamins are not miracle pills. Nor are they necessarily benign products that can't do you any harm. However, while most health professionals take a firm "food first" approach, evidence is growing that for at least some of the people, some of the time, supplements can be helpful.

(Note: According to the U.S. Food and Drug Administration [FDA], the term "dietary supplement" refers to any product taken by mouth that contains a so-called "dietary ingredient" and whose label states it is a dietary supplement. These "dietary ingredients" may include vitamins, minerals, herbs, amino acids, enzymes, metabolites, and extracts. For the purpose of this article, however, the term "supplement" will refer only to vitamin and mineral supplements.)

What supplements aren't

While they may be hawked as magic bullets, curing everything from the common cold to heart disease, in reality, no supplement can provide a miracle cure, nor can popping pills make or keep you healthy. Supplements will not compensate for bad eating habits, counteract the damage done by poor blood sugar control, or make up for a sedentary lifestyle.

Supplements also cannot take the place of food. Isolated vitamins or minerals in a supplement do not provide the same benefits as whole foods. For example, while both a calcium supplement and a glass of skim milk will help keep bones healthy, only the milk also provides protein, potassium, riboflavin, vitamin B_6, and a number of other nutrients.

There may also be subtle interactions between nutrients in foods that help the body absorb and use the vitamins and minerals they contain. This action may not be duplicated when the vitamins and minerals are isolated in pill form. And food may contain substances with important health benefits that scientists have not yet uncovered.

Supplemental hazards

While it is extremely difficult to take in too much of a vitamin or mineral through food, there is a danger of overdosing with supplements, especially when a pill or two packs 10 to 20 times the Recommended Dietary Allowance for a nutrient. Excessive amounts of water-soluble vitamins (such as B vitamins and vitamin C) are usually excreted in the urine, but fat-soluble vitamins (A, D, E, and K) can be stored in the body and build up to toxic levels. It is also easy to take too high a dose of minerals since many are needed in only small amounts.

Consider just a few examples of the consequences of vitamin and mineral overdosing:

■ In a study of vitamin D intake, researchers found that four out of 39 study participants were getting far too much. Rather than helping their bones, these participants were actually losing bone density due to the toxic effects of excessive vitamin D.

■ While the mineral zinc is needed for a healthy immune system, regular daily intake in excess of 50 mg (milligrams) can decrease immune function

and lower levels of high-density lipoprotein (HDL) cholesterol (the "good" cholesterol); a daily intake exceeding 40 mg may impede the body's absorption of calcium.

■ Large doses of vitamin C can cause diarrhea, nausea, and vomiting.

In the world of supplements, it's generally best to err on the side of caution and take them only in amounts close to the Recommended Dietary Allowances unless you have detailed advice from your doctor to do otherwise.

Another potential problem in taking supplements lies in the complicated interactions between nutrients that take place in the body. In some cases, large doses of one nutrient can rob the body of another. For example, calcium can inhibit absorption of iron. So if you take a calcium supplement right after, say, a steak dinner, you may lose out on valuable iron. (To get around this, take calcium supplements after meals or snacks that don't contain much iron.)

Even moderate amounts of some vitamins and minerals can interfere with some drugs. For example, vitamins C and E can interfere with blood-thinning medicines.

Finally, there is always the possibility that taking supplements will provide a false sense of security and provide a convenient excuse for failing to eat healthfully.

How much do we need?

It would be convenient to look at what quantity of vitamins and minerals we need, subtract what we get from food, and then consider whether or not to cover any shortfalls with supplements. Unfortunately, it's not always easy to know what we need.

Traditionally, the Recommended Dietary Allowances (RDA's), issued by the Food and Nutrition Board of the U.S. Institute of Medicine, have been used for estimating nutrient need and nutritional adequacy. By definition, the RDA's are intended to reflect the level of intake of essential nutrients judged to be adequate to meet the known nutrient needs of practically all healthy people. Essentially, the RDA's were designed to prevent nutritional deficiency diseases. For example, the RDA that was used for vitamin C for years was set at a level (with a considerable margin for error) to prevent the deficiency disease scurvy. However, most current nutrition research centers on preventing and managing chronic disease. So the current RDA for vitamin C was established with an eye not only toward preventing scurvy but also toward the antioxidant protection the vitamin can offer.

In response to the growing understanding of the role of good nutrition in preventing chronic disease—and public hunger for such information—entire new sets of values, the Dietary Reference Intakes (DRI's), are being compiled and released by the Food and Nutrition Board. The DRI's, which take into account the role of nutrients in chronic disease, include (if sufficient data are available) the following reference values for each nutrient: a Recommended Dietary Allowance (RDA); an Estimated Average Requirement, used in establishing the RDA; a Tolerable Upper Intake Level (UL); and an Adequate Intake (AI), which is an estimate of the daily intake thought to be safe and sufficient and is used when there is not enough information to establish an RDA.

Dietary Reference Intakes are being developed for seven nutrient groups. As of the end of 2001, DRI reports had been issued for four: (1) calcium, vitamin D, phosphorus, magnesium, and fluoride; (2) folate and other B vitamins; (3) vitamins C and E and selenium; (4) vitamins A and K and the minerals arsenic, boron, chromium, copper, iodine, iron, manganese, molybdenum, nickel, silicon, vanadium, and zinc. (To learn more about the DRI's, visit the Institute of Medicine Web site, http://www.iom.edu. Click on Ongoing Studies; on the Ongoing Studies page, click on Food and Nutrition Board; on the Food and Nutrition Board page, click on Dietary Reference Intakes.)

When the report on DRI's for folate and other B vitamins was issued in 1998, recommendations were made for the first time that large groups of people take supplements or eat fortified foods. Specifically, to reduce the risk of having a child with neural tube defects, women of child-bearing age were advised to obtain 400 micrograms of supplemental folic acid in addition to eating a diet rich in the B vitamin folate. (Folic acid is a synthetic form of folate found only in supplements and fortified foods.)

In addition, the report advised those over age 50 to take supplemental vitamin B_{12} or use fortified foods. This is because as many as 30% of older adults cannot properly absorb food sources of B_{12}, partly because they don't have enough acid in their stomachs to "free" the B_{12} from the food it is bound to.

In general, older adults may do well to get their supplemental B_{12} from a daily multivitamin and mineral tablet rather than a pill containing just vitamin B_{12}. This is because older people are more vulnerable to nutrient deficiencies (for reasons ranging from a decreased ability to absorb nutrients to a lower intake of food), and they are more likely to develop the chronic diseases that adequate vitamin intake may help prevent. What's more, preliminary research indicates that there may be a link between intake of minute amounts of nutrients and mental capacity. A daily multivitamin may fill in any gaps left by inadequate food intake or absorption problems.

Other factors besides age can alter nutrient needs. Pregnancy, for example, increases the need for a num-

COMMON MYTHS ABOUT SUPPLEMENTS

MYTH: Vitamins can increase energy.
FACT: Calories provide energy. Vitamins have no calories and thus cannot provide energy.

MYTH: "Natural" supplements are better than others.
FACT: The body doesn't distinguish between "natural" or "organic" supplements and supplements from any other source.

MYTH: Supplements can prevent or cure disease.
FACT: While selected supplements may be helpful for some people, the nutritional mainstay for promoting health and preventing disease is a healthful diet.

MYTH: Supplements can help you lose weight effortlessly.
FACT: Advertising aside, scientific evidence gives no credence to such things as "fat-burning pills." If you want to lose weight, you must take in fewer calories than your body burns.

MYTH: Expensive supplements are better than generic or "house" brands.
FACT: Cost is not necessarily a guide to effectiveness. When choosing a multivitamin, look for a supplement that contains amounts in the range of the Recommended Dietary Allowance for a broad number of nutrients. Make sure the label contains the USP (US Pharmacopeia) seal ensuring that the supplement has met quality standards for disintegration, dissolution, strength, and purity.

ber of nutrients, and supplements are almost routinely prescribed for pregnant women. Some drugs can cause nutrient losses, so people taking those drugs may benefit from taking supplements. And some people simply cannot or will not get enough of a nutrient from food alone. For example, to take in 1200 mg of calcium a day (the amount recommended for those over 50) in a healthful fashion, a person would need to eat three to four servings a day of low-fat or fat-free milk, yogurt, or cheese. This amount may be difficult to fit into some diabetes meal plans, and some people may simply be unwilling or unable to consume this amount of dairy products. Taking supplements is preferable to omitting needed calcium. (Note: While healthy people with diabetes need the same amount of calcium as healthy people who don't have diabetes, those with kidney disease may need to limit calcium intake).

Keep in mind, however, that, like most other major health organizations, the American Diabetes Association does not routinely recommend supplements. According to the 2001 Clinical Practice Recommendations issued by the Association, "When dietary intake is adequate, there is generally no need for additional vitamin and mineral supplementation for the majority of people with diabetes."

The remainder of this article will explore what we know about some specific vitamins and minerals.

Antioxidants

Oxidation is a chemical process that occurs inside the body as part of normal metabolism. Oxidation produces compounds called *free radicals*, which, when present in excess, are believed to damage cells, sometimes leading to cardiovascular disease and cancer. There is some evidence that people with diabetes may be more vulnerable to oxidative damage, which may help explain the increased risk of coronary heart disease that accompanies diabetes.

Antioxidants are substances—including some vitamins, minerals, and other compounds—that are believed to slow down or prevent oxidation. Among the vitamins that are antioxidants are the carotenoids (of which beta-carotene is the most familiar example), vitamin E, and vitamin C.

Beta-carotene. Early studies showed a link between supplemental doses of beta-carotene, the plant form of vitamin A, and a reduced risk of cardiovascular disease. However, several subsequent well-designed studies have not borne out this finding. And two studies investigating the use of supplemental beta-carotene to reduce the risk of developing lung cancer in smokers found a slightly higher rate of lung cancer in participants taking supplements.

While this certainly puts the safety of beta-carotene supplements in question, it doesn't mean that beta-carotene in the amounts found in food is dangerous. In fact, the opposite is true. Diets rich in food sources of beta-carotene and of other carotenoids such as lycopene (found in red fruits and vegetables such as tomatoes) and lutein (found in broccoli and green, leafy vegetables) have been associated with a reduced risk of cancer and other diseases. While studies haven't always been designed well enough to say for sure that it was beta-carotene and/or other carotenoids that lowered cancer risk, there appear to be substances in fruits and vegetables that lower cancer risk.

This is one area in which the clear moral of the story—at least for now—is to forget about supplements and stick to a diet rich in fruits and vegetables.

Vitamin E. In several studies, vitamin E supplements have been linked to a lower risk of heart disease. One theory is that vitamin E prevents low-density lipoprotein (LDL) cholesterol (the "bad" cholesterol) from oxidizing and causing arterial plaque buildup. Some studies, however, have had ambiguous results, and one recent study showed no benefit from taking vitamin E supplements. Even studies with positive results have not been designed to ensure that vitamin E, and not some other dietary or lifestyle factor, is responsible for the lower risk.

The current RDA for adults is 15 mg of the form known as alpha-tocopherol; this amount is equivalent to 15 international units (IU). For lactating women, the RDA is set at 19 mg. The UL for adults is 1,000 mg.

Vitamin C. Vitamin C is another antioxidant with promise. Studies have suggested that people who eat diets high in vitamin C may have lower rates of cancer and cardiovascular disease. It is unclear, however, whether supplements would carry the same benefits (and again, it cannot be said for certain that it is vitamin C and not some other factor in food that is responsible). While the current RDA for vitamin C is set at 90 mg for adult males and 75 mg for adult females (levels for smokers and for pregnant and breastfeeding women are higher), some health-care groups would like to see the RDA raised. But even if the RDA were raised to 200 mg, as one group has proposed, it would still be easy to get all the vitamin C you need from food. One cup of orange juice, for example, has about 100 mg of vitamin C.

If you do take supplemental vitamin C, many experts recommend not exceeding 500 mg a day. At that level, body tissues are saturated with vitamin C, and much of the vitamin is excreted in the urine. The UL for adults is 2,000 mg. As mentioned earlier, higher doses have been associated with some side effects.

Folate

In addition to possibly preventing some birth defects, folate appears to play some other protective roles in the body. Of particular interest is research indicating that folate consumption might offer protection against heart disease. People born with a medical condition in which their bodies are unable to properly process the amino acid homocysteine build up high levels of homocysteine in their blood. Because these individuals are also prone to strokes or heart attacks early in life, researchers speculate that high homocysteine levels may lead to heart disease and stroke in these people, as well as in people who don't have this congenital condition.

Because people who have higher blood levels of folate also have lower levels of homocysteine, and because it is known that folate is involved in processing homocysteine, scientists believe that folate may help lower homocysteine levels in the blood. However, no studies have yet proven that lowering homocysteine levels through diet or supplementation can ward off heart attacks or strokes.

Calcium and vitamin D

As noted earlier, relatively high levels of calcium are recommended to help maintain healthy bones. However, the body cannot absorb calcium without vitamin D, and getting enough vitamin D can sometimes be a problem. While the body can make vitamin D from exposure to sunlight, in northern areas of the United States and in Canada, the sun isn't strong enough during the winter for the body to make adequate vitamin D. And older bodies are much less efficient at both making vitamin D from the sun and processing the vitamin D from food or supplements.

Vitamin D is not widely distributed in the food supply. Although it is added to liquid milk, it is not added to other dairy products such as yogurt or cheese. Many people, especially those over age 70—for whom the recommended daily intake of vitamin D is 600 IU—may find they need to obtain vitamin D through supplements. Multivitamins typically contain 400 IU, which may be sufficient for most people. Those over age 70 who drink little or no milk may also want to choose a calcium supplement with added vitamin D. Bear in mind, however, that, as noted above, too much vitamin D can be toxic. According to the DRI's, the safe upper limit for vitamin D is 2,000 IU.

Magnesium

There are strong indications that a magnesium deficiency may be associated with diabetic complications such as insulin resistance and high blood pressure. Researchers have also puzzled over whether magnesium deficiency is a risk factor for the development of diabetes. Historically, it has been difficult to determine whether or not an individual is deficient in magnesium because there were no simple tests to assess body stores. New technology, however, has been developed that makes this process easier. When these new methods are used, it appears that many people with Type 2 diabetes do have low levels of magnesium.

There are several possible links between diabetes and low body stores of magnesium. Magnesium can be lost in the urine if diabetes is poorly controlled. Diuretics given to control high blood pressure may also cause losses. And because insulin is involved in moving magnesium into cells, it is possible that this process does not work as well in people with diabetes. In addition, other complications of diabetes may affect dietary intake and/or absorption of magnesium.

In 1992, an American Diabetic Association consensus conference recommended testing magnesium levels in those at particular risk of magnesium deficiency and supplementing where necessary. Those at risk of magnesium deficiency include people with chronic heart failure or those who have had heart attacks, people with ketoacidosis, people with calcium or potassium deficiencies, people taking diuretics and some other drugs, and pregnant women.

Chromium

Chromium is a mineral involved in carbohydrate and fat metabolism. While many claims about chromium—such as its ability to promote weight loss or build muscle mass—are overblown, its possible usefulness in managing Type 2 diabetes is still being assessed by researchers.

One group holds that chromium supplements can help control blood glucose levels. Others say that supplements are beneficial only in those who are deficient in chromium, which most Americans are not. This debate is complicated by the fact that it is difficult to assess chromium status. There is also great debate over how much chromium we actually need and how much is present in our food supply. The Institute of Medicine has not issued an RDA for chromium, because scientists do not have enough data to establish one. Instead estimated AI's have been issued: 35 micrograms for men and 25 for women; the levels were 5 micrograms less for those over 50. Given all the unknowns about chromium, people with diabetes may wish to discuss with their doctor whether or not they should take a chromium supplement.

Summing up supplements

For most people, the bottom line may be to start with a balanced diet that is high in fruits, vegetables, and low-fat dairy products, then consider taking a broad multivitamin and mineral supplement "just in case." That's a fairly safe, conservative approach. Depending on your diet, age, geography, and other considerations, you may need to consider supplemental calcium and possibly vitamin D. And you might want to talk with your doctor about taking extra vitamin E or another vitamin or mineral supplement. Remember, though, that some supplements can interact with certain drugs or may become toxic at high doses, so it's a good idea to be careful and clear any supplement with your doctor first. ❑

THE ABC'S OF HERBAL SUPPLEMENTS

by Belinda O'Connell, M.S., R.D., L.D.

G ot the sniffles? Take some echinacea. Feeling down? How about some St. John's wort? Anxious and can't sleep? Have you tried melatonin or valerian?

These days, it seems as if everyone is using botanical therapies for whatever ails them, whether it's a common cold or something more serious. Use of herbal supplements has grown dramatically over the past few years: Recent surveys show that between 30% and 50% of adults in the United States use herbal supplements, at a cost of billions of dollars each year. Since herbal supplements are not typically covered under insurance policies, this money comes directly out of consumers' pockets.

Why are people willing to spend this money? What benefits do they believe they get from herbal products that they do not get from synthetic drugs purchased over the counter or prescribed by doctors? Are herbal therapies safe?

This article attempts to answer these questions and gives you some guidelines for safe use of plant-based supplements. Such supplements are correctly called "botanical" supplements, since the term "botanical" covers all plants. ("Herbal" refers to only a small group of plants.) However, this article refers to all plants with medicinal value as "herbs" or "herbal supplements" because these are the terms with which most people are familiar.

Widely available but barely regulated

In surveys, Americans say they use herbal medicines because they believe they are more effective, have fewer side effects, and are safer than prescription drugs. They like that herbal supplements are "natural" and that they can pick and choose what to take themselves: They don't need a prescription or a doctor's permission to

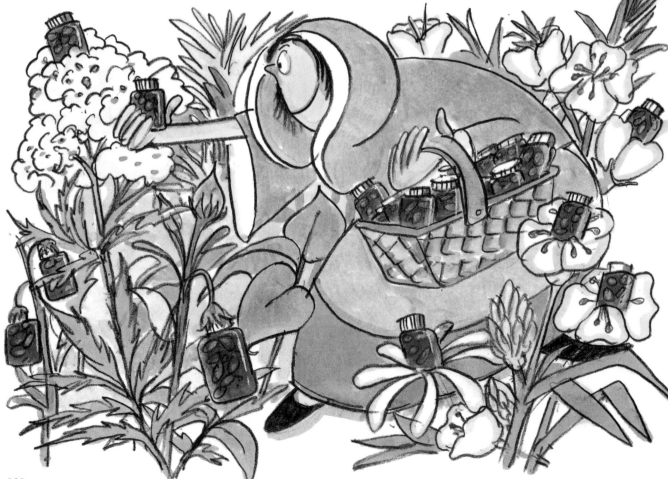

try supplements. Many people also resort to herbs out of frustration when it seems nothing else is helping their condition. The general attitude seems to be, "It can't hurt, and it might help, so why not try it?"

In fact, there are some good reasons to hold off on using most herbal supplements for now, or to at least carefully investigate the products you choose to use.

Because they use herbal supplements as medicine, many people think the federal government regulates them in the same way it does synthetic prescription or over-the-counter drugs. They think all herbal products are tested for safety and effectiveness and can be trusted to be free of dangerous contaminants. However, this is not the case. The government treats herbal supplements in a completely different way from how it treats synthetic drugs, and currently it provides little regulatory oversight of their production.

Herbal products are regulated under the 1994 Dietary Supplement Health and Education Act (DSHEA). The primary goal of this act is to ensure that the supplement industry provides consumers with factual, nonmisleading information on dietary supplements. DSHEA focuses on the marketing and sale of these products, not on whether they are tested for safety or effectiveness. Under this act, supplement manufacturers are not required to perform any tests of product composition, quality, strength, or effectiveness.

This lack of oversight has had a number of unfortunate results. For one thing, many supplements contain little of the active herbal component listed on the label. Some have been found to be contaminated with dangerous substances such as lead, other heavy metals, and potent prescription drugs, including steroids and digoxin, a drug used to treat congestive heart failure and irregular heartbeat. And some supplements currently available at your local pharmacy and grocery contain herbal components known to have serious negative side effects such as organ failure and death. (Some herbal products to beware of include belladonna, blue cohosh, borage, broom, chaparral, comfrey, ephedra, germander, kombucha tea, lobelia, magnolia–stephania preparation, mistletoe, pennyroyal, poke root, sassafras, skullcap, willow bark, wormwood, and yohimbe.)

These dangerous products are available because, under the DSHEA, the government cannot restrict the sale of any product unless it can prove that it is unsafe *when used according to package directions*. This is extremely time-consuming and difficult to prove, and so far, the Food and Drug Administration (FDA) has not physically removed any supplements from retail shelves because of safety concerns. In general, when concerns about contamination or safety have arisen, the FDA has issued warnings and requested voluntary recalls of the supplement by the manufacturer.

If the DSHEA doesn't regulate quality and safety of supplements, what does it do? The DSHEA defines what a supplement is and what products fall into that category. It requires that all dietary supplements have a Supplement Facts label similar to the Nutrition Facts label for foods. It also regulates what health claims can be used on a supplement label and what types of additional advertising (such as books, newsletters, and testimonials) can be used in marketing supplements. In addition, under the DSHEA the FDA is able to place restrictions on the amount of potentially dangerous herbs, such as ephedra (also called ma huang), included in supplements.

The FDA is also able to require specific warning labels on certain herbal supplements. For example, products containing ephedra must have the following warnings on the label: "Taking more than the recommended serving may result in heart attack, stroke, seizure, or death. Do not use this product for more than seven days." The label must also list contraindications (reasons not to use the product), including pregnancy, diabetes, high blood pressure, and heart disease.

Purity, quality, and standardization

Since the government doesn't regulate the manufacture of supplements, you really have no way of knowing whether you are getting what you paid for, and in many cases, you are not. Tests conducted by independent laboratories and consumer advocacy groups consistently find that many herbal supplements contain little or none of the advertised active ingredient and that some are contaminated with dangerous materials.

Even when an herbal supplement does contain the advertised herb in the amount listed on the label, it is likely that there are significant variations in activity from one brand of supplement to another and within one brand from season to season. This is because the potency of herbal preparations can vary widely with time of harvest and with climate, soil, storage, and manufacturing conditions. At this time, there are no universal guidelines to ensure that all supplements, regardless of brand, contain the same quantity of active components and are of the same potency. A supplement that has been tested and shown to have a certain amount of what is believed to be the active ingredient of an herb is said to be "standardized" to that amount of ingredient.

To counter the problems of purity and potency, several groups within the herbal product industry are stepping into the gap left by the government and pushing for increased self-regulation of supplement production. These organizations are calling for increased standardization, improved labeling, and voluntary adoption of "Good Manufacturing Practices," or GMP's, similar to those required by the government of the food and pharmaceutical industries. (The FDA has been charged with establishing GMP's but has not yet drawn up standards.) It is hoped that these changes within the industry will eventually lead to the increased availability of herbal products consumers can trust to be pure and safe and to contain the ingredients listed on the label.

Until then, anyone who chooses to use herbal supplements should plan to do some research on the products under consideration. The following industry trade organizations and independent companies—which test herbal products for quality—may be helpful when doing such research: the National Nutritional Foods Association (NNFA), the U.S. Pharmacopeia, and ConsumerLab.com. (See page 143 for contact information.)

NNFA. The National Nutritional Foods Association is a private organization that represents the interests of retailers and manufacturers in the dietary supplement and natural products industry. It has developed a self-regulatory program called the TruLabel program, with the goal of ensuring the availability of high-quality products for the consumer. It promotes quality assurance, safety, and good manufacturing guidelines for the industry. Manufacturers of registered products are randomly tested by independent laboratories to ensure that labels on herbal products accurately indicate the contents of the supplement.

In 1999, the NNFA began its Good Manufacturing Practices compliance program. This program specifies good manufacturing practices related to personnel, plant and grounds, sanitation, equipment, storage, and distribution. Manufacturing facilities are inspected by independent third parties, and only those that pass the inspection process are allowed to use the NNFA GMP seal of approval.

U.S. Pharmacopeia. The U.S. Pharmacopeia is a non-profit private organization that acts much like a governmental or public institution. It establishes standards for purity and quality of medicines and herbal and nonherbal supplements. This organization administers the "NF" and "USP" symbols of quality used on labels. Federal law requires products that display these symbols to follow the standards specified in the publications *United States Pharmacopeia* and *National Formulary*. This is enforced by the FDA within the United States. Only certain supplements are eligible for the USP or NF designation at this time.

ConsumerLab.com. ConsumerLab.com is a private company that provides information for the consumer about the purity and quality of herbal and dietary supplements. It is an independent third party that tests the quality of herbal and dietary supplements. The company posts this information on its Web site for free use by consumers. ConsumerLab.com administers two seals of quality: The Approved Quality Product Seal is designed for supplement labels and can be used by manufacturers whose products pass the quality testing program. The Approved Quality Retailer

WHAT CLAIMS ARE ALLOWED?

In general, supplement labels may contain statements about the effect of an herb on body structure or normal body functions. They may not contain statements that refer to diseases. Here are some examples of what's allowed and what's not.

STATEMENTS ALLOWED	STATEMENTS NOT ALLOWED
Use as part of diet to maintain healthy blood sugar levels.	Controls blood sugar in persons with insufficient insulin.
Helps absentmindedness and mild memory problems associated with aging.	Prevents or treats Alzheimer disease and other senile dementia.
Helps maintain cholesterol levels that are already within the normal range.	Lowers cholesterol.
Helps maintain or build strong bones.	Prevents osteoporosis.
Supports healthy immune system function.	Prevents or treats colds.
Helps relieve symptoms of premenstrual syndrome and normal healthy attitude during PMS.	Prevents severe depression associated with the menstrual cycle.

Seal can be used by retailers who agree not to sell products that have failed the company's testing. **Standardization pros and cons.** In general, the increased level of standardization provided by these types of regulatory programs is beneficial. Herbal supplements that are standardized are likely to have more predictable effects.

But standardization—or making sure a supplement has a set amount of an active compound—does not guarantee that a product is potent or effective. That's because, in many cases, it is not known exactly which compounds in the herb have beneficial effects. There may be more than one active ingredient in an herb. So standardized products are not necessarily more beneficial or more potent than nonstandardized products.

The industry is still divided as to whether standardization is the way to go. Some people feel that standardization is important to provide more reliable products and to increase consumer trust of supplements. Others feel that the beneficial aspects of herbs may be lost when they are extracted and highly purified. It seems reasonable to think that herbs may be like food in the sense that whole foods have health benefits not provided by individual nutritional supplements.

Supplement labels

As mentioned earlier, herbal and nutritional supplements are required to have a Supplement Facts Panel similar to the Nutrition Facts Panel required for foods. The Supplement Facts Panel provides basic information on ingredients, including a complete ingredient list, botanical names, parts of the plant used, and the amounts of active ingredients per serving. However, because not all supplement manufacturers use the same names for botanical ingredients, figuring out exactly what you are taking can be difficult. The use of a variety of names for one plant also makes it difficult to compare products and look up information on the safety and appropriate use of herbs.

The two types of names you will most commonly see on herbal supplement labels are the botanical name of the plant and the common name. (You may also see proprietary or trademarked names created by the manufacturer.) Botanical names describe the plant in a scientific manner. Generally, botanical names have two parts: the genus and the species. In the name *Momordica charantia,* for example, *Momordica* is the genus, and *charantia* the species. The botanical name is in Latin and is always in italics.

Many herbs are known by more than one common name. For example, two common names used for *Momordica charantia* are bitter melon and bitter gourd. Common names used for herbs have historically varied a great deal from place to place. Recently, however, the American Herbal Products Association (an

HOW TO CHOOSE AN HERBAL SUPPLEMENT

When shopping for an herbal supplement, take some time to read the label before you buy. Here are some hints to help you find a product that is safe and that contains what the label says it does:

■ Look for nationally known food and supplement companies. These companies are more likely to have Good Manufacturing Practices (GMP's) in place and follow industry guidelines for quality and purity.

■ Look for products that have recognized symbols of quality. Examples include the USP and NF symbols, the TruLabel symbol, and the ConsumerLab.com symbol. Also look for products that have been assessed by independent third parties such as ConsumerLab.com.

■ Avoid foreign products unless their quality is known. Foreign products, especially those from China and India, are more likely to be adulterated or have dangerous contaminants.

■ Look for appropriate label claims. Avoid companies that make sensational claims or have misleading labeling. Companies that do not follow government regulations for advertising are not likely to follow voluntary standards for quality manufacturing processes either.

■ Look for products that have standardized extracts and for labels that clearly identify the quantities of active ingredients. Common measurements that you may see include gram (g), milligram (mg), and microgram (mcg or µg).

■ Look for products that have an expiration date. Capsules and tablets generally have the longest shelf life. Store these products in a cool, dark place at home. Fresh herbs can be frozen in airtight containers, but capsules and tablets should not be frozen.

■ Look for products that provide a toll-free customer service phone number. Ask if their products undergo third-party testing or have any published studies supporting their use. Ask if products are tested for uniformity, bioavailability (or how much of the active components are absorbed and used by the body), and the presence of contaminants.

industry trade organization) designated standard common names that should be used when labeling products for retail sale. This should help to clear up some of the confusion.

Supplement labels must also specify directions for use and a recommended serving size. All supplement labels must include the name and address of the business selling the product and, if the label makes any health or benefit claims, must carry the disclaimer, "This statement has not been evaluated by the Food and Drug Administration. This product is not intended to diagnose, treat, cure, or prevent any disease."

With a disclaimer like this, it's a wonder so many people take herbal supplements. The disclaimer does explain, however, why label claims are often vague and difficult to interpret.

Label claims

Supplement manufacturers have the difficult job of convincing you of the benefits of their product while staying within the guidelines set by the government that limit what they may say. The DSHEA allows supplement manufacturers to make health claims on labels that describe the supplement's effects on general health and well-being or the role of the product in maintaining normal structure and functions of the body. They are strictly prohibited from making disease-related claims, meaning they cannot suggest that a supplement is capable of treating, preventing, or curing a specific disease. Examples of claims that are permitted and prohibited are listed on page 140.

The government recently changed the original Dietary Supplement Health and Education Act to increase the number of conditions about which supplement manufacturers are allowed to make claims. For example, supplement labels can now make claims about PMS (premenstrual syndrome), absentmindedness, and noncystic acne, because these are considered nonserious conditions associated with normal life stages, not diseases. Supplement labels are also now allowed to make claims similar to those allowed for common over-the-counter medicines such as digestive aids, antacids, and short-term laxatives.

But it is often difficult to determine just when a symptom or condition crosses the line between normal and pathological. Exactly when does normal absentmindedness turn into Alzheimer disease? What is the difference between "feeling stressed" and having an anxiety disorder? When does occasional sleeplessness become chronic insomnia? And when do mild mood disorders associated with the menstrual cycle become serious depression? The government's labeling guidelines are designed to help protect the consumer, but in practice they can make things more confusing.

"Natural" is not harmless

One of the most common misconceptions people hold about herbal products is that because they are "natural" and less potent than synthetic medicines, they are less likely to have side effects. This is not true. There are plenty of examples of products found in nature that are poisonous. And as many experts point out, anything that is potent enough to have a positive effect is also strong enough to have negative side effects. (Unfortunately, with herbal products, consumers are often unaware of what these side effects may be.)

When debating the virtues of "natural" supplements, keep in mind that many common synthetic drugs were originally discovered and derived from "natural" plant sources (examples include aspirin and digoxin). In addition, many herbs are now consumed not in their native form but in processed forms such as pills and tablets. Those herb products that are relatively unprocessed are less likely to have consistent effects because of normal variations in active components.

Many herbs do appear to be fairly safe when consumed as directed on package labels. Serious side effects have occurred most commonly when an individual took more than the recommended amount of an herb or mixed supplements with other supplements or prescription drugs. When using supplements, always follow label guidelines for use and dosages.

Research

Herbal products have been used for hundreds of years by nearly all traditional cultures of the world. In many regions, these plant-based medicines are still the only medical treatments available. The staying power of these herbs suggests that many have some therapeutic benefit, but overall there is little scientific proof that herbal products are effective.

Because there are very few good studies on herbs, there is little hard data on the best ways to use them. Currently, there is no consensus, even among experts in the field of herbal medicine, as to what doses and combinations of products are most effective. Even in cases where there is some research and experts' recommendations are similar, it may be difficult to find reliable products because of the lack of standardization in producing herbal medicines.

Lack of standardization also makes it difficult to conduct good research studies. When supplements vary in potency and in the quantity of active ingredients, study subjects may get variable doses, and researchers may find it difficult to repeat or confirm one another's results. Most of the research studies on herbal products so far have been very small and have not been blinded or placebo-controlled studies, so their results are not considered highly reliable. (The most rigorous studies are what are called double-blind, placebo-controlled studies. This means that there is a group of people that gets the active substance being tested and a control group that gets a "dummy" or inactive pill. No one knows who is in which group until after the study is completed.)

Another reason that studying the effects of medicinal herbs is difficult is that the manner in which traditional cultures approach health and wellness is not easy to quantify using Western medical methods. Many traditional cultures believe, for example, that there are vital energies that flow through the body and that illness is due to a "blockage" in the flow of this vital energy. Therapies such as acupuncture, massage, and use of herbs are believed to clear such blockages. A certain herb, for example, may be believed to improve the energy flow to the kidneys.

Not only do Western scientists tend to view how the body works and why illnesses occur differently, but, while they may be skilled at conducting technically well-designed research studies, they often do not understand herbal products well enough to ensure they are using, storing, and processing the herbs properly. The best research studies may need to wait until traditional healers and Western scientists find a way to collaborate. The U.S. National Institutes of Health has created a special branch called the National Center for Complementary and Alternative Medicine to help promote collaboration and research in the field of alternative medicine.

Cost-benefit evaluation

Herbal supplements do not come cheap, and since insurance companies do not generally cover them, consumers pay the entire cost from their own pockets. This means they have fewer dollars to spend on treatments that may have a greater impact on their overall health. For instance, money spent on herbs could be put toward fresh fruits and vegetables or an exercise or smoking cessation class. (A diet high in fruits and vegetables, exercise, and stopping smoking have all been proven to lower the risks of certain diseases.)

In addition to the price tag, there can be other costs associated with taking herbs. For example, the cost of treating a medical condition when conventional treatment has been delayed in favor of ineffective herbal treatments can be high. Treating a person for side effects or adverse interactions between herbal medicines and synthetic drugs can also be expensive.

Should I take herbal supplements?

The decision to take or not take herbal supplements is up to you and your health-care team. If you choose to try a supplement, think of it as an experiment, not a proven medical treatment, and take appropriate precautions. Be smart about your use: Follow the guidelines in this article and work with your health-care

INDEPENDENT QUALITY REGULATORS

This is a list of private organizations that have taken on the task of regulating the quality and content of herbal supplements. Since there are no government standards by which to compare herbal products, each of these organizations has developed its own standards and its own mark of quality to award to products that meet those standards.

NATIONAL NUTRITIONAL FOODS
ASSOCIATION
(800) 966-6632
www.nnfa.org
The NNFA's TruLabel program recognizes products, such as health foods and dietary supplements, whose manufacturers are members of the NNFA. To meet the standards, the products must undergo and pass tests to assess the purity and safety of their ingredients. The NNFA also provides GMP (Good Manufacturing Practices) certification to the manufacturers themselves.

U.S. PHARMACOPEIA
(800) 822-8772
www.usp.org
This organization awards USP and NF insignia to drugs and dietary supplements that meet the criteria for quality and safety laid out in the publications *United States Pharmacopeia* and the *National Formulary*, respectively.

CONSUMERLAB.COM
(914) 722-9149
www.consumerlab.com
ConsumerLab.com grants its Approved Quality Product Seal to products that maintain set safety and quality standards, and its Approved Quality Retailer Seal to stores that do not carry products that have failed tests for the standards.

team. Expect to do some research about specific herbs and different brands of supplements.

Set a specific time frame for use of a supplement. Chronic consumption of herbal supplements over extended periods is expensive, potentially dangerous, and not likely to be of therapeutic benefit. (What is considered "chronic" varies with the specific supplement and may be as little as a week or two. In general, most herbs should not be used for more than three to six months.) Even in countries such as Germany where herbal medicines are used much more commonly than in the United States, these medicines are prescribed in specific doses, for specific time periods, and are used under the care of a physician.

Be on the lookout for side effects and other problems. Have reasonable expectations. Herbs will not likely replace, or even significantly reduce, your need for medicines or insulin at this time. Do not approach the use of herbal supplements in a random manner: Keep records of the positive and negative effects of the supplement, and be more careful than usual in monitoring your blood glucose. ❑

GUIDELINES FOR USING HERBAL SUPPLEMENTS

Do not assume that because they are "just herbs" you do not need to take herbal supplements seriously. In fact, because supplements are not tested rigorously before being put on the market, they may require even more caution on the part of the consumer. Here are some steps to take to make sure you and your family avoid dangerous side effects or drug interactions:

■ Research the supplements you are interested in taking. Know which herbs are in a supplement and the amounts of each.

■ Always discuss supplement use with your doctor. Do not try to self-treat conditions requiring medical care. Be sure to tell your doctor or health-care provider about all of the medicines, herbs, and vitamin supplements you are taking.

■ Keep records of your supplement use. Record doses, date started, side effects, blood glucose levels, what you expect the supplement to do for you, and how well it performs.

■ The long-term use of most supplements is generally not recommended. If a product is not giving you the benefits you expected, stop taking it.

■ Add only one new product at a time. It is generally easier to track the effects of one supplement than several taken simultaneously. If you use more than one supplement or if you use a combination formula, check the labels to ensure that you are not taking more than the recommended dose of any one herb.

■ Follow the dosage guidelines on supplement labels. To be on the safe side, start with a half-dose and work your way up to a full dose over a week or more. Do not take more than the recommended dose since side effects are more likely to occur with increased doses.

■ Do not combine supplements and prescription drugs without the knowledge of your doctor. Many herbal supplements can interact with synthetic medicines, altering the way they work. In some cases, these changes can lead to dangerous increases or decreases in the synthetic drug's activity.

■ Never discontinue synthetic drugs without consulting your doctor first. Herbal supplements are generally not appropriate substitutes for prescription drugs. If you have concerns about the drugs you are using or are experiencing unpleasant side effects, discuss them with your doctor. He or she may be able to prescribe a different drug that works better for you.

■ If you experience side effects when using herbal supplements, stop using them and contact your doctor. Negative side effects from herbal supplements can be very serious. Always pay attention to changes in how you feel and to minor side effects that occur when you start using an herbal supplement; these symptoms may be a sign of a more serious problem.

■ Do not use herbal supplements if you are pregnant or nursing. Because the effects of herbal preparations on a fetus or infant are not known, the safest course of action is to not use them when pregnant or nursing. If you are of childbearing age and wish to use herbal products, you should use an appropriate method of contraception.

■ Do not give herbal supplements to infants or young children. Even herbs that seem safe and that you have used yourself may contain contaminants that a child is less able to tolerate than an adult.

■ All medicines, including vitamins, herbs, and synthetic drugs, should be safely stored in their original containers (which can provide information in case of overdose or adverse reaction) out of the reach of young children.

■ Stop using all herbal supplements (or check with your doctor) before surgery, anesthesia, and other medical procedures. Several herbs are believed to decrease the ability of the body to form blood clots and could be dangerous for those undergoing surgery. Others have been found to alter the effect of anesthesia or decrease seizure threshold. Avoid using these before major medical procedures where anesthesia or pain medication may be required.

HERBAL SUPPLEMENTS IN DIABETES MANAGEMENT

by Belinda O'Connell, M.S., R.D., L.D.

More than 1200 plant compounds have been tested for their ability to lower blood sugar levels. Many have been found to contain chemical components that have hypoglycemic activity (the ability to lower blood sugar) when tested in test tubes or in animal models. However, there is very little research on such compounds using human subjects, and what research does exist is generally not of high quality.

A few herbal remedies for diabetes have been tested in humans and have been found to have mild blood-sugar-lowering properties. These compounds have not had very powerful effects, and at this time are not felt to be adequate for the management of diabetes when used alone. The most promising of these botanicals include bitter melon (*Momordica charantia*), fenugreek (*Trigonella foenum-graecum*), gurmar (*Gymnema sylvestre*), goat's rue (*Galega officinalis*), bilberry (*Vaccinium myrtillus*), ginseng (chiefly *Panax*), nopal (*Opuntia streptacantha*), and garlic and onion (*Allium sativum* and *Allium cepa*).

Bitter melon

Also called bitter gourd, bitter cucumber, balsam pear, karela, and charantin, bitter melon is the most widely used traditional remedy for diabetes. It is commonly used in Asia, especially in India, and in Africa. Bitter melon is frequently eaten as a vegetable and looks like a misshapen, bumpy cucumber. As a treatment for diabetes, it is typically the juice or an extract of the unripe fruit that is used. Dried or powdered forms of bitter melon are not believed to have the same activity.

Several compounds isolated from bitter melon are believed responsible for its blood-sugar-lowering properties. These include charantin and an insulin-like protein called polypeptide-P, or plant insulin. Bitter melon is thought to act both on the pancreas and in nonpancreatic cells, such as muscle cells.

There are no well-designed studies using bitter melon in humans. Most studies have not used controls or placebos, and those that have did not always randomly assign people to treatment groups. These precautions are needed to ensure that the results obtained are real and not merely due to chance. Most of the studies that have been done are short-term studies.

In one study, polypeptide-P isolated from bitter melon was injected (in a manner similar to that used with commercial insulins) into subjects with Type 1 diabetes and Type 2 diabetes. It decreased blood glucose levels from an average of 305 mg/dl before treatment to 168 mg/dl after four hours in subjects with Type 1 diabetes, and from 140 mg/dl to 95 mg/dl after one and a half hours in subjects with Type 2 diabetes. There were no significant changes in the control subjects. The results in subjects with Type 2 diabetes were generally not considered significant, most likely due to the small number of subjects and the variability of bitter melon's effects in different people.

Another small study tested the effect of eating powdered whole bitter melon for one week in people with Type 2 diabetes. Fasting blood sugar levels and blood sugar levels measured after consuming 50 grams of pure glucose (this is called a *glucose tolerance test* and is commonly used in research studies) were significantly lower after eating bitter melon. The average fasting blood sugar level fell from 248 mg/dl to 155 mg/dl.

Two other studies, which used fresh bitter melon juice, had similar results. One study found that there were "responders," people whose blood sugar levels during a glucose tolerance test were lower after treatment with bitter melon, and "nonresponders," or people for whom the bitter melon did not have any beneficial effects.

Current preparations of bitter melon are generally not standardized, making recommendations for a specific effective dose difficult. Typically, however, 50 to 200 milliliters (about 2 to 5 ounces) per day of the fresh juice; 3 to 15 grams of the dried, powdered fruit; or 300 to 600 milligrams (divided into three separate doses of 100 to 200 milligrams each) of a standardized extract per day have been used.

There are currently no studies that look at the effects of bitter melon over an extended period of time, and there are no studies of bitter melon's safety, though it is commonly consumed as a vegetable in India and is generally believed to be safe. More research is needed before it can be considered as a potential treatment for diabetes.

Bitter melon is a component of some herbal formulas advertised for people with diabetes. If you use the fresh fruit, prepare it with care: A mildly toxic chemical has been isolated from the seeds and the outer rind. There also are reports of toxicity in children and bleeding and contractions in pregnant women, so this plant should be avoided by individuals in these groups. Whatever formulation you choose, work closely with your doctor and health-care team. This precaution is important because there is the potential for hypoglycemia when this herb is combined with medicines that lower blood glucose. Positive effects on blood sugar should be noted fairly quickly. If changes are not seen within four weeks, the herb should be discontinued.

Fenugreek

Fenugreek is a common spice, and in small concentrations is categorized by the U.S. Food and Drug Administration as "Generally Recognized As Safe." Its seeds or a defatted powder made from the seed have been used as a treatment for diabetes. Fenugreek is one of the better researched herbal treatments for diabetes, with both human and animal studies suggesting it has hypoglycemic activity. There is also research suggesting that fenugreek may improve blood cholesterol and triglyceride levels. (Triglycerides are a type of fat that circulates in the blood. High levels are thought to increase the risk of heart disease.)

Fenugreek has been found to improve blood glucose levels in both Type 1 and Type 2 diabetes. In one study, subjects with Type 1 diabetes were randomly assigned to receive either defatted fenugreek seed powder or a placebo (inactive substitute) for 10 days. After the first 10 days, subjects then received the other treatment for another 10 days. Fenugreek significantly decreased fasting blood glucose levels, improved glucose tolerance test results, and decreased blood cholesterol and triglyceride levels. Blood insulin levels did not change with the treatment.

In people with Type 2 diabetes, three studies have demonstrated positive effects of fenugreek on blood glucose and cholesterol levels. All of these studies used placebos and had more than 20 subjects. In the longest study, lasting three months, people with higher initial blood glucose levels did not respond as well as those with lower initial blood glucose levels. In people who had a positive response, average fasting and postprandial (after-meal) blood glucose levels decreased by about 35 mg/dl. This was statistically significant.

Fenugreek seeds are very high in fiber, and it is believed that at least part of fenugreek's effects are achieved because the fiber decreases absorption of dietary carbohydrates. In the study involving people with Type 1 diabetes, the fiber content of the diet containing fenugreek was very high, containing about 80 grams of fiber per day. (For comparison, most Americans get less than 15 grams of fiber per day.)

Other compounds believed to contribute to fenugreek's activity include proteins, saponins, and alkaloids. Names you may see listed on herbal supplements include fenugreekine and trigoneline.

The dose of fenugreek used in studies has varied a great deal—from 5 grams to 100 grams per day—and

is generally divided into at least two equal portions. Since the larger amounts would be impossible to consume in a capsule, they have generally been incorporated into foods in the studies. Some herbal supplements designed for people with diabetes include much smaller quantities of fenugreek, often combined with other herbs, in capsule form. Plain dried fenugreek seed powder is also available in capsules, as a bulk powder, and in a chewable wafer form.

Common side effects seen with high doses of fenugreek include diarrhea and upset stomach. It has also been reported that it may decrease blood coagulation, so people using anticoagulant medicines ("blood thinners") or aspirin should use this herb only under the supervision of their doctor. In animals, extracts of fenugreek have been shown to stimulate uterine contractions in late pregnancy, so this herb should not be used by pregnant women. Because of its high fiber content, it may also alter absorption and effectiveness of other medicines taken at the same time. This herb should not be taken at the same time as other medicines.

Gurmar

Gymnema sylvestre leaf has been used as a traditional treatment for diabetes in India. Because chewing the leaf decreases the sensitivity of taste buds to sweet tastes, gymnema has also been called gurmar, which means "sugar destroyer." This effect is reported to last several hours. In people who have had extracts of gymnema applied to their tongue, this decrease in sensitivity to sweets caused a short-term decrease in food consumption. It seems unlikely that consuming gymnema in a capsule or pill would have the same effect.

The active ingredient in gymnema is believed to be a mixture of molecules called gymnemic acids. You may see gymnemic acids listed on the labels of herbal supplements marketed to people with diabetes. Gymnema is believed to improve the function of pancreatic beta cells (the cells in the body that make insulin).

In animals with diabetes, gymnema has appeared to help regenerate or increase the number of functional beta cells present in the pancreas, but when gymnema was given to animals that had had their pancreas removed, there was no effect. This suggests that gymnema requires some residual beta-cell function to work. Gymnema may also decrease glucose absorption from food and improve the ability of the body to use glucose for energy.

There is minimal research on gymnema at this time, and the studies there are in humans have not been well designed. One study, which used subjects with Type 2 diabetes, found that consumption of a concentrated extract of gymnema decreased blood glucose levels and blood cholesterol levels. Gymnema also increased blood insulin levels in these people. Another study using people with Type 1 diabetes found that long-term consumption of gymnema decreased blood glucose levels, glycosylated hemoglobin (HbA$_{1c}$) levels, and insulin requirements. These results are intriguing, but gymnema cannot be recommended as a treatment for diabetes until we have better studies and more of them. One manufacturer of gymnema supplements is currently planning a larger clinical trial to test the effects of gymnema in people with Type 2 diabetes in the United States.

A typical daily dose of gymnema is 400 to 600 milligrams of an extract (standardized to at least 24% gymnemic acids). Gymnema has no known toxic effects, but its safety has not been directly tested, and it should not be taken by children or pregnant or nursing women. Gymnema does not appear to cause hypoglycemia in people who do not have diabetes.

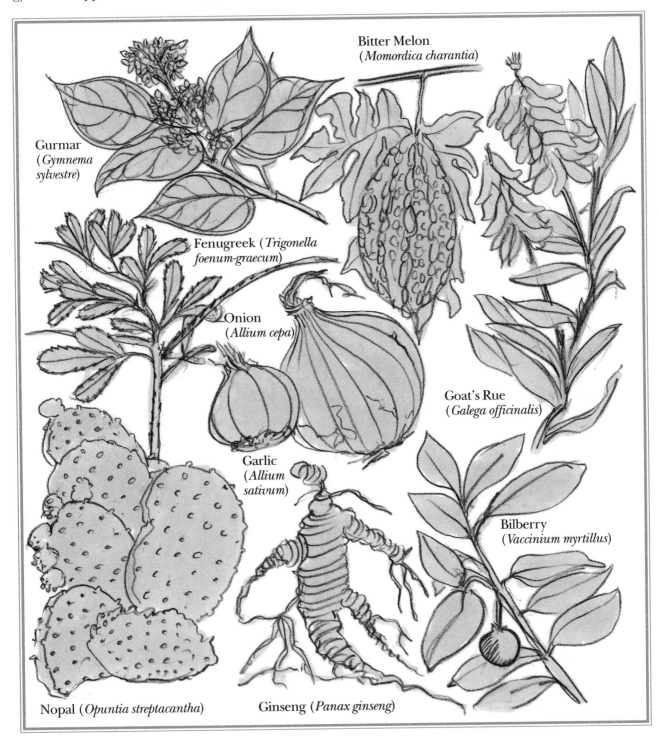

Bitter Melon (*Momordica charantia*)

Gurmar (*Gymnema sylvestre*)

Fenugreek (*Trigonella foenum-graecum*)

Onion (*Allium cepa*)

Goat's Rue (*Galega officinalis*)

Garlic (*Allium sativum*)

Bilberry (*Vaccinium myrtillus*)

Nopal (*Opuntia streptacantha*)

Ginseng (*Panax ginseng*)

Goat's rue

Goat's rue is another traditional remedy for diabetes, and it has been shown to have hypoglycemic activity in humans. It appears to act in a manner similar to the synthetic drug metformin (brand name Glucophage), an oral hypoglycemic drug used to treat Type 2 diabetes. Metformin lowers blood sugar by decreasing the production of glucose from the liver. Goat's rue may also inhibit glucose absorption from the intestinal tract. In obese animals, dried goat's rue added to the diet led to decreases in body weight and body fat.

However, one of the active ingredients in goat's rue, galegine, when purified is too toxic to be used as a medicine, and there have been reports of poisoning from goat's rue in grazing animals. It is not recommended as a treatment for diabetes at this time due to its potentially toxic effects.

Bilberry

The leaves of bilberry, also known as European blueberry, are reported to contain chromium and have been used as an antidiabetic tea. In animals, extracts of the leaf decreased blood glucose and blood triglyceride levels. The berries are a rich source of antioxidants (compounds that may decrease the risk of heart disease, cancer, and other chronic diseases) and may improve circulation. They have been suggested as a treatment for diabetic retinopathy.

Chronic consumption of bilberry leaf or capsules is not recommended, as it can be toxic. Potential side effects include anemia, severe weight loss, and excitability. Consumption of high doses can be fatal. Bilberry may also interact with anticoagulant medicines, potentially causing increased bleeding.

Ginseng

Ginseng has long been used as a botanical remedy in the Orient. Today, it is also one of the most commonly used herbal supplements in the United States, where it is sold chiefly as an energy booster. Americans spent more than $86 million on ginseng in 1997. However, ginseng supplements have been found to be one of the less reliable supplements on the market. Tests conducted by independent laboratories frequently find little or no ginseng in the supplements, so purchasers of these products need to do their own background research to avoid spending money on "placebo," or inactive, pills.

The term ginseng has been used to refer to more than one plant group. There is the *Panax* genus, which includes Korean, Japanese, and American ginseng, and there is the *Eleutherococcus* genus, which includes Siberian ginseng. It is generally felt that the Asian and American ginsengs act similarly, but that

Siberian ginseng is not a true ginseng and cannot be used in place of *Panax* ginseng. The main active ingredients in ginseng comprise a group of molecules called ginsenosides.

There are only a few small studies looking at the hypoglycemic effects of ginseng, and most of the information we have is with Type 2 diabetes. One study did not specify the type of ginseng used but reported decreases in fasting blood glucose levels and HbA_{1c} in people newly diagnosed with Type 2 diabetes on diet therapy only. The second study used American ginseng (*Panax quinquefolius*) and tested the short-term effect of a large dose of ginseng (3 grams) on blood glucose levels after consuming 25 grams of glucose. In people with diabetes, consuming ginseng 40 minutes before or with the glucose decreased postprandial blood sugar levels. (These results were marginally significant.)

Typical doses vary from 200 to 600 milligrams per day of a standardized extract, taken in one or two equal doses. Ginseng is generally believed to be safe, but side effects of its use include increased blood pressure, excitability, nervousness, headache, insomnia, diarrhea, nausea, and worsening of asthma. Ginseng may also have mild estrogen-like properties, sometimes causing postmenopausal bleeding or amenorrhea, the absence of menses. It may also interact with the medicines digoxin, warfarin, and diuretics, increasing or decreasing their effectiveness.

Nopal cactus

The stem or leaf of nopal cactus has been used in traditional Mexican medicine to treat Type 2 diabetes. Short-term, uncontrolled studies of this herb in humans have measured decreases in blood glucose, blood cholesterol, and triglycerides. The active ingredient in nopal is not known, but researchers hypothesize that fiber from nopal helps to decrease glucose absorption from the intestine, and that other compounds help to increase the effectiveness of insulin.

Most studies use cooked or fresh nopal, but extracts from the fresh plant are also used. A typical dose is 500 grams of fresh or cooked nopal eaten before or with the meal. There are no known risks associated with eating nopal other than those you would find with an increase in fiber from any source.

Garlic and onions

Garlic is one of the top-selling herbal supplements in the United States. It is best known for its potential protective effects in cardiovascular disease. It has been claimed that garlic can decrease blood cholesterol levels, decrease high blood pressure, and decrease the likelihood of blood clots forming, properties that are all beneficial in preventing heart disease. Numerous studies have examined these effects. In general, it appears that garlic does have a positive effect on these risk factors, but the consensus of the scientific community is that more research is needed before garlic can be recommended as a common treatment.

Garlic and onions have also been used as folk medicines to treat diabetes. There is much less research on this potential role of garlic, but a few studies do suggest that it (and onions) may have some mild blood-sugar-lowering properties. It is believed that garlic and onions lower blood sugar levels by decreasing the rate at which insulin is inactivated and degraded by the body, effectively increasing quantities of circulating insulin and decreasing blood glucose levels. Overall, these effects do not appear to be strong enough to warrant use of garlic or onion as a blood-sugar-lowering agent.

Garlic appears to be generally safe and well tolerated when taken as a supplement. Common side effects include mild stomach discomfort and an unusual body odor (even with the "odorless" forms of garlic). The primary safety concern about garlic relates to its ability to decrease blood clotting. In people who take aspirin or anticoagulant therapies, garlic may lead to increased bleeding. People who use these drugs should discuss with their doctor the safety of taking a supplement containing garlic. Garlic supplements should also be discontinued several weeks before surgery to prevent any problems with blood clotting. They should not be used by pregnant women, because they may cause contractions.

The active ingredients in garlic and onions are sulfur-containing molecules. (These compounds are what give garlic and onions their distinctive smell.) There are more than 20 molecules that are believed to contribute to garlic's effects, but the best understood are allicin, also called diallyl disulfide oxide, and APDS, or allyl propyl disulfide. You may see any of these names on garlic supplement labels.

Common doses for blood-sugar-lowering effects are quite high, and probably not realistic for the general population. Typical doses used to decrease blood cholesterol levels are 600 to 900 milligrams, in tablet or capsule form, or one to three fresh cloves per day. Look for products that are standardized and list the active ingredient allicin on the label. Heat and acid destroy the active ingredients in garlic and onions, so slow-release forms or enteric-coated forms of supplements may be more effective.

Safe supplement use

Because the safety and effectiveness of the herbal supplements covered in this article are unproved, people who are interested in using them are in a sense acting as human "experiments." They need to approach the treatments they use very carefully, preferably with the

POTENTIALLY DANGEROUS PLANT PRODUCTS

Many plants have potentially dangerous side effects when consumed. These may include (but are not limited to) dizziness, abdominal pain, nausea and vomiting, fainting, hallucinations, increased or decreased heart rate, blurred vision, rash or hives, increased bleeding or bruising, confusion or difficulty concentrating, decreased appetite, changes in sleep patterns, drowsiness or insomnia, sensitivity to sun, laxative effects, nervousness, and allergic symptoms, including problems breathing.

The following list highlights some potentially dangerous herbal products. However, it is not all-inclusive. The fact that an herb is not listed here does not mean it is safe.

POTENTIALLY FATAL
Ackee fruit
Bilberry (in amounts greater than
  480 milligrams per day)
Ephedra or Ma huang
Lupine
Mistletoe
Scenecio herb

AVOID IF YOU HAVE HIGH BLOOD PRESSURE
Ginseng
Juniper
Licorice
Yohimbine

AVOID BEFORE ANESTHESIA
St. John's wort

AVOID IF YOU TAKE ANTICOAGULANTS ("BLOOD THINNERS")
Garlic
Ginger
Ginkgo
Ginseng

guidance and support of their health-care team. If you would like to try an herbal supplement, here are some guidelines to keep in mind:

■ Discuss your plans with your primary health-care provider, and ask whether any of the supplements you'd like to try might interact with drugs you currently take or have other negative side effects.

■ Do not use herbal preparations if you are pregnant or nursing. The effects of herbs on a fetus or baby are unknown. Do not give children herbal supplements without first consulting their pediatrician.

■ If you get your doctor's OK to try herbal supplements, keep a log of all the supplements you are taking and the specific doses you are taking.

■ Try only one new supplement at a time so that you can more effectively gauge its effects.

■ Follow the dosage guidelines on the supplement label. Make sure you don't take more than the recommended dose.

■ Monitor your blood sugar levels more frequently, and keep careful records of your numbers. This is the only way to know what effect the supplement is having on your blood sugar levels.

■ Pay attention to any symptoms, such as headaches, nausea, rash, or changes in sleep patterns or mood, that may be due to a supplement. If symptoms persist, stop the supplement and see your doctor.

■ Store herbal supplements in their original containers with safety seals intact and out of the reach of children. Having the original container is important in case of accidental overdose or side effects.

■ Set a time limit for trying a supplement, usually three to six weeks. If it hasn't had any effect within that limit, stop using it.

Herbal remedies are unlikely to replace existing diabetes drug treatments any time soon. It is possible, however, that some will be shown to be effective in helping to control blood sugar levels or as a basis for designing new drug treatments for diabetes. ❏

HERBAL THERAPIES AND DIABETES COMPLICATIONS

by Belinda O'Connell, M.S., R.D., L.D.

For many people with diabetes, the most problematic aspect of having diabetes is not the day-to-day tasks of living with diabetes but the symptoms of (or fear of) complications of diabetes. Complications of diabetes are other medical conditions, including eye disease (retinopathy), kidney disease (nephropathy), nerve disorders (neuropathy), and heart disease, that can develop as a result of long-term diabetes.

Exactly what causes diabetes-related complications and why some people seem to have a greater risk of developing them is still uncertain, although a person's level of blood glucose control and blood pressure control clearly play a major role. It is likely that a combination of other factors, including genetics and blood lipid (fat) levels, as well as other factors not yet identified, are also involved. The good news is that even if the specific causes of diabetes complications are not known, much is known about treating and preventing them.

Preventing complications

Several large research studies have definitively shown that keeping blood glucose levels as close to normal as possible can delay or prevent the development of complications in people with either Type 1 or Type 2 diabetes. In the Diabetes Control and Complications Trial, which enrolled only people with Type 1 diabetes, "tight" blood glucose control was shown to

decrease the development of neuropathy by 60%, retinopathy by 76%, and early indications of kidney disease by 39%. Tight control also slowed the progression of kidney disease and retinopathy.

Similar results were seen in the United Kingdom Prospective Diabetes Study (UKPDS), which examined the impact of blood glucose control and blood pressure control on the development of complications in people with Type 2 diabetes. The UKPDS found that maintaining control of blood glucose levels in people with Type 2 diabetes resulted in a 25% decrease in all *microvascular* (small-blood-vessel) complications, including kidney disease, eye disease, and nerve disorders.

The UKPDS also found a direct relationship between blood glucose level and risk of complications: With each percentage point decrease in glycosylated hemoglobin (HbA_{1c})—from 8% to 7%, for example—the risk of complications decreased 35%. (The HbA_{1c} test gives an indication of a person's overall blood sugar control over the previous two to three months. The American Diabetes Association recommends that most people with diabetes attempt to keep their HbA_{1c} result under 7%. Any result over 8% should prompt a review of a person's diabetes management routine.)

In addition, the UKPDS found that controlling blood pressure is very important in preventing and delaying the progression of diabetic complications.

Treating complications

Expanding our knowledge about how to prevent complications is important, but there is still a need to learn how to treat complications in people already experiencing them. In some cases, bringing blood glucose levels closer to the normal range and maintaining them there can relieve symptoms and slow progression of existing complications. (To read more about treating symptoms of nerve damage, see "Treating Neuropathy While Waiting for a Cure" on page 192.)

Some of the new, experimental treatments for complications of diabetes include nutritional and herbal supplements. (In this article, in addition to herbal supplements, we will also cover other alternative therapy supplements.) But so far, there has been very little research done on such supplements as therapies for complications. For the most part, therefore, they have not been proven safe or effective treatments. But because many supplements are already being marketed and sold in pharmacies, natural food stores, and other retail establishments, as well as being investigated in research studies, we feel it would be helpful to review what is known about some of these treatments and their effects and side effects.

Heart disease

Many supplements may be of potential benefit in the treatment or prevention of heart disease, a common *macrovascular* (large-blood-vessel) complication of diabetes. However, at this time, few supplements have been well researched or accepted as beneficial treatments for heart disease. Among those discussed here are fish oil, fenugreek (*Trigonella foenum-graecum*), garlic (*Allium sativum*), red yeast (*Monascus purpureus*), antioxidants, and several herbs that inhibit blood clotting.

Fish oil. Regular consumption of fish is associated with lower rates of cardiovascular disease. It is believed that the cardioprotective benefits of fish are due to oils present in the fat of the fish. Fish oil is a rich source of omega-3 fatty acids such as DHA (docosahexanoic acid) and EPA (eicosapentanoic acid).

Omega-3 fatty acids decrease production of compounds in the body that cause inflammation and increase blood clotting and blood pressure. Fish oil and omega-3 fatty acid supplements have been found to decrease blood triglycerides, a type of blood fat associated with increased cardiovascular disease, by as much as 30% to 50%. In some research studies, they are also associated with a decreased number of both initial and fatal heart attacks.

However, several studies have documented small but consistent increases in LDL cholesterol (commonly referred to as "bad" cholesterol) with fish oil supplements. And fish oil supplements may raise blood glucose levels in people with Type 2 diabetes. For these reasons, fish oil supplements should be used only after consulting with your doctor.

Typical doses of fish oil used in research studies are between 3 and 6 grams per day. Up to 3 grams per day is generally considered safe, but because fish oil supplements may inhibit blood clotting, their use can lead to increased bleeding in people who take drugs or herbs that decrease blood clotting. People using drugs or herbs such as warfarin (brand name Coumadin), vitamin E, ginkgo extract, and garlic should check with their health-care provider before using fish oil supplements. In addition, fish oil supplements should be avoided before surgery.

Fenugreek. The ability of fenugreek seed to lower blood sugar is discussed on page 146. Fenugreek also appears to decrease blood cholesterol and triglyceride levels. It is believed that fiber, nicotinic acid, and other compounds in the fenugreek seed contribute to its tendency to lower cholesterol.

The doses of fenugreek used in research studies have varied a great deal, but most commonly fall between 5 and 30 grams of the powdered, defatted seed. Common side effects include diarrhea and upset stomach. Because it is high in fiber, fenugreek may alter the absorption of other drugs, so it should be taken separately. Fenugreek may also decrease the ability of the blood to clot, causing increased bruising or bleeding. People who take drugs such as warfarin or aspirin should check with their doctor before using this herb. Fenugreek has also been found to stimulate uterine contractions, so it should not be used by pregnant women.

Garlic. One of the most commonly used supplements in the United States, garlic has been the focus of numerous research trials probing its potential effects on blood cholesterol, high blood pressure, and blood clotting. (The blood-sugar-lowering properties of garlic are discussed on page 149.) Results of research studies have been mixed, with some showing positive effects, and others showing no effect of garlic supplementation. Overall, garlic may have a mild positive effect on blood cholesterol levels, causing decreases of 5% to 10%. There is less known about garlic's effects on high blood pressure.

Garlic contains many compounds that may contribute to its effects, but the most well understood are the sulfur-containing compounds allicin (diallyl disulfide oxide), APDS (allyl propyl disulfide), and S-allyl cysteine. Common doses used to decrease cholesterol levels are 600–900 milligrams per day in tablet or capsule form, or one to three cloves of fresh garlic per day. Garlic supplements are generally considered relatively safe. But because garlic may inhibit blood clotting, people who take anticoagulant drugs or herbal supplements known to decrease blood clotting should check with their health-care provider before using garlic. Garlic supplements should also be discontinued several weeks before surgery. Pregnant women should avoid garlic supplements because of the risk of increased bleeding or contractions.

Red yeast. A traditional Chinese food additive and medicine, red yeast is produced by fermenting rice in a particular type of fungus. (It is sometimes called red yeast rice.) It is sold under the brand name Cholestin in the United States, and it contains naturally occurring *statins,* chemical compounds similar to the active ingredients of many prescription drugs used to lower blood cholesterol levels. Statins act by inhibiting cholesterol production by the body. A recent research study found that Cholestin supplements decreased total cholesterol levels by 16% and LDL ("bad") cholesterol levels by 22%. Research studies have generally used 2.5 grams of Cholestin per day. There have been no significant side effects reported in short-term studies.

While the research on Cholestin is promising, there are still many questions about the supplement's long-term safety, as well as concerns about the production and standardization of Cholestin. Because potential side effects could be serious—remember, this supplement contains the same compound as many prescription cholesterol-lowering drugs but is less well tested and regulated—people considering taking Cholestin should discuss it with their doctor first.

Antioxidants. During the process of normal metabolism, the body produces damaging compounds known as free radicals. Because free radicals are very reactive, they can interact with many cellular components very quickly, causing a large amount of damage to a cell and even killing it. Free radicals are believed to play a role in many chronic conditions, including cancer and heart disease, as well as in the bodily changes associated with aging. Free radicals may also play a role in common complications of diabetes such as neuropathy and eye disease.

Antioxidants are compounds that are able to neutralize or stop free radicals. Many compounds present in fruits, vegetables, and herbs, such as vitamin E and beta-carotene, act as antioxidants. Other antioxidant compounds (and antioxidant-containing herbs) that you may see listed on supplement labels include flavonoids, quercetin, coenzyme Q10, hawthorne (*Crataegus laevigata* and *Crataegus monogyna*), phenols, green tea extract, grapeseed extract, garlic, bilberry (*Vaccinium myrtillus*), and alpha-lipoic acid.

There is very little research on the effectiveness of these compounds in treating and preventing disease when taken as individual supplements. (In fact, certain antioxidant supplements have increased, rather than decreased, the incidence of cancer when taken

in pill form.) However, there is a great deal of research showing the benefits of a diet high in fruits and vegetables. So at present, the best approach for people who want to reap the benefits of antioxidants is to increase their intake of fruits and vegetables.

Herbs that inhibit blood clotting. Several herbs appear to decrease the "stickiness" of blood platelets—special, disk-shaped cell fragments that play a role in blood clotting. People who have had a heart attack or who have cardiovascular disease are often prescribed drugs that decrease the ability of their blood to clot, and this decreases their chances of a heart attack. Herbs that may have similar effects on blood clotting include ginger, garlic, ginkgo extract, and ginseng.

Because decreasing the ability of the blood to clot can lead to uncontrolled bleeding and can potentially increase risk of certain types of strokes, these herbal supplements (and others with similar actions) should only be used under the close guidance of a physician. They should be avoided by people who use drugs or other supplements that also decrease blood clotting. (Examples include aspirin, warfarin or coumarin, and vitamin E.) Ginger, garlic, ginkgo extract, and ginseng should be discontinued several weeks before surgery. Because ginseng may also increase blood pressure, people with high blood pressure should use it only under the care of their physician.

Peripheral neuropathy

People with diabetic peripheral neuropathy are understandably eager for new treatments. This microvascular complication can cause pain and numbness in the feet, legs, hands, and arms, depriving many people of sleep and raising their risk of developing foot ulcers. While existing treatments do bring symptomatic relief to some people, they don't work for everyone, and they may stop working for those they initially help. Treatments with potential benefit for easing symptoms of peripheral neuropathy include alpha-lipoic acid and evening primrose oil (*Oenthera biennis*). One with demonstrated benefit is capsaicin (*Capsicum frutens*).

Alpha-lipoic acid. Also called thioctic acid, alpha-lipoic acid is a potent antioxidant compound that has been studied as a treatment for diabetic peripheral neuropathy. It may also help improve insulin sensitivity. There are several studies that show that alpha-lipoic acid, taken orally or intravenously, has a favorable effect on some but not all measures of nerve function and symptoms of neuropathy. Some people appear to respond to alpha-lipoic acid more than others, and in some studies, intravenous alpha-lipoic acid appears more effective than oral. There is little information on the long-term effectiveness of oral alpha-lipoic acid or on the potential role of alpha-lipoic acid as a preventive agent.

The effective dose of alpha-lipoic acid in oral trials ranged between 1200 milligrams per day and 1600 milligrams per day. No significant side effects were noted with oral use of up to 1800 milligrams per day. However, there is a potential for hypoglycemia in people who use insulin or oral blood-glucose-lowering medicines. One study in animals also found taking alpha-lipoic acid to be fatal in animals who were deficient in the B vitamin thiamine. (People who are at risk for thiamine deficiency include the elderly, alcoholics, and people on kidney dialysis.)

At this time, alpha-lipoic acid has not been proven an effective treatment for diabetic neuropathy and is not recommended for such use. Additional studies, however, are currently under way.

Capsaicin. An irritant that makes hot peppers hot, capsaicin is noted both for its ability to relieve pain and its popularity as a condiment (in the form of chili peppers) in many countries around the world. Topical application of creams containing capsaicin have been shown in research studies to decrease the pain associated with peripheral neuropathy. Such creams work by depleting levels of *substance P*, a neuropeptide involved in the transmission of painful impulses from the peripheral nerves to the spinal cord.

Use of capsaicin-containing creams initially causes irritation and an increased burning sensation; these effects should decrease over time, generally within five days of use. Most over-the-counter capsaicin creams contain very low concentrations of capsaicin (in the range of 0.025% to 0.25%) and have been found to have mild and variable effects. Creams containing higher concentrations of capsaicin (over 1%) may be more effective and are currently being studied by researchers.

For maximal effect, capsaicin creams need to be applied regularly, up to four to five times per day, for several days. After application, careful washing of the hands is needed to avoid accidental irritation of the eyes, skin, and mucous membranes.

Evening primrose oil. Derived from the seeds of a native American wildflower, evening primrose oil has been suggested as a potential treatment for cardiovascular disease and diabetic neuropathy because of its high concentration of gamma-linolenic acid, an omega-6 fatty acid. The potential benefits of gamma-linolenic acid appear to be due to its effect on the production of compounds in the body that regulate inflammation.

Only a few studies have looked at evening primrose oil or gamma-linolenic acid supplements in people with diabetes. These studies suggest that evening primrose oil and other sources of gamma-linolenic acid may help to improve some measures of nerve function in people with peripheral neuropathy. Effects were generally greater in subjects whose blood glucose levels were closer to target range at the study's outset.

Gamma-linolenic acid and evening primrose oil appear to be relatively safe when consumed in doses under 3 grams per day or 100 milligrams per kilogram of body weight per day. Typical doses used in research studies range from 0.5 gram to 6 grams per day of evening primrose oil and 0.5 gram to 3 grams per day of gamma-linolenic acid. Other good sources of gamma-linolenic acid include borage oil and black currant oil. However, use of borage oil is not recommended due to the presence of several potentially toxic compounds.

Retinopathy

Bilberry, also called European blueberry, and ginkgo have both been proposed as potential treatments for diabetic retinopathy, but neither is currently recommended for this use.

Bilberry. Bilberry was used by pilots in the British Royal Air Force during World War II to improve their

RECORDING FORM FOR HERBAL SUPPLEMENT USE

When you use an herbal supplement, keeping records will help you determine whether it's having an effect. Records can also come in handy in the event of side effects. Here's an example.

PRODUCT NAME, ACTIVE INGREDIENTS	BRAND, LOT #, COMPANY, PHONE #	GUIDELINES FOR USE	PRECAUTIONS	DATE STARTED	SIDE EFFECTS	REASON FOR TAKING HERB, EFFECTS ON BLOOD GLUCOSE LEVEL
Mega-Herb Tea, peppermint, chamomile, slippery elm	Herbal-licious Products, Lot 101, ABC Herbs, (800) 555-5555	Brew one cup of tea three times a day. Drink between meals.	Do not use if you have gallstones.	1/23/01	Mild indigestion.	Hope to ease cold symptoms; no noticeable effects on blood glucose level.

night vision. Bilberry may also improve blood flow to the small arteries of the eyes and decrease the "leakiness" of arteries and veins sometimes seen in diabetic retinopathy, thereby decreasing fluid accumulation, or edema. The active compounds in bilberry are believed to be flavonoids and anthocyanosides, which are potent antioxidants.

The bilberry leaf has been used as a blood-sugar-lowering agent by Native Americans but has been found to be toxic with long-term consumption and in high doses. Potential side effects from bilberry fruit include gastrointestinal distress and decreased ability of the blood to clot. Its use is not recommended at this time due to lack of evidence and the potential for serious side effects.

Ginkgo. A popular herb product in the United States, ginkgo extract (the name is also spelled gingko), from *Ginkgo biloba,* is most commonly taken to "enhance memory," although there is no actual proof it can preserve, improve, or restore memory function. Ginkgo is reported to improve blood flow, decrease blood clotting, and act as an antioxidant. It has been studied as a treatment for peripheral vascular disease, a condition in which the legs and sometimes the arms become clogged with fatty plaque buildup (atherosclerosis), and it appears to improve ocular blood flow. However, at this time, there is no information available on its potential role in treating diabetic retinopathy.

Potential side effects of ginkgo include increased bleeding, allergic reactions, gastrointestinal upset, and headaches. People using anticoagulants, herbs, or vitamins should use ginkgo only under a doctor's care.

Impotence

The herb yohimbe (*Pausinystalia yohimbe*) has long had a reputation as an aphrodisiac and a treatment for impotence, but clinical trials generally do not support its use. In fact, the U.S. Food and Drug Administration (FDA) has had yohimbe on its unsafe herb list since 1977. While there is no information on the long-term safety of yohimbe, potential side effects of short-term use include anxiety, nausea, vomiting, changes in blood pressure and heart rate, dizziness, headache, and kidney failure. Yohimbe may interact with over-the-counter stimulants such as caffeine, with phenylephrine (an active ingredient in many cold and allergy medicines), and with many kinds of antidepressants. It should not be used by people with high blood pressure, kidney or liver disease, psychiatric disorders, or a history of gastric or duodenal ulcers.

All complications

One way high blood glucose levels are believed to contribute to complications is by increasing the amount of glucose that is converted to *sorbitol* in the cells of the body. When blood glucose levels are high, glucose can also build up in the cells, including those in the lens of the eye, retina, nerves, and blood vessels. The extra glucose is converted to sorbitol, which can then be changed further into *fructose.* Water is chemically attracted to sorbitol and fructose and tends to accumulate inside cells that have high levels of them. This causes swelling of the cells, cellular damage, and, over time, the symptoms of diabetic complications. (Note that eating foods that contain either sorbitol or fructose does not have the same effect and therefore does not raise the risk of developing diabetic complications.)

There are several experimental drugs and some herbal supplements that may prevent this type of damage. These compounds are called aldose reductase inhibitors, or ARI's, and they act by inhibiting the action of aldose reductase, the enzyme that converts glucose into sorbitol. In animal studies and in vitro (test tube) studies, several compounds and herbs have been shown to inhibit the enzyme aldose reductase. Some of these include flavonoids, quercetin, and extracts from licorice root. However, none of these compounds have been studied in humans.

The usefulness of licorice or licorice extracts (glycyrrhizic acid) may be limited because of potential side effects, which include high blood pressure, fluid retention, and low potassium levels. Licorice is also known to interact with some antihypertensive drugs, heart drugs, and steroids. It should not be used by people with kidney, liver, or heart disease. Most licorice candy sold in the United States is actually flavored with anise oil and other flavoring agents and does not contain true licorice extracts.

Overweight

While being overweight is not considered a complication of diabetes, it is a condition that often accompanies Type 2 diabetes, and it can make controlling blood glucose levels more difficult. In many cases, losing even a small amount of weight (about 10% of body weight) can significantly lower both blood glucose and blood cholesterol levels. Diabetes experts generally recommend that people who would like to lose weight do so by increasing their physical activity and by following a nutritious diet that is moderate in fat and calories.

There are numerous herbal and nutritional supplements sold through mail-order companies and in grocery stores, pharmacies, and natural food stores that are marketed to people who are trying to lose weight. None of these "special formulations" have been tested in scientific studies, and none have been shown to be effective in helping people lose significant amounts of weight or maintain weight loss. Any weight loss that does occur initially with these products is due to increased water loss and mild appetite suppression.

Some of the individual components of these products have been studied under research conditions, but none has been proven to be a safe and effective way to lose weight.

Common ingredients found in herbal weight-loss preparations include various diuretics and laxatives, guarana (*Paullinia cupana*), ephedra (*Ephedrae herba*), and garcinia (*Garcinia cambogia*).

SUGGESTIONS FOR FURTHER READING

A surge of interest in herbal therapy has increased the amount published on the topic. Some resources are listed below.

ARTICLES
"HERBAL ROULETTE"
Consumer Reports, November 1995, pages 698–705.

"HERBAL RX: THE PROMISES AND PITFALLS"
Consumer Reports, March 1999, pages 44–48.

BOOKS
AMERICAN HERBAL PRODUCT ASSOCIATION'S BOTANICAL SAFETY HANDBOOK
Michael McGuffin
CRC Press, L.L.C.
Boca Raton, Florida, 1997

ENCYCLOPEDIA OF POPULAR HERBS
Robert S. McCaleb, Evelyn Leigh, and Krista Morien
Prima Communications, Inc.
Roseville, California, 2000

TYLER'S HERBS OF CHOICE
The Therapeutic Use of Phytomedicinals
James E. Robbers and Varro E. Tyler
The Haworth Herbal Press
Binghamton, New York, 1999

TYLER'S HONEST HERBAL
A Sensible Guide to the Use of Herbs and Related Remedies, 4th edition
Steven Foster and Varro E. Tyler
The Haworth Herbal Press
Binghamton, New York, 1999

NEWSLETTERS
THE AMERICAN HERB ASSOCIATION QUARTERLY NEWSLETTER
American Herb Association
P.O. Box 1673
Nevada City, CA 95959

CONSUMER REPORTS ON HEALTH
(800) 333-9784
www.consumerreports.org
A general health publication that sometimes covers herbal products.

ENVIRONMENTAL NUTRITION NEWSLETTER
(800) 829-5384
A general nutrition publication that sometimes covers herbal products.

HERBALGRAM
(512) 926-4900

NUTRITION ACTION HEALTH LETTER
(202) 332-9110
www.cspinet.org
A general nutrition publication that sometimes covers herbal products.

ORGANIZATIONS
AMERICAN BOTANICAL COUNCIL
(512) 926-4900
www.herbalgram.org
Publications about herbs are available for purchase. (Members receive a discount.) Brief descriptions, uses, pictures, and suggested doses of some common herbs are available on the Web site, which also has many links to other relevant sites.

HERB RESEARCH FOUNDATION
(800) 748-2617
www.herbs.org
Sells information packs about many herbs and health conditions. (Members receive a discount.) Green papers, which contain information on a few herb-related topics, can be viewed on the foundation's Web site.

U.S. NATIONAL CENTER FOR COMPLEMENTARY AND ALTERNATIVE MEDICINE
(formerly the National Institutes of Health Office of Alternative Medicine)
(888) 644-6226
http://nccam.nih.gov
Clearinghouse sponsored by the federal government that distributes free educational materials put together by the National Institutes of Health. The Web site provides access to such resources as answers to frequently asked questions, fact sheets, and consensus reports.

Diuretics. Diuretics cause increased urination and fluid loss. Those found in weight-loss preparations include dandelion root (*Taraxacum officinale*), bearberry (*Arctostaphylos uva-ursi*), juniper (*Juniperus communis*), chickweed (*Stellaria media*), and stinging nettle (*Urtica dioica*).

Because overuse of diuretics can lead to dehydration and loss of magnesium and electrolytes such as potassium and sodium, these products should be used only under the care of a doctor. (Electrolyte imbalances can cause serious abnormalities in heart contractions.) People with diabetes, heart disease, or high blood pressure are at greater risk of complications and drug interactions with the use of diuretics.

Laxatives. Laxatives include aloe (*Aloe barbadensis*), senna (*Cassia senna* and *Cassia angustifolia*), and buckthorn (*Rhamnus frangula*). Note that the aloe with laxative properties is not the same as aloe gel, the clear, mucilaginous substance used in lotions, shampoos, and similar products. Both come from the same plant, but they are found in different parts of the plant.

Overuse of laxatives can cause dehydration and loss of many trace minerals and electrolytes that are needed for normal metabolism. In addition, overuse of laxatives can result in decreased spontaneous bowel function and dependence on laxatives.

Guarana. A caffeine-containing appetite suppressant, guarana is made from a shrub native to Brazil and Uruguay, where it is used to make a hot beverage. It has potentially negative side effects at high doses, including anxiety, nausea, irregularities in heartbeat, and seizures. Guarana should be avoided by people with gastric reflux (a condition in which stomach acid backs up into the esophagus), gastric ulcers, or high blood pressure and by people who take the drug theophylline.

Ephedra. Also called ma huang and herbal fen-phen, ephedra contains numerous alkaloids, including ephedrine and pseudoephedrine. These compounds are central nervous system stimulants and can alter the strength of heart contractions, heart rate, and blood pressure. There is a small amount of research that suggests that ephedra, when taken in combination with caffeine, may slightly increase weight loss—about 1½ pounds more over several months—when compared to a placebo treatment. But these mild effects on weight loss do not outweigh the potential negative side effects of ephedra.

There have been hundreds of adverse side effects of ephedra reported to the FDA, including heart attack, stroke, and death. The FDA has issued warning statements about the use of ephedra as a weight-loss agent, and the agency restricts the amount of ephedra allowed in a single dose of a supplement. Ephedra is not recommended as a weight-loss supplement for anyone, and it could be especially harmful for people with high blood pressure, heart disease, diabetes, thyroid disease, enlarged prostate, angina, or a history of stroke. Ephedra can cause uterine contractions and should not be used by pregnant women.

Garcinia. Derived from the fruit of a tree native to India and other areas of Southeast Asia, garcinia is a source of hydroxycitric acid and is reported to decrease appetite and food intake, inhibit fat and cholesterol synthesis, and promote weight loss. (It is sometimes, though incorrectly, called Malabar tamarind; it is not the same as tamarind.)

Results of human studies have been mixed, with a recent, well-designed study showing no effect on weight loss when compared to placebo treatment. There are no long-term studies of the safety or effectiveness of garcinia or of hydroxycitric acid, though short-term studies have reported no notable side effects with doses up to 1500 milligrams per day.

Using supplements safely

If you are currently using or would like to try the supplements discussed in this article or other herbal therapies, remember that the manufacturing and production of supplements is not regulated closely by the federal government. This means that supplements can and often do contain variable quantities of active ingredients. Some supplements have even been found to be contaminated with dangerous compounds. Until these issues are corrected, herbal supplements, even if shown to be effective in a research setting, may not be safe or effective for general use. Here are some tips for avoiding serious problems:

■ Research the products you are considering using.

■ Discuss the potential safety concerns of the product with your doctor and other members of your health-care team.

■ Follow health-care team guidelines for use—or advice not to use.

■ Determine the benefits you hope to receive, and keep track of the dose taken and any apparent side effects. Record this information in a log or journal. (A sample recording form is shown on page 153.)

■ Stop all supplements if benefits are not seen within several weeks or if you notice any side effects. Report all side effects to your health-care team.

Research into potential therapeutic agents for complications of diabetes is exciting, and we all hope for as many effective treatments as soon as possible. In the meantime, however, the best research we have to date on preventing and treating complications indicates that the best defense against complications is maintaining blood glucose levels as close to normal as possible and bringing blood pressure down to near-normal levels. Work with your health-care team to achieve these goals. You will feel better now—and later. ❏

CARDIOVASCULAR HEALTH

WHAT IS YOUR RISK OF HEART DISEASE?
A SELF-TEST

by Prudence E. Breitrose, M.A.

Think of the people you know who have had a heart attack, and then think about those who haven't. Do you know someone who smokes like a chimney, doesn't watch her weight, eats whatever she likes, and is still going strong at 83? And do you also know someone who looked after himself, kept his weight down, exercised regularly, didn't smoke, and suffered a heart attack long before retirement age?

When you think about people like these, you may conclude that it's hard to assess the risk of having a heart attack, right? Wrong. At least, mostly wrong. Yes, there are surprise heart attacks and surprise survivors, but these are the exceptions rather than the rule. When we look at large populations, we can see how the actual risk adds up for the *average* person by counting the number of risk factors—such as having diabetes, high cholesterol, or high blood pressure, smoking, and not getting enough exercise—that an individual has.

But what about shortcuts? Every so often you read about some new discovery that seems to promise instant immunity against heart disease—a daily glass of wine, fish oil, or orange juice. And yes, it's true that those things may be able to help. But there's no magic pill or magic food that can work on its own. Heart disease is a complicated condition, and preventing it requires paying attention to known risk factors.

This quiz will help you to assess how well you are doing with regard to various risk factors. For each question, circle the letter of the choice that best describes you. At the end, we suggest four things you can do to reduce your risk or keep it low.

What's your risk?

First, here are the risk factors that are hard (or even impossible) to change.

1. What's your sex and, for women, the status of your hormones?
A. I am a man, or I am a woman before menopause
B. I am a woman after menopause, and I do not take hormone replacements
C. I am a woman after menopause, and I do take hormone replacements

2. How many of your close relatives (parents, grandparents, uncles, aunts, siblings) had heart attacks before the age of 65?
A. A whole bunch
B. More than one
C. One
D. None

Here are some risk factors that you *can* change:

3. What is your total cholesterol level?
A. Over 240 mg/dl
B. 220 to 239 mg/dl
C. 200 to 219 mg/dl
D. Under 200 mg/dl

4. What is your high-density lipoprotein (HDL) cholesterol (the "good" cholesterol) level?
A. Under 35 mg/dl
B. 35 to 42 mg/dl
C. 43 to 50 mg/dl
D. Over 50 mg/dl

5. What is your systolic blood pressure (the higher number)?
A. Higher than 160 mm Hg
B. 141 to 160 mm Hg
C. 121 to 140 mm Hg
D. 120 mm Hg or lower

6. What is your diastolic blood pressure (the lower number)?
A. Higher than 100 mm Hg
B. 91 to 100 mm Hg

C. 81 to 90 mm Hg
D. 80 mm Hg or lower

7. Do you smoke cigarettes and, if so, how much?
A. More than a pack a day
B. Half a pack to one pack a day
C. Less than half a pack a day or smoke a pipe
D. Don't smoke

8. When it comes to physical activity, how do you rate?
A. A couch potato
B. Occasionally active
C. Moderately active on most days
D. Very active on most days

9. How thick is the roll of fat when you pinch your side at your waistline?
A. As thick as my wrist, or thicker
B. Between the size of my thumb and the size of my wrist
C. About the size of my thumb
D. Smaller than the size of my thumb

10. How is excess fat distributed on your body?
A. I look like an apple (wider at the waist than around the hips)
B. I look like a pear (wider below the waist, in the buttocks and thighs)
C. I do not look like a piece of fruit
D. I don't have much excess fat

11. What kind of stress do you feel and how often?
A. I am often angry
B. I feel tense and rushed much of the time
C. I feel tense and rushed occasionally
D. I'm generally pretty calm

How did you rate?

Let's look first at the factors you may not be able to do much about.

QUESTIONS 1 AND 2.
In the general population, men have a higher risk of developing heart disease than women who are of childbearing age. After menopause, when estrogen production drops off, a woman's risk may become as high as a man's. For people who have diabetes, however, the relative risks are a little different. For one thing, having diabetes raises the risk of heart disease for both sexes. And women with diabetes are just as likely to develop heart disease as men with diabetes, even before menopause. Hormone replacement therapy (HRT) may reduce the risk for some women after menopause. Women past menopause who are not on

HRT may want to talk to their doctor about its pros and cons. (See also "Hormone Replacement: More Than Just Estrogen" on page 388.)

A family history of heart attacks may raise your risk for heart disease. But if there's also a family tendency to have high cholesterol or high blood pressure or to be overweight, there are steps you can take to break out of the family pattern.

So if your answers for questions 1 and 2 appear to put you at a higher risk, don't assume there's nothing you can do. If you scored only C's and D's on questions 3 through 11, your total risk may be quite low.

Now let's look at the factors that you can do something about:

QUESTIONS 3 AND 4 (Blood Cholesterol).

Cholesterol comes in two main types: high-density lipoprotein (HDL) cholesterol, the "good" kind, and low-density lipoprotein (LDL) cholesterol, the "bad" kind. HDL cholesterol plays an important role in lowering the level of LDL cholesterol in the blood.

High levels of total cholesterol and low levels of HDL cholesterol can contribute to the buildup of plaque in the arteries, narrowing the opening through which blood flows. When plaque builds up in the tiny coronary arteries that supply blood to the heart muscle, the heart doesn't get enough oxygen to do its work, and the result can be angina (chest pain). Even small plaques can rupture, which can result in a total blockage of blood flow through the vessel. If the heart muscle supplied by the blocked artery has no other source of blood, it will die, and the individual will have a heart attack. If an artery supplying blood to the brain gets blocked, the result is a stroke.

Fortunately, total cholesterol levels can be brought down through changes in diet such as reducing the amount of saturated fat you eat. Total cholesterol also usually comes down as people lose weight. If those two measures don't work, talk to your doctor about medicine to reduce cholesterol levels.

Changing your diet can't improve your HDL level, but there are other ways you can raise it. If your HDL is too low (30 or 40 mg/dl), you may be able to bring it up by losing weight or by increasing your physical activity. And HDL cholesterol is naturally higher in women before menopause and in those who take hormones after menopause.

QUESTIONS 5 AND 6 (Blood Pressure).

Systolic blood pressure is the pressure while the heart is actually pumping, and diastolic blood pressure is the pressure between beats. Both numbers are important. Blood pressure goes up when the blood vessels don't stretch as far as they should to accommodate the flow of blood. When blood vessels lose flexibility, the

heart has to work harder, which strains the heart itself and also creates wear and tear on the arteries.

High blood pressure can almost always be brought down, often by things you can do yourself. For most people, blood pressure drops sharply as they lose weight. For others, it responds well to a reduction in dietary salt and other forms of sodium. Consuming more potassium from bananas and other fruits and vegetables can also help lower blood pressure. If these measures don't work, there's a wide choice of drugs that can be lifesavers, provided you take them.

QUESTION 7 (Smoking).

Don't. Please. Cigarette smoking is one of the main causes of heart attacks, killing many more people than lung cancer or other lung diseases. How? By constricting the arteries, speeding up the heart, and adding to the blockage of blood vessels. How to quit? It's not easy, but many people succeed when they follow a quitting program (like the ones offered by the American Cancer Society and the American Lung Association) and/or use a nicotine patch or nicotine gum. You need to follow the directions for nicotine products exactly. If you have any doubts or questions, check with your doctor.

QUESTION 8 (Physical Activity).

There's good news for couch potatoes and others who don't yet enjoy moving their bodies: You don't need to "work out," jog, or even go for long brisk walks to reduce your risk of heart disease. Although these are still probably the best options, you can get many of the same health effects by moving at a moderate intensity for a total of about 30 minutes a day. Such movement might include walking to the store, mowing the lawn, cleaning windows, climbing stairs, or dancing. Anything that moves your body will do. It doesn't have to be all at once, but you will need to keep track of your activity to make sure it adds up to 30 minutes a day.

QUESTIONS 9 AND 10 (Body Fat).

How much you weigh may not be as important as what that weight is made of. A 300-pound man could be in great shape if he's constructed mostly of muscle. A 150-pound man could still be too fat if he has more fat than muscle on his body. The pinch test tells you how much excess flab you are carrying around.

Excess fat is considered especially harmful if you have "male-pattern obesity," that is, if you are shaped more like an apple than a pear. Women who carry their excess fat around the buttocks and thighs, rather than around the waist, are considered somewhat better off than apple-shaped women.

QUESTION 11 (Stress).

Excessive stress plays a smaller role in the onset of heart attacks and strokes than many people think.

However, there are two exceptions: If you are constantly seething with anger and hostility, your risk may go up. And if you often feel rushed and anxious, you are less likely to look after yourself in other ways. You may even be tempted to smoke, drink, or turn to junk food in an attempt to relieve your stress. The solution? Read on.

Adding it up

Did you get a lot of C's and D's? Congratulations.

What about A's and B's? Well, obviously it's a good idea to start thinking about some changes, especially if your A's and B's popped up in questions 3 through 7, where we put the Big Three risk factors: cholesterol levels, high blood pressure, and smoking. Individually, each of these factors is serious enough. If you have more than one, then alarm bells should ring because the damage can accumulate quickly. It may help to think of it this way:

■ high total cholesterol = increased risk
■ high cholesterol + high blood pressure = double that risk
■ high cholesterol + high blood pressure + smoking = quadruple that risk

Now for the good news. If you smoke, your risk will start to go down on the day you quit. And the other risk factors can be tackled all at once, through changes described below.

The "Hot Four" behaviors

Entire books have been written on each of the risk factors we describe in this article. Yet you can make a big difference in your life by paying attention to only four types of behavior. If you take these four steps every day (and quit smoking cigarettes), your general health will improve, and your score in the heart risk quiz will slip comfortably downward in the alphabet, as those A's and B's turn into C's and D's.

1. Cut down on saturated fat and **trans** *fat.* Saturated fat can raise levels of blood cholesterol and increase your risk of heart disease if eaten in excess. Choosing low-fat or nonfat dairy products, removing the skin before eating chicken, and eating red meat only in moderation are all ways to cut back on saturated fat in your diet. (For more tips, see "Cutting Back on Saturated Fat" on page 281.)

Recent research suggests that *trans* fats, or hardened unsaturated fats, may be even worse for you than saturated fat. *Trans* fats are found in stick margarines, solid vegetable shortening, most commercial baked goods, and foods that have been deep-fried in vegetable shortening. *Trans* fats are created when vegetable oils are "hydrogenated," or hardened, to make them firmer and more resistant to becoming rancid. Using the softer tub margarines on toast and using liquid vegetable oils for cooking and baking will help cut down on your *trans* fat consumption.

2. Read labels. The Nutrition Facts labels on prepared foods tell you what a serving size is and how many calories, how much saturated fat, and how much sodium each serving contains. Some people use these labels to help keep track of their daily consumption of fat, sodium, and calories. Others use them to compare the nutrient content of different brands of the same product.

Labels are especially useful in helping you spot hidden saturated fat. Most saturated fats are found in animal products, but they also turn up in tropical oils such as palm oil and coconut oil, so it's important to read the label. *Trans* fats are not currently listed on food labels, but the word "hydrogenated" almost always means they're there.

3. Eat more vegetables and whole grains. There is more and more evidence accumulating about the benefits of eating vegetables and whole grains. It's not just the fiber in these foods (which has been shown to lower blood cholesterol levels) or the fact that when you fill up on vegetables and whole grains, you tend to eat less meat. We now know that there are many compounds in plants that can promote health by helping the body fight off both heart disease and cancer. For example, vegetables rich in vitamins C and E provide antioxidants that are believed to help prevent damage to the insides of the arteries. Folic acid, found in such foods as beans, spinach, and orange juice, appears to prevent the buildup of a substance called homocysteine, which can also damage arteries. And many fruits and vegetables are excellent sources of potassium, which can help control blood pressure.

So take a minute to think about your eating habits. Do you eat at least five servings of fruits or vegetables a day? Do you eat a variety of vegetables, including orange and dark green ones? Do you eat bread made with whole grains? If not, think about how you could add more fruits, vegetables, and whole grains to your diet—preferably prepared without a lot of added fat.

4. Get more active. For most people, getting more active can't hurt. And in almost all cases, it will help. People who are really active can cheat the calendar: Their bodies act much younger than the bodies of people their age who don't exercise. Activity can help you control your weight, blood cholesterol, blood pressure, and level of stress, and it makes you feel more cheerful. As an added bonus, activity also helps you control your blood sugar.

While you're thinking about it, take a quick inventory of your usual physical activity. Do you exercise vigorously for at least 20 minutes at least three times a week? Or do you keep track of your moderate activity throughout the day? Do you get at least 30 minutes of brisk walking or other moderate activity as part of your daily routine? If you know you've been slacking off on exercise, think about how and when you could do a little more, and mark your next "exercise appointment" on your calendar.

Working with your doctor

As you can see, there's a lot you can do by yourself. But there's also a lot you can do where you'll need your doctor's help. Prescription drugs for blood pressure and cholesterol control can be lifesavers. For women past menopause, the question of whether to take hormone replacements is a critical one, and your doctor can lay out the pros and cons. Your doctor can also advise you about nonprescription drugs such as small doses of aspirin to help prevent formation of blood clots, or even a (purely medicinal) glass of wine. And your doctor can advise you on safe and useful amounts of physical activity.

But remember that most of your heart health is in your own hands. It's up to you to make changes and to find ways of living that will keep you healthy and add to your enjoyment of life at the same time. ❏

HOW EMOTIONS AFFECT YOUR RISK OF A HEART ATTACK

by Prudence E. Breitrose, M.A.

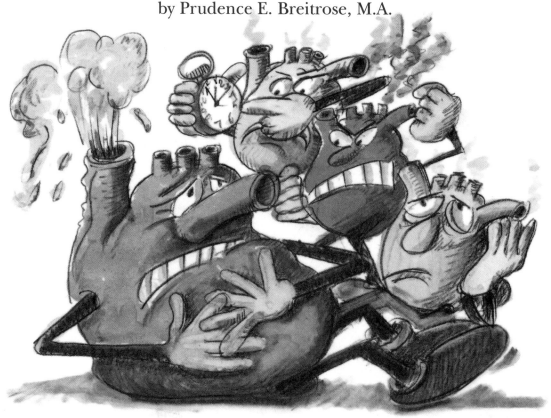

A high-powered executive clutches his chest and collapses as a particularly stressful moment carries him into the great beyond. Or the surviving member of a loving couple turns up his or her toes and expires, gently dying of a broken heart. These are images we all grew up with. But are they true? Do these things really happen?

These devices may help movie plots along nicely, but nowadays we are much more scientific, aren't we? If we are going to have heart attacks, they will be caused by measurable risk factors such as high cholesterol levels, high blood pressure, overweight, and smoking, won't they? And as for dying of a broken heart, it only happens in poems or romance novels. Right?

Well, not exactly. That pendulum is swinging again. Researchers have been finding that there is, after all, a connection between our emotions and our bodies. Many now suspect that psychological stress, anger, and depression—and our responses to these emotions and problems—can indeed increase the risk of a heart attack.

Stress

Let's look first at stress. There is no doubt that stress can have a powerful temporary effect on the way our bodies work. That's what it's for. We were given the "stress response" in order to give us the extra strength to deal with emergencies. The stress response speeds up the heart; directs more blood to the brain, for quick thinking; directs more blood to the legs and arms, for speed and strength; and pumps out the extra hormones needed for a quick response.

This system was terrific for cavemen (and cavewomen), who presumably encountered animal predators and other such acute threats and needed the strength to fight back or run away. But the "fight-or-flight" response isn't so useful in modern times, when sources of stress tend to be chronic. And there is evidence that stress can be harmful to health in a number of ways.

For one thing, stress can increase the heart's need for blood, just as physical exercise does. At the same time, however, it can reduce the amount of blood flowing through the coronary arteries. This can obviously spell bad news for a heart that already has less-than-perfect circulation.

This was evident from a study at Duke University, which was reported in 1996. Researchers took 126 people with established coronary artery disease and gave them mental tests that raised their stress level. Some of the subjects experienced inadequate blood flow to the heart during these stressful moments. And it turned out that those subjects had a much higher rate of a heart attack in the following months and years than the people who didn't react so strongly to stress.

Another study, at Johns Hopkins, involved 148 people who did not have heart disease but were at high risk for getting it because they had brothers or sisters who had experienced heart problems before age 60. The researchers deliberately raised the subjects' stress levels with fiendish mental tests designed to confuse them. Those who were most stressed by the tests were 19 times more likely to experience a temporary shortage of blood to the heart than the others.

Evidence from yet another study shows that stress may actually lead to a buildup of plaque in people's arteries. This study took place in Finland, where 901 men were given a series of mental tests designed to cause stress. The men who were the most stressed out were found to have more plaque in the lining of their arteries. And research indicates that it's a buildup of plaque that leads to most heart attacks and a large percentage of strokes.

What's the connection between stress and clogged arteries? Researchers don't have the whole picture yet, but they do know that the hormones that bring about the body's quick reaction at times of stress (or anger) can also promote the buildup of plaque. They also know that stress can raise blood pressure, and frequent and prolonged episodes of high blood pressure can damage the insides of the arteries.

Depression

What about depression? More than 50 years ago, a doctor named Benjamin Malzberg noticed that patients admitted to the New York State Psychiatric Hospital for severe depression had more than six times as much heart disease as the general population. More recent studies bear out this observation. In one long-term study in Baltimore, doctors kept track of 1,151 people for 15 years after checking them out for depression. At the end of that period, they found that heart disease was much more common among those who showed signs of depression at the beginning of the study. Why? We don't yet know exactly, but people who are depressed tend to have higher levels of stress hormones, which can damage arteries and may also contribute to disturbances in the heart's rhythm.

Depression also tends to affect how well a person takes care of his health. As you know, you can do a lot to prevent heart disease by looking after yourself: watching your diet, getting regular exercise, and so on. People who are depressed (or stressed out) are more likely to neglect themselves and perhaps to take up damaging habits such as smoking, drinking, or overeating.

Rate your stress level

While a certain amount of stress is inevitable in anyone's life, how you react to stress is to a large degree under your control. How much stress do you have in your life? How is it affecting you? And what can you do about it? Take this quiz to find out where you stand. Then we'll give tips for lowering your stress level.

YES NO

☐ ☐ Does stress give you aches in the head, back, stomach, or neck?

☐ ☐ Do you get a clenched jaw or tight muscles?

☐ ☐ Do you feel you never have enough time?

☐ ☐ Do you often feel impatient?

☐ ☐ Do you often lose your temper?

☐ ☐ Do you often feel angry, irritated, or impatient?

☐ ☐ Are you always in a hurry?

☐ ☐ Do you find it hard to sit still?

☐ ☐ Do you tend to eat and speak fast?

☐ ☐ Do you find it hard to relax?

YES NO
☐ ☐ Do you find it hard to concentrate?
☐ ☐ Do you get tired easily?
☐ ☐ Do you often feel anxious or worried?
☐ ☐ Do you have trouble putting across your point of view?
☐ ☐ Do you have trouble being assertive without being aggressive?
☐ ☐ Do you have phobias or panic attacks, or frequently experience acute anxiety?

Dealing with stress

If you answered yes to a whole bunch of these questions and are under severe stress, it's a good idea to get professional help. Ask your health-care provider to refer you to a stress-control program. If you suffer from panic attacks or severe phobias, tell your doctor. These can now be treated successfully, usually through a combination of medication and behavioral therapy. If you have only moderate stress, you can probably make it more manageable on your own by following these suggestions:

Clear at least 15 minutes of time for yourself every day. Do something you like. Or use this simple relaxation technique:

■ Set a timer for 15 minutes.

■ Lie back in your most comfortable chair and close your eyes.

■ Allow your muscles to relax.

■ Relax your mind by imagining calm, natural scenes such as leaves rustling in a slight breeze or a summer day at the lake.

Practice deep breathing. Make sure that your stomach goes in and out with each breath, not just your chest.

Take a walk on most days. Exercise makes you feel calmer. There's a bonus for people who can walk with a dog: Owning a pet can be very good for stress.

If you find that your day is simply too short to do everything you want to do, make a plan. Decide which activities are essential and which you can skip if you run out of time. Remember to leave some time for yourself!

Practice communicating better, especially if anger is one of your problems. Here are some tips for improving your communication skills:

■ Express your own point of view, without blaming anyone else.

■ If you anticipate a difficult scene or confrontation, practice what you will say first.

■ Listen to what the other person is saying, and if it isn't clear, go over it again.

■ Choose your battles. Don't try to win every argument.

If you can't change reality, change how you think about it. It may sound hard, but it isn't! When a trou-bling thought is gnawing at you, simply say to yourself, "There's nothing I can do about that. I'll think of something pleasant instead, like my vacation." It works!

Finally, avoid putting things in your body that can increase tension, such as excessive caffeine or alcohol.

Dealing with depression

Everyone feels sad or blue sometimes. For example, if you have been turned down for a job, lost a friend, crashed your car, or just heard that your kid flunked out of college, that can be profoundly depressing. But that sort of depression usually clears up, either because the situation improves, or because the passage of time helps heal the wound.

The more damaging type of depression is the sort that doesn't seem to have any particular reason. This is very common, and fortunately, with modern methods, can usually be treated. But first, do you have it? Here's a brief quiz.

YES NO
☐ ☐ Have you lost interest in hobbies or activities that used to give you pleasure?
☐ ☐ Do you have trouble sleeping, or are you sleeping much more than normal?
☐ ☐ Do you feel more irritable than before?
☐ ☐ Do you feel sad or apathetic?
☐ ☐ Are you worried about dying? Are you worried about the death of loved ones?
☐ ☐ Do you get terribly worried about world events?
☐ ☐ Do you have trouble concentrating?
☐ ☐ Do you feel tired or short of energy?
☐ ☐ Do you feel guilty much of the time?
☐ ☐ Has your weight gone up or gone down significantly?

If you answered yes to a lot of these questions, we suggest that you talk to your doctor about getting treatment. If you just have a few yes answers, here are some suggestions for improving your mood:

■ Read through our suggestions for dealing with stress. Those steps can help you feel more in control of your life. And that's often the first step toward easing depression.

■ Try to be with people. We are social beings, and living in isolation can make anyone feel down. Make plans to participate in activities that will require you to talk to people.

■ Get a pet. A pet can do two things: It will show you affection (if it's the right sort of pet), and it will demand attention. The fact that another creature is depending on you can help lift you out of your gloom.

■ Exercise! Physical activity helps in a number of ways: It can make you feel good about yourself, help pass the time pleasantly, help you to sleep better, make you look better, and give you more energy. Exercise can also actually pump a natural "upper" into the brain to make you feel good.

■ Avoid getting overwhelmed. If you feel your life is getting out of control, bring it back into a shape you can deal with. Break large tasks down into small ones so you feel good about completing something, not depressed because you can't finish the task.

■ Be aware of what you are thinking about yourself, and if it is negative, stop it! Many people are surprised to find how much power they have over what's going on in their heads. If you find yourself having depressed thoughts, change them!

■ Don't blame yourself for feeling depressed. It happens!

Feeling better

Emotional problems—stress, anxiety, depression—can't take all the blame for heart disease. And they may not even affect your chances of a heart attack unless you already have some other risk factors such as high cholesterol or high blood pressure. But even if these psychological problems didn't present any physical danger, it would be worth getting rid of them. Life would just be a whole lot more pleasant without them! ❑

REINING IN HIGH BLOOD PRESSURE

by J. Christopher Lynch, Pharm.D., Barbara K. Lynch, R.D., L.D., C.D.E., and Vivian Fonseca, M.D.

High blood pressure, also called hypertension, is a deadly disease that commonly occurs in people with diabetes. It is estimated that 24% of American adults have hypertension and that people with diabetes are twice as likely to have hypertension as people who don't have diabetes. Not only are people with diabetes more likely to develop hypertension, they are two to four times more likely to suffer the condition's most serious consequences: stroke and acute heart problems

such as heart attacks and unstable angina—in which there occurs a loss of blood flow to part of the heart, resulting in chest pain.

Hypertension and diabetes are also strong risk factors for the development of congestive heart failure, a long-term condition in which the quantity of blood pumped by the heart is insufficient to meet the body's needs for oxygen and nutrients. Any disease that affects the heart or interferes with circulation can lead to congestive heart failure.

Hypertension is often called "the silent killer" because most people with high blood pressure have no symptoms of the damage being done to their body. For this reason, it is very important that you have your blood pressure measured regularly.

Hypertension is commonly associated with atherosclerosis, a narrowing of the arteries leading to the heart and brain. In people with diabetes, chronic high blood glucose levels have also been shown to be related to the progression of atherosclerosis. Eventually, atherosclerosis causes the heart to have to work harder to deliver blood to all parts of the body. Not only does this result in increased blood pressure, but it also results in damage to the heart.

The American Diabetes Association (ADA) has laid out guidelines for identifying hypertension in people with diabetes. The ADA's blood pressure goal for most adults with diabetes is blood pressure less than 130/80 mm Hg. For adults who have achieved that goal and can tolerate what it takes to lower blood pressure further, the goal is blood pressure less than 120/80 mm Hg.

To understand these goals, or any blood pressure reading, it is important to understand what the numbers mean. The top (higher) number represents the *systolic* pressure: This is the pressure in an artery during a contraction of the heart (a heartbeat). The bottom (lower) number represents the *diastolic* pressure: This is the pressure in an artery between heartbeats. Blood pressure is measured in units of millimeters of mercury (mm Hg). This represents the height of the column of mercury in the traditional measurement device.

The higher the blood pressure, the greater the risk for stroke, heart disease, kidney disease, and eye disease. The ADA recommends that you have your blood pressure checked at every regular diabetes visit. If it is high, your doctor will discuss ways to lower it, including lifestyle changes and possibly blood-pressure-lowering drugs.

Lifestyle changes

Your lifestyle habits—including whether you smoke, how you eat, how much you exercise, and how you deal with stress—can all affect your blood pressure. For many people, changing one or more lifestyle habits can help to lower blood pressure.

Stop smoking. The most important lifestyle change you can make is to stop smoking tobacco. The nicotine in tobacco causes constriction of the blood vessels, increasing the risk for microvascular (small blood vessel) disease. This vascular constriction can seriously aggravate hypertension and worsen other complications of diabetes, including loss of sensation in the feet, legs, hands, and arms (a form of diabetic neu-

ropathy, or nerve damage) and impotence. If you smoke you are also more likely to have a heart attack and less likely to survive one.

Nicotine is extremely addictive, and quitting smoking can be difficult or impossible without help. While there are several prescription and over-the-counter drugs available to help you quit, they all work much better if you combine them with some sort of education program. If you need help finding a program near you, contact your local chapter of the National Lung Association or the American Cancer Society.

The good news for smokers is that heart disease risks revert to those of a nonsmoker within a relatively short period after stopping smoking. Regardless of how long you smoked or the number of cigarettes you smoked daily, within weeks of quitting tobacco, your risk of having a heart attack will diminish.

Weight control. Being overweight makes it two to six times more likely that a person will develop hypertension. Overweight is also a risk factor for developing Type 2 diabetes. Weight loss does not come easily, but it's worth the effort, and you may not need to lose as much as you think: Often, a 5% to 10% reduction in body weight has health benefits. Losing weight usually involves changing your eating habits. To know which of your habits may need changing, it helps to keep a written record of your food intake. Knowing where you have a problem is the first step in making a change.

One common problem that leads to overeating is not feeling satisfied, or sated, after a meal. It takes 20 to 30 minutes for a person to have a feeling of fullness after eating, making the first few minutes after a meal one of the danger times for overeating. To get through this time without eating more, try getting up from the table and doing something for 20 to 30 minutes. It may help to make a list of activities or chores and post it on the refrigerator. Your list might include calling a friend, taking out the trash, putting in some laundry, feeding a pet, tightening a loose screw in the door, or anything that will keep your mind occupied for 20 to 30 minutes.

Another common problem is eating for reasons other than hunger. Boredom and anxiety, for example, often lead to overeating, so it is important to pay attention to why you are eating. If it has been four hours since you last ate, it may well be time for a snack or meal. But if it has been only two hours since your last meal and you are bored, try giving yourself positive self-messages to stave off the impulse to eat. You might say to yourself, for example, "I am in control; I can wait." You might also try having a diet drink or getting busy with a chore to distract yourself. As you practice tuning in to your mind and your body, you will learn to distinguish between physical hunger and emotions such as anxiety that might prompt you to eat.

Dietary changes. Not only may changing the amount you eat help lower your blood pressure, but changing what you eat may also have positive effects. A three-year study called the Dietary Approaches to Stop Hypertension (DASH), reported in 1997, found striking reductions in blood pressure for people who followed a meal plan high in fruits and vegetables and low-fat dairy products and low in fat, saturated fat, and cholesterol. The meal plan was also rich in magnesium, potassium, calcium, protein, and fiber. (For more details on this meal plan, see "The DASH Diet" on this page.)

After eating this diet for as little as two weeks, study participants saw their systolic blood pressure reduced by an average of about 6 mm Hg and their diastolic blood pressure reduced by about 3 mm Hg. Participants with higher blood pressure at the outset of the study saw even greater reductions.

While the DASH diet is generally appropriate for people with diabetes, you may need to tailor it to your particular calorie and carbohydrate needs. A registered dietitian who is familiar with diabetes can help you do this.

Sodium restriction. Consuming too much sodium, a component of table salt, may increase your blood pressure. It has been common practice for many years to advise people with hypertension to restrict dietary sodium. But not all people are equally sensitive to sodium and its effect on blood pressure. Some health authorities recommend no more than 3,000 milligrams of sodium per day for the general population, while other authorities recommend no more than 2,400 milligrams per day. In its "Nutrition Recommendations and Principles for People With Diabetes Mellitus," the American Diabetes Association advises people with mild to moderate hypertension to limit sodium to 2,400 milligrams per day or less and for people with hypertension and nephropathy (kidney disease) to limit sodium to 2,000 milligrams per day or less. (The

THE DASH DIET

The Dietary Approaches to Stop Hypertension (DASH) study examined the effect of diet on blood pressure. After eight weeks, it was clear that the people following the diet described below—heavy on grains, fruits, vegetables, and low-fat dairy products with a low saturated fat and total fat content—experienced the greatest drops in blood pressure, compared to people following two other diets.

The number of servings of grains, fruits, and vegetables called for by the DASH diet may seem enormous, but the portion sizes are actually quite small. A person on a 2,000-calorie-per-day diet would eat 7–8 servings of grains, 4–5 servings of vegetables, 4–5 servings of fruit, 2–3 servings of low-fat or fat-free dairy foods, 2 or fewer servings of meat, poultry, and fish, and 2–3 servings of fats and oils per day, as well as 4–5 servings of nuts, seeds, and dry beans and 5 or fewer servings of sweets per week.

The DASH diet may need to be adapted for those following a diabetes meal plan. If you would like to follow the DASH diet, you should work with a dietitian to tailor it to your carbohydrate and calorie needs.

To get a copy of the DASH diet from the U.S. National Heart, Lung, and Blood Institute, write to the NHLBI Information Center, P.O. Box 30105, Bethesda, MD 20824-0105. People with Internet access can read more about the DASH diet at the Web site www.nhlbi.nih.gov.

At right is an approximation of the DASH diet.

FOOD GROUP	DAILY SERVINGS	1 SERVING EQUALS
GRAINS AND GRAIN PRODUCTS	7–8	1 slice bread ½ cup dry cereal ½ cup cooked rice, pasta, or cereal
VEGETABLES	4–5	1 cup raw leafy vegetable ½ cup cooked vegetable 6 ounces vegetable juice
FRUITS	4–5	1 medium fruit ½ cup fresh, frozen, or canned fruit ¼ cup dried fruit 6 ounces fruit juice
LOW-FAT OR NONFAT DAIRY PRODUCTS	2–3	8 ounces milk 1 cup yogurt 1½ ounces cheese
LEAN MEATS, POULTRY, OR FISH	2 or less	3 ounces cooked meats, skinless poultry, or fish
NUTS AND OTHER ALTERNATIVES TO MEAT	½	1½ ounces or ⅓ cup nuts 2 tablespoons seeds ½ cup cooked legumes

ADA defines mild to moderate hypertension as a systolic pressure between 140 and 159 mm Hg and a diastolic pressure between 90 and 99 mm Hg.)

If you are just learning to count carbohydrates or follow an exchange meal plan, your doctor or dietitian may not spend much time discussing sodium restriction with you. Nonetheless, we recommend that you make an effort to lower your sodium intake by making it a habit to read food labels and becoming better informed about sources of dietary sodium; by avoiding foods with a high sodium content; and by refraining from adding salt to your food at the table, particularly if salt was already added to it during cooking. Learn to season your food with herbs, spices, and other flavorful, low-sodium ingredients.

Exercise. Any number of studies have shown that regular exercise lowers the risk of developing high blood pressure and helps reduce blood pressure in those who already have hypertension. To reap the benefits of exercise, the U.S. Surgeon General's guidelines for physical activity state that "all adults should accumulate at least 30 minutes of moderate-intensity physical activity on most and preferably all days of the week." Most Americans currently do less than that and would benefit from an increase in exercise and physical activity.

If you do not engage in much physical activity now, however, you need to start with what you are capable of doing and build up to 30 minutes of physical activity a day. For example, if you can only walk 10 minutes at a time now, start with that and gradually increase the number of walks per week and the length of your walks—but only by one or two minutes each week. Take your time. It may take a month or more to reach your 30-minute-per-day goal, but with patience and persistence, you will get there.

Remember, if you have any numbness in your feet or any other foot problems, consult your doctor before undertaking a walking program. In addition, all people with diabetes should check their shoes for pebbles or other foreign objects before putting them

DRUGS FOR HIGH BLOOD PRESSURE

These drugs are commonly used to treat hypertension in people with diabetes.

DRUG CLASS	EXAMPLES (with brand name)	ADVANTAGES	SIDE EFFECTS/ DISADVANTAGES
THIAZIDE DIURETICS	HYDROCHLOROTHIAZIDE (HydroDiuril)	Low cost. Proven to decrease rates of heart attacks and strokes.	May cause short-term worsening of blood glucose control. Short-term increase in cholesterol.
BETA-BLOCKERS	ATENOLOL (Tenormin) PROPRANOLOL (Inderal)	Proven to decrease rates of heart attacks and strokes.	May worsen impotence. May hide signs of low blood sugar.
ACE INHIBITORS	CAPTOPRIL (Capoten) ENALAPRIL (Vasotec) LISINOPRIL (Prinivil, Zestril)	May slow the progression of certain kinds of kidney disease. Very slight beneficial effects on blood glucose and cholesterol.	Cough. Severe allergic reaction.
CALCIUM CHANNEL BLOCKERS (Only long-acting versions of these drugs should be commonly used.)	DILTIAZEM (Cardizem, Dilacor) NIFEDIPINE (Procardia, Adalat) VERAPAMIL (Verelan, Calan, Isoptin)	Diltiazem may be beneficial in certain kinds of kidney diseases. Has no effect on blood glucose or cholesterol.	Some calcium channel blockers cause edema (leg swelling).
ALPHA-BLOCKERS	DOXAZOSIN (Cardura) PRAZOSIN (Minipress) TERAZOSIN (Hytrin)	May help improve some prostate problems. Small positive effect on blood glucose.	Dizziness. Hypertension worsens quickly if doses are missed.

on and should check their feet for blisters or hot spots after taking a walk.

Different types of exercise affect your body in different ways. Aerobic exercise—which is exercise that raises your heart rate and breathing rate—is the most beneficial to your heart and lungs. Walking, swimming, bicycling, and water aerobics are all good, low-impact ways to get started with aerobic exercise. Strengthening exercises, such as weight lifting, are good for building muscle tone and strong bones but offer little benefit to your heart or blood pressure.

Relaxation techniques. Relaxation has proven to be a very effective tool in the treatment and prevention of high blood pressure. Simple relaxation techniques can produce modest but consistent decreases in blood pressure. Relaxation need not be complicated: Doing something quiet that you enjoy for 20 minutes twice each day can be quite effective. Some quiet activities that you may find relaxing include taking a warm bath, doing yoga, meditating, or reading a book or magazine.

Alcohol. People with diabetes should consume alcohol only in moderation. Excessive alcohol consumption may cause hypoglycemia (low blood sugar), neuropathy (nerve damage), and obesity and may increase blood cholesterol levels. Excessive alcohol consumption for many years will also have a toxic effect on the heart muscle, adding to the risk of congestive heart failure.

Alcohol also adds calories without nutritional value to your diet. We recommend limiting your intake to two alcoholic drinks per week, with a drink equaling 4 ounces of wine, 12 ounces of beer, or 1½ ounces of liquor. To avoid low blood sugar, remember to always consume alcohol with food.

Goal-setting. Setting goals that are specific, attainable, and forgiving is necessary to making long-range lifestyle changes. Learn to reward yourself with non-food rewards such as a new compact disk, a night at the movies, or a manicure. Monitor your progress. Keep records and review them. Evaluate what worked and what didn't, then think about what you will try the next time a given situation comes up. Never give up. Set new goals and try again.

The support of family and friends is very important in reaching your goals. But to get what you need, you may need to spell out what kind of support feels best to you. If your family's idea of support is nagging you to exercise and watching your food choices like hawks—and yours isn't—you are likely to resent their efforts. So let them know what you need, and when they deliver, let them know you appreciate it.

Many people also find joining a support group—where they meet with others facing similar challenges—to be helpful in meeting their goals and just

coping with everyday problems. To find a diabetes support group in your area, contact your local American Diabetes Association affiliate.

Medication

In addition to making lifestyle changes, most people with diabetes and hypertension will also have to take one or more drugs every day to control their blood pressure. Numerous factors influence your health-care provider's decision about which antihypertensive drug might be right for you. Ethnicity, age, and other medical conditions you might have—such as congestive heart failure, angina, impotence, or gout—may factor in to the drug selection process.

Some of the more common classes of drugs used to treat hypertension are presented on the opposite page. Many people with diabetes and hypertension will initially be treated with one of a group of medicines called ACE inhibitors. These drugs not only lower blood pressure; they also help slow the progression of certain types of kidney disease in people with diabetes. If you are unsure if you are taking an ACE inhibitor, ask your doctor or pharmacist.

It has been estimated that not taking antihypertensive drugs as prescribed accounts for inadequate blood pressure control in two-thirds of people who take them. Many people stop taking their prescribed antihypertensive drugs because of inconvenience or side effects such as sedation or impotence. If these are issues for you, talk to your health-care providers about this immediately. In many cases, your doctor can prescribe an alternative antihypertensive.

The cost of the drugs may also make you less willing to take blood pressure medicines. If paying for a prescribed drug is a problem, ask your doctor or pharmacist if there is an another medicine that is lower in price or has a generic equivalent. Generics should be purchased when available, since they offer equal efficacy at a lower price. You should know that all drug manufacturers in the United States also offer assistance programs to help you obtain medicines that you cannot afford. Information on these programs may be available from your physician or pharmacist.

Managing your hypertension

The most important thing you can do to control your hypertension is to get involved in your care and treatment. People who take an active role in managing both their diabetes and hypertension are more likely to meet their treatment goals for both conditions.

One way to take an active role in managing hypertension is to measure your own blood pressure between doctor visits. Many pharmacies have an automatic blood pressure machine near the prescription area for customers to use. If your pharmacy doesn't have one, ask the pharmacist to check your pressure for you. Your doctor, if it might be beneficial for you, may advise you to purchase a home blood pressure monitor. You can expect to pay less for a manual squeeze-bulb monitor than for a compact monitor that can be worn on the wrist. It is important for you to check your monitor's performance regularly against the monitor at the doctor's office. Regardless of how you obtain your readings, be sure to record the results and take them with you to your doctor appointments.

For more information about hypertension, check out the Web site of the U.S. National Heart, Lung, and Blood Institute at www.nhlbi.nih.gov. To hear recorded messages about high blood pressure prevention and treatment, call toll-free (800) 575-WELL (575-9355). ❑

WHY HIGH TRIGLYCERIDES SPELL TROUBLE

by Robert S. Dinsmoor

People with diabetes, especially Type 2 diabetes, have a higher-than-normal risk for heart and blood vessel disease. For this reason, they are often told to keep a close eye on their cholesterol levels. But what about levels of triglycerides, another type of blood fat? Doctors don't yet know exactly what role triglycerides play in heart and blood vessel disease, but make no mistake: High triglyceride levels are bad news. Here's what is known about the role of triglycerides in diabetes and heart disease and, more important, what you can do to keep your triglycerides at a healthy level.

Macrovascular disease

Type 2 diabetes puts people at greater risk for *macrovascular disease,* or disease caused by atherosclerosis, the narrowing of the large blood vessels of the body. People with Type 2 diabetes are about two to four times more likely to develop heart disease due to narrowed coronary arteries. They are also about two to three times more likely to develop cerebrovascular disease, such as strokes and "ministrokes" resulting from a diminished blood supply to the brain. In addition, they are more prone to peripheral vascular disease, or diminished circulation to the extremities, especially the feet. To make matters worse, when atherosclerosis occurs in people with diabetes, it develops at an accelerated rate.

Why is macrovascular disease more prevalent in diabetes? Researchers don't yet have all the answers to this question, but they have identified a number of factors that may play a role. People with Type 2 diabetes are more likely to have hypertension (high blood pressure), obesity, and dyslipidemia (a blanket designation for decreased HDL cholesterol levels and increased LDL cholesterol and triglyceride levels), all of which are known risk factors for heart disease.

People with Type 2 diabetes also tend to have high levels of *fibrinogen,* a substance that promotes blood clotting, as well as excess amounts of *plasminogen activator inhibitor-1* (or PAI-1), which slows the breakdown and removal of blood clots. The end result of all this is that people who have Type 2 diabetes are more likely to develop blood clots, which can suddenly block already narrowed coronary arteries and cause heart attacks.

No one knows exactly why these changes accompany Type 2 diabetes, but many scientists believe that the chief culprit is insulin resistance—the body's inability to use insulin properly to utilize glucose. In response to insulin resistance, the pancreas churns out more and more insulin. The combination of insulin resistance and high blood levels of insulin tends to lead to hypertension and can change the way in which the body handles fats.

Cholesterol

Since the 1950's, medical researchers have become increasingly aware of the importance of blood cholesterol levels in cardiovascular disease. The liver produces most of the cholesterol in the bloodstream, and the rest comes from the foods we eat, particularly foods high in saturated fat.

Over the past few decades, researchers have discovered that not all cholesterol is created equal. One type, for example, is known to raise the risk of cardiovascular disease, and another type lowers it. Cholesterol is transported in the blood as part of fat-protein "packages" called lipoproteins.

Low-density lipoprotein, or LDL, transports cholesterol throughout the body. Since LDL tends to deposit cholesterol on artery walls, contributing to atherosclerosis, LDL cholesterol is often called the "bad" cholesterol.

High-density lipoprotein, or HDL, sweeps up excess cholesterol throughout the body before it can build up on artery walls and transports it to the liver, which breaks it down. Since high levels of HDL cholesterol appear to reduce the risk of atherosclerosis, HDL cholesterol has been dubbed the "good" cholesterol.

According to the American Diabetes Association (ADA), people with diabetes with an LDL cholesterol level greater than or equal to 130 mg/dl are at high risk for heart disease, people with a level of 100–129 mg/dl are at borderline risk, and people with a level below 100 mg/dl are at low risk for heart disease.

The HDL cholesterol levels that confer high, borderline, and low risk differ for men and women with diabetes. For a man, an HDL cholesterol level of less than 35 mg/dl puts him at high risk for macrovascular disease, a level of 35–45 mg/dl puts him at borderline risk, and a level greater than 45 mg/dl puts him at low risk for macrovascular disease. For a woman, an HDL cholesterol level of less than 45 mg/dl puts her at high risk for macrovascular disease, a level of 45–55 mg/dl puts her at borderline risk, and a level greater than 55 mg/dl puts her at low risk for macrovascular disease.

Triglycerides

Triglycerides are the body's main storage form of fat. The name triglyceride comes from the chemical structure of the fat: A triglycFeride molecule is composed of three fatty acids attached to a glycerol molecule.

Like cholesterol, triglycerides enter the body as food and are also manufactured by the liver. Also like cholesterol, they are carried though the bloodstream by lipoproteins, with the least-dense lipoproteins carrying the greatest amount of triglycerides. In other words, HDL's carry the least amount of triglycerides, while lipoproteins called very-low-density lipoproteins (VLDL's) carry the greatest amount of triglycerides.

While cholesterol levels are an important indicator of a person's risk for cardiovascular disease, they don't tell the whole story. Some people with normal or only moderately high levels of total and LDL cholesterol experience heart attacks. Triglyceride levels may supply at least some of the missing pieces of this puzzle.

Since the late 1950's, some scientists have suspected that high triglyceride levels play a role in heart disease risk, but this theory has only gained widespread acceptance since the late 1980's. In fact, scientists are still trying to determine the exact role of triglycerides in heart disease risk. They know that people with Type 2 diabetes tend to have high triglyceride levels (as well as low levels of HDL cholesterol). However,

researchers aren't yet sure whether triglyceride is just an innocent bystander associated with other lipid abnormalities, or whether it's a risk factor for heart disease unto itself.

One intriguing observation is that elevations in triglyceride levels may somehow change the size and density of LDL cholesterol. In fact, various studies have made the following associations:

■ People who have high triglyceride levels and low HDL cholesterol levels tend to have smaller, denser LDL particles.

■ People with diabetes tend to have more of these smaller, denser LDL particles.

■ People with these smaller, denser LDL particles tend to have a greater risk of heart attacks, even when other risk factors such as total cholesterol levels, body-mass index, and diabetes are taken into consideration.

Despite the uncertainties, the general consensus is that high triglyceride levels are bad news and that lowering them is a very, very good idea. Over the past decade, a number of studies have also shown that high triglyceride levels are associated with increased risk of coronary artery disease and that lowering triglyceride levels can decrease the risk of heart attacks, death from heart attacks, strokes, and ministrokes by roughly a quarter.

Lowering triglyceride levels

According to the ADA, a triglyceride level greater than or equal to 400 mg/dl puts people with diabetes at high risk for macrovascular disease, a level of 200–399 mg/dl puts them at borderline risk, and a level below 200 mg/dl puts them at low risk for macrovascular disease, although a level below 150 mg/dl is desirable. In addition to raising the risk of cardiovascular disease, very high triglycerides can cause inflammation of the pancreas, or pancreatitis.

How can you find out your triglyceride level? It should be part of your yearly blood lipid profile. The ADA recommends annual testing of blood lipids, including fasting serum cholesterol levels, triglyceride levels, HDL cholesterol levels, and calculated LDL levels. (Failing to fast for at least 12 hours before a lipid profile can cause false high results.) If your lipid levels fall into the low-risk category, you only need to be tested every two years. If your doctor doesn't routinely go over your lipid profile results with you, ask about them at your next appointment.

If your triglyceride levels are high, there are a number of lifestyle changes you can make to help bring them down. Some of these same measures will help improve your other lipid levels and other risk factors for cardiovascular disease as well:

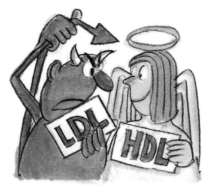

Intensify your blood glucose control. Bringing blood glucose levels closer to the normal range can lower triglyceride levels and may moderately raise HDL cholesterol and lower LDL cholesterol levels.

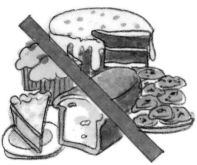

Limit refined carbohydrate intake. A diet high in simple sugars (such as table sugar, honey, corn syrup, and molasses) and refined carbohydrates (such as baked goods made with white flour) is associated with high triglycerides. Make an effort to eat whole grains and whole-grain products and to limit the amount of sweets you eat in general.

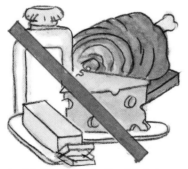

Limit saturated fat intake. A diet high in saturated fats tends to raise LDL cholesterol levels, which is why the ADA, the American Heart Association, and many other major health organizations recommend getting no more than 10% of your daily calories from saturated fat. (For a person who eats about 2,000 calories a day, 10% of calories from saturated fat works out to about 22 grams of saturated fat.) Foods high in saturated fat include butter, cheese, whole milk, red meat, poultry (particularly the dark meat), processed meats, coconut and coconut oil, and palm and palm kernel oils.

While people who don't have diabetes may wish to substitute calories from carbohydrate for calories from saturated fat, people with diabetes may do better to substitute monounsaturated fat for saturated fat. Studies have shown that monounsaturated fat doesn't tend to raise lipid levels. Foods high in monounsaturated fats include olive, canola, and peanut oils.

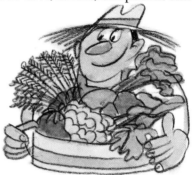

Eat more fiber. A study recently reported in *The New England Journal of Medicine* compared the effects of a lower-fiber diet with those of a higher-fiber diet in 13 people with Type 2 diabetes. Both diets contained exactly the same number of calories and the same composition of carbohydrate, protein, and fat, and both followed general ADA dietary recommendations. However, the higher-fiber diet incorporated 50 grams of fiber daily (from ordinary foods, not from supplements), while the lower-fiber diet contained 25 grams. The high-fiber diet not only lowered average blood glucose levels, but it also significantly improved lipid levels, lowering subjects' triglyceride levels by 10%. Whole grains, dried beans, many vegetables, and fruits eaten with their skins are good sources of fiber.

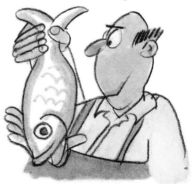

Eat more fatty fish. Regularly eating fatty fish—such as salmon, mackerel, sardines, lake trout, and albacore or bluefin tuna—is associated with lower rates of cardiovascular disease. The health benefits of fish are believed to come from the omega-3 fatty acids found in fish; omega-3 fatty acids are a type of polyunsaturated fat that have been found to lower triglyceride levels.

Taking fish oil supplements may also be helpful. A meta-analysis of 18 trials conducted over a 10-year period, reported in the September 2000 issue of the journal *Diabetes Care,* showed that fish oil supplements lowered triglyceride levels in people with Type 2 diabetes without significantly affecting blood glucose levels. However, according to the researchers, it was not possible to determine the ideal dose of fish oil from the pooled data. And in some of the studies, the fish oil supplements appeared to cause a small increase in LDL cholesterol levels.

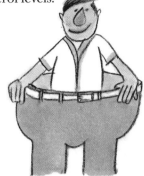

Lose weight. If you're overweight, lose weight. Excess weight is a risk factor for heart disease. Talk to your doctor and dietitian about safe, effective ways to lose weight. Keep in mind that any excess calories consumed are converted by the body into triglycerides.

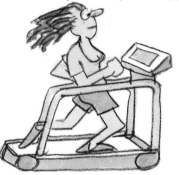

Exercise. Increasing your level of physical activity can lower your blood sugar levels, raise HDL levels, and help you maintain weight loss. Inactivity itself is a risk factor for heart disease. Check with your health-care team before starting a formal exercise program.

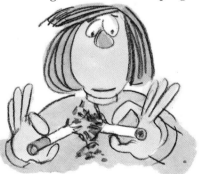

Don't smoke. Smoking appears to increase triglyceride levels and should be avoided for this and many other reasons.

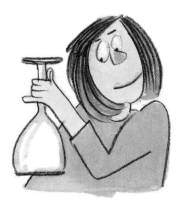

Drink in moderation or not at all. In people who already have high triglyceride levels, alcohol may raise them even further. Some experts say that moderate alcohol consumption, on the order of one to two drinks per day, should do no harm in people whose triglyceride levels are under control. (A drink is defined as 12 ounces of beer, 4 ounces of wine, or 1½ ounces of hard liquor.)

Drugs

In many cases, lifestyle changes alone cannot restore normal lipid levels, and drugs are needed to supplement—but not replace—dietary and other efforts. There are several different types of drugs that can help, and each type differs in its specific effects on HDL cholesterol, LDL cholesterol, and triglycerides. The proper choice of drug, therefore, depends at least in part on a person's overall lipid profile. (Other considerations include the presence of liver or kidney disease.)

Statins. Officially called HMG-CoA reductase inhibitors but nicknamed "statins," these drugs lower cholesterol levels by making the liver absorb more cholesterol from the bloodstream. They also lower LDL cholesterol levels, moderately raise HDL cholesterol levels, and lower triglyceride levels. Currently available statins include atorvastatin (brand name Lipitor), fluvastatin (Lescol), lovastatin (Mevacor), pravastatin (Pravachol), and simvastatin (Zocor).

Nicotinic acid. Also called niacin, this B vitamin (sold at prescription doses under such brand names as Niaspan and Niacor), slows the release of fatty acids from fat cells, effectively lowering both LDL cholesterol and triglyceride levels. Nicotinic acid should not be confused with nicotinamide, another B vitamin with no lipid-altering effects.

While preparations of niacin are sold over the counter as dietary supplements, attempting to self-treat high lipid levels with such supplements is not recommended. Self-prescribing large doses of niacin is likely to lead to side effects, which may be minimized by supervised use and lipid level monitoring to assure use of the lowest effective dose.

TRIGLYCERIDES AND TYPE 1 DIABETES

Should people with Type 1 diabetes be concerned about their triglyceride levels? Yes and no. According to the American Diabetes Association, individuals with Type 1 diabetes whose blood sugar levels generally fall within the normal range tend to have healthy lipid levels. However, all people with diabetes are advised to have their lipid levels tested regularly, and if the levels are abnormal, they should be treated with diet and possibly lipid-lowering drugs. In people with Type 1 diabetes, keeping blood glucose levels close to normal may be one of the most important steps for maintaining or restoring normal blood lipid levels.

Even when taking prescribed doses of nicotinic acid, some people experience unpleasant facial flushing and lightheadedness. Although these side effects can be minimized by starting with a small dose and gradually increasing it, some people can never tolerate it and have to use other drugs. In addition, use of nicotinic acid can cause high blood sugar levels in some people and may be inappropriate for those people.

Fibrates. Drugs known as fibrates lower blood fats by decreasing the liver's production of triglycerides and VLDL's and increasing the rate at which triglyceride-rich lipoproteins leave the bloodstream. Fibrates effectively raise HDL cholesterol levels and lower triglyceride levels. Currently available fibrates are gemfibrozil (Lopid), fenofibrate (Tricor), and clofibrate (Atromid-S).

No matter what drug you take, your doctor will want to monitor your progress with periodic blood tests. Initially you may need to have blood tests every one to two months to see how you are responding to the lipid-lowering therapy. Once your triglycerides have come down to goal levels, you may only need to have your blood checked every six months. If your triglycerides do not come down to desired levels with the first drug you try, your doctor may increase your dose, prescribe a different drug, or prescribe a combination of drugs. Be sure to ask your doctor about side effects you should look out for and to report any side effects you experience.

Taking steps to lower your triglycerides is one more way you can lower your risk of heart disease. Ask your doctor to work with you in developing a plan to keep your triglycerides low and your heart and arteries as healthy as they can be. ❑

DIABETES COMPLICATIONS

Coping With Complications

by J. Shawn Faulk, M.S., R.D., C.D.E.

COMPLICATIONS. It may be the scariest word you hear after learning that you have diabetes. Your fears are understandable. We know that diabetes is the leading cause of blindness in adults ages 20 to 74 and the leading cause of end-stage kidney disease. About 60% to 70% of people with diabetes have some degree of nerve damage, and more than half of all lower limb amputations in the United States are done on people with diabetes.

Maybe you aren't familiar with all the statistics, but you do know that Aunt May had to have a leg amputated because of her diabetes, Grandma Edith had diabetes and required dialysis before her death, and your neighbor with diabetes is legally blind. And what about the man in your doctor's waiting room who said he could hardly eat because of gastroparesis?

OK, so some fear is warranted. In spite of what I have learned as a dietitian and diabetes educator, I would have to admit that in my 28 years with diabetes, I have battled fear many times. Sometimes it is the panic that comes with an acute complication: I have had laser surgery in both eyes, and I have gastroparesis and some degree of peripheral and autonomic neuropathy. And in 1990, after four months of dialysis, I had a kidney transplant. More often, I feel the more subtle but persistent anxiety related to challenges that may lie ahead. Will I maintain the vision I do have? Will I someday lose a finger or a foot? Will I ever need another new kidney?

How do those of us with diabetes direct those fears so they don't control our lives? If complications do occur, how do we cope without letting them become who we are?

Diabetes fatalism

Of the many internal battles that plague people with diabetes, one of the most dangerous is *diabetes fatalism.* People with diabetes fatalism pour their energy into worrying about the inevitability of complications and the devastating impact they will have rather than channeling their concern into taking positive steps to prevent or limit those complications or developing ways to enjoy life even if they do occur. While it's almost impossible to never think about complications, succumbing to diabetes fatalism can affect your behavior in negative ways and lead to a dangerous mind-set that contributes to the very complications that frighten you. Diabetes fatalism can prevent you from caring for your diabetes before complications set in, and it can keep you from making the best of things if complications do develop.

How do you recognize this danger zone? Diabetes fatalism has some clearly identifiable characteristics that can be active at any stage of diabetes—before any complications begin, after a few have appeared, or when a complication poses significant challenges to your life. The first step in coming to terms with the threat or actuality of diabetes complications is to recognize these faulty beliefs and see how they prevent you from taking better care of yourself, both physically and emotionally.

Apathy. If you have decided that diabetes complications will set in regardless of what you do to take care of yourself, it becomes very easy to give up and just let things happen. Why deny yourself all those opportunities to enjoy chocolate cake if you believe that following a meal plan won't make a difference? You've given up doughnuts for breakfast. Isn't that enough?

The truth is that taking control of diabetes does help, both in preventing complications and limiting them if they start. So keep appointments with your medical team members—your discussions with them will remind you of the payoffs for good diabetes self-management. Track your lab results, noting improvements and lapses, and use them as a baseline to set new short-term goals. Stay in contact with other people with diabetes who you look to for inspiration. And always try to make your exercise program a priority, no matter what your fitness level is. It will help your physical and mental well-being and energize you to take action.

Denial. The prospect of possible blindness, renal failure (kidney disease), stroke, or amputation can be overwhelming. Such complications seem unacceptable and incomprehensible. Denying the possibility that these complications could ever happen to you makes it easier to downplay the importance of careful diabetes self-management. After all, you don't feel the consequences of poor diabetes control until it is too late. If you felt shooting pain every time your blood sugar rose above 200 mg/dl, it probably would never get that high. But most of us function just fine with elevated blood sugar levels. In fact, having higher-than-normal blood sugar can even become comfortable if low blood sugar is a concern. Unfortunately, while you may be able to trick your mind into thinking that chronically high blood sugar is acceptable, your eyes, kidneys, heart, and nerves won't be fooled.

Complacency. You can tell yourself that letting your blood sugar control slide isn't really doing any damage. You may find yourself saying, "I'm just going to splurge *today*" or "I think I'll take a break and not test my blood sugar *today*" or "*Today*, I'm too tired to exercise." While taking a short "diabetes vacation" is fine once in a while, taking too much time off can be harmful. Complacency can lead you to let those days add up into weeks, months, and even years of half-hearted diabetes control.

Loss of identity. When faced with a chronic illness, another common response is to let that illness define who you are. Complications can overtake your mind, your purpose in life, and your individuality. Instead of being a unique person who happens to have diabetes, you risk feeling like a walking collection of medical diagnoses and complaints.

I have experienced this loss of identity in my own struggles with diabetes complications. Instead of being Shawn Faulk, dietitian and diabetes educator, surrounded by friends and family, I allow myself to become the nameless kidney recipient who can't drive at night, can't feel her feet, and takes over 20 pills a day. Recently, when I expressed those thoughts to a friend, he reminded me that he was aware of my diabetes and complications when we became friends. He then pointed out how irrelevant they were compared to all the other things that kept our friendship strong. He wasn't going to allow me to create a world focused on my losses and self-pity. It was a giant step toward putting things back in perspective.

Guilt. Guilt is a plague, and diabetes is fertile ground for those harmful feelings. Diabetes may trigger feelings of guilt because you haven't followed your diabetes regimen to the letter, or because you ate those cookies last night. Even worse, you may fear that you are a burden to your family, that your medical expenses are too high, or that you may have contributed to your own complications. Guilt can become a powerful and destructive force that, like a thief, steals away your optimism and energy, taking with it the very traits that can help you regain control of your life.

A facade of freedom. Rebelling against diabetes by dismissing the many necessary self-care tasks is another danger of diabetes fatalism. "What is the point of living if I can't eat and do what I want? No one can restrict my freedom," you may want to cry out. But remember, when you convince yourself that freedom means giving up your healthy diabetes-care routine, the freedom you find is short-lived and hollow.

The reality is that the self-care we give ourselves now, no matter how tiresome or inconvenient it is, protects our freedom in the future. If complications set in, you may lose some of the freedom to do the things that you enjoy or that help you remain independent. For instance, if your vision becomes restricted, you may lose the freedom to drive. If you lose a foot, you may lose the freedom to play tennis or go dancing. Giving up your self-care responsibilities today will only steal from your real freedom in the future.

Surrender. One would think that the first inkling of a complication would cause you to snap out of your diabetes fatalism and realize how important it is to take charge. Instead, complications can confirm our worst fears and bolster the faulty beliefs that pushed us into the danger zone. Once the downward spiral has begun, you may feel there's nothing you can do to stop it. So you do nothing, more complications appear, and your tainted belief system is confirmed once more. In other words, you surrender.

Fatalism prevention

No matter what the stage of your diabetes or complications, it is never too late to make changes. Here are some of the steps involved in preventing diabetes fatalism, taking charge of your health, and keeping diabetes from overwhelming you.

Recognize the problem. The first step in coping with diabetes complications (or fear of them) is to recognize your own behavior and thoughts about diabetes. Do you have a pessimistic outlook when it comes to your health? Have you given up on yourself? It is only by stepping back and honestly assessing what you do that you can begin to reverse harmful behaviors.

Make a plan. If you are worried that some of your behaviors are destructive, make a concrete plan to break the cycle. First, write down a list of the things you would like to change. For instance, you may decide to test your blood sugar three times a day and to meet with a dietitian to learn how to better balance your meals and your medication. Once you have made your list, pick one goal to work on first. Start small: Trying to become "the perfect diabetes patient" overnight is an overwhelming and impossible task. A more realistic goal is to simply become a *better* diabetes patient.

Use teamwork. Managing diabetes and diabetes complications is hard work, and no one should have to do it alone. That's why it is important to stay connected to the diabetes community. This means making and keeping your regular appointments with your doctor, diabetes educator, dietitian, and other health-care professionals. It also means seeking out peer support. Staying in touch with a network of people who have diabetes can help keep you up to date on diabetes information, provide encouragement and support from people who share your concerns and struggles, and offer you inspiration and enthusiasm to renew your efforts.

Be your own advocate. Learn to stand up for yourself and seek out the best care available. Self-advocacy is a necessary survival skill in today's health-care environment. Among other things, self-advocacy means knowing your insurance coverage, asking questions and demanding answers, learning everything you can about your disease, networking, and taking an active part in your health care. In short, it's anything that helps ensure your health-care needs are met.

When complications arise

If you're in good health now, you can work with your doctor to try to prevent diabetes complications. Despite your best efforts, though, complications can still set in.

Having diabetes complications does not mean an end to the joy and meaning in life. Many people lead productive lives in spite of their complications. Coping does require some changes, however, in both attitude and self-care.

Let fear motivate you. Fear can be a good thing if it inspires you to take action. Sometimes fear can drive you to seek more information about diabetes, which may help you to seek out the best treatment. Fear can also encourage you to explore your own attitudes and behaviors, possibly helping you to reverse self-destructive patterns. It is only fear without hope that feeds diabetes fatalism.

When Emily was newly diagnosed with Type 2 diabetes, she knew little about diabetes care. But she was all too familiar with the devastating effects the disease had had on family members. Her mother was on dialysis when she died, an uncle had lost a limb due to diabetes complications, and another uncle had had a stroke in his forties and had difficulty walking because of the painful neuropathy in his feet.

Emily was terrified of diabetes, but rather than letting her fear paralyze her, she sought my help. We talked about ways to stay healthy, starting by reducing her carbohydrate and fat intake, beginning an exercise program, and keeping regular clinic appointments. When I saw her two months later, her blood sugar was down to 97 mg/dl, she had lost 15 pounds, and she felt great about herself and the changes she had made. And seeing that she could take control of her diabetes helped her to feel a lot less frightened.

Forgive yourself. Remember, guilt is destructive, and it is an obstacle to any forward motion. Maybe you have slipped up on your self-care occasionally, but guess what: People with diabetes are human, too. We just pay more dearly for some common human frailties. So forgive yourself for past actions, for your rebelliousness and denial, and even for having diabetes.

My friend Jerry, now blind as a result of diabetes, used to spend so much time beating himself up for years of eating and drinking what he wanted, when he wanted it, that he had little time or energy left to adjust to and cope with his new challenges. And since he couldn't get around easily, he hibernated for almost three years, too embarrassed to go out in public. To his surprise, when I introduced him to several friends with diabetes, he learned that none of us was perfect, but that we had forgiven ourselves and set new goals. He was able to take our examples to heart and finally forgive himself. Now he goes out with friends and family, is in much better control, and allows himself to feel good about it.

Stay educated. The most powerful fear is fear of the unknown. Without all the necessary information, it's easy to jump to worst-case scenarios and assume that the tingling in your feet will quickly lead to amputations and wheelchairs or that the subtle signs of autonomic neuropathy mean you will never exercise again. In reality, most complications can stabilize indefinitely, especially if you step up your efforts to control your diabetes. Consulting your doctor about any symptoms you have is the only way to learn what they signify and how they may affect you later. Addressing small things by learning the facts will help keep them small.

With knowledge, even the big things can be made smaller. There was a time when fear of end-stage kidney disease immobilized my life. For the first time, I felt total despair. That was before I knew that transplantation was an option for me and learned about its rate of success. Every day, new drugs are approved, new treatment options are offered, and new resources become available. If we don't expose ourselves to and seek out information, we may miss opportunities to improve our care and, ultimately, our quality of life.

Discover peer fellowship. Relationships with other people who have diabetes offer an instant bond that transcends any other diabetes support system. Because they share your experiences, peers offer trust and an instant credibility that cannot be duplicated by even the most well-meaning friends, family, or medical team members.

Friends with diabetes provide camaraderie and compassion. Isolation, whether it be physical, mental, or emotional, magnifies negativity. Meeting others facing the same challenges helps diminish feelings of hopelessness and helplessness and stirs a natural compassion. True compassion comes from common experience. True compassion has no judgment.

Peers also offer the opportunity to laugh at yourself. I'll never forget taking an evening walk with my fiancé who also has diabetes. Wham! He walked straight into a telephone pole he didn't see because it was dark and he is blind in his right eye. Luckily, he wasn't hurt. When I started to laugh, he looked at me and said, "Anybody but you..." and started laughing, too. I was allowed to laugh because the week before, I had walked right into the wall of a dark theater! People with diabetes give each other permission to laugh at situations we don't allow others to laugh at. Laughter helps to dilute the sense of loss at a time when we are grieving over the loss of good health. It helps to put the loss in perspective and reminds us that life still has a lot to offer.

Accept that diabetes is not fair. It is not fair that you face potential complications because of your diabetes. It is not fair that you carry an extra burden of self-care: blood sugar testing, injections or medicines, frequent doctor appointments, and the expenses of your medical care. It is not fair that you can do all the right things and still have erratic blood sugar levels. Diabetes is not fair. Life is not fair.

It wasn't until my kidney transplant that I accepted the truth and clarity of those words. Learning to accept them gave me tremendous freedom from the questions "Why me?" and "Who do I blame?" Freedom from these questions will allow you to focus on your actions in the moment.

Seek professional help when necessary. I realize now that the despondency I felt when I was on dialysis was part of a clinical depression I did not seek help for. There are a number of antidepressants available that can be helpful when a person is feeling overwhelmed by negativity and pessimism. Talking with a mental health professional who has expertise in diabetes can be even more helpful. He or she can make a huge difference in helping you gain perspective and providing you with guidance and support so you can make healthy, positive changes.

Redesign your dream. In the transplant community, we use those words to describe our adjustment to life as an organ recipient. We don't stop dreaming, but our dreams may change. Whether it's kidney failure or

GETTING SUPPORT

To find a diabetes support group in your area, call your local hospital, diabetes center, or affiliate of the American Diabetes Association. You can call the national office of the American Diabetes Association at (800) 232-3472 or (800) 342-2383 to find an affiliate near you. You can also find local sources of support through the Association's Web site, www.diabetes.org.

Books
To read more about coming to terms and coping with your diabetes, look for these books in your local library or bookstore.

LIVING WITH DIABETIC COMPLICATIONS
A Survival Guide for Patients by a Patient
Judy Curtis
Companion Press
Shippensburg, Pennsylvania, 1993

PSYCHING OUT DIABETES
A Positive Approach to Your Negative Emotions
Richard Rubin, June Biermann, and Barbara Toohey
Lowell House
Los Angeles, 1992

another diabetes complication, your own expectations of yourself will be the highest and the most difficult to adjust. But accepting your limitations gives you the opportunity to recognize and develop talents and strengths you may never have tapped otherwise.

John, for example, worked in construction before his transplant. Circulation problems and the need for a less demanding schedule led him to a vocational rehabilitation class in computer programming. The transition from outdoor work to a desk job wasn't easy, but now John has a new career that he loves with steady hours and more time for his family. In many ways, the transplant opened doors, even while it closed some others.

Moving on

I have found, professionally and personally, that attitude and sense of empowerment are closely linked when it comes to diabetes and diabetic complications. Even though you may continue to have down times (let me remind you that you are human!), you can recognize those times for what they are and recognize your ability to make choices and changes. With education, peer fellowship, and the support of the medical community, you offer yourself the best quality of life possible. ❑

KEEPING AN EYE ON RETINOPATHY

by Jeanne L. Rosenthal, M.D.

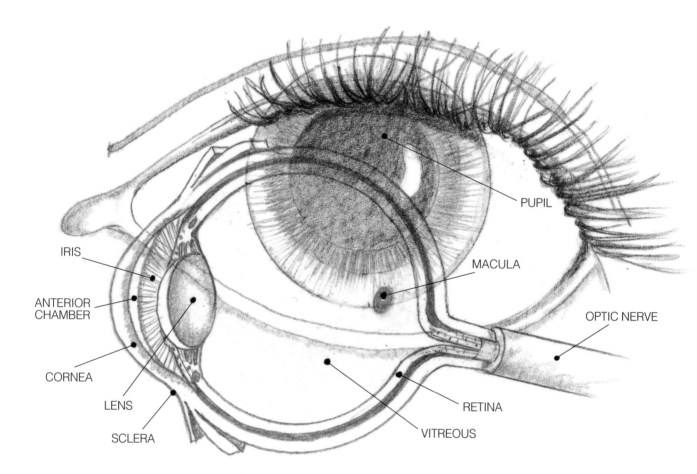

Are you afraid you'll lose your sight because of diabetes? It's possible, but it's not inevitable, and keeping your blood sugar levels under control is the most important step you can take to lower your risk of diabetes-related eye problems. In fact, studies have shown that keeping your blood sugar levels at near-nondiabetic levels can reduce your risk of diabetic retinopathy (the most common form of diabetic eye disease) by up to 76%. Controlling your blood sugar can also raise the chances that treatment for retinopathy will be successful, if you need it. To learn more about diabetic retinopathy and what you can do to prevent it, let's have a look at how your eyes work.

Surveying sight

The eye is shaped like a ball. It is essentially hollow, although it is filled with a gelatinous substance. The front of the eyeball is clear tissue called the cornea. Behind the cornea is a small, fluid-filled area called the anterior chamber. The back surface of the anterior chamber is the iris, the colored part of a person's eye. The iris is a ring of muscle tissue with a hole in the center. The opening in the center of the iris is called the pupil; it appears black when you look at an eye from the front. Just behind the iris is the lens, which is clear in healthy eyes. Behind the lens is a relatively large cavity filled with a clear gel called the vitreous. The retina is a thin layer of tissue that lines the back and sides of the large cavity like wallpaper. The outside surface of the eyeball, or the "white" of the eye, is a layer of connective tissue called sclera.

Light enters the eye through the cornea. The iris adjusts the size of the pupil to let in the right amount of light for maximum clarity. The lens focuses the light on the retina.

The parts of the eye work much like the parts of a camera: The camera lens focuses an image on the film in the back of the camera, and the amount of light that reaches the film is controlled by opening and closing the aperture.

The retina is a highly complex tissue made up of 10 layers of different types of cells. It senses the light entering the eye and sends the information to the brain via the optic nerve. The brain uses this information to form an image. Any damage to the retina, like damage to film in a camera, will make the image unclear.

Recognizing retinopathy

Diabetes affects the blood vessels in the retina in the same way that it affects blood vessels in other parts of the body, which is that it damages the vessel walls. In the eye, diabetes primarily affects the walls of the tiny capillaries that bring oxygen and nutrients to the retina and remove carbon dioxide and waste products. High levels of glucose in the blood weaken the walls of the capillaries, causing small, balloonlike pouches called microaneurysms to form. This type of damage also causes the capillary walls to leak blood, fluid, or fatty material into the retinal tissue. During a dilated eye exam, an ophthalmologist can see this leakage, as well as other signs of retinopathy such as swelling in the retina.

The early stage of retinopathy is called *background diabetic retinopathy*. Usually, no treatment is necessary for this stage unless the center of the retina, called the macula, is affected. The macula is the area of the retina responsible for central vision, which is the sharpest vision and important for tasks such as driving and reading. Background retinopathy that affects the macula often causes blurred vision, blind spots called scotomas, or distorted vision. Objects may appear larger or smaller in the affected eye than in the other eye, or they may appear tilted. Laser treatment of the leaking areas can usually stop vision loss and can sometimes restore vision. The laser seals the leaking spots, which allows the blood and fluid to be reabsorbed.

If background retinopathy progresses, it can lead to enough damage to capillaries that blood does not flow through them properly. In areas of the retina where blood flow is poor, function is impaired or stops altogether. These areas of reduced blood flow to the retina are analogous to tiny strokes in the brain. The difference is that in the brain, therapy can sometimes help other areas take over the function of the area damaged by the stroke. But in the retina, healthy areas are not able to take over for the damaged areas. Hampered circulation to the retina may noticeably impair vision, depending on where it occurs.

The major problem that areas of poor circulation in the retina cause, however, is the stimulation of a healing process in which the body grows new blood vessels to try to reestablish circulation. The process of new blood vessel growth is called *neovascularization*. Although new blood vessel growth may sound like a good thing, it is not. The new blood vessels grow in a disorderly fashion, are weak, and rupture easily, allowing more blood to leak into the retina.

When neovascularization occurs in the retina, a person is said to have *proliferative diabetic retinopathy*, a condition that threatens vision. This stage of disease is treated with a laser in a "scatter" pattern to areas outside the macula. This procedure suppresses the growth of new blood vessels; following treatment, existing vessels often regress or are reabsorbed.

If laser treatment is not done soon enough or if it is unsuccessful, new blood vessels can grow into the vitreous. When this happens, the fragile vessels may bleed into the vitreous, causing a person to have very poor vision or to see spots that look like hairs or bugs. The new blood vessels can also cause scar tissue to form in the vitreous. The scar tissue can pull the retina out of its normal position lining the back of the eye. This is called *traction retinal detachment*. The areas where the retina is detached have very poor vision. These complications can only be treated with a surgical procedure called *vitrectomy*, in which the blood and scar tissue are removed from the eye with very fine instruments.

Preventing problems

Finding diabetic retinopathy and treating it early increases the likelihood that treatment will be successful and that no vision will be lost. For this reason, the American Diabetes Association recommends that people with diabetes have a yearly dilated eye exam. The exam should be performed by an ophthalmologist or an optometrist who is knowledgeable and experienced in managing diabetic retinopathy. (Some but not all optometrists are qualified to give dilated eye exams.)

Even though the treatment of diabetic retinopathy can usually prevent vision loss, it would be better to prevent it altogether. For many people, this is possible by tightly controlling blood sugar levels, exercising regularly, and controlling blood pressure. The Diabetes Control and Complications Trial clearly showed that lowering blood sugar levels can reduce the risk of developing diabetic retinopathy and other complications of diabetes. Tight control can reduce the rate of diabetic retinopathy by as much as 76%. Your glycosylated hemoglobin (HbA$_{1c}$), which is a measure of your average blood glucose level over the past two to four months, indicates your level of control. If your HbA$_{1c}$ is above 8%, ask your doctor or diabetes educator what you can do to lower it.

Not everyone can or should maintain near-normal blood glucose levels, but any reduction in HbA$_{1c}$ lowers the risk of diabetic retinopathy. Discuss with your doctor what your target blood glucose range should be. In addition, make sure you have an annual dilated eye exam as part of your regular diabetes care regimen. Together, these measures improve your chances of avoiding retinopathy altogether, catching it early if it develops, and treating it successfully, to preserve as much vision as possible. ❏

ADJUSTING TO VISION LOSS

by Ann S. Williams, M.S.N., R.N., C.D.E.

Imagine yourself as one of the following people. What would you do? Where would you turn for help?

YOU ARE a single parent of two teenagers. You did not receive a formal education beyond high school, and you are determined that your children will have more opportunities than you did. You are a valued employee in a small business, and your boss is quite flexible about letting you schedule your working hours around your teenagers' busy schedules. You get up at 5:30 every morning, and your days are filled with activities until you go to bed at about 11:00. So over the past several years, when you found yourself feeling tired a lot of the time, you blamed your busy schedule. It was not until your eyesight became blurry that you took time to see a doctor. You were completely surprised when the doctor said that you have Type 2 diabetes, that you have probably had it for several years at least, and your blurry eyesight is due to diabetic retinopathy. Although laser treatments have successfully prevented further deterioration, the initial damage cannot be repaired. You now have permanent visual impairment: You are not legally blind, but you have low vision and can no longer drive or read regular print.

YOU ARE a 21-year-old college student. You have had Type 1 diabetes for as long as you can remember. You have been very active in high school and college sports, have had excellent grades throughout your school career, and are planning to attend graduate school. Like many high school students with diabetes, you did not maintain control of your blood sugar during your teen years. However, recently you have managed your diabetes more carefully. Without any warning, while in class one day, you experience a sudden retinal detachment. A few months of intensive eye surgeries follow, but your ophthalmologist is unable to save your eyesight. Within a year, you have become totally blind.

YOU ARE a busy attorney in a large urban practice. You have had a successful career so far and are considering

retirement. You have had Type 2 diabetes for 18 years. You noticed three years ago that colors seemed less vivid than they once did, and that your vision had become blurry. Your primary-care doctor referred you to an ophthalmologist, who found that you had both cataracts and proliferative diabetic retinopathy. Now, three years later, your cataracts have been removed, and you have had laser surgery five times to treat the retinopathy. Your remaining vision is stable, but you are now legally blind.

Visual impairment and diabetes

In recent years, advances in the management of diabetes and of diabetic eye disease have given us the ability to prevent most vision loss due to diabetes. But as these true stories show, diabetes still causes vision loss in many people.

In fact, the federal government's Centers for Disease Control and Prevention estimates that 12,000 to 24,000 people in the United States become legally blind from diabetic retinopathy every year. Cataracts and glaucoma also occur at a greater rate among people with diabetes. In addition, the risk of age-related macular degeneration, which is not believed to be caused by diabetes, increases, like diabetes, as people grow older. One recent estimate indicates that as many as 2 million people may currently be living with both diabetes and low vision or blindness in the United States. So, if you have both diabetes and visual impairment, you are not alone. Fortunately, a lot of help is available to you.

Rehabilitation services

The purpose of low-vision and blindness rehabilitation services is to teach people with vision impairment how to use adaptive tools and nonvisual techniques to care for themselves and to live as active

RESOURCES

The following organizations can help you find low-vision or blindness services. Your state's government can also help. Check the Government Listings pages in your phone book or call Information to find the agency that handles low-vision and blindness services.

AMERICAN ASSOCIATION OF DIABETES EDUCATORS
A professional organization for diabetes educators. It has a Visually Impaired Persons Specialty Practice Group. For referrals to a diabetes educator near you, call (800) TEAM-UP-4 (832-6874). For other information, call (800) 338-3633. You can also obtain referrals and information through the AADE's Web site, http://www.aadenet.org.

NATIONAL FEDERATION OF THE BLIND
Publishes "Diabetes Resources: Equipment, Services, and Information," a comprehensive list of diabetes resources, available in large print and Braille and on audiocassette (recorded at slow speed, 15/16 ips). Order from NFB Materials Resource Center by calling (410) 659-9314. The list can also be accessed through the Web page www.nfb.org/diabres.htm.

The NFB also publishes a quarterly newsletter, *Voice of the Diabetic,* which is available free of cost in standard newsprint and on audiocassette (recorded at slow speed, 15/16 ips). To subscribe, call (573) 875-8911 or use the form available at www.nfb.org/voice.htm.

AMERICAN FOUNDATION FOR THE BLIND
Provides information on services for blind and visually impaired persons and maintains a referral list. Phone (800) AFB-LINE (232-5463) or (212) 502-7600, or check the Foundation's Web site, www.afb.org.

NATIONAL LIBRARY SERVICE FOR THE BLIND AND PHYSICALLY HANDICAPPED, LIBRARY OF CONGRESS
Through the Talking Book program, provides recorded books and equipment to play the books to visually impaired people and others who have a disability that prevents use of print materials. For more information call (202) 707-5100 or visit the Web page www.loc.gov/nls.

and involved lives as they wish. A variety of low-vision and blindness rehabilitation services are available throughout the United States. Typically, services include at least the following:

Low-vision services. Certain tools and techniques allow people to make the most of the vision they have. Tools include high-powered magnifiers, bright, filtered or tinted lighting, and closed-circuit televisions that provide enlarged images of reading materials. Techniques for people who have gaps in the visual field include learning special eye movements to make images fall on the parts of the eye that still have usable vision.

Daily living skills. Cooking, cleaning, putting together matching outfits, and doing other ordinary tasks of daily living require learning nonvisual methods and developing the other senses. For example, a person might use touch, temperature sense, and smell to cook safely. He or she might use touch and a systematic approach for cleaning effectively and for personal grooming tasks such as shaving or applying makeup. Labels distinguishable by touch can indicate the color of an article of clothing.

Orientation and mobility training. Moving safely from one place to another is possible with impaired vision. Memory and touch are usually enough to move about in the home. Outside the home, a white cane or a guide dog and public transportation allow a person to get around safely.

Communication. Learning nonvisual communication does not always mean learning to read and write Braille. Some people learn Braille and others do not. However, nearly everyone learns to dial a phone by touch. For keeping records, such as phone numbers or blood glucose levels, audiotapes work well. The Talking Books program of the National Library Service for the Blind and Physically Handicapped provides reading material (including *Diabetes Self-Management*) in audio format. People who are used to reading print may need to improve their listening skills to enhance learning from speech and recorded materials.

Additional rehabilitation services that may be available include the following:

Computer services. Large screens or audio systems make computers easier to use. Some rehabilitation centers have computer specialists and a variety of equipment for people to try to help them identify the adaptations that best meet their needs.

Employment services. Such services help people who want to work find and keep employment that is appropriate to their education, skills, and intelligence.

DO YOU NEED REHABILITATION SERVICES?

Temporary visual changes are common when people are experiencing unstable blood glucose levels. People who are having low blood glucose sometimes have temporarily dim vision, double vision, or flashing lights in the visual field. People with high blood glucose can sometimes have blurred vision because of changes in the fluid pressure in the eye. This is especially common around the onset of diabetes symptoms and during times of fluctuating blood glucose. Once blood glucose levels are under control, it can take as long as six to eight weeks for vision to stabilize. If you have visual changes that go away when your blood sugar stabilizes, you do not need low-vision or blindness rehabilitation services. You do, however, need to learn how to maintain greater consistency in your blood glucose control.

A person's vision is measured by comparing it to full vision. When someone with 20/70 vision is standing 20 feet away from an object—say an eye chart or a street sign—he or she can see the object as clearly as a person with full vision (20/20) standing 70 feet away. Likewise, a person with 20/200 vision sees as clearly 20 feet away as a person with full vision standing 200 feet away. In general, low-vision services are provided to people whose corrected vision (meaning vision when wearing glasses or contact lenses with a current prescription) in their best eye is between 20/70 and 20/200. At this level, a person has some usable vision, but it is difficult to use it effectively.

Blindness rehabilitation is usually provided to people who are legally blind, meaning their corrected vision in their best eye is 20/200 or worse, or who have a visual field of 20 degrees or less. (People with normal vision have a visual field of 180 degrees.)

Some people receive low-vision or blindness rehabilitation services even though they do not meet these criteria. For example, if a person's job requires fine visual discrimination, low vision services may be needed with vision of 20/50. If you have irreversible visual loss that interferes with your ability to perform tasks that are important in your life, contact the low-vision or blindness rehabilitation services in your area for help.

Rehabilitation counseling. Such counseling aims to help people go through the process of adjusting emotionally to the many losses, changes in body image, role changes, and new ways of doing things that accompany vision loss. Counseling may be provided in individual or group settings. Some programs also have peer counseling, which is support provided by other visually impaired people with diabetes.

Finding services near you

Low-vision and blindness rehabilitation services are usually not connected to doctors' offices and hospitals, so health-care professionals sometimes are not aware of these services. As a result, people who need the services do not always hear about them. However, information is easy to find when you know where to look.

Every state in the United States has a state government agency that provides rehabilitation services to blind people. Many areas also have private agencies that provide low-vision and blindness rehabilitation services. In addition, the Department of Veterans Affairs provides comprehensive services to visually impaired veterans throughout the United States. By calling the information office for your state government, you can learn how to contact your state's blindness rehabilitation agency. The state agency should have information about local private agencies and veterans' services. Another source of information is the American Foundation for the Blind, which has a referral list of local blindness services. (See "Resources" on page 183 for contact information.)

Diabetes self-care

Imagine again that you are one of the people described at the beginning of this article. You are independent and have always taken care of your own personal needs. Even though your visual ability has changed, you will certainly want to continue doing your own diabetes self-care.

Fortunately, visually impaired people, diabetes educators, and equipment manufacturers have worked together in recent years to develop many tools and techniques that make this possible. All routine diabetes self-care tasks can be done safely and effectively by people who have low vision or blindness. Large print, Braille, and audiotapes let you keep blood sugar records. Adaptive tools and techniques include syringe magnifiers, tactile insulin measurement devices, talking blood sugar monitors, talking scales for weighing oneself, talking thermometers, audiotapes for learning about new developments in diabetes care, and nonvisual methods for measuring food portions, labeling and sorting multiple medicines, inspecting one's own feet, and exercising safely.

To learn to use these tools and techniques, your best bet is to find a diabetes educator near you who teaches adaptive diabetes education to visually impaired people. Since 1989, the American Association of Diabetes Educators (AADE) has had a Visually Impaired Persons Specialty Practice Group (VIP-SPG) composed of diabetes educators who take a special interest in helping people who have diabetes and visual impairment meet their diabetes-care needs. Although their numbers are relatively few, members of the VIP-SPG are located throughout the United States. (See "Resources," on page 183, for contact information.)

The National Federation of the Blind (NFB) also has a special division, called the Diabetes Action Network, devoted to the special needs of people who have diabetes and visual impairment. The Diabetes Action Network publishes a quarterly newsletter, *Voice of the Diabetic*. It contains information, news, and personal stories about living with diabetes and visual impairment. It is available in print and audiotape formats, and is free of charge. In addition, NFB maintains a comprehensive list of resources for people with diabetes entitled "Diabetes Resources: Equipment, Services, and Information." This list has resources for all diabetes self-care needs but pays special attention to products, such as adaptive equipment, for visually impaired people. It is available in large print, Braille, or audiotape formats. (See "Resources," on page 183, for contact information.)

Life goes on

Imagine one more time that you are one of the people described at the beginning of the article. What can you expect your life to be like following rehabilitation? It is very likely that you would go through a period of grieving and also a period of intensive learning of adaptive skills. Then, most likely, you would find that you could continue the activities that are most important to you.

Your personality and temperament would probably stay largely the same. For example, suppose that when you had good eyesight, you enjoyed getting out a lot, meeting new people, and socializing. With a visual impairment, you would use the skills you learned in orientation and mobility training to continue to get out and socialize. You would learn to be more attentive to sounds and other nonvisual cues to help you communicate well. On the other hand, if you preferred being home alone or inviting one close friend to your home, you could use the daily living skills you learned to feel comfortable doing just that. If you enjoyed reading, you could continue to read, using large print, Braille, or audiotape books. If you held a job outside the home, it is likely that you could learn adaptive techniques to continue your job. If you liked to do gourmet cooking, you could use your senses of touch and smell to continue to do so. If you prefer not to use a stove, you could learn nonvisual use of a microwave or learn how to get to nearby takeout restaurants.

As a visually impaired person, you could do almost everything you did before—you would just do things in different ways. You would be the same person on the inside. Although your life would probably be somewhat different from what you had previously imagined, it is very likely that you would find ways to have as full and satisfying a life as you had before. ❑

HYPERGLYCEMIC CRISES
What They Are and How to Avoid Them
by Robert S. Dinsmoor

One type results in about 100,000 hospitalizations a year with a mortality rate of under 5%. The other is thought to cause fewer hospitalizations, yet the mortality rate is about 15%. Severe hyperglycemic conditions, known as *diabetic ketoacidosis* (DKA) and *hyperosmolar hyperglycemic state* (HHS), involve very serious imbalances in blood chemistry and usually require that a person be hospitalized until normal blood chemistry is restored. Because they can occur in anyone with diabetes, everyone should know what causes them, how to prevent them, how they are treated, and when to seek medical attention.

The body in balance

Glucose metabolism is a complex balancing act. In people who don't have diabetes, a number of interconnected processes help the body to use glucose and keep blood glucose levels in the normal range. The body constantly balances glucose extracted from foods and produced by the liver with glucose utilization by the body's tissues. When there is ample glucose in the bloodstream, the liver converts some of it into glycogen for storage. When the body needs more energy, such as during a prolonged period of fasting or activity, the liver converts stored glycogen back into glucose so that it can be used by the body's tissues. The liver also can create glucose from amino acids and fats.

Insulin lowers blood glucose levels both by slowing down the liver's glucose production and by helping the body's tissues to use glucose for energy. If the blood glucose level goes too low, other hormones, called counterregulatory hormones, work against the action of insulin to raise blood glucose levels. These hormones include glucagon, epinephrine, growth hormone, and cortisol. All work by prodding the liver to release glucose and by limiting glucose utilization by the body's tissues.

In diabetes, this delicate balance is disrupted. People with Type 1 diabetes do not produce insulin, so they must inject it. They may have deficient or altered counterregulatory responses as well. People with Type 2 diabetes either do not produce enough insulin or do not respond properly to insulin, or both. They, too, must take steps to control their blood glucose with diet, exercise, or diabetes pills or insulin. If blood glucose control measures don't work, high blood sugar is one of the possible, undesired results.

DKA

What sets the stage for diabetic ketoacidosis (DKA) is hyperglycemia (high blood sugar), especially when there is not enough insulin to handle it. In the absence of insulin, at least two things happen: The liver begins to produce more glucose, and the body's fat and muscle cells are unable to use glucose for energy and begin to starve. The body reacts to starvation by releasing counterregulatory hormones, which signal the liver to break down fat cells for energy. But because the liver and fat cells are unable to use the glucose in the bloodstream, they are unable to properly and completely break down the fat. Instead, they stop at a chemical "halfway point," producing chemical by-products called *ketones*.

Soon, the bloodstream gets flooded with excessive amounts of these ketones, rendering it more and more acidic. At the same time, the kidneys begin filtering large amounts of glucose from the blood and producing large amounts of urine. As the person urinates more frequently, the body becomes dehydrated and loses important minerals called *electrolytes,* which include sodium, potassium, and calcium. Having the proper amount of electrolytes is critical to many body functions, including the contraction and relaxation of the heart muscle. If not treated, all of these serious imbalances can eventually lead to coma and death.

HHS

Hyperosmolar hyperglycemic state (HHS) most commonly affects elderly people. Like DKA, HHS starts with hyperglycemia and insulin deficiency. As in DKA, people with HHS urinate frequently and become dehydrated. However, unlike in DKA, HHS impairs the ability of the kidneys to filter glucose from the bloodstream, so the hyperglycemia worsens.

Individuals developing HHS don't experience the same buildup of ketones in the blood as do those with DKA. Diabetes experts believe that this is probably because most people with HHS have Type 2 rather than Type 1 diabetes, so they probably have enough insulin secretion left to prevent the breakdown of fats. Even so, because of the extreme dehydration, HHS can be life-threatening and even more difficult to treat than DKA.

Common triggers

Either of these conditions can occur in anyone with diabetes, whether it be Type 1 or Type 2 diabetes. However, DKA more commonly affects people with Type 1 diabetes and HHS more commonly affects those with Type 2. Both DKA and HHS may be triggered by insulin deficiency or by any major stress to the body, which can cause the counterregulatory hormones to surge and elevate blood sugar levels.

The most common trigger for a hyperglycemic crisis is an infection, such as strep throat, pneumonia, an infected foot ulcer, an intestinal virus, or a urinary tract infection. Other triggers include stroke, heart attack, trauma, alcohol abuse, certain drugs (such as corticosteroids and certain blood pressure medicines), and the skipping or lowering of one's insulin dose.

In rare instances, mechanical problems with insulin pumps, such as blocking or kinking of the tubing, can stop insulin delivery and result in extreme hyperglycemia. People who use a rapid-acting insulin analog such as lispro (brand name Humalog) in an insulin pump need to be particularly alert to pump malfunctions. Since lispro stops working more quickly than Regular insulin does, hyperglycemia can occur more quickly.

Crisis prevention

DKA and HHS can be prevented by keeping hyperglycemia from happening in the first place. Prevention involves carrying out all parts of your diabetes regimen, monitoring your blood glucose level regularly, and learning to adjust your insulin dose properly, if you use insulin.

Because infection is a common trigger, it's important to be aware of signs of infection (such as high blood sugar) and to seek treatment promptly. In addition, when you're sick, it's important to take your usual doses of insulin or diabetes pills, monitor your blood glucose frequently, and test your urine for ketones. (See "Sick-Day Management" on this page for more specifics.)

It's also important to be aware of symptoms of hyperglycemia, which include thirst, increased appetite, frequent urination, weight loss, and dehydration, since both DKA and HHS typically start with hyperglycemia. These symptoms may be present for several days before either condition develops. Signs of dehydration include dryness of the mouth, cracked lips, sunken eyes, weight loss, and flushed, dry skin. As the situation worsens, vomiting, weakness, confusion, and coma may occur. People with DKA may experience abdominal pain and a "fruity" odor on the breath, due to the presence of ketones.

Children and adolescents. DKA is the most common diabetes-related cause of hospitalization and death in children with diabetes. Unfortunately, hospitalization for DKA is often the way a child is first diagnosed with diabetes. To prevent DKA in children and adolescents, parents need to find a balance between giving children responsibility for their diabetes care and taking a supportive and active role in helping them maintain good monitoring and medicine habits. (Although some children are mature for their age, responsibility and good judgment are not hallmarks of childhood and adolescence.) Parents should also anticipate when high levels of blood glucose may occur, such as when a child is sick, and be ready to take a more active role in such situations to avoid problems.

SICK-DAY MANAGEMENT

Any illness, and particularly one that causes vomiting, diarrhea, and dehydration, can trigger either diabetic ketoacidosis (DKA) or hyperosmolar hyperglycemic state (HHS). To avoid having a garden-variety flu turn into something much worse, here are some guidelines to follow when you're sick:

■ Plan ahead. The best time to discuss sick-day management with your health-care team is before you become sick. You should agree on how to manage your blood sugar, when to test for ketones, and, most important, when to seek medical help. Keep adequate supplies of test strips, ketone strips, and insulin on hand (if insulin is part of your sick-day treatment), and make sure to store them properly.

■ When you are sick, let a friend, neighbor, or relative know, so that he or she can check in on you and call for help if you are unable to help yourself.

■ If you have symptoms of a cold or flu, check your blood glucose level and test your urine for ketones, and continue checking both every four hours. (In fact, you should set an alarm clock to wake you every four hours during the night.) If your blood glucose level is below 250 mg/dl and your urine shows no ketones, stick with your usual insulin or pill regimen and continue checking your blood and urine every four hours until the symptoms have passed. If your blood glucose level rises above 250 mg/dl, if your urine tests positive for ketones, or if you are vomiting repeatedly, call your health-care provider.

■ Treat the underlying illness. Be sure to consult your health-care team and follow their directions for treating any sickness. This may mean taking a course of antibiotics if you have a bacterial infection or taking acetaminophen or other medicines for a fever. The sooner your illness resolves, the sooner your blood sugar levels go back to normal.

■ If you have vomiting or diarrhea, drink plenty of fluids. Some good choices for fluid replacement are Gatorade or similar products or one standard bouillon cube dissolved in 8 ounces of water. To prevent more vomiting, it is best to sip these fluids a little at a time rather than drinking a large amount all at once.

■ Ask your physician to recommend medicines or techniques to minimize nausea and vomiting. Stopping vomiting can be an important step for preventing dehydration.

■ Never skip an insulin dose because of loss of appetite, nausea, or vomiting. Even though you're not eating or keeping food down, your blood glucose may still be high because of the action of the counterregulatory hormones. Frequently monitor your blood and urine, and adjust your insulin dose as needed, with the help of your health-care team.

■ Maintain contact with your health-care team and be prepared to tell them about your blood sugar levels, urine ketones, and the type and quantity of fluids you have consumed.

■ Signs that your condition may be getting worse include continued vomiting, becoming short of breath, or becoming excessively sleepy. Let your health-care provider know: He or she may recommend that you go to an emergency room.

A common cause of DKA in children is failing to take insulin. This can happen for any number of reasons, including having poor organizational skills, not understanding the consequences of skipping injections, or disliking or resenting the unrelenting regimen, the sense of being different from other children, or the discomfort of sticking oneself with needles. Children and adolescents may also skip injections because they seek to lose weight or gain attention. A parent's support and understanding can help a lot in these situations. Consulting a mental health professional who specializes in children with diabetes or other chronic diseases can also be a big help, for both the child and the whole family.

Weight issues. When people start taking insulin, many notice some weight gain, and typically they blame it on the insulin. The fact that skipping some insulin doses causes weight loss seems to prove the theory, and some people take to habitually skipping insulin to control their weight. This is a risky practice that can lead to short-term, acute complications such as DKA, and long-term complications of the eyes, nerves, and kidneys.

The weight-gain culprit when starting insulin therapy is not the insulin alone. When blood sugar levels are high, excess sugar is lost in the urine. When insulin therapy is started, the sugar is used or stored by the body instead of being dumped into the urine. The storage of glucose as fat is what causes the weight gain.

A person who uses insulin can safely lose weight without skipping insulin doses. This is best done with the help of a registered dietitian, who can design a healthy, reduced-calorie diet that doesn't compromise blood glucose control. Since exercise is key to maintaining weight loss, people wishing to lose weight should ask their doctor for advice on starting an exercise regime or ask for a referral to an exercise physiologist.

When a child or adolescent desires to lose weight, parents should not hesitate to consult the diabetes-care team. Even in a child who is overweight, weight *maintenance,* not weight *loss,* is often the preferred approach. But often, body image is the real problem, not body weight, and it's a problem that should be taken seriously since it can lead to eating disorders and to both acute and long-term diabetes complications.

Safe alcohol use. Alcohol can cause dehydration, which can contribute to DKA and HHS. However, alcohol can be consumed safely in moderation by many people with well-controlled diabetes. In most cases, "moderation" is defined as no more than two servings of alcohol a day for men and no more than one serving of alcohol a day for women.

To prevent hypoglycemia, do not drink after exercise or on an empty stomach. To prevent weight gain, remember to include the calories in your drink in your meal plan. People who take certain medicines, includ-ing metformin (brand names include Glucophage, Glucophage XR, and Glucovance), may need to limit their alcohol intake to prevent liver problems.

HHS. HHS typically takes much longer to develop than DKA. Studies have shown that HHS most commonly affects older people who either live alone or live in a nursing home, where their confusion may go unnoticed. Unfortunately, decline in mental status in an older person may be mistakenly attributed to "senile dementia." Once considered an inevitable consequence of growing old, dementia is now known to be a pathological condition. Therefore, any impairment in memory, thought processes, reasoning, or language or any personality changes in an older person should be brought to the attention of that person's medical provider. It is also important to take note of any symptoms of hyperglycemia or dehydration in an older person with diabetes.

Lactic acidosis. Although it is not a hyperglycemic crisis, lactic acidosis is another diabetes-related crisis worth knowing about, particularly if you take any drug containing metformin. Lactic acidosis is a potentially deadly condition caused by a buildup of lactic acid in the tissues. Such a buildup can be due to dehydration, lack of oxygen, prolonged exercise, hyperventilation, diarrhea, vomiting, kidney disease, or liver disease. If you take metformin and notice symptoms of lactic acidosis, such as lightheadedness, tiredness, weakness, muscle pain, slowed or irregular heartbeat, feeling cold, or unusual stomach pain, you should call your physician.

Treatment

Although your doctor may be able to talk you through the treatment of a mild case, both DKA and HHS usually call for a trip to the emergency room. If caught in time, these conditions can sometimes be reversed in six to 12 hours. If they are advanced, it may require a two- to three-day hospital stay. To treat either condition, doctors must carefully monitor and treat several chemical imbalances at once.

Here's a summary of how hyperglycemic crises are treated:

■ Intravenous saline solution (water and sodium) is given to reverse dehydration. This improves circulation and helps the kidneys function properly again.

■ Insulin is given to lower the blood glucose level, stop the breakdown of fats, and thus stop the production of ketones.

■ Potassium is also replaced. Potassium is lost in the urine, a problem that is compounded when insulin is administered, because it can cause a person's cells to suddenly soak up large amounts of potassium from the bloodstream. Because a very low blood potassium level (called hypokalemia) can interfere with the ability of the heart to function properly, potassium replacement is extremely important.

■ In the case of DKA, depending on how acidic the blood is, doctors may also inject sodium bicarbonate to restore it to a normal level of acidity.

Throughout this treatment, doctors and nurses may check the person's pulse, blood pressure, mental status, temperature, blood glucose level, acid levels, and serum potassium and phosphate levels to make sure the treatment is working properly. Sometimes electrocardiograms are performed to make sure that the heart is beating properly.

An experience worth missing

Diabetic ketoacidosis and hyperosmolar hyperglycemic state are both serious and life-threatening conditions. Even though they can be treated successfully in many cases, especially if caught early, they're both worth skipping in the first place. The best way to prevent them is to keep close tabs on your blood glucose levels, to observe the "sick-day management" rules when you become ill, and to seek medical help if you cannot control your blood glucose level with self-care efforts. ❑

HYPOGLYCEMIA
RESEARCH UPDATE
by Wayne L. Clark

The hallmark of diabetes, and the root cause of most of the damage it does, is too much glucose in the blood. In Type 1 diabetes, the islet cells of the pancreas do not produce insulin, and the only therapy is to replace the insulin. Many people with Type 2 diabetes also need insulin, because the pancreas does not produce enough to meet the body's needs. For these people, that means taking insulin by injection or by infusion through an insulin pump.

Ironically, the very therapy that keeps so many people alive can create the most significant acute complication of diabetes. Hypoglycemia is the opposite of the original problem: not too *much* glucose in the blood, but too *little*. Everyone who takes insulin most likely knows the feelings caused by hypoglycemia: sweating, racing heart, shaking, hunger, dizziness, and emotional changes. More than just an inconvenience, if not treated, hypoglycemia can sometimes be deadly.

Hypoglycemia has become a more prevalent problem since the discovery that tight blood sugar control can reduce or eliminate long-term diabetic complica-

tions. (Tight control has been defined as keeping blood sugar levels as close to normal as possible with frequent monitoring and, at least for people with Type 1 diabetes, three or more daily injections or an insulin pump.) The Diabetes Complications and Control Trial (DCCT), which involved only people with Type 1 diabetes, and the more recent United Kingdom Prospective Diabetes Study, which enrolled only people with Type 2 diabetes, provided conclusive proof that the lower blood sugar levels are maintained, the lower the incidence of long-term complications. So the trend in diabetes control has emphasized lower blood sugar levels, and the incidence of hypoglycemia has increased.

In fact, the DCCT participants who maintained tight control were three times more likely to experience hypoglycemia. The good news/bad news trade-off is a short-term complication against long-term complications, and the balance is critical.

Another surprising finding of the DCCT was that the conventional wisdom that hypoglycemia is usually caused by not eating enough, taking too much insulin, or getting too much exercise may not be correct. In the study, most episodes of hypoglycemia were independent of those factors, suggesting a fundamental defect in the body's handling of blood glucose regulation in Type 1 diabetes.

In its 1997 Research Task Force report the Juvenile Diabetes Research Foundation International (JDF) named hypoglycemia as one of the five most important research focus areas. JDF-funded researchers are working on a number of fronts to solve the mysteries of this seemingly simple but very complex process.

Why hypoglycemia occurs

The first step in preventing hypoglycemia is understanding exactly what it is and how it works. With this knowledge, medical researchers may be able to find ways to correct the functional defects that allow hypoglycemia to happen.

This is what we know: People with diabetes have a dysfunctional *counterregulatory response* to blood sugar levels. In people who do not have diabetes, a decrease in blood sugar levels triggers the release of *glucagon* from the pancreas. Glucagon is a hormone that causes the liver to convert stored glucose, called *glycogen,* into glucose and release it into the blood, thus raising the blood sugar level. If that doesn't work, or doesn't work well enough, the adrenal glands release another hormone, *epinephrine* (also called adrenaline), which causes the liver to convert more glycogen to glucose.

The glucagon response is missing in people with Type 1 diabetes, so the epinephrine response kicks in. (In people with Type 2 diabetes, the glucagon response can be—but isn't always—missing or impaired.) The epinephrine response is a "back-up" system, and it's the source of the sweating and shaking symptoms commonly associated with low blood sugar. When it works, the epinephrine response triggers the release of enough glucose to correct the hypoglycemia or at least bring the blood sugar up long enough for the person to treat it by consuming carbohydrate.

But this response is not the ideal way to control blood sugar levels, and worse, it appears to become less effective over time. It seems that episodes of hypoglycemia somehow create a predisposition for more episodes. It also appears that hypoglycemia lowers the blood sugar level that triggers the counterregulatory response, so that over time, the blood sugar level must fall further before the body responds.

As this threshold lowers, the warning symptoms of hypoglycemia don't occur until the blood sugar level is very low, making it more difficult to treat it in time. This *hypoglycemia unawareness* is most commonly seen in people with diabetes who have frequent episodes of hypoglycemia, those who have had recent episodes of hypoglycemia, and those who routinely keep their blood sugar levels low to practice tight control.

Hypoglycemia also interferes with blood sugar control because it can be such a frightening experience. People may not attempt tight control for fear of hypoglycemia, and parents of young children especially will often let their children run "high" in order to avoid the feared, middle-of-the-night hypoglycemic episode.

Focusing on the brain

Researchers have zeroed in on the brain as they look for the primary defect in the counterregulatory system of people with diabetes. The brain is especially sensitive to changes in blood sugar levels, and some researchers think one particular area of the brain, the hypothalamus, may be the key.

Stephanie Amiel, M.D., of King's College in London is using an imaging method called positron emission tomography (PET) to track glucose as it travels through the brain. By labeling glucose with radioactive tracers, she can follow its path throughout the body. She wants to see where in the brain glucose accumulates, where it is metabolized, and how this changes in people with diabetes who are experiencing hypoglycemia. The findings of her JDF-funded research may help determine where and how the brain seemingly "adapts" its ability to take up glucose.

At Yale University School of Medicine, Robert S. Sherwin, M.D., is conducting JDF-funded research into the neurochemistry and function of the brain during hypoglycemia. The project employs a microdialysis technique to analyze the fluid between brain cells at various levels of hypoglycemia while the subjects undergo memory testing.

Another aspect of the Yale team's project involves using an imaging technique called noninvasive nuclear magnetic resonance spectroscopy to investigate what is happening in the brains of people while they are hypoglycemic. The researchers want to measure the rate of glucose metabolism and the action of *neurotransmitters,* the substances that transmit nerve impulses in the brain. A third phase of the project uses another type of imaging study, called functional MRI tests, to measure the effect of hypoglycemia on the changes that occur in various regions of the brain during cognitive tasks such as memorization.

Charles Mobbs, Ph.D., a JDF researcher at Mount Sinai School of Medicine in New York City, is studying the glucose sensitivity of the neurons in the hypothalamus of people with diabetes, with the suspicion that their impaired responsiveness may be due to impaired action of the enzyme *glucokinase.* If this is the case, it may be possible to develop a drug to restore the glucokinase action to normal.

At the Veteran's Administration Puget Sound Health Care System in Seattle, Dianne Figlewitcz Lattermann, Ph.D., is conducting JDF-funded research into specific nerve cells in the brain that she suspects may be responsible for the decreased response to hypoglycemia. So-called *noradrenergic* neurons, which help stimulate the brain during stress, may be impaired by hypoglycemia and consequently less able to function normally during subsequent episodes.

In addition, glucose transport across the *blood–brain barrier*—a mechanism that prevents many substances from leaving the blood and entering the brain—appears to be altered by hypoglycemia. In what may be a primitive protective response, the entrance of glucose into the brain increases during a hypoglycemic episode. If the brain "hoards" glucose this way, it may not recognize the next drop in blood sugar and may not initiate the counterregulatory response.

Stephen Davis, M.D., at Vanderbilt University in Nashville, Tennessee, suspects that the stress hormone *cortisol* may be at least one factor responsible for "blunting" the counterregulatory response. It is known that exercise can induce hypoglycemia, and also that exercise releases cortisol. Dr. Davis believes that the release of cortisol in response to physiologic stress—whether it be exercise or an episode of hypoglycemia—causes the brain to adapt and inhibit the counterregulatory release of glucagon and epinephrine.

Other areas of research

Some researchers believe that the brain is not the only organ responsible for the faulty counterregulatory response. Some suspect the liver. And, at the State University of New York at Stony Brook, Eugenio Cerosimo, M.D., Ph.D., is examining the role of the kidney in the body's defense against hypoglycemia. Normally, the kidney's production of sugar increases when blood glucose levels drop. This reaction may be diminished in people with diabetes.

More than half of hypoglycemic episodes, and the majority of severe episodes, occur at night. Often, people are unaware of these episodes. There is also a strong correlation between low blood sugar at night and increased hypoglycemia during the day. All this has led a number of researchers to consider whether sleep reduces the counterregulatory response.

William V. Tamborlane, M.D., and his colleagues at Yale helped to confirm this theory in their work with adolescents. They found that the counterregulatory response to mild hypoglycemia is reduced during deep sleep. The investigators are now continuing their work to determine why.

It is certain that severe hypoglycemia can sometimes cause coma, permanent brain damage, and even death. Less is known about the effects of less severe or chronic hypoglycemia. Dorothy Becker, M.B., B.Ch., at the Children's Hospital of Pittsburgh believes that it is important to protect children from mild hypoglycemia because it causes a temporary decrease of up to 20% of cognitive capacity. The effect is seen in "mental efficiency" tasks involving memory, attention span, and visual–spatial relationships. Dr. Becker and her colleagues are exploring the use of lactate as a substitute fuel in the absence of glucose as a means of giving children "insurance" against the cognitive deficits of low blood sugar.

Meanwhile, at the University of Western Australia, Timothy Jones, M.B., B.S., is using cognitive testing, electroencephalograms (tracings of brain waves), and MRI scans to measure the brain function of a group of children whose hypoglycemic history is known, to see if and how hypoglycemia has affected them.

Advancing technology

Achieving tight control while avoiding hypoglycemia requires a balance that is difficult to maintain. Easier and more accurate methods of monitoring blood sugar levels, along with better ways to deliver insulin, could make it easier. There is a great deal of research and development activity focused on devices to do both.

What if you didn't have to draw blood to get a blood sugar level? Glucose is found not only in blood, but in the fluid between most cells. This *interstitial fluid* can be found very close to the skin and can be sampled with much less discomfort than is experienced when drawing blood with a lancet. Various techniques are being developed to tap and measure the glucose in interstitial fluid, including laser piercing, ultrasound, and microlancets.

For example, the GlucoWatch Biographer, which was developed by Cygnus, Inc., leaches glucose through the skin and gives a blood sugar reading every 20 minutes for 12 hours. It was approved for marketing by the U.S. Food and Drug Administration in March 2001. Michael Pishko, Ph.D., at Texas A&M University is conducting JDF-funded research into the use of ultrasound to extract interstitial fluid, and other researchers are experimenting with skin patches that pull fluid from the skin and can then be "read" in a meter.

Other researchers are looking at various *biosensors* that react to glucose. Biosensors are compounds that can be implanted in a device, and their reactions can be monitored either visually or by radio signals. Sensors based on glucose oxidase and similar compounds are being tested in a variety of configurations. Joseph Lucisano, Ph.D., and his team at Glysens, Inc., in San Diego have developed one such sensor system and have used it to measure and transmit blood glucose levels in dogs. In ongoing research under a JDF Special Grant, they are exploring the possibility of achieving similar success in human trials.

Homme Hellinga, Ph.D., at Duke University is genetically engineering a protein that reacts to glucose and contains a fluorescent molecule. His JDF project has the goal of developing a means to measure the fluorescence and use it to continuously measure blood sugar levels.

On a different tack, Jaime Castano, Ph.D., at Reti Tech, Inc., in El Sobrante, California, is developing tests of visual sensitivity based on the known changes that blood sugar causes in the retina of the eye. Ultimately, these tests could be used for home monitoring.

For many, the ultimate goal of better blood sugar measurement is its application to a "closed loop" system: one that both measures blood glucose levels and administers the appropriate amount of insulin. Already, both pieces of such a system exist; the challenge is to marry them.

The insulin pump manufacturer MiniMed, Inc., has developed the Continuous Glucose Monitoring System, which uses a Teflon catheter that stays under the skin and measures blood glucose levels every five minutes for up to three days. (Currently, the MiniMed system must be prescribed by a doctor.) Yale's Tamborlane is conducting a JDF-funded clinical trial examining how the device may help children and adolescents maintain desired blood sugar levels without the risk of hypoglycemia.

The insulin pump has made blood sugar control more effective and more convenient for many people with diabetes, and if it could respond automatically to blood sugar levels it would become a "virtual pancreas." MiniMed's implantable pump, already approved for use in Europe, combined with the right sensor, could make an implantable closed loop system a reality.

Meanwhile, another company, Animas Corporation, is developing an implantable, optical sensor to measure glucose levels and has developed its own insulin pump.

Hypoglycemia will be conquered only when scientists achieve a better understanding of how it works. Then, taking advantage of new treatments and prevention strategies, people with diabetes will be able to manage their fear of low blood sugar and have an easier time maintaining an appropriate balance between high and low. ❑

FOR MORE INFORMATION

To learn more about the Juvenile Diabetes Research Foundation International, call (800) JDF-CURE (533-2873), or check out the organization's Web site at www.jdf.org.

TREATING NEUROPATHY WHILE WAITING FOR A CURE

by Wayne L. Clark

It's easy to name the single factor responsible for diabetic neuropathy, the nerve degeneration that can plague people with diabetes in a variety of ways: If there were no high blood sugar, there would be no diabetic neuropathy. It's much more difficult to tell people with diabetes how to cope with the condition, and even more difficult for researchers to uncover the reasons for it.

Diabetic neuropathy is caused by *hyperglycemia*, the high blood sugar levels that are associated with diabetes, and it includes a number of somewhat different syndromes. It is estimated that 60% or more of people with diabetes of long duration have some degree of neuropathy, which can develop within 10 years of the onset of the disease. The condition occurs both with Type 1 diabetes and with Type 2 diabetes, and it may already affect many people with diabetes at the time they are diagnosed.

The most common form is *peripheral diabetic polyneuropathy,* which can affect the feet, legs, arms, and hands. This kind of neuropathy is responsible for the seemingly paradoxical symptoms reported by many people with diabetes: lack of sensation or numbness in the extremities, and burning or stabbing pain.

Autonomic neuropathy, in contrast, may affect the digestive system, the sexual organs, the urinary tract, the heart, and even the sweat glands. Symptoms take a variety of forms, including sexual dysfunction.

Autonomic neuropathy may be partly responsible for the high rates of cardiovascular mortality associated with diabetes. People with diabetes often develop *congestive heart failure* (CHF), a condition in which the heart is unable to pump sufficient blood to meet the needs of the body. CHF typically develops in people who have had one or more heart attacks, but people with diabetes who develop CHF often lack a history of heart attacks, because they've had "silent" heart attacks during which they don't feel pain because of neuropathy.

Focal neuropathies may affect the eyes, facial muscles, hearing, pelvis and lower back, thighs, or abdomen. As the name implies, they are focused on very specific nerves or areas. The effects are often described as twinges, jabbing pains, twitches, or palsies.

What happens to the nerves

The damage that high blood glucose levels cause to the nerves is a complex and not clearly understood cascade of cellular events that is sometimes described as a "dying back" of the nerve fibers.

"Think of a nerve as an electrical cord," says Eva Feldman, M.D., Ph.D., a neurologist at the University of Michigan and Director of the Juvenile Diabetes Research Foundation (JDRF) Center for Complications of Diabetes. "The nerve fiber itself is the wire inside the cord, and it is surrounded by insulation. In diabetic neuropathy, the nerve fiber itself becomes damaged at its farthest points, and the insulation also becomes damaged. Also, the cell body that supplies the nerve becomes dysfunctional and dies."

In other words, the longest nerves, such as those that go to the toes, are affected first. The destruction of their insulation compounds the damage, like a short-circuit in a wire with broken insulation. Eventually, the cells that supply the nerve with food and fuel die.

There is a common culprit behind the various specific types of damage in neuropathy: *oxidative stress.* Too much glucose, the fuel that feeds cellular processes, causes the cellular machinery to run out of control. The result is oxidative stress and the creation of *free radicals* that damage the nerve cells and the blood vessels that supply them. The interruption of blood flow further accelerates the stress. Oxidative stress also impairs the action of *neurotrophic factors,* which help nerves regenerate.

What you can do

The good news is that there is an approved product to treat the cause of neuropathy, and you already have it: insulin. Controlling blood sugar using insulin—or oral drugs in the case of Type 2 diabetes—can not only delay the onset of neuropathy but can also reportedly improve symptoms for those already affected. The Diabetes Complications and Control Trial, a major study whose results were published in 1993, demonstrated conclusively that there was at least

a 60% decrease in neuropathy when blood sugar levels were kept close to the normal range.

For control of neuropathic pain, it has been suggested that keeping blood glucose level stable is even more important than keeping it at any particular level, since swings in blood glucose may aggravate the pain. This means that newer diabetes control regimens, such as the use of an insulin pump, may provide an advantage by "evening out" blood sugar levels.

There is some symptomatic relief available now for those who have painful neuropathy. A number of drugs can help, as can some other methods of pain control. While none of these drugs or treatments treat the actual disorder, they can mask the symptoms.

Most promising for many people has been the adaptation of the drug gabapentin (brand name Neurontin) and other anticonvulsant drugs such as carbamazepine (Tegretol) from their original uses as anticonvulsants to treat epilepsy.

"Neurontin has proven to be a very helpful drug to treat diabetic neuropathy with minimal side effects and drug interactions," says Leann Olansky, M.D., Professor of Medicine at the University of Oklahoma Health Sciences Center.

"A number of antidepressants do work, and I think it's important to have more than one thing in your armamentarium," she says. "For some people, for instance, amitriptyline [Elavil] is not a good choice because it leads to increased appetite, weight gain, sedation, and other side effects. So it's good to have other choices."

Most doctors frown upon the use of barbiturates—drugs sometimes prescribed for anxiety and sleep disorders—for treating neuropathic pain. But narcotics—the most powerful painkillers available—may have a place. "Narcotics, if they're used intelligently, can be helpful," Dr. Olansky says. "If a person is having trouble sleeping, for instance, and taking a narcotic at night allows them to get rest, then that's worth doing. Once you start getting round-the-clock narcotics, that's not ideal.

"Everything needs to be taken in context in managing medications: what the patient stands to gain, and what the downside is. Sometimes using different drugs in combination will provide the most help."

Many people with diabetic neuropathy have used over-the-counter topical capsaicin creams for local relief of pain. Capsaicin is responsible for the "hot" in hot peppers. When using a capsaicin cream, it is important to follow label directions and watch for skin irritation.

Another nonpharmaceutical approach to treating neuropathy pain is transcutaneous electrical nerve stimulation (TENS). TENS units are small, battery-operated devices that deliver tiny electrical currents through electrodes taped to the skin. Dr. Olansky says this process, which blocks the pain message from getting to the brain, is helpful for some people. "Again, it's good to have more than one modality available, and TENS does work for some people," she says. "The problem is, TENS works a lot better if it's used sparingly, and people tend to use it more and more, and it becomes less effective."

Paradoxically, pain management may be needed by some people even as their neuropathy improves. Pain that increases as blood sugar is brought into a more normal range is actually a good sign, because improved nerve health may allow the person to feel pain that simply couldn't be felt before. Increased pain may also be caused by nerves that "misfire" as they make new connections.

Autonomic neuropathies can also be treated symptomatically. The drug sildenafil (Viagra) is helpful in treating impotence and metoclopramide (Reglan) for treating gastrointestinal problems. Autonomic neuropathy can also cause unexpected drops in blood pressure on standing and unexplained rapid heart-

MORE ON NEUROPATHY

To learn more about neuropathy and its potential treatments, consult the following resources:

NATIONAL INSTITUTE OF DIABETES AND DIGESTIVE AND KIDNEY DISEASES
"Diabetic Neuropathy: The Nerve Damage of Diabetes"
July 1995
This booklet describes the causes and common symptoms of diabetic neuropathy, the tests used to diagnose it, and various treatments. It can be read online at www.niddk.nih.gov/health/diabetes/pubs/neuro/neuro.htm.

"Keep Your Nervous System Healthy"
May 2000
This booklet, one in a series on preventing diabetes problems, explains how diabetes affects the nervous system and how to prevent such problems. It does not describe treatments for neuropathy. It can be read online at www.niddk.nih.gov/health/diabetes/pubs/complications/index.htm or ordered as described below.

For free copies of this and other booklets and fact sheets on diabetes-related topics, call, write, fax, or e-mail the National Diabetes Information Clearinghouse, 1 Information Way, Bethesda, MD 20892-3560. Phone: (800) 860-8747; fax: (301) 907-8906; e-mail: ndic@info.niddk.nih.gov.

JUVENILE DIABETES RESEARCH FOUNDATION INTERNATIONAL WEB PAGE
www.jdf.org
This Web site contains information on neuropathy (from the Home page, click on "Life With Diabetes") and on research sponsored by the JDRF (from the Home page, click on "Clinical Trial Information"). The JDRF's clinical trials page also has a link to the database of ongoing research trials sponsored by the U.S. National Institutes of Health, www.clinicaltrials.gov.

AMERICAN DIABETES ASSOCIATION WEB PAGE
www.diabetes.org
For an overview of the symptoms of and treatments for neuropathy, log on to the Association's Home page, click first on "Basic Diabetes Information," then on "Complications," and then on "Neuropathy."

THE UNCOMPLICATED GUIDE TO DIABETES COMPLICATIONS
Marvin E. Levin and Michael A. Pfeiffer, eds.
American Diabetes Association
Alexandria, Virginia, 1998
Provides easy-to-understand explanations of common and not-so-common diabetes complications.

NUMB TOES AND ACHING SOLES
Coping With Peripheral Neuropathy
John A. Senneff
MedPress
San Antonio, Texas, 1999
Describes just about every treatment anyone has ever tried for peripheral neuropathy, from prescription drugs to relaxation techniques. Each description is followed by comments from people who have tried the treatment, both satisfied and unsatisfied customers.

THE NEUROPATHY ASSOCIATION
(800) 247-6968
www.neuropathy.org
Nonprofit member organization provides support and education and promotes research into the causes and cures for peripheral neuropathy. The Association publishes a newsletter, *Neuropathy News,* and the booklets "Explaining Neuropathy" and "Exercising With Neuropathy," as well as a relaxation audiotape.

beat, and there are drugs available to help with both problems.

The best first line of treatment for all diabetic neuropathies, every medical professional makes a point to remind us, is still control of blood sugar levels. It's something over which a person can exercise direct control. There's another important self-care issue in neuropathy as well, as Dr. Olansky points out.

"Smoking makes *all* the complications of diabetes worse," she says. "So it's very important for people who have neuropathy to stop smoking. It's something else they can do to help themselves."

Prevention of complications

Early detection and intervention will become increasingly important as new treatments become available. The earlier therapy is started, the greater the likelihood of saving and regenerating nerve tissue. The problem is, the early signs and symptoms of diabetic neuropathy are often overlooked.

Neuropathy is dangerous because it is subtle, and that makes awareness paramount. The feet that are most likely to ulcerate and possibly be amputated are not the painful feet but the numb feet. Symptoms of advanced neuropathy—such as balance problems or difficulty with fine-motor tasks such as buttoning a shirt—may be vague. The reason for such symptoms may not become apparent until an observant health-care provider takes a full history.

There are a growing number of sophisticated diagnostic tools to help diagnose diabetic neuropathy and measure its severity, but as a practical matter they are primarily of interest to researchers. But there are simple, noninvasive ways to screen the average person with diabetes for neuropathy, and they should be part of every routine examination. Doctors can check muscle strength and reflexes to test if nerves are as responsive as normal, and they can do a monofilament screening by applying a nylon filament (a threadlike strand of nylon) to selected sites on the feet to test for evidence of sensory deficiency.

New knowledge about who is at risk for diabetes may help people be aware of their risk for neuropathy earlier. One reason is that the definition of diabetes itself is being challenged, as the line between impaired glucose tolerance (IGT) and diabetes becomes less clear. IGT is a condition in which blood sugar levels are higher than normal, but not high enough for a diagnosis of diabetes. However, people with IGT are considered at higher risk of developing diabetes.

What this means for people already diagnosed with diabetes and for people at risk of developing diabetes is that vigilance and early detection is critical. "New guidelines lower the threshold for defining impaired glucose tolerance," Dr. Feldman says. "We published a study in collaboration with other centers in which we found that in our patient population, when someone is sent to us with numb, aching feet of unknown cause, one-third have impaired glucose tolerance. So early diagnosis is key, and I believe that IGT is the first step toward frank diabetes and that we need to diagnose early and treat early signs of neuropathy."

New help on the way

Even the best control cannot eliminate episodes of high blood sugar altogether, and currently available treatments offer only symptomatic relief, so researchers are looking for other ways to stop the oxidative stress or its consequences. The goal is to cure the disorder or even prevent it. Dr. Feldman and her colleagues, for instance, at the JDRF Center for Complications of Diabetes, are taking a multifactorial approach to what appears to be a process that has metabolic, vascular, and neurodegenerative components.

They hope to demonstrate that neuropathy can be stabilized, reduced, or even prevented by combining ways to combat these three components. Control of blood sugar is first and foremost to limit the cause of the process. When too much sugar circulates throughout the body, it interacts with *aldose reductase,* an enzyme in the cells surrounding the nerves. The metabolic disarray caused by this interaction might be stopped by the use of drugs called aldose reductase inhibitors. Antioxidant therapy would be employed to fight the destruction caused by oxidative free radicals, and neurotrophic factors would be stimulated or added to the body to encourage the regeneration of nerve tissue.

Neurotrophic factors are proteins that promote the survival of nerve tissue and may also promote its regeneration. The action of neurotrophins was first described half a century ago, but only in the past few years have some types been tested in clinical trials of neuropathy treatment.

One of the potential ways neurotrophic factors might be used is being investigated at the University of Pittsburgh by David Fink, M.D., and Joseph Glorioso, Ph.D., at the JDRF Center for Gene Therapy Approaches to Diabetes. They are working on a gene therapy approach that would "infect" nerve cells with the genes that produce neurotrophic growth factors. The ultimate objective of this research would be to give the nerve cells back the ability to protect themselves and regenerate.

Progress in treating and preventing diabetic neuropathy may ultimately help people with other neurodegenerative diseases. There are neuropathies that are caused by other syndromes, and there also is a spontaneously occurring idiopathic neuropathy that is age-related. Then there are the other, often devastating degenerative diseases of both the peripheral and central nervous system.

"There's an underlying common thread in nerve damage," Dr. Feldman says, "whether it's in the brain, such as in Alzheimer's disease, Parkinson's disease, and Huntington's, or in the peripheral nerves. In all these disorders, it appears that cells undergo a similar process of programmed cell death. It's likely due at least in part to oxidative stress. So if we understand and clearly treat one neurodegenerative disease, such as diabetic neuropathy, it will have clear applicability to other neurodegenerative disorders." ❑

TREATING IMPOTENCE

by Neil Baum, M.D.

Henry is 43 years old and has Type 2 diabetes. In the past two years, he has developed a progressive inability to attain and maintain an erection. He and Cynthia, his wife of 20 years, have a loving relationship, and previously they enjoyed a mutually satisfying sex life. But lately, Henry's sexual dysfunction—and his reluctance to do anything about it—has caused anxiety and tension in their relationship.

After two years of suggesting, cajoling, and nagging Henry to see his doctor, Cynthia put her foot down and made an appointment herself. Henry's primary-care doctor listened carefully as the couple described the problems they'd been having. After examining Henry, the doctor told them about various treatment options for impotence. They were advised to first try Viagra, the new oral medicine for impotence, and were reminded to keep the lines of communication open. If Viagra didn't seem to work for them, the doctor said, come back in, and they would discuss what to do next. Since trying Viagra, and making an effort to talk more openly about their sexual needs and preferences, Henry and Cynthia both report feeling happier about their sexual relationship.

Henry's erection problems place him in good company. Not only is impotence fairly common among men with diabetes, it is the most common type of sexual dysfunction among all men, affecting 20 to 30 million American men. Whether it is caused by diabetes

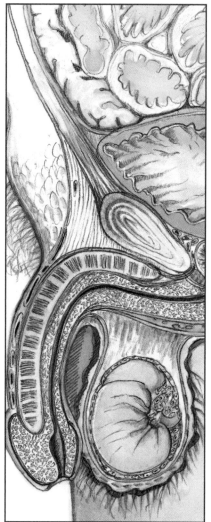

or not, impotence can be devastating for a man, undermining his self-confidence, self-esteem, and concept of himself as a man. In the past, impotence tended to be guarded as a shameful secret, but nowadays more and more men are seeking medical treatment for it. This is at least in part because the newer impotence treatments are less invasive and easier to use.

In this article, we discuss the relationship between impotence and diabetes, current methods of diagnosis, as well as a variety of treatment options.

The normal erection

An erection is primarily vascular in nature. In order for an erection to occur, more blood needs to enter the penis through the arteries than leaves the penis through the veins. The nervous system is also involved in the creation of an erection. With sexual arousal or stimulation, nerve signals are sent from the brain to the penis, where nerves release nitric oxide for the conversion of the chemical GTP to cyclic GMP. Cyclic GMP causes the smooth muscles in the penis to relax. When the smooth muscles relax, the blood vessels dilate and supply more blood to the *corpora cavernosa*, the erectile tissue within the penis. As more blood flows in, this spongy tissue becomes firm and expands, swelling and lengthening the penis. At the same time, the expanding tissue traps blood in the penis by compressing small veins and preventing the outflow of blood from the penis (see "How an Erection Occurs," on page 198). The more nitric oxide and cyclic GMP available to the smooth muscles in the penis, the longer the erection lasts. An erection subsides when cyclic GMP is broken down to GMP by an enzyme called phosphodiesterase 5. When this happens, the smooth muscles contract, and blood is no longer trapped in the penis.

Defining impotence

Impotence is the chronic or persistent inability to achieve and maintain an erection satisfactory to complete sexual intercourse. It is common and natural for a man to not be able to achieve or sustain an erection at one time or another, but this does not mean that he has impotence. Instead, impotence is diagnosed when physical or psychological factors result in the persistent inability to maintain an erection sufficient for intercourse. To distinguish impotence from other problems associated with sexual dysfunction, such as a lack of sexual desire or problems with ejaculation and orgasm, medical professionals also use the term *erectile dysfunction* to mean impotence.

Diabetes and impotence

There are an estimated 5 million men diagnosed with diabetes in the United States, and it has been estimated that 50% to 65% of these men will experience erectile dysfunction. On average, men with diabetes develop impotence 10 to 15 years earlier than men without diabetes. It is not uncommon for someone seeking treatment for impotence to find out he has diabetes and that this may be the underlying cause of his erectile dysfunction.

Impotence can result as a complication of diabetes in two ways. First, hardening of the arteries (arteriosclerosis) is accelerated in men with diabetes, resulting in restriction of blood flow to the penis. Second, nerve damage (neuropathy) prevents the normal transmission of nerve impulses to the blood vessels in the penis. This type of complication (called *peripheral neuropathy*) can also cause loss of sensation or pain in the legs and feet when nerves to the lower extremities are damaged. In men with diabetes, impotence does not usually appear all at once; it usually progresses as a slow, steady decline in sexual function. As nerve fibers and blood vessels become permanently damaged, impotence becomes permanent and complete.

Good blood sugar control has been shown to prevent or slow down the onset of complications related to diabetes, including the onset of erectile dysfunction. Other risk factors associated with erectile dysfunction in diabetes include obesity, high blood pressure, and high cholesterol levels. Psychological factors such as anxiety, guilt, depression, stress, and fear of sexual failure cause 10% to 20% of all cases of impotence.

In spite of his erectile dysfunction, a man whose impotence is caused by diabetes may be normal in all other aspects of sexuality. His sex drive, or libido, may be just as strong as before he had problems attaining or maintaining an erection. Like many other men with impotence, men with diabetes can still be stimulated to ejaculation and orgasm even though the penis is soft.

Diagnosis

A man can be evaluated for impotence by his primary-care physician or by the doctor who manages his diabetes. Sometimes a doctor will refer a man to a urologist when specialized or additional tests are needed. An evaluation usually involves a review of a man's medical history, a physical examination, and laboratory tests to diagnose the cause of impotence.

Medical history. To help guide him to appropriate testing, a doctor will try to determine the man's sexual and psychological status. The man may be asked about the degree and frequency of erection problems and the presence or absence of erections upon waking in the morning. The absence of erections in the morning suggests a physical cause, while the presence of erections suggests a psychological cause for erection difficulties. To examine psychological factors, a doctor may also ask whether the man feels particularly stressed or fatigued or whether there have been any significant changes in his life—such as divorce, a death of a loved one, or financial problems—that may cause stress.

A review of a man's medical history can reveal the cause of difficulty achieving or maintaining erections. For example, prostate surgery can injure nerves and arteries near the penis, causing impotence. Injury to the penis, spinal cord, prostate, pelvis, or bladder can also damage nerves, arteries, erectile tissue, and smooth muscle in the penis. Men with cardiovascular disease are also more likely to experience impotence.

Use of some medicines can cause impotence as a side effect. Certain medicines used to treat high blood pressure and heart disease, including thiazide diuretics and beta blockers such as propanolol, are common offenders. The cardiovascular drugs that are least likely to cause impotence are the angiotensin-converting enzyme (ACE) inhibitors and the calcium channel blockers. Other drugs associated with erectile dysfunction include antidepressants, antihistamines, appetite suppressants, certain drugs used to treat stomach ulcers, and pain medicines. Cigarette smoke, excessive alcohol intake, and illicit drugs can also damage nerves and blood vessels involved in an erection.

Physical examination. During the physical examination, the doctor will look for changes in secondary sex characteristics (including changes in breast, penile, and testicular size) and changes in hair, skin, or voice

HOW AN ERECTION OCCURS

Cross section of the penis. In the relaxed state, blood flows from the artery that feeds each of the corpora cavernosa, through the sinusoids, and empties via the emissary veins that lie within the tunica albuginea. In the erect state, the smooth-muscle walls of the sinusoids relax, allowing blood to expand the sinusoids, which results in swelling of the penis and compression of the emissary veins. Any further flow of blood into the penis causes rigidity.

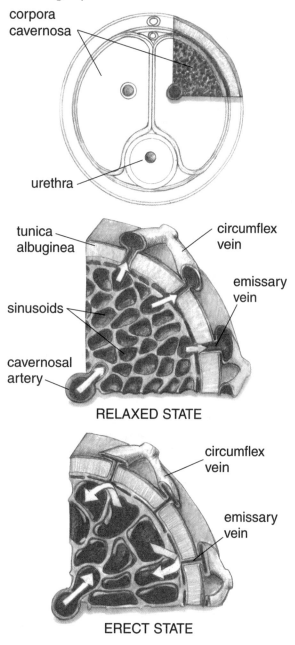

corpora cavernosa

urethra

tunica albuginea

circumflex vein

emissary vein

sinusoids

cavernosal artery

RELAXED STATE

circumflex vein

emissary vein

ERECT STATE

patterns that can indicate a hormonal imbalance as the cause of erection problems. A testosterone deficiency can cause impotence, breast enlargement, loss of pubic hair, and smaller, softer testes.

The testes and penis will be examined for physical abnormalities that may cause impotence or may interfere with effective treatment. For example, Peyronie disease, a curvature of the penis caused by plaque formation, may pose a problem for some forms of impotence treatment if the curvature is severe. A digital rectal exam will be performed to evaluate the prostate gland; abnormalities in the prostate gland may affect blood flow or nerve transmission to the penis.

A physical examination also includes an evaluation of the blood vessels and nerves surrounding the pelvis and in the lower extremities. The vascular system can be examined by feeling the pulse in the legs and feet. Blood vessels of the penis can be evaluated by ultrasound examination. Measurement of blood pressure in the legs can reveal problems in the arteries in the pelvis and groin that supply blood to the penis.

Drugs that dilate the arteries of the penis can also be injected for diagnostic purposes. If the injection doesn't cause an erection or if the man can't maintain an erection, the penile veins may be leaky and unable to hold blood in the penis.

A neurologic examination in the lower extremities can reveal the presence of peripheral neuropathy. In particular, nerve tests can be conducted to determine whether the nerve supply to the penis appears normal.
Laboratory tests. Laboratory tests, including urinalysis and blood work, can help determine whether other health problems may be responsible for the appearance of erectile dysfunction. For example, a blood cell count can identify anemia or infection, both of which can affect normal sexual function. Low sexual desire may be caused by low testosterone in the blood, which suggests a problem with the endocrine system.
Nocturnal penile tumescence. Healthy men have involuntary erections during sleep. Monitoring erections via a nocturnal penile tumescence (NPT) test can reveal whether impotence has a physical or psychological basis. However, tests of nocturnal erections are not completely reliable, and scientists have not set standards for their use in diagnosing impotence.

Treatment

When choosing the appropriate course of treatment, doctors usually begin with the least invasive option and progress to more invasive ones if early attempts are not successful. Currently, a variety of options are available to treat impotence, including oral drug therapy, external vacuum devices, penile suppositories, penile injection therapy, penile implant surgery, and vascular surgery. For men with diabetes or other health concerns, special considerations may make one option more preferable than others.

Viagra. Since the beginning of recorded history, men have been looking for a pill that will treat impotence. Finally, it seems that the grail has been found. In March 1998, the U.S. Food and Drug Administration (FDA) approved the pill sildenafil citrate (brand name Viagra) as an oral treatment for impotence. Viagra works by blocking the enzyme phosphodiesterase 5, which normally breaks down cyclic GMP and causes an erection to subside. By preventing the action of this enzyme, Viagra allows cyclic GMP to accumulate, which causes the smooth muscles in the penis to relax, resulting in an increase in blood flow to the penis and sustained erections.

Viagra was originally tested for treatment of angina, or chest pain due to a restricted blood supply to the heart muscles. Early studies showed that Viagra was not very effective for angina but produced erections in many of the men who participated in these studies. What a wonderful side effect! Early tests for treating impotence in the United States and Europe found success rates for Viagra of 70% to 80%. In one study of 4,500 men, many of whom had diabetes, 60% of the men with diabetes were able to engage in sexual intercourse after taking Viagra.

Viagra is available in three doses (25, 50, and 100 micrograms) and it is taken by mouth 30 to 60 minutes prior to engaging in intercourse. The drug remains effective for about four hours. Men are advised to take Viagra on an empty stomach and without alcohol to promote absorption of the drug into the bloodstream. Viagra can be used once in a 24-hour period.

There are few side effects associated with the use of Viagra. A few men report headaches, flushing, nausea, indigestion, and nasal congestion. Rarely, men report transient visual changes such as a blue halo around lights, which subsides after a few hours. Viagra is not associated with prolonged erection, or *priapism*, which is occasionally seen in men treated with injections or urethral suppositories.

Viagra is not appropriate for men who use nitrates, including nitroglycerin, for treating heart disease. The combination of these drugs can lower blood pressure to potentially dangerous levels.

Prostaglandin. Prostaglandin is a naturally occurring chemical that promotes relaxation of the smooth muscles in the penis and a subsequent increase in the arterial inflow to the erectile bodies. Prostaglandin can be administered by urethral suppositories or through direct needle injection into the erectile bodies.

Prostaglandin-containing suppositories can be inserted into the penis via the medicated urethral system for erection (MUSE). MUSE may be an option for men with diabetes who do not respond to Viagra. The suppositories contain alprostadil (a synthetic form of prostaglandin) in the form of a pellet that is inserted into the urethra (the tube in the penis that transports urine from the bladder to outside the body) through a sterile inserter. An erection usually occurs 5 to 10 minutes after insertion of the pellet and lasts for 30 to 60 minutes. MUSE is available in four strengths (125, 250, 500, and 1,000 micrograms) and should be stored in the refrigerator prior to use. MUSE can be used twice in 24 hours. In clinical studies, 65% of men with impotence had a positive response to medicated urethral suppositories.

The side effects of MUSE include penile pain, a decrease in blood pressure, minor urethral bleeding, and priapism (an unwanted, sustained erection). Any erection that lasts longer than four hours is an emergency that requires immediate medical attention. The penile pain associated with MUSE is usually mild and rarely causes men to discontinue using urethral suppositories.

Drugs can also be delivered by self-injection into the corporal bodies of the penis, where blood flow accumulates for an erection. An erection occurs in 5 to 10 minutes and lasts about 20 minutes. Self-injection should be limited to two times per week. The American Urological Association recommends alprostadil as the drug of choice for injection therapy. If this drug is not effective, then a combination of papaverine hydrochloride, phentolamine, and alprostadil can be tried. It may take some trial and error to learn proper injection technique and to determine the optimal dose for each man.

The possible complications of self-injection therapy include pain at the site of injection, internal scar formation that can worsen impotence, and priapism, which occurs in approximately 3% of men receiving injections.

Vacuum constriction devices. External vacuum devices are safe, simple to use, and relatively inexpensive. The vacuum device consists of a plastic cylinder, a hand-held vacuum pump, and an elastic constriction band. The plastic cylinder is placed over the penis and held against the body to form an airtight seal. As air is pumped out of the cylinder, negative pressure builds up and creates a partial vacuum around the penis, which causes the body's blood to enter the corpora cavernosa. The blood is then held in the penis by sliding the elastic constriction band to the base of the penis. After the tension ring is placed around the base of the penis, the vacuum chamber is removed. The man can safely engage in intercourse for 30 minutes, and then the elastic ring must be removed. Unlike other treatments, the vacuum can be used any time an erection is desired. However, most men request an alternative to the vacuum device because it is cumbersome to use.

Vacuum constriction devices should be used with caution in men with diabetes, especially those with severe blood vessel or nerve damage. All men must make sure not to leave the constriction band on for longer than 30 minutes since cutting off the blood supply can result in damage to the penile skin and underlying tissue. Vacuum devices may also not be appropriate for men with bleeding disorders or those who take blood-thinning drugs.

The main complaints about vacuum devices are discomfort from the tight elastic ring and the inconvenience of using the equipment that is needed to create the erection. Occasionally, minor bruising may occur with the use of vacuum devices, and a man's partner may complain that his penis is colder than normal.

Penile implants. When simpler, reversible, and less expensive treatments are inadequate in treating impotence, penile prosthetic implants can be surgically placed inside the penis to aid or create erections.

Implants consist of two cylinders that are placed into the corpora cavernosa. One type consists of semi-rigid rods that can be bent down but once inserted create a permanent erection. A second type consists of an inflatable cylinder that can be filled with fluid when an erection is desired. In this type of implant, a pump placed in the scrotum moves fluid from a reservoir in the abdomen or scrotum into the cylinder to create an erection. The erection is reduced by releasing a valve in the scrotum. A third type of implant consists of a self-contained, inflatable implant, in which each cylinder contains a pump, fluid, and release valve. Squeezing the head of the penis forces fluid to transfer forward and cause rigidity. Bending the penis in another way causes the fluid to flow back into the storage area, ending the erection.

Surgery to install a penile implant is permanent and is therefore a last resort. Surgery generally requires one day of hospitalization and is now also done on an outpatient basis. The recovery period at home is one week, and the man is able to engage in intercourse four to six weeks after surgery. Disadvantages associated with this mode of treatment include risk of infection, which is normally associated with any type of surgery, and malfunction or deterioration of the equipment, which may require subsequent surgery.

Vascular surgery. The American Urological Association considers surgical means to restore blood flow to the penis experimental. Procedures to reroute blood flow around blockages in arteries have not generally been successful. Surgery to repair leaky veins has also only presented a temporary solution.

Other treatments. In some cases, therapy for erectile dysfunction involves raising a man's sex drive. Two options for increasing libido are testosterone supplements and yohimbine extract.

A deficiency in testosterone, although rare, may cause impotence by lowering sex drive in men with diabetes. Low levels of testosterone in the bloodstream can be detected by a blood test. The treatment for testosterone deficiency is an injection of testosterone every one or two weeks or the application of a testosterone patch to the scrotum or other hairless area of skin every day. The side effects of testosterone treatment include prostate growth and an excess of red blood cells, which, in rare cases, can lead to stroke in some individuals. People with diabetes may also need to monitor blood glucose levels more carefully, as hormones such as testosterone may lower blood glucose levels and affect insulin requirements.

Yohimbine, the second option mentioned above, is a natural substance derived from the bark of the yohimbe tree that has traditionally been used as an aphrodisiac. Some doctors prescribe the drug when they suspect psychological problems are the cause of erection difficulties. The drug appears to increase the blood supply to the penis. Although it is relatively well tolerated and relatively inexpensive, its effectiveness is equal to a placebo or sugar pill for the treatment of erectile dysfunction. The response of men with erectile dysfunction to yohimbine is at best marginal.

Talk therapy. At any stage of sexual difficulty, men with erectile dysfunction may benefit from counseling from a trained therapist. Psychological stress or anxiety about physical failure can worsen the problem. A psychiatrist, sex therapist, or social worker may be able to help couples resolve interpersonal issues contributing to a man's impotence.

On the horizon

At this time, several drugs are under investigation as treatments for impotence in the United States. Apomorphine, an oral drug that causes a signal in the brain to trigger an erection, is currently being tested. Phentolamine, which is already used in combination with alprostadil or papaverine in penile injections, is under review by the FDA as an oral drug (to be marketed as Vasomax) for impotence. It is believed to work by blocking the chemical adrenaline, causing relaxation of smooth muscles and dilation of arteries in the corporal bodies. The alpha blocker prazosin (to be marketed as Alibra) has also been tested in combination with alprostadil, but it, too, has not yet received FDA approval.

Working together

For many, it remains a difficult subject to discuss, but impotence no longer has to be considered the tragedy that puts an end to sexual intimacy. The multitude of options now available for treating the physical causes of impotence raises the hope that at least one will work well for every man. Finding the most effective one for each man involves assessing the cause of impotence, considering both partners' preferences, and being willing to put up with some trial and error.

While some men prefer to seek help alone, without their partner's input or even knowledge, most doctors believe that a man's chances of overcoming impotence are greater when he works together with his partner. As Henry and Cynthia learned, seeing the doctor together, choosing an impotence treatment that appealed to both of them, and communicating openly about their feelings helped them feel they were working as a team. After all, a medical treatment for impotence is only one part of rebuilding a sexual relationship. Demonstrating love and affection for one another and letting your partner know you still care can help both of you through the rough times and can help buffer the emotional impact of impotence. ❏

WHEN DIABETES AFFECTS THE STOMACH

by Virginia Valentine, R.N., M.S.N., C.D.E.

Y ou have probably heard of nerve damage, or neuropathy, that affects the feet and legs. Did you know that there is also a form of neuropathy that affects the stomach and intestines? Called *gastropathy*, it comprises all the conditions caused by slow emptying of the stomach. These problems have been referred to as *gastroparesis* in the past, but now the term gastroparesis is reserved for the condition when the stomach is severely affected and is very slow to empty solid foods. Such complications affecting the gastrointestinal tract are far more common than most people with diabetes and their health-care providers realize.

Symptoms of gastropathy

Symptoms that a person might experience with delayed stomach emptying include constipation, abdominal pain, nausea and vomiting, and diarrhea. In some studies of people with diabetes, only 24% of respondents reported no gastrointestinal symptoms.

Despite the high incidence of gastropathy, however, it is very common for people with diabetes who are experiencing its symptoms not to complain of them to their doctor or diabetes team. Often, they don't realize that these problems could be related to their diabetes. But as many as 30% of people with Type 2

TESTS FOR EVALUATING THE STOMACH

If you are experiencing symptoms of slowed stomach emptying, your doctor may advise you to have one of the following tests done. All require fasting overnight before the test. To avoid hypoglycemia during the test, people who use insulin should take half of their morning insulin dose before the test.

TEST NAME AND PURPOSE	HOW IT'S DONE	PREPARING FOR THE TEST	PROS AND CONS
Endoscopy. Looks at the lining of the gastrointestinal tract to see if ulcers or other abnormalities are present.	A tube is inserted through the mouth to view the lining of the esophagus, stomach, and top 10 inches or so of the small intestine. The test causes minimal discomfort; it may take less than an hour. Some people have a sore throat afterward.	Requires fasting overnight. Prior to the test, the person is given a drug to relax.	This test is expensive, but it informs the medical team whether there are any changes in the lining of the gastrointestinal tract.
Upper gastrointestinal (GI) series. Evaluates the structure of the esophagus, stomach, and top section of the small intestine. Areas of abnormal muscle tone show up as pouches or narrowed areas.	The person drinks a substance that shows up as opaque on x-rays, which are taken every few minutes to watch the progress of the fluid as it works its way through the gastrointestinal tract. It takes several hours.	Requires fasting overnight, and then drinking a substance that is similar in texture to Maalox.	Not very expensive. A drawback is that it may take several days to rid the body of the substance.
Gastric emptying (gastric scintigraphy). Measures how soon food leaves the stomach.	The person eats a small meal (usually scrambled eggs) that has a small amount of a radioactive substance added, which can be measured from outside the body. The amount of food leaving the stomach is tracked over several hours.	Requires fasting overnight, then eating a small meal.	Expensive and not available in all areas. It involves a small amount of radiation exposure. Having an elevated blood glucose level, over 200 mg/dl, or a very low level at the time of the test affects the gastric emptying rate. The test results may be normal in symptomatic people.
Electrogastrography (EGG). Measures the electrical activity of the stomach wall muscle.	Electrodes are placed on the skin over the stomach.	Requires fasting overnight and remaining very still during the test.	Can be difficult to interpret, but may do a good job of measuring a mismatch between contractions in the stomach and top section of the small intestine. The procedure is painless.

diabetes and up to 40% to 50% of people with long-standing Type 1 diabetes have delayed emptying of solids from the stomach.

Normal digestive function

To understand gastropathy, it is useful to review normal functioning of the stomach.

The stomach is just one part of the digestive tract—a long and complex tube that begins with the mouth and ends...at the other end. This tube is surrounded by muscle and nerves to move food from the mouth to the stomach, and then through the small bowel and colon to the anus. The function of the esophagus is to move food from the mouth, where it is chewed into small pieces, to the stomach. The stomach breaks food into tiny particles and mixes them into *chyme*, a blend of nutrients and stomach juices that is then emptied into the small intestine, where the nutrients are absorbed for use by the body. Finally, the colon assists in the absorption of water and moves waste out of the body.

The process of digesting and absorbing the nutrients from food is a complex process that requires healthy function of both muscles and nerves in the gastrointestinal tract. The branching nerve that supplies the stomach and controls the passage of food through the digestive tract is called the *vagus nerve*.

What causes gastropathy?

Complications of the stomach in people with diabetes are thought to be caused by *autonomic* neuropathy. This is neuropathy that affects the nerves that govern the functions of the body that are automatic, not those nerves that are under your voluntary control. Autonomic functions include breathing, heart rate, the functioning of the gastrointestinal tract, and other internal functions.

The cause of diabetic neuropathy, whether it affects the stomach or the feet, is high blood sugar. When stomach nerves and muscles are affected by neuropathy, the stomach cannot push food through the system in the normal rhythmic waves (called *peristalsis*). There may also be a loss of coordination between the motion of the stomach and the opening at the end of the stomach (the *pylorus*), which allows the digested food into the small intestine.

Self-evaluation for gastropathy

The first sign of a problem with slow emptying of the stomach may be erratic blood sugar levels. If food doesn't leave the stomach and get absorbed as blood glucose, there may be a mismatch in timing between your insulin or oral diabetes medicine and your blood sugar level following meals. Moreover, your diabetes medicines may not get fully absorbed and therefore not reach effective levels when the stomach is not working. If you have low blood sugar after meals, or if your blood sugar is fluctuating for unknown reasons, these may be signs of gastropathy.

Another way to decide whether you might have gastropathy is to review your symptoms. For example, you might ask yourself the following questions:
- Has my appetite changed?
- Do I feel full after eating a small amount?
- Do I feel bloated after eating?
- Do I feel nauseated after meals or in the morning?
- Am I having unexplained vomiting of undigested food?
- Am I having stomach cramping or pain?
- Am I having diarrhea or constipation?
- Have I gained or lost weight recently?

Diagnosis and treatment

If you suspect that you are having delayed stomach emptying, you should discuss it with your doctor and diabetes-care team. Gastropathy is not always easy to diagnose. This is because some people with delayed stomach emptying may not have any symptoms, while others with symptoms may not show delayed stomach emptying in diagnostic tests. Nonetheless, your doctor may recommend any of several diagnostic tests (see "Tests for Evaluating the Stomach" on page 202), or he may start you on a drug to help the stomach work better to see if that eases any symptoms you may have.

There are a number of drugs, called *prokinetic* drugs, that can help your stomach work better. "Prokinetic" means they stimulate the muscular waves to move food through the stomach. Some of these drugs may also reduce nausea. Drugs used to help people with gastropathy include the following:

Metoclopramide (brand name Reglan) increases stomach muscle contractions to promote gastric emptying, and it also helps resolve nausea. Some people have side effects such as drowsiness, tremors, other involuntary physical movements, and breast tenderness.

Domperidone (Motilium) improves nausea and gastric emptying without the side effects of Reglan, but it is not commercially available in the United States. It seems to be well tolerated with few side effects.

Erythromycin is an antibiotic that also improves stomach emptying. Its possible side effects include nausea, vomiting, and abdominal cramps.

Cisapride (Propulsid) improves gastric emptying and has been used for treatment of gastropathy. However, it was withdrawn from pharmacies because it was found to cause fatal heart rhythm abnormalities in people with heart disease or those taking certain other drugs. Cisapride remains available in the United States to a limited number of people for whom other drug treatment has failed.

DIETARY ADVICE FOR PEOPLE WITH GASTROPATHY

For most people, a healthful diet includes lots of fruits, vegetables, and whole grains. When you have delayed stomach emptying, however, these high-fiber foods can aggravate gastropathy, as can high-fat foods, hence the advice to avoid the foods in the left column and substitute those in the right column. It is also wise to work with a dietitian to make sure you are getting all the nutrients you need in your meal plan.

AVOID THESE	SUBSTITUTE THESE
High-fat meats	Low-fat meats, chicken without the skin, fish, eggs
Most vegetables	Tomato or vegetable juice, well-cooked carrots, mushrooms, strained baby vegetables
Most fruits	Canned peaches, strained baby fruits, fruit juices, applesauce, bananas
Potatoes with skins	Mashed potatoes, rice, pasta, baked French fries
Whole grain breads	White bread (including French or Italian bread), English muffins, flour tortillas, crackers, pancakes, waffles, cereals (such as Cream of Wheat, grits, quick oats, Cheerios, Cocoa Krispies, Froot Loops, Kix, puffed wheat, Rice Krispies, Special K), puddings, gelatin, angel food cake, graham crackers, plain sherbet, sorbet, vanilla wafers

Dietary and lifestyle guidelines

Most people with gastropathy find that they have less trouble with the condition when following these dietary and lifestyle guidelines:
■ Eating a low-fat diet (fat slows down the process of gastric emptying)
■ Eating a low-fiber diet (indigestible fiber and skins from vegetables can collect in the stomach and form a ball called a *bezoar*)
■ Eating small, frequent meals
■ Switching to liquids when having difficulty with gastric emptying (see section below)
■ Stopping smoking

Some types of food to avoid and possible substitutes are listed in "Dietary Advice for People With Gastropathy" on this page. Keeping blood sugar within the near-normal range is also very important to protect autonomic nerves from further damage.

Further adjustments and fine-tuning

People with gastropathy often notice that their stomach function is very different from day to day. Some days, everything is working fine, but on other days, they can't seem to eat anything. At such times, they will have to switch to liquids. Most people with gastropathy notice that they have difficulty with solid food but can tolerate liquids just fine. Some examples of liquids or soft foods that might be better tolerated include Jell-O (regular or sugar-free), yogurt, fruit juices, broth or clear soups, and liquid nutritional supplements.

If you have gastropathy, you should add more starches and even sugar to your diet for adequate caloric intake as well as for flavor and variety. These foods are generally well tolerated by the stomach and can be eaten if your diabetes medicines are adjusted to cover them.

A "basal–bolus" insulin regimen is often required to achieve blood glucose control. This regimen allows people to cover foods with short-acting insulin such as lispro (which may be taken after the meal so that the insulin peak matches the glucose rise), and have the flexibility of basal, or background, insulin coverage. That way, they can skip a meal and let their stomach rest without developing high or low blood sugar. Basal insulins include Ultralente human insulin, NPH, and Lente human insulin. NPH should be given in a small dose in the morning so that it has very little peak. Lunch can then be covered with rapid- or short-acting insulin.

A new, long-acting insulin analog, called insulin glargine (Lantus), was approved by the U.S. Food and Drug Administration in April 2000 and represents another option for a basal–bolus regimen. Glargine works in the body for 24 hours, so it can be injected once a day. Additionally, it has almost no peak, which means that the risk of hypoglycemia is lower. Glargine is approved for use by people with either Type 1 diabetes or Type 2 diabetes.

Regaining predictability and control

The key to understanding how well your medicines and food are working together is, of course, to check blood glucose frequently. Many people find that checking at least four times a day, and sometimes as many as six or eight times a day, is essential for adjusting their food and medicine to get good control. This system provides better quality of life because you regain control and predictability of your diabetes. It is important to learn how to cover carbohydrates with insulin and to take the right amount of insulin so you will be able to "correct" high blood glucose when not eating. Work with a dietitian who is knowledgeable about diabetes, and allow your diabetes-care team to assist you with achieving good diabetes control and a diet that works for you.

Gastropathy is a Catch-22 in that delayed stomach emptying can make blood sugar control more difficult, and high blood sugar can slow stomach emptying. Gastropathy is therefore a problem that requires commitment and effort by the person experiencing it and by his or her health-care team. ❏

LIVING WITH KIDNEY DISEASE

by J. Shawn Faulk, M.S., R.D., C.D.E.,
and Tina Kress, R.N., B.S.N., C.C.T.C., C.P.T.C.

Diabetes means a lifetime of challenges, and some challenges that may grow increasingly formidable over the years. We begin with the daily disciplinary demands: testing blood sugar levels, following meal plans, taking insulin or drugs, and exercising regularly. In time, 30% of those with diabetes will also face long-term complications and their associated challenges.

Among those complications is *diabetic nephropathy*, or diabetic kidney disease, the leading cause of kidney failure in the United States. Diabetic nephropathy occurs in up to a third of those with Type 1 diabetes or Type 2 diabetes, but it develops to kidney failure in a much larger percentage of Type 1 patients than Type 2 patients. It increases the risk of death ninefold, but prevention, detection, and treatment continue to offer more effective ways to decrease its toll of illness and death.

In coping with any aspect of diabetes, acquiring knowledge is the first step. Knowledge offers empowerment. One of the authors of this article, Shawn Faulk, has diabetes, but most of her knowledge was acquired after her diagnosis of kidney failure, when it was too late for preventive measures. It doesn't have to be that way. Learning about diabetic kidney disease and its prevention and treatment will help provide the tools for successfully coping and living with its challenges. We hope this article helps in that process.

What follows is a description of living with kidney disease from both a professional and a personal perspective.

Stages

The kidneys normally filter waste products, water, and chemicals from the blood, send the filtered material to the bladder as urine, and return the cleansed blood to the bloodstream. Nephropathy progressively damages their ability to carry out these tasks and may lead to a life-threatening condition called end-stage renal (kidney) disease (ESRD). Researchers have described five stages in the progression to ESRD in people who have diabetes. Because the early stages are so insidious (symptoms do not occur until it is well advanced), people with diabetes need a self-care protocol that includes taking steps to ensure early detection, and they need to understand the stages of progression and the options available once a diagnosis is made.
STAGE 1:
Hyperfiltration. At this stage, above-normal amounts of blood flow through the kidneys and, thus, through the nephrons, the filtering units of the kidney. Blood levels of creatinine and the nitrogen in urea (blood urea nitrogen, or BUN), waste products commonly measured to assess kidney function, may fall to below normal levels during this stage. Although filters are overworked, hyperfiltration alone will not lead to kidney failure. No real physical damage can be detected, and blood sugar control can halt further progression. Some people stay in Stage 1 indefinitely; in others, the disease advances to Stage 2 after many years.
STAGE 2:
Microalbuminuria. Years of hyperfiltration may eventually lead to the leaking of tiny amounts of protein

into the urine. In a healthy kidney, waste products such as urea are filtered out of the blood, while red blood cells and protein too large to pass through the filters remain in the blood, where they belong. Once damage has occurred, however, minute amounts of protein called *albumin* can be detected in the urine; this is called *microalbuminuria*. Often, a mild but significant rise in blood pressure also occurs. Testing for microalbuminuria should be part of your annual checkup. A routine urinalysis will not detect such small amounts of protein. A special lab test must be used. Stage 2 can last for many years, and detection can help prevent development into the more serious stages.

STAGE 3:

Overt diabetic nephropathy. At this stage, protein leakage has increased to the point where it can be found with routine urinalysis, even though creatinine and BUN levels may remain within normal limits or show slight increases. Because so much protein is being lost in the urine, levels of blood protein fall. Blood proteins help to keep body fluids in the circulatory system. When levels fall, fluid leaks out of the blood vessels and accumulates in tissue, most typically in the ankles because of the effects of gravity. This type of swelling is called *edema*.

Stage 3 is usually seen after 15 to 17 years of Type 1 diabetes. In Type 2 diabetes, it is often detected sooner after diagnosis. This is probably because Type 2 diabetes is often not diagnosed until well after its onset, and by the time the diagnosis has been made, kidney damage could already have occurred. People with Type 2 diabetes may linger in Stage 3 much longer than people with Type 1 diabetes. It is highly unlikely that this stage would be missed with regular visits to your health-care team.

STAGE 4:

Advanced clinical nephropathy. In Stage 4, the kidney has lost most of its ability to remove the blood's waste products. Creatinine and BUN levels rise, and these and other toxins begin to accumulate in the blood. In addition, because a normal kidney aids the bone marrow in its production of red blood cells, advanced nephropathy leads to a low red blood cell count, or anemia, with accompanying fatigue.

STAGE 5:

End-stage renal disease. At this stage, the kidneys no longer have the ability to filter, and a toxic condition called *uremia* occurs. Symptoms of uremia (the accumulation of toxins in the bloodstream) include nausea, vomiting, weakness, fatigue, loss of sleep, difficulty concentrating, and fluid weight gain with obvious edema.

Sustaining life with ESRD requires dialysis or transplantation.

Prevention

Measures to prevent diabetic nephropathy or to slow its progression are most effective from the onset of diabetes to Stage 3, but tools of prevention can also be effective in slowing the progression of Stages 4 and 5. These tools include tight blood sugar control, early detection, blood pressure control, ACE inhibitors, and a low-protein diet.

Blood sugar control. The value of tight blood sugar control cannot be underestimated. Hyperfiltration and nephron destruction are directly linked to high blood sugar. The results of the Diabetes Control and Complications Trial, published in 1993, showed that intensive blood sugar control can reduce the incidence of microalbuminuria and slow the progression of kidney disease in those with Type 1 diabetes, and there is evidence that this is also true for Type 2 diabetes. Consistent glycosylated hemoglobin (HbA_{1c}) test results of less than 8% (levels for people who don't have diabetes are 4% to 6%) substantially reduce the risk for microalbuminuria.

Early detection. If signs of kidney disease are detected early, aggressive action can be initiated at stages that might otherwise be ignored. Screening for microalbuminuria should begin by at least the fifth year after diagnosis of Type 1 diabetes and be done annually thereafter. Screening should be done upon diagnosis of Type 2 diabetes. If microalbuminuria is present, a 24-hour urine test for total protein and creatinine clearance usually follows. The amount of protein in the urine will indicate the severity of the damage to the kidneys; the amount of creatinine is a good estimator of how well the kidney filters are working.

Blood pressure control. Normalization of blood pressure can delay the progression of kidney disease considerably. People who have high blood pressure are more likely to develop kidney disease, and high blood pressure is two to three times more common in people with diabetes than in the general population. To complicate matters, damage to the kidneys from kidney disease makes high blood pressure worse, which causes more kidney damage, and so on.

High blood pressure should be treated aggressively, with a goal of blood pressure less than 130/80 mm Hg for persons with adequate kidney function and less than 120/80 mm Hg for persons with compromised kidney function. Blood pressure medicines, a low-salt diet, and weight loss will help to control blood pressure. Tobacco and alcohol, both of which tend to raise blood pressure, should be avoided.

ACE inhibitors. The class of blood pressure drugs known as ACE inhibitors (angiotensin-converting enzyme inhibitors) may help slow kidney disease both in people who have high blood pressure and people who do not. ACE inhibitors protect against the deterioration of kidney function in diabetic nephropathy by reducing both hyperfiltration and the constriction of the blood vessels in the kidney. Constriction decreases the kidneys' waste-filtering capabilities. Where some of these filtering capabilities have already been lost, ACE inhibitors can partially reverse the damage or prevent more damage, even in people with normal blood pressure. They should be considered a first-line therapy in the presence of microalbuminuria.

Low-protein diet. Another line of defense is the low-protein diet. It is well documented that high protein intake increases the workload of the kidneys and may contribute significantly to the progression of diabetic kidney disease. Since the protein intake of many Americans can be four times the recommended daily amount, adherence to a low-protein diet can be very difficult. Protein allowances can be as low as the equivalent of one whole chicken breast spread over the day. Starch and vegetable proteins appear to be more beneficial than animal proteins in the treatment of nephropathy. People at any stage of diabetic kidney disease should meet with a registered dietitian to design a meal plan tolerable to the individual.

Treatment

When people with diabetic kidney disease develop ESRD, they must undergo either dialysis or transplantation. People can be sustained on dialysis indefinitely; however, it can be physically, mentally, and emotionally debilitating, and it is generally hoped that dialysis will serve as a bridge to transplantation.

Dialysis

Dialysis removes from the blood the waste products and extra fluid that have accumulated there because the kidneys are not working properly, or at all. There are two main types of dialysis, *hemodialysis* and *peritoneal dialysis,* and which of the two is chosen depends partly on the physician's recommendations and partly on the recipient's wishes.

Hemodialysis. In hemodialysis, blood is pumped through a needle inserted into a surgically enlarged vein (usually in the arm) to an artificial kidney machine outside the body. In the machine, the blood flows over an artificial membrane that acts as a filter and cleanses it. The cleansed blood is then returned, via another needle, to the same enlarged vein. Most people receive three treatments per week lasting three to four hours each at a local dialysis unit. Some people choose to do hemodialysis in their home, in which case a caregiver or household member must be trained to perform the treatment. People often choose hemodialysis when they prefer to have someone else responsible for their direct dialysis care.

Some people on hemodialysis complain of feeling very fatigued after treatment, then better for part of the next day, and then worse again as toxins begin to accumulate in the blood. Other disadvantages of hemodialysis are the required travel to and from the dialysis center, a fixed treatment schedule, two needle sticks for each treatment, and a restrictive diet.

Although food choices for people with diabetes have become more flexible in recent years, food choices for a person with ESRD are limited. Six factors are considered: calories, fluid, protein, potassium, phosphorus, and sodium. Once dialysis has begun, calorie and protein needs increase. Fluid and sodium are restricted to prevent excess fluid retention and congestive heart failure. Potassium and phosphorus are not filtered adequately by hemodialysis, and foods containing them must be limited to avoid serious health consequences.

Peritoneal dialysis. This form of dialysis uses your *peritoneal membrane* (the lining of your abdomen) as the filter. A tube called a catheter is surgically placed through the wall of your abdomen to allow passage of a special dialysis solution into the peritoneal cavity. Over several hours, the solution, called *dialysate,* draws waste products and excess fluids out of the bloodstream, and the used dialysate is then drained out through the catheter and discarded.

The two most common methods of peritoneal dialysis are continuous ambulatory peritoneal dialysis (CAPD) and continuous cycling peritoneal dialysis (CCPD), both of which are done at home. In CAPD, a bag attached to the catheter feeds dialysate into the peritoneal cavity. Several hours later, the dialysate is drained back into the bag and discarded, and the process begins again, with a fresh bag, three or more times that day. This is all done manually by the person undergoing treatment, who can schedule normal activities around the dialysate exchange sessions. In CCPD, the catheter is connected to a machine at night, and the machine does three or more exchanges automatically while the person sleeps. The catheter is disconnected in the morning, with a fresh batch of dialysate left in the peritoneal cavity all day until the person reconnects to the CCPD machine that evening. This method is generally chosen by people with a demanding day schedule.

Advantages to peritoneal dialysis include more freedom, a less restricted diet (diet is still important, but since peritoneal dialysis is performed daily, guidelines are not as restrictive), no needles, and a more steady physical condition. Peritoneal dialysis does require self-motivation, however, and storage space for supplies. There is an increased risk of infection because of the external catheter, and many people are uncomfortable with the distended belly caused by two liters of solution in the abdomen. And because the dialysis solution contains dextrose, people with diabetes may have more difficulty controlling blood sugar levels and weight. Those with vision problems will need to assess whether they have adequate vision to perform exchanges, but assistive devices are available.

During her time on dialysis, Shawn Faulk chose peritoneal primarily for the freedom it offered in schedule and diet. Also, she feared that the hours required in a hemodialysis unit would keep her too focused on her condition. But other people consider their unit a reliable support system and enjoy the social interaction with ESRD peers. Peritoneal worked for Shawn because she had family support and adequate vision.

Transplantation

Transplantation provides the best potential quality of life for people with diabetes and kidney failure and is the recommended course of treatment. A kidney transplant offers release from the rigors of the dialysis regimen and the diet restrictions associated with it and from the complications associated with both kidney disease and dialysis. Consequently, kidney transplant recipients experience not only improved energy levels and blood sugar control, but also an improved sense of mental, emotional, and physical well-being. One-year graft survival rates are at an all-time high: 89% for cadaver donor kidneys, or kidneys from someone who recently died, 94% for living donor kidneys, and 70% to 90% for a kidney and a pancreas transplanted at the same time. (Note: These are the survival rates of the transplanted organs themselves, not the recipients of the organs. The recipient survival rates are even higher.)

The surgical procedure is relatively simple, hospital stays are often less than a week, and physical and mental status improve rapidly. Unfortunately, the number of donors is far less than the number of people needing a new kidney, and the wait can be as long as three years, or even more.

In living donation, a kidney is donated by either a relative or a nonrelated person. Although it is sometimes easier to find a good match within the family, *immunosuppressive drugs* have become so effective that donation from an unrelated person has a high degree of success. These drugs suppress the immune system so it won't identify the new organ as an invader and reject it; the drugs must be taken indefinitely.

The biggest advantage to living donation is reducing the wait for a new organ; some people are able to skip dialysis entirely. Potential donors are evaluated to make sure the surgery will not compromise their future health in any way. Donors live perfectly normal lives with their one remaining kidney.

The only way for people with Type 1 diabetes to achieve consistently "perfect" blood sugar control is with the successful transplant of a pancreas that will produce the insulin their own pancreas cannot. (Pancreas transplants will not work for people with Type 2 diabetes because their bodies can't respond properly to insulin.) Simultaneous kidney/pancreas transplants have become increasingly common with improved procedures and success rates. Usually the pancreas and kidney are transplanted from a single cadaver donor, although a couple of transplant centers in the country will transplant part of a pancreas from a living related donor.

A successful pancreas transplant brings independence from insulin injections. But it has associated costs: a suppressed immune system and the side effects of the drugs used to maintain that suppression, both of which are discussed below. Therefore, most pancreas transplants have traditionally been done for people with long-standing diabetes who already need a kidney transplant. Those who are unable to detect life-threatening low blood sugar levels or who experience other advanced diabetes complications may be eligible for a pancreas transplant alone.

Tradeoffs for transplantation

The life of a transplant recipient is, of course, not problem-free. A kidney transplant alone does not cure diabetes or eliminate the possibility of more diabetes complications, and adjusting to the transplant is a challenge in itself. But the highest costs of transplantation (literally and figuratively) have to do with the immunosuppressive drugs necessary to keep the body from attacking the new organ. A suppressed immune system cannot play its usual role of defending the body against illness and infections, meaning that it is easier to get sick; infection is a particular problem for people who take immunosuppressive drugs.

There are also the side effects and expense of the drugs. Individual experiences vary, but common side effects are weight gain, hair growth, mood swings, acne, and shaky hands. The degree to which these side effects are experienced is individual and dose-related. That means that side effects are greatest shortly after transplant when drug doses are high, but gradually subside as the doses are lowered. Some recipients see increased cholesterol levels and blood pressure. A smaller percentage experience weakened bones (severe cases may require a hip replacement) from long-term use of corticosteroids, one type of immunosuppressant.

An ongoing issue for recipients of any organ type is the cost of immunosuppressant drugs, which can run as high as $20,000 a year. Lifetime insurance coverage of some kind is a necessity. Under a 1973 law,

Medicare covers kidney transplants for ESRD patients. Medicare generally also covers 80% of transplantation-related drug costs for the first three years after a kidney transplant; coverage for those 65 or older was extended to 44 months in 1999 and to the life of the transplant in 2000 (the changes in coverage also applied to other transplant recipients whose transplant was paid for by Medicare and who either met the age criterion or qualified for disability under Medicare). Transplant recipients who do not qualify for Medicare coverage based on age or disability, or who are not covered through their employee health plans, may be forced to stay at the poverty level to qualify for Medicaid or some type of medical assistance program. Such recipients need to use all of their patient advocacy skills to maintain diligent and comprehensive health care.

Faulk received a donated kidney from her sister after four months of dialysis, and her drug costs were covered by Medicare for one year (Medicare coverage was later expanded to three years). When her Medicare coverage ended, she was allowed 18 months grace under a work experience program that allowed her to test her ability for long-term employment. At that time, the Americans With Disabilities Act was not in force, and she was denied health insurance through her employer. Creative networking and assistance programs offered by pharmaceutical companies filled her medicine needs until she could obtain coverage, but the experience created high levels of stress and the fear of losing her sources.

In spite of the tradeoffs, testimonies for quality of life following transplantation are abundant. Talks with dozens of transplant recipients yield a theme that is almost universal: "I feel productive and energetic again," "Now I feel like I really have a future," "I've been given a second chance at life."

Before and after stories are dramatic. Before Faulk's transplant, she didn't have the energy to walk around the block, she experienced the frequent pain and vomiting of advanced *gastroparesis,* in which the stomach loses its ability to empty normally, and she was often found unconscious from undetected low blood sugar levels. (When kidneys are unable to do their usual job of filtering, insulin levels are unpredictable.) With the exceptional pretransplant and posttransplant support and care of the Sharp Memorial Transplant Team in San Diego, her life became more productive and fulfilling than ever before. Since her transplant almost eight years ago, she has been able to complete her master's degree, pursue her career as a registered dietitian and diabetes educator, go to aerobics class four to five times per week, and devote volunteer hours to helping, she hopes, to improve the quality of life for others with chronic disease.

SUPPORT ORGANIZATIONS

To find out more about the prevention, detection, and treatment of diabetic kidney disease, call the organizations on this list or pay a visit to their Web sites.

AMERICAN ASSOCIATION OF
KIDNEY PATIENTS
(800) 749-AAKP (749-2257)
www.akp.org

AMERICAN DIABETES ASSOCIATION
(800) DIABETES (342-2383)
www.diabetes.org

INSULIN-FREE WORLD FOUNDATION
(888) RING-IFW (746-4439)
www.insulin-free.org

NATIONAL KIDNEY FOUNDATION
(800) 622-9010
www.kidney.org

Coping with ESRD

There are many different ways of coping, and no single method is the best for everyone. In general, though, it helps to start by acknowledging the grief and loss of a failed organ. Shock, denial, bargaining, and anger are all natural reactions that we have to work through. Depression is rampant among people with ESRD, and if feelings of anger or hopelessness develop to such an extreme level that they interfere with physical, mental, or emotional health, then it is time to seek professional help.

For most, a support network is essential. People with ESRD find support from family members, friends, dialysis and transplant social workers, and, most important, ESRD peers. Peer fellowship is so valuable that the San Diego Transplant Association, with which both authors are allied, has developed a Transplant Mentor Program. Through referral, the association is able to match anyone with organ failure, either before or after transplantation, with someone who has already had the experience of going through the transplant process.

Another powerful coping skill is "giving back." Almost everyone with organ failure is passionate about supporting transplantation, the "gift of life." Ways to give back include mentoring others with organ failure, volunteering at dialysis units and transplant centers, participating in organizations like the

San Diego Transplant Association and the National Kidney Foundation, and helping to educate the general public about organ donation. By sharing your experience, you can truly can help make a difference for someone else.

Going on

As you can see, dealing with diabetic nephropathy is fraught with challenge, but it has its rewards. First, there are now successful treatment options that offer not only the gift of life, but the gift of quality of life. Those faced with organ failure are stimulated to rec-

ognize what is important in their lives and the lives of those around them, and they learn to refocus their energies in those directions. In the process, they meet dozens of others who have similar priorities, people who have learned to live in the moment, appreciate simple pleasures, and are grateful for each day. And they are given special gifts, including understanding and compassion, that offer personal fulfillment and add some sense of purpose to their struggles. People in the transplant community have a unique perspective on life. They are thankful to have been given a second chance. ❑

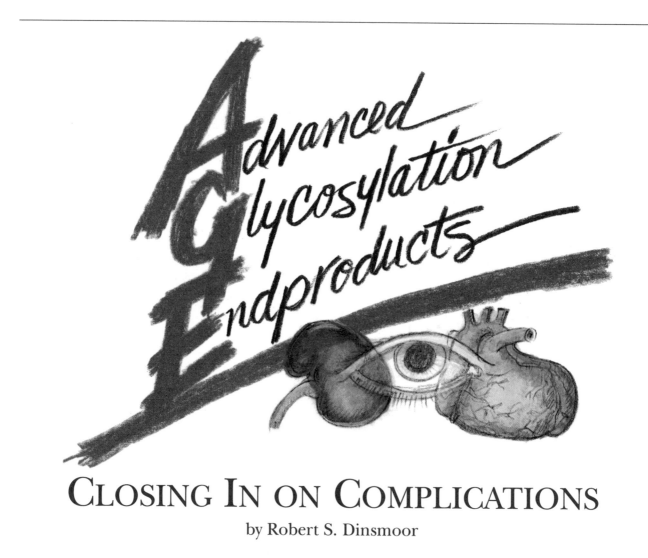

CLOSING IN ON COMPLICATIONS

by Robert S. Dinsmoor

Scientists know a lot about diabetes, but one of the mysteries that remains is how high blood glucose levels lead to diabetic complications. Now some researchers think they are getting closer to finally coming up with an answer to this question, and at least part of the answer seems to involve AGE's.

AGE's (advanced glycosylation endproducts) are substances created as a result of blood glucose binding to the body's proteins. They accumulate in everyone over time, gradually altering the body's tissues. However, in people with diabetes, AGE's accumulate much more quickly and are thought to play a key role in the development of diabetic complications. AGE's have also been found to be more abundant in people who smoke.

Some scientists believe they may be able to slow and perhaps even reverse diabetic complications using drugs that inhibit the formation and accumulation of AGE's. They have even begun conducting clinical trials of such drugs. For example, the drug pimagidine (aminoguanidine) has been tested in people with diabetes who have kidney disease.

Diabetic complications

Until insulin became commercially available in 1921, the most common cause of death among people with diabetes was diabetic ketoacidosis. Once insulin became widely available, diabetic ketoacidosis rarely happened, and the main cause of death became heart disease. This is at least in part because diabetes doubles a person's risk of developing heart disease and stroke. Currently, heart disease affects 20% of people with diabetes who are 65 years and older.

One of the main causes of heart disease is atherosclerosis (hardening of the arteries), which is known as a *macrovascular*, or large blood vessel, disease. Some of the complications that can result from macrovascular disease include stroke, peripheral vascular disease (narrowing of the blood vessels in the legs and sometimes arms), and foot ulcers.

People who have had diabetes for many years also run a high risk of developing a number of complications resulting from *microvascular* diseases, or diseases of the small blood vessels. These complications include the following:

■ Diabetic kidney disease, which affects 40% of people with diabetes and can, in some cases, lead to complete kidney failure.
■ Diabetic retinopathy or retinal disease, which affects 50% of people with diabetes 10 years after diagnosis and 80% of people with diabetes 15 years after diagnosis. In its most advanced form, it can cause blindness.
■ Diabetic neuropathy or nerve disease, which can cause pain or numbness in the extremities and impair the function of many internal organs. Some 60% to 70% of people with diabetes are believed to have at least some degree of neuropathy.
■ Cataract, or clouding of the lens of the eye, which occurs more commonly and at a younger age in people with diabetes.

What causes complications?

In the beginning, scientists did not know what caused these complications to occur in people with diabetes. Some speculated that they were caused by higher than normal levels of glucose in the blood. In the ensuing decades, however, the relationship between high blood glucose levels and diabetic complications remained controversial.

This controversy was finally laid to rest by the landmark Diabetes Control and Complications Trial, or DCCT. This study, the results of which were published in 1993, showed that people with Type 1 diabetes who kept their blood glucose levels relatively close to normal drastically lowered their risk of developing diabetic retinopathy, diabetic nephropathy, and diabetic neuropathy and also improved many of the risk factors for developing heart disease and peripheral vascular disease. Further research showed that these benefits could be extended to people with Type 2 diabetes as well.

However, it has also become clear that blood glucose levels don't tell the whole story about the risk of complications. Scientists have long noted that some people who maintain very good blood glucose control nonetheless develop complications, while others with poor blood glucose control never develop any complications.

Since the 1980's, scientists have come a long way toward discovering how high blood glucose levels lead to diabetic complications. They now know that glucose in the blood binds to proteins in the body in a process called *nonenzymatic glycosylation*. In nonenzymatic glycosylation, glucose and protein interact in a series of chemical reactions. Some of the products of this process break down again as blood glucose levels fall. However, one type of product that does not break down—and that tends to accumulate in the body—is *advanced glycosylation endproducts,* or AGE's. Some researchers believe that a chemical reaction called oxidation may help to create these irreversible AGE's.

AGE's combine with other molecules to form irreversible bonds, called *cross-links,* between proteins. Again, oxidation appears to play a role in helping AGE's form these cross-links. As these cross-links accumulate, they change the nature of the body's cells, tissues, and blood vessels, making them stiff and dysfunctional.

This reaction, which actually changes the color of the body's tissues, has also been called the "browning" reaction and is very similar to what happens when meat turns brown during cooking, bread gets toasted, and coffee beans are roasted. In fact, when you overcook a steak, the reason it gets so tough and hard to cut is the formation of these cross-links. Although this process occurs gradually in all people as they age, it is greatly accelerated in people with diabetes.

Years ago, scientists discovered by accident that people who smoke also have higher levels of AGE's in their bodies' proteins. They soon came to realize that the process of curing tobacco browns it and creates highly reactive sugars that enter the bloodstream through the lungs when a person smokes. In fact, the level of AGE's in a smoker who doesn't have diabetes is similar to that of a nonsmoker with diabetes. And, of course, people with diabetes who smoke have even higher levels. This may account for the higher rate of diabetic complications seen in people with diabetes who smoke.

How AGE's contribute to complications

Scientists are still unraveling all of the ways that AGE's can cause the complications of diabetes.

Macrovascular complications. Atherosclerosis, the root of macrovascular complications, may begin with damage to the *endothelium*, the inner coating of the arteries that has direct contact with the bloodstream. Blood platelets tend to build up on the injured area, forming a substance called plaque. Lipids in the blood, especially so-called "bad" low-density lipoprotein (LDL) cholesterol, also contribute to plaque. If the plaque enlarges enough, it may severely block the passage of blood through the artery.

AGE's contribute to macrovascular complications in at least two basic ways: First of all, they oxidize LDL. Oxidized LDL is picked up by certain white blood cells called macrophages, which then become engorged and turn into "foam cells." These bloated foam cells tend to stick easily to the endothelium. Second, AGE's can cause cross-links to occur in the collagen and other proteins that line the blood vessel walls. Both of these changes set the stage for the subsequent gradual buildup of atherosclerotic plaque on the walls of blood vessels.

Diabetic nephropathy. AGE's may also damage the glomeruli of the kidneys, promoting diabetic nephropathy. Each kidney contains anywhere from 400,000 to 1 million glomeruli, which are tufts of tiny blood vessels called capillaries within the kidneys that filter waste products, chemicals, and water from the blood to produce urine. Within the first two years of developing diabetes, people with diabetes have an increase in the width of the glomerular basement membrane, the surface across which this filtration occurs.

In people who eventually develop advanced nephropathy, the core between the capillaries of the glomeruli, called the *mesangium*, begins to expand, compressing the capillaries. This compression decreases the surface area available for filtration, so the kidneys become less efficient at filtering the products from the blood. At some point, the process becomes self-perpetuating and inevitable, and eventu-

ally the mesangium and the capillaries become a mass of scar tissue. A person in whom this happens will eventually develop end-stage renal disease, requiring dialysis or kidney transplantation.

Exactly how AGE's contribute to diabetic nephropathy is not known. However, when researchers inject AGE-altered proteins into mice, the result is a widening of the basement membrane and expansion of the mesangium, two changes related to the progression of kidney disease. Furthermore, kidney disease itself appears to increase the level of AGE's in the body, which do not seem to be removed by standard dialysis. This not only causes a vicious circle, accelerating kidney disease, but may also explain why people with diabetes with advanced kidney disease also develop atherosclerosis so rapidly.

Researchers are currently working on developing new dialysis techniques, with the goal of removing AGE's during the dialysis process. Some of these techniques have shown promise in early studies.

Diabetic retinopathy. In the earliest stage of diabetic retinopathy, called background retinopathy, AGE's are believed to cause damage to the capillaries in the retina. These damaged capillaries begin to swell up in places (causing *microaneurysms*) and cause "dot and blot" hemorrhages, tiny leaks of fluid into the retina. These fluids can collect and cause the retina to swell. If this swelling occurs in the central part of the retina (the *macula*), the condition is called *macular edema*, which can cause blurry vision.

In the proliferative stage, abnormal new blood vessels grow over the surface of the retina. These new blood vessels may rupture and leak blood into the *vitreous humor*, the clear gel that fills the center of the eye, causing severe vision loss. Sometimes scar tissue forms, which may pull on the retina and cause it to become detached from the back of the eye.

Diabetic neuropathy. Nerves carry electrical impulses throughout the body, much like electrical wire. They are surrounded by a sheath of cells called *Schwann cells*, in a fashion similar to the way insulation coats electrical wire. Diabetic neuropathy occurs when the Schwann cells swell and squeeze the nerves, keeping them from functioning properly. It is not known exactly how AGE's contribute to the process, but it is possible that they may affect the tiny blood vessels that feed the nerves, or they may even alter the Schwann cells directly.

Cataract. Even in people who don't have diabetes, changes take place in the lens of the eye as they age. Lenses that were once clear and colorless become yellow and opaque over time, causing cataracts. Again, this is the result of cross-linking in the tissue of the lens, a process that happens faster in people with diabetes.

Interrupting the process

The DCCT showed conclusively that keeping blood glucose levels near normal can greatly reduce a person's risk of developing diabetic complications. However, tight blood glucose control is difficult to achieve, and some people develop complications in spite of excellent blood glucose control.

Fortunately, research into AGE's is yielding potential ways of preventing or even reversing diabetic complications, both by preventing new cross-links or breaking existing cross-links between proteins. One way to do this may be found in promising new experimental drugs called AGE inhibitors.

One AGE inhibitor that has undergone testing is pimagedine. In animals, pimagedine has been shown to decrease AGE's and to slow the progression of diabetic nephropathy, diabetic retinopathy, and diabetic neuropathy. Meanwhile, scientists have been working on a new generation of AGE inhibitors designed to break existing cross-links. While these results are very preliminary, they do suggest that it may one day be possible not only to prevent, but to reverse, diabetic complications.

Antioxidants may inhibit the formation of AGE's as well. In a study reported in 1991, Italian and Belgian scientists showed that vitamin E inhibited the formation of AGE's. Thirty people with Type 1 diabetes were divided into three groups: One group received no vitamin E, one group took 600 mg (milligrams) of vitamin E each day, and a third group took 1200 mg daily.

When tested after one and two months, there were fewer AGE's in the groups taking vitamin E, and the group taking the larger dose of vitamin E had the fewest AGE's.

Researchers have also shown that vitamin E reduces the oxidation of LDL and decreases the adherence of foam cells, changes that would lower the risk of atherosclerosis and heart disease. In fact, studies have also shown that people with heart disease who take vitamin E have a much lower risk of nonfatal heart attacks. There is also preliminary research in animals that suggests that antioxidants may help slow the progression of diabetic retinopathy as well.

Medical research is slowly unraveling how AGE's form and how they contribute to the development of diabetic complications. Promising new drugs are being developed, but until they are available, people with diabetes must stick with the tools they have for preventing complications. Controlling blood glucose levels has been shown conclusively to lower this risk substantially. In people who smoke, kicking the habit can slow the development of complications. Finally, taking antioxidants such as vitamin E supplements is relatively safe and may also lower the risk of complications.

However, it is always wise to consult your doctor before taking any supplement. Even the relatively nontoxic vitamin E may have side effects when consumed in large amounts; for example, it may cause bleeding problems, especially in individuals taking anticoagulant drugs. ❏

FOOT HEALTH

FOOT SMARTS
Pitfalls and Preservation
by Orna Feldman

You may be planning to jump feet first into a project or put your best foot forward. But if you have diabetes, it's best to take care that your feet don't become your Achilles heel. The fact is that people with diabetes are prone to foot problems. The problems can be serious, leading not only to reduced mobility but also to one of the most feared of complications—amputation.

Although the rate of amputation in the United States has been on the increase, the good news is that half the amputations that occur could be prevented. Experts say that many people with diabetes can avoid serious problems in the first place by taking good care of their feet, in consultation with their doctor or other health-care professional. When limb-threatening infections do occur, amputation does not always have to follow. At Foot Care Specialists at Boston Medical Center, which is renowned for pioneering treatments that protect at-risk lower extremities, doctors have succeeded in dramatically reducing the amputation rate.

In 1980, one-third of their patients admitted with limb-threatening infections underwent amputation. By the late 1990's, only 4% underwent the procedure. Just as good basic foot care may prevent serious problems, catching and treating foot problems early raises the chances of successful treatment.

Diabetes and foot problems

Diabetes poses a special challenge to feet. It can cause arteries in the legs and feet to become hardened and clogged, which prevents blood from circulating properly. Diabetes also can affect the nerve endings in the feet, resulting in a loss of sensation. (Nerve damage as a result of diabetes will be discussed in more detail later.) Diminished feeling in your feet means the appropriate information isn't being sent back to your brain—the alarm system isn't working—making it difficult to take action to remedy any problems.

Diseased arteries. As you get older, your arteries may become diseased in two ways. They may become hard

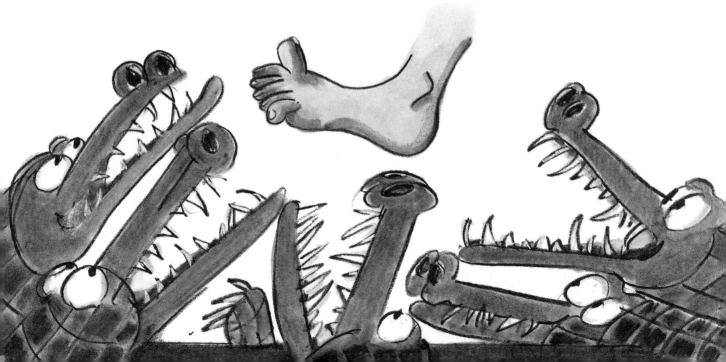

and inflexible. And they may become clogged with plaque—a condition called *atherosclerosis*—narrowing the opening through which blood flows. People with diabetes tend to produce higher-than-normal levels of cholesterol and triglycerides, making them prone to getting clogged arteries earlier than other people. If you're 40 years old and have had diabetes for 10 years, your arteries can be similar in condition to those of a 50-year-old without diabetes.

Diabetes is often accompanied by high blood pressure, which tends to speed the development of vascular problems. Many people with diabetes are also overweight, which boosts cholesterol and triglyceride levels and increases blood pressure. In addition, the arteries of people with diabetes tend to become clogged below the knee more frequently than in other locations.

What is the impact of these conditions on your feet? The effect is that blood circulates poorly in the lower extremities, which slows and impairs the healing process if your foot becomes injured. That's why a seemingly minor infection—starting with a blister on a heel, small cut or scratch, callus, corn, or toenail injury, for example—can spread quickly through the foot and sometimes even into the bone.

To keep problems at bay, it's important to recognize the signs of poor circulation. Look for the telltale signs: dry skin, hair loss on feet, feet that are cold to the touch, redness when your feet are hanging down, paleness when your feet are raised above the level of your heart, and no pulses in your foot.

Another indication of diminished circulation in the lower extremities is *claudication*. Claudication develops when muscles aren't getting enough blood. People with claudication experience pain, cramping, or an odd sensation when walking and have to stop and rest. The pain is most common in the calf but can also occur in the foot, thigh, hip, or buttocks, depending on where blood vessel blockage or narrowing is located and how severe it is. The pain is always relieved with rest. The shorter the distance a person can walk without problems, the more severe the claudication.

A second symptom of claudication is a deep ache when the foot is at rest. Often occurring at night, the pain may make you hang your feet over the side of the bed or stand up to take a walk. If you experience this kind of rest pain, your problem has become severe. Discuss with your doctor the need for a vascular consultation as soon as possible.

If you have any of the signs or symptoms of claudication, your doctor or podiatrist can do tests to evaluate the adequacy of the blood flow through the arteries in your legs. One test involves inflating specially designed blood pressure cuffs that are placed at the thigh, calf, ankle, forefoot, and toe. As the cuffs are deflated, the blood pressure is measured, similar to a blood pressure reading on the arm.

Peripheral neuropathy. Another major complication of diabetes that affects feet is *peripheral neuropathy*. This is the most common form of diabetic neuropathy, or nerve damage caused by chronic high blood sugar. If your sensory nerves are damaged, you will lose feeling in your feet and won't be able to sense temperature changes, pressure, or pain. This may sound ideal, but actually it's a problem, since a cut or wound on your foot won't hurt and may go unnoticed. You may continue walking, which creates additional damage with every step and prevents the wound from healing.

Peripheral neuropathy also can affect motor nerves, which carry commands for movement from the brain to the muscles in your extremities. When motor nerves become severely damaged, some of the muscles may become weak and waste away. This can make it very difficult to walk and balance properly and can lead to foot deformity.

The symptoms of neuropathy can be continual or sporadic. You may lose feeling in your feet, even to the point of numbness. You may also feel shooting pain, tingling, pricking, or burning sensations on your skin. The severity can range from quite mild to excruciating. Another sign of neuropathy is a painless ulcer. The important thing is not to deny the problem but to seek attention right away.

Bringing blood sugar levels under control can sometimes reverse the symptoms of neuropathy. If you have lost sensation in your feet, however, it's important to be aware of what has happened, otherwise you may neglect your feet and an injury could result. Regular foot inspections—every day, if not several times a day—are critical. If you can't inspect your feet yourself, because you're overweight or your eyesight is impaired, for example, ask for help. Things to look out for include dry skin, blisters, cuts, red areas, toenail injuries, warts, or anything out of the ordinary. If you can't bend over to see the bottom of your feet, try placing a hand mirror on the floor so you can see your feet reflected in the mirror.

Caring for your feet

Daily foot inspections are important for everyone with diabetes, not only for those with peripheral neuropathy. The earlier that foot problems are caught, the sooner they can be treated. Besides foot inspections, there are several steps you can take to protect your feet.

Shoes. Proper shoes are critical, since poorly fitting shoes inflict pressure, and thus trauma, on the foot. Dr. Gary Gibbons, a vascular surgeon and executive director of Foot Care Specialists, considers the matter of shoes vital and estimates that amputations would drop by 20% if people with diabetes simply wore proper shoes and changed them twice a day.

The best shoes are supportive and cushioned, such as walking or athletic shoes with soft, breathable uppers, shock-absorbing soles, and support around the heel. Avoid wearing thong sandals, clogs, flip-flops, or pointy shoes, which squeeze the toes. Remember that you should break in new shoes gradually; this helps prevent blisters from forming. (For

HELPING TO HEAL FOOT ULCERS

Foot ulcers are notoriously hard to heal, but help may be on its way. In recent years, several pharmaceutical companies have developed products intended to improve wound healing, particularly healing of ulcers of the feet and legs. These products either require a doctor's prescription or must be applied by a health-care professional. If you have an ulcer that is slow to heal, ask your doctor if one of the following products would be useful for you.

APLIGRAF. A living skin product, Apligraf was approved by the U.S. Food and Drug Administration (FDA) in May 1998 for the treatment of venous leg ulcers and in June 2000 for the treatment of diabetic foot ulcers. Apligraf is developed through tissue technology, contains two types of skin cells, and looks and feels like human skin. When applied to a wound, it facilitates new tissue formation and wound closure. Apligraf must be applied by a doctor in a hospital outpatient facility or a wound-care center. After being placed in position, it is secured by a nonadherent dressing. For venous ulcers, compression bandages are also applied to the area to decrease swelling and promote blood flow to the wound. Within several weeks, the healing site takes on characteristics of the person's own skin—such as skin color.

In clinical studies, Apligraf healed more than twice as many venous ulcers lasting more than one year as standard compression therapy, and it healed them faster. In a large clinical study involving diabetic foot ulcers, more than half of ulcers were fully closed after 12 weeks of treatment with Apligraf, compared to two-fifths of ulcers treated with conventional therapy. The most frequently observed side effect was suspected infection of the wound.

DERMAGRAFT. A bioengineered human skin replacement treatment, Dermagraft was developed to help heal diabetic foot ulcers and prevent their recurrence. It is produced by growing a certain type of human skin cells on miniature scaffolds. The cells secrete structural proteins and growth factors, leading to the formation of human dermal tissue, or the layer of skin called the dermis. This tissue is implanted into ulcers, where it encourages the growth of a healthy dermis, which in turn encourages the regrowth of the epidermis, thus closing the wound.

Dermagraft was approved by the FDA in 1998 as a "treatment investigational device," allowing it to be made available on a special, case-by-case basis at selected medical centers.

FIBRACOL. A wound dressing made of collagen and calcium alginate fibers, Fibracol was approved by the FDA in July 1993 for management of moderately to heavily draining wounds. An improved product, Fibracol Plus, twice as absorbent as its predecessor and featuring 80% more collagen, was introduced in 1999. Collagen, the most abundant protein in the body, gives structure to skin and bone and plays an important role in wound healing. Alginate forms a gel when it comes in contact with fluid from the wound, creating a moist wound environment that encourages healing. In clinical studies, Fibracol wound dressing closed chronic wounds effectively and closed them faster than other wound dressings.

REGRANEX. A topical gel that facilitates the healing of foot ulcers, Regranex was approved by the FDA in December 1997 and is now available by prescription. The active ingredient in Regranex Gel is becaplermin, a genetically engineered growth factor that imitates natural proteins in the body. When applied to a clean ulcer, Regranex causes wound-healing cells to migrate to the ulcer site, encouraging faster tissue growth at the open wound.

In clinical studies, a once-daily application of Regranex Gel combined with good ulcer care healed more diabetic ulcers than placebo gel combined with good ulcer care. In one study, involving 118 people, 48% of those treated with Regranex had complete ulcer closure, compared with 25% of those who received a placebo gel. In another study, involving 382 people, 50% of those treated with Regranex had complete ulcer closure, compared with 35% of those who received a placebo gel.

—*The Editors*

more on choosing shoes, see "Picking the Shoe to Fit the Occasion" on page 224.)

Changing shoes several times a day is also very important, because that way, if a shoe is putting pressure on a particular spot on your foot, it won't be doing it for hours on end. Also, after three or four hours of wear, the cushioning in shoes loses some of its resiliency. This causes the foot to slide inside the shoe, thereby increasing friction, a cause of blistering and skin ruptures. Another advantage to alternating shoes throughout the day is that it gives you more opportunities to inspect your feet.

Paying attention to your socks is also important. Avoid socks that are too tight, since they constrict circulation, and socks with holes or thick seams, since they can irritate your skin and cause sores. Changing into dry socks when those you're wearing become damp is also a good idea. This is especially true if your feet sweat a lot. Sport socks, which often have an extra layer of cushioning in the sole and heel, offer your feet added protection from hard walking surfaces. For people with a history of foot ulcers, wearing a synthetic sock liner is advisable, since it reduces the friction between sock and skin.

Skin care. Since the skin is the body's barrier against infection, any rupture in it calls for immediate attention. This is particularly true if you have diabetes, since poor circulation reduces your body's infection-fighting and healing capabilities. Small cuts can lead to larger wounds, and the goal is to eliminate out-of-control infections that may necessitate amputation.

If you get a cut or scratch, use a mild antiseptic after you wash the affected area. Never use a strong antiseptic, such as iodine, Mercurochrome, boric acid, Epsom salts, creosol, or carbolic acid. Avoid using adhesive bandages (such as Band-Aids) on your feet; the adhesive may tear thin or weakened skin when it is pulled off. Instead, use a dry, sterile dressing, and secure the dressing to itself (not to the skin) with paper tape or a gauze bandage. If the affected area doesn't improve within a couple of days, call your doctor. Also contact your doctor if redness, increased warmth, or a yellowish drainage occurs. Just because it doesn't hurt doesn't mean it shouldn't be seen professionally.

Dry skin poses a risk because it leads to cracks, which can bleed and become infected. The dryness of people's skin varies. If the skin on your feet is not too dry, use a soothing cream or lotion on them once a week. If the skin is quite dry, use cream every day. The best creams for foot care are those containing urea; look for one that has 10% to 25% urea. Put the cream on your heel and work it toward your toes. Don't put cream between your toes; this will over-moisturize the skin in this area, which tends to stay damp anyway, weakening its ability to protect against bacterial infections.

If the skin around your heels is dry and cracking, try putting cream on the area before going to bed. Cover the area with a piece of clear plastic wrap and wear a sock over it during the night. You can repeat this procedure two or three times a week, but don't do it more often unless you have specific instructions from your doctor to do so. Overuse of this type of dressing can lead to skin breakdown. If the dryness is severe and persists, consult your doctor, podiatrist, or dermatologist.

The word on washing your feet is to do it daily, using warm, soapy water. Whatever you do, don't soak your feet, and never use a whirlpool. Soaking dries the skin and makes it more susceptible to cracking and breaks. Also, don't use hot water; the heat helps spread bacteria and can cause burns in people with nerve damage. After you've washed your feet, rinse them well and dry them carefully, especially between the toes, where infections are prone to develop.

Toenail care. If you can care for your toenails yourself, cut them straight across using a toenail clipper. Use an emery board to smooth rough edges. If you have ingrown toenails or if your nails are thick or hard or growing in a distorted manner, go to a podiatrist for help. Ingrown toenails that become infected can become a serious problem if not treated appropriately.

If you have poor circulation or vision, have lost sensation in your feet, or have severe arthritis in any of your limbs, ask a friend or family member for help with your toenails, or go to a podiatrist.

Vascular surgery

Despite all the care you take, you may continue to have problems with your feet. A common foot problem among people with diabetes is the development of an ulcer, or painless sore that does not heal. Ulcers frequently become infected, and the infection may penetrate to the bone. Treatment of ulcers involves removing all the dead tissue in an ulcer, using antibiotics to control infection, and relieving pressure from the area of your foot with the ulcer. You may have to use crutches or a wheelchair or even stay in bed to keep weight off the ulcer and allow for proper healing.

Since poor blood circulation to the feet can delay the healing of an ulcer, your doctor may refer you for vascular evaluation. Depending on the results of tests to evaluate your blood flow, you may need to have a portion of an artery reconstructed through either angioplasty, in which a balloon at the tip of a catheter inserted into the artery is inflated to clear the blockage, or bypass surgery. To help the vascular surgeon determine whether you need vascular treatment, *arteriography* may be used. In this diagnostic procedure, dye is injected into your arteries, and x-rays and subsequent computer analysis highlight the clogged areas. Another diagnostic tool your surgeon may use to examine your blood circulation is ultrasound, or venous Doppler. This test can give important diagnostic information without requiring a dye injection or x-rays. However, ultrasound is not a substitute for arteriography when the latter test is called for.

Experts agree that surgery is needed if impaired circulation causes severe pain in your feet and legs, prevents sores or ulcers from healing, or causes gangrene—which is greenish-black dead tissue that may develop anywhere on the leg or feet. Several procedures may be used to restore circulation, including angioplasty and implantation of a stent (a small, tube-shaped device that holds a section of the blood vessel open). Another option is a distal bypass graft, an innovative microsurgical procedure that bypasses the blockage. Distal bypass grafts are now routinely performed, even to very small arteries in the feet.

The success rate of distal bypass surgeries, which are covered by Medicare and Medicaid, is impressive: circulation is immediately restored in the extremities of 98% of people who otherwise would have lost part of their foot or leg. After three years, the success rate approaches 94%, and after five years it is 87%. These success rates are national benchmarks for this type of treatment in people with diabetes. It is important to remember, however, that the earlier circulation problems are detected and treated, the higher the likelihood that treatment will be successful.

Another key to success, say practitioners at Foot Care Specialists, is a team approach. "Management of diabetic foot ulcers is complex and often requires a multispecialty collaborative approach," says Dr. Geoffrey Habershaw, chief of podiatry at Boston Medical Center and Clinical Director of Foot Care Specialists. The team includes vascular surgeons, internists, infectious disease specialists, orthopedists, diabetologists, and podiatric doctors. By working together, the team brings multiple skills to bear on each person and can treat complicated cases in a more comprehensive way.

The longer an ulcer is present, the more likely it will lead to amputation. But even if your foot complications are severe, it's worth your time to seek out a second opinion. "We believe that almost all foot amputations are avoidable, and we encourage anyone who has been told he needs an amputation to get a second opinion," says Dr. Gibbons.

For people with diabetes, foot care takes a bit more time and attention than for those who don't have diabetes. But the extra attention is worth it. You'll be able to ward off many of the effects of foot complications or protect your feet despite the complications. The bottom line is that healthy feet will preserve your lifestyle and ultimately get you where you want to go. ❏

FOOT RESOURCES

There are many potential sources of help and information for people with diabetes-related foot problems. Your doctor or podiatrist is your first best resource when it comes to caring for your feet. We list here some other options you may wish to investigate:

■ To get a second opinion or more information about serious and persistent foot problems, call the Foot Care Specialists at Boston Medical Center at (617) 414-6840.

■ For a list of board-certified podiatrists in your area, call the American Board of Podiatric Surgery at (415) 826-3200.

■ For the most up-to-date, comprehensive review and recommendations for the diagnosis and treatment of diabetic foot wounds, see the Consensus Statement published in *Diabetes Care,* Volume 22, Number 8, August 1999, pages 1354–1360.

■ A free brochure about foot care is available for the asking. Called "Diabetic Foot Problems and Treatments," it is published by the American College of Foot and Ankle Surgeons. The text of this brochure (and others that may be of interest) can be accessed through the College's Web site, www.acfas.org/patbrlist.html. You may also get a copy by calling or writing to the following address:
Foot Health Institute
c/o American College of Foot and Ankle
  Surgeons
515 Busse Highway
Park Ridge, IL 60068-3150
(888) THE-FEET (843-3338)

■ Another free booklet, called "Take Care of Your Feet for a Lifetime," is published by the U.S. National Institute of Diabetes and Digestive and Kidney Diseases. It and related materials can be accessed at the Web site of the National Diabetes Education Program:
http://ndep.nih.gov/materials/pubs/feet/feet.htm

The materials can also be obtained by calling or writing to the following address:
National Diabetes Information Clearinghouse
1 Information Way
Bethesda, MD 20892-3560
(800) 860-8747 or (301) 654-3327

TREATING AND PREVENTING FOOT ULCERS
Keeping One Step Ahead

by Elizabeth Warren-Boulton, R.N., M.S.N.

Anyone with diabetes is at risk for foot problems, and the longer you've had diabetes, the higher your risk. One of the most dreaded foot problems is a foot ulcer. Luckily, foot ulcers are also one of the most preventable diabetes-related foot problems—*if* you know what to look for and make a point of looking for it every day.

The beginnings of a foot ulcer are often so subtle they go unnoticed. Changes in the shape and structure of the feet tend to develop very gradually, and small breaks in the skin may not even be felt, especially if a person has a diminished sense of touch in the feet. But seemingly small changes and minor injuries can turn into major disabilities if they are ignored. For this reason, both you and your doctor need to engage in ongoing preventive efforts

How ulcers form

Healthy skin helps perform many vital functions in the body, including regulation of body temperature, prevention of dehydration, sensation of touch and pain, and protection against injuries and infection. The outer surface of the skin, called the *epidermis,* consists of layers of cells that contain *keratin,* a hardened protein substance, and forms an effective protective covering from the outside environment. Underlying this tough outer layer is the *dermis,* which contains hair follicles, sebaceous glands (which secrete the oil that keeps skin from drying out), sweat glands, nerve endings, blood vessels, and connective tissue. A skin ulcer is a loss of an area of the epidermis, some of the dermis beneath it, and sometimes even some of the underlying tissue.

Ulcers can occur anywhere on the foot. They often occur at the site of an injury or at points of high pressure, particularly the areas that bear your weight when you stand or walk. Common ulcer sites include under the toes, on the ball of the foot, at the heel, between the toes, and wherever there are corns or calluses. Foot deformities are associated with ulcers because they can cause increased pressure on certain areas of the foot. With hammertoes, for example, the tops and the bottoms of the toes as well as the balls of the feet are at risk, as shown in the illustration on page 223.

Two complications associated with diabetes—neuropathy (nerve damage) and peripheral vascular disease (blood vessel disease)—can reduce the skin's ability to perform its usual functions well, setting the stage for the development of a foot ulcer.

Neuropathy. Although there are several ways in which neuropathy can affect the foot of a person with diabetes, the most important (with regard to ulcers) is the loss of sensitivity to pain and temperature, making the foot vulnerable to injury. The most common cause of injury is simply walking, and ill-fitting shoes often contribute to the problem. People who still have feeling in their feet respond to foot pressure or pain while walking either by changing their stride to avoid irritating an area, by resting, or by checking their shoes for problems. But because many people with diabetes have lost the sensation of pain and pressure, they have no indication that something's wrong and do not try to stop the irritation. If it continues, a blister or tear may form or the area may become red and swollen. When a bony part of the foot is subjected to repeated pressure, the skin overlying the area may increase keratin production to form a callus.

Walking injuries can occur in many ways: People with little sensation in their feet have been known to walk around with objects such as pebbles, coins, or paper clips—even shoehorns—in their shoes without noticing them. Sharp objects such as nails can poke through the soles of shoes and cause puncture wounds. Walking barefoot on a hot beach or other hot surface can burn and tear your skin. Spending extensive time outdoors in the cold can cause frostbite to your toes.

When you don't have complete feeling in your feet, it's possible to injure them in ways besides walking, and any injury can lead to an ulcer. For example, improper toenail trimming can lead to gouged skin, ingrown nails, infected nails, or nails that grow into an adjacent toe. Hot or cold temperatures can cause thermal injuries to feet with no sensation. Soaking your cold feet in hot water or placing your feet in front of the fire or radiator can cause severe burns if you can't feel when it's time to remove your feet from the heat. You can also cause chemical injury to your skin by using callus and corn removers or by soaking your feet in a strong antiseptic solution such as iodine, Lysol, boric acid, or Epsom salts.

When diabetes causes damage to the nerves that control muscle movement, the result can be weakened muscles in the foot, leading to deformity and injury. Toes can become bent and misshapen, and hammertoes can develop. This type of nerve damage can also cause thinning of the protective fat pads on the soles of the feet. The imbalance caused by structural deformity leads to more joint distortion. A serious condition called Charcot foot can develop, in which the midsection of the foot collapses, causing a rounded, rocker-bottom shape to the foot. This causes weight-bearing on bony points that do not normally bear weight, which can lead to calluses and possibly ulcer formation.

A callus is often a warning sign that something is irritating your foot. Calluses are usually protective and can be trimmed safely by a podiatrist. But as calluses thicken, they become rigid and unyielding, adding more pressure at the site. Prolonged irritation can lead to inflammation (a hot spot), bleeding, and infection underneath the callus, forming a "pre-ulcer." If untreated, the soft tissue over the bone breaks down, causing swelling and a discharge with a bad smell. The callus and dead tissue sloughs off, leaving an open ulcer usually surrounded by a ridge of callus.

Autonomic neuropathy (damage to the nerves that control the involuntary functions, including the function of glands, organs, and the heart) can also contribute to foot injuries and ulcer formation. In the foot, sweat and sebaceous glands get less nerve stimulation from damaged nerves and, as a result, secrete less fluid. This leads to dryness, cracking, and fissures in the skin. Less nerve stimulation can also decrease blood flow, impairing your body's defenses against the bacteria that enter breaks in the skin.

Peripheral vascular disease. While neuropathy leads to ulcers by increasing the chance of foot injuries, peripheral vascular disease leads to ulcers by slowing the rate at which injuries heal. Increased blood viscosity (thickness), which contributes to the formation of blood clots, can cause circulation problems in the arteries in the legs and feet. *Atherosclerosis,* or deposits of fats and other cells that form plaques that narrow and harden blood vessel walls, also obstructs the flow of blood. When peripheral vascular disease is present, oxygen, nutrients, and antibiotics are not delivered to the foot efficiently, making infections hard to treat.

Treating foot ulcers

Treatment of a foot ulcer focuses on healing the ulcer and preventing amputation. Both you and your doctor play important roles in the treatment process. Today's medicine can heal most foot ulcers, but it won't work without your help.

Your doctor's role. When you have a foot ulcer, your doctor will probably x-ray your foot to check for struc-

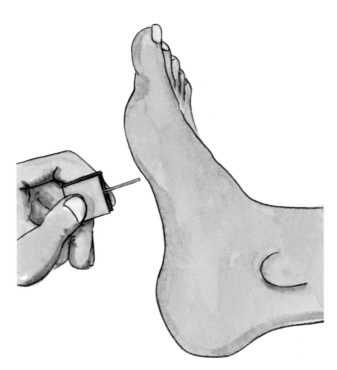

LEAP FOR YOUR FEET

To determine whether you've lost any feeling in your feet, doctors use a simple device: It is a filament—a thin, flexible, threadlike piece of nylon—designed to exert a specific amount of pressure. If you cannot feel the light touch of the filament on your foot, your doctor knows you've lost some ability to feel pain there and can tell you how to protect your feet from injuries and other problems.

You can perform the same simple screening test at home with a free kit that includes a filament made to exert the same amount of pressure as your doctor's and instructions on how to perform accurate tests. If the home test indicates that you have lost some sensation, you should see your doctor.

The test kit is part of the Lower Extremity Amputation Prevention (LEAP) Program. The program also teaches people to inspect their feet daily, to prevent and treat dry skin, to wear proper shoes, and to be responsible for foot care.

For a test kit and more information, contact the LEAP Program at this address:
LEAP Program
Bureau of Primary Health Care
Division of Programs for Special Populations
4350 East West Highway, 9th Floor
Bethesda, MD 20814
(888) ASK-HRSA (275-4772)
www.bphc.hrsa.gov/leap

FOOT CARE RESOURCES

For a list of board-certified podiatrists in your area, call the American Board of Podiatric Surgery at (415) 826-3200 or send an e-mail request to info@abps.org.

For a brochure about foot care, contact:
AMERICAN PODIATRIC MEDICAL ASSOCIATION
9312 Old Georgetown Road
Bethesda, MD 20814-1698
www.apma.org
(800) FOOTCARE (366-8227)

To find out about specially fitted shoes, contact:
PEDORTHIC FOOTWEAR ASSOCIATION
7150 Columbia Gateway Drive, Suite G
Columbia, MD 21046
(410) 381-7278
www.pedorthics.org

For a free booklet called "Take Care of Your Feet for a Lifetime," contact:
NATIONAL DIABETES INFORMATION CLEARINGHOUSE
1 Information Way
Bethesda, MD 20892-3560
(800) 860-8747
http://ndep.nih.gov/materials/pubs/feet/brochure/index.htm

To obtain the names and phone numbers of certified diabetes educators in your area, call the American Association of Diabetes Educators at (312) 424-2426 or visit the Association's Web site: www.aadenet.org.

For diabetes-related activities and information, call your local chapter of the American Diabetes Association or visit the Association's Web site: www.diabetes.org

ture and joint changes and for infection and foreign bodies. Then dead tissue will be removed so only healthy tissue remains. The size and depth of an ulcer, which may not be obvious until the dead tissue has been removed, will be carefully measured to help track your healing progress.

Before dressing the wound, your doctor may use an antibiotic cream to protect it from infection and to promote healing. Other therapies, including special skinlike grafts and gels with growth factors or collagen, are also available. When these grafts or gels are placed over the clean ulcer and carefully bandaged in place, they can reduce the time it takes for ulcers to

heal completely. Your doctor may also prescribe an oral antibiotic, because persistent or recurring ulcers can spread infection to surrounding tissue and bone.

All pressure needs to be removed from the ulcer to allow it to heal, so your doctor will instruct you not to put any weight on the affected foot. This usually means staying in bed for a period of time, then using crutches or a wheelchair. Sometimes, a cast that spreads pressure over an increased surface area of the foot and leg can keep weight off the site, allowing you to walk and the ulcer to heal.

Because a good blood supply is so important to the healing process, an evaluation of the blood vessels in your leg and foot may be necessary. A vascular surgeon may use ultrasound to analyze blood pressure and blood flow in your foot and leg or may perform an *arteriogram* (an x-ray of arteries that have been injected with dye) to identify any clogged vessels. If circulation to the foot needs to be restored to improve healing, surgery can open blocked vessels or bypass the blockage.

Your role. Wounds heal best when your blood sugar is in the normal range, so keep your blood glucose under the best control you can. Although any sustained lowering of the blood glucose level helps, a hemoglobin A_{1c} of less than 7% is recommended (hemoglobin A_{1c}, or HbA_{1c} for short, is a measure of average blood glucose control). Blood sugar values should range between 80 mg/dl and 120 mg/dl before breakfast and between 100 mg/dl and 140 mg/dl at bedtime. Controlling both blood sugar and blood pressure reduces the risk for cardiovascular disease, which can hinder wound healing when blood vessels in the legs are affected. For people with diabetes, the recommended goal for blood pressure is 130/80 mm Hg or lower. Because each person is different, the goals you and your doctor set may be slightly different from these recommended levels.

Blood glucose control entails day-to-day decisions about food, exercise, taking diabetes drugs, and monitoring blood sugar. An ulcer may increase blood sugar levels because of infection or reduced physical activity, so talk to your doctor about any changes you should make in your usual diabetes self-care routine.

Wound cleaning and dressing changes may be required for several weeks until the ulcer space is filled with healthy new tissue. Home health-care providers often can assist with this process initially and instruct you and your family members in the correct technique. They can also teach you to identify problems that require professional attention. You will improve your chances of full recovery by keeping your appointments for ulcer treatments and review of healing and by keeping your doctor abreast of any problems you're having.

The month or so after an ulcer has closed over is a critical point in the healing process. Follow your doctor's recommendation not to put any weight on the affected foot. Once your doctor has told you it's OK for you to walk on it, take special care to avoid foot injuries and to wear proper shoes and any necessary shoe modifications. This will help prevent a recurrence of the ulcer. Preventive care of the other foot is important because it will be at high risk for problems, too.

Preventing trouble

Whether you've had a foot ulcer or not, it's important to take steps to prevent an occurrence or recurrence. If you've never had an ulcer, the first step is to ask your doctor or nurse educator if your feet are at high risk for ulcers. People who have one or more of the following are considered to have high-risk feet: loss of pain and temperature sensation in the feet, poor circulation in blood vessels in the foot, severe foot deformity, and having already had a foot ulcer or amputation. If you have high-risk feet, be sure your feet are examined at every visit to your doctor (in fact, all people with diabetes should have their feet examined at every visit), and see a podiatrist for routine care of calluses, corns, or thickened nails. Remember to change your shoes at least twice a day to change the pressure spots on your feet.

You may need special shoes or shoe inserts to prevent serious foot problems. If you have Medicare Part B insurance, you may be able to get some of the cost of the special shoes or inserts paid for. If you qualify, your doctor or podiatrist can tell you how to get them.

If you have low-risk feet, they should be thoroughly examined at least every year by your doctor. Your doctor will test for the presence or absence of the sensation of touch, probably by lightly pressing a monofilament (a special nylon fiber) to different parts of the foot. Some people learn how to test their own feet with a monofilament to detect changes as early as possible.

Regardless of your risk status, gently wash and dry your feet every day, then inspect them all over for signs of injury, redness, or swelling. Look also for signs of poor circulation, including coolness and a shiny appearance, the absence of hair on the top of the foot and the toes, and thickened toenails. Frequent fungal infections are another sign of poor circulation. To prevent foot injuries and infections, apply lotion to prevent dryness and cracked skin on the tops and bottoms of your feet. Do not put lotion in the moist areas between your toes. Wear well-fitted, cushioned, supportive shoes, and get specially made shoes if necessary. Before you put your shoes on, check inside them for foreign objects, and make sure the lining is smooth. Call your doctor if a cut, sore, blister, or bruise on your foot does not begin to heal after one day.

Another important preventive measure is to keep your blood sugar under control with a target hemoglobin A_{1c} below 7%. Controlling blood glucose levels plays a major role in preventing or delaying the onset of nerve damage (as well as eye and kidney disease), thereby keeping the feet healthy and decreasing the risk for foot ulcers. Talk with your doctor, diabetes educator, and dietitian about the best ways to achieve and maintain this goal. ❑

HAMMERTOE

Foot deformities can cause increased pressure on parts of the foot, sometimes leading to skin erosion and ulcers. A hammertoe, shown here, causes increased pressure on the top and tip of the toe as well as on the ball of the foot, at the base of the toe.

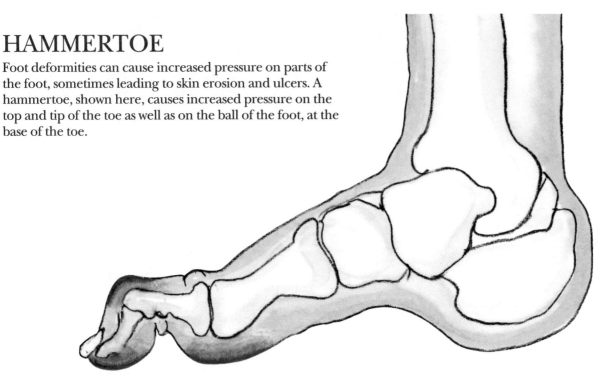

PICKING THE SHOE TO FIT THE OCCASION

by Dennis J. Janisse, C.Ped.

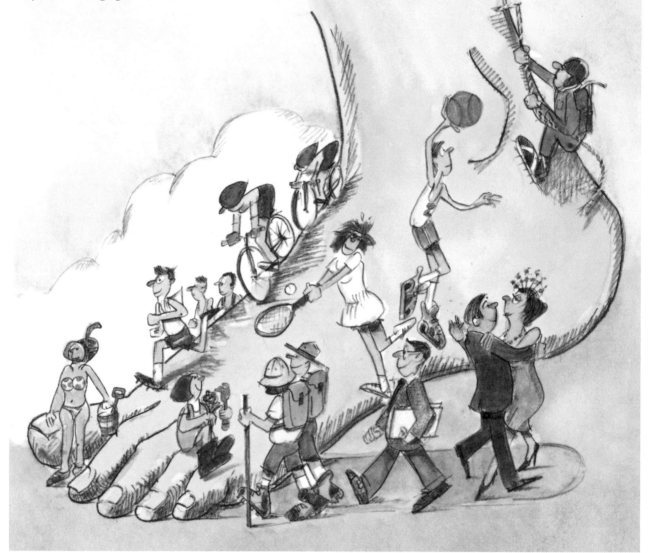

Wearing the right footwear is very important for people with diabetes, especially if you already have foot problems. But even if you don't, the right shoes can be a key factor in preventing diabetes-related foot complications. Of course you want to choose shoes that are comfortable and that fit your feet well, but you also want to make sure that your shoes fit the occasion for which you'll be wearing them. Different shoes are designed for different situations, and in this article we help you learn to pick the shoe that's right for just about any occasion.

The basics

Let's start with a little bit about how shoes are made. There are two basic parts to a shoe: the *sole*, which is the bottom part of the shoe, and the *upper*, which covers the top and sides of the foot. The sole can have up to three parts. The *insole* is the top of the sole and is the part that touches your foot. The *outsole* is the bottom layer of the sole, which touches the ground. Some shoes also have a middle layer of sole material, or *midsole*, which provides additional cushioning. The upper includes the *toe box*, which covers the toe area; the *vamp,* which covers the instep; the *tongue,* which is the part under the laces; the *counter,* which fits around the heel; and the *collar,* which is the top edge of the counter.

A good shoe for a person with diabetes will depend, to some extent, on the condition of the individual's feet. However, anyone would do well to look for the following qualities in their shoes:

Plenty of room in the toe area. A relatively high toe box is important to allow room for the toes, without excessive rubbing or pressure.

Laces. Laces or Velcro closures not only allow the shoe to be adjusted, they also make for a better fit. Ladies' pumps have no laces and not even much of a vamp, so to prevent them from falling off a person's foot they have to fit too snugly.

A strong counter. This offers heel support and stability for the back part of the foot.

Padded collar and tongue. It's always a good idea to avoid rubbing or pressure on any part of the foot because this can lead to blisters, ulcers, and even deformity. A padded collar and tongue help minimize rubbing or pressure on the top and sides of the foot.

Minimal seams in the upper. Seams can rub and lead to skin breakdown; styles with seams should be avoided.

Shock-absorbing sole. To prevent excess pressure on the bottom of the foot, the sole should provide shock absorption. Choose outsole materials such as crepe, Vibram, or EVA rather than leather or hard rubber. The insole should also offer some shock absorption.

Low heel. High heels lead to excessive pressure on the metatarsal heads, the bones at the base of the toes. This is a particularly sensitive area of the foot in people with diabetes and is often one of the first areas where ulcers occur. The lower the heel, the less pressure on this potential problem area.

Soft, breathable upper. Choose natural materials such as leather or deerskin, or try nylon mesh or canvas, which are used in athletic shoes. Vinyl is not breathable and should be avoided.

Proper shoe shape. Remember to match the shape of the shoe to the shape of your foot. Don't wear a shoe that puts pressure on some part of your foot or forces it into an unnatural shape.

Proper shoe size. Don't be locked into one particular shoe size. Sizes vary tremendously depending on the style and the manufacturer, and the size for you is the one that fits your foot. When trying on shoes, remember to consider the width: Not everyone can fit into the medium width of most shoes. You may need a narrower or wider shoe. Having your feet measured will give you a good starting point to use when determining which size shoe to buy, but keep in mind that shoe sizes are not absolute measurements. Keep in mind, too, that

your feet may change size over time. You won't know for sure whether shoes fit until you try them on.

Everyday shoes

What's the best type of shoe for ordinary, everyday activities like shopping and running errands? Most people do well with what are usually called *walking shoes* or *comfort shoes.* These are casual, reasonably priced shoes that are available in a variety of widths. They usually come in neutral colors such as black or tan and have fewer seams and less detailing than typical athletic shoes. Walking shoes are lightweight, have a flexible sole, offer good shock-absorbing materials in the outsole, and often have a removable insole. A removable insole can be replaced with a new one if the old one wears out or with a custom-made insert, called an *orthosis,* which may be necessary for someone with foot deformities. Walking shoes are also constructed so that prescription modifications can be made. The outsole on most walking shoes is shaped to make walking easier and to relieve pressure on the metatarsal heads; such a sole is often referred to as a rocker sole because it helps to "rock" the foot as you walk. This type of shoe is especially good for older people, many of whom have problems picking up their feet when they walk or maintaining their balance.

A recent study showed that among those 65 and older, shoes were often to blame for falls that caused injuries. Some falls were caused by athletic running shoes, which have heavy rubber outsoles and often have rubber tips on the toes. Such soles can stick to carpeting, throwing a person off-balance and causing a fall. Falls can also be caused by synthetic or leather outsoles, which can be slippery on wet surfaces. And too much cushioning insole material can also make an older person unstable. Walking shoes, on the other hand, offer good traction and support without heavy rubber soles or rubber tips on the toes, and they don't have an excessive amount of cushioning material.

Walking or comfort shoes are great for just about anyone with diabetes, even those with more severe foot problems. Manufacturers who currently offer this type of shoe include Soft Spots, SAS, Clinic, New Balance, Easy Spirit, and Canfield (made by P.W. Minor & Sons).

Athletic shoes

If you're going to participate in sports, such as running, tennis, or biking, you'll want to buy a more specialized athletic shoe. Be sure to check with your doctor before starting any kind of serious exercise or athletic program. The state of your diabetes and the condition of your feet will be important factors for your doctor to consider in determining which types of athletic activities are best for you. Once you've decided to pursue a particular activity, you'll want to purchase your shoes at a shoe store that specializes in athletic footwear and has experienced, knowledgeable salespeople who can help you pick the right shoe for your foot and your activity. The salesperson can also help you get a good fit. He or she should know, for example, which brands of athletic shoes come in multiple widths and which brands tend to run wider or narrower.

Walking. If you walk for exercise, the walking shoes described above would be a good choice. Walking shoes with a more athletic look are also widely available in athletic shoe stores. If you're going to be walking indoors, at a mall or fitness center, for example, or on any wet surface, be sure the outsoles are made of rubber rather than synthetic materials, which can slip on smooth or wet surfaces.

Running. Running puts much greater stress on the foot than walking. This means that running shoes need to offer better shock absorption than walking shoes. Running shoes also differ from walking shoes in that they offer more stability in the heel and counter area, greater flexibility in the ball of the foot, and more control over how the foot rolls. They also weigh less, have better traction, and have more breathable uppers.

Running shoes use a combination of leather and nylon or mesh in the uppers. The outsoles are made of hard carbon rubber or blown rubber (rubber with air blown into it for a lighter weight), with a good tread design for traction. Extra shock absorption is usually found in the midsole, with materials such as polyurethane, EVA, silicone gel, and ambient air. The sole is also wider at the heel to increase stability.

More research and design has been done in the area of running shoes than in all other areas of athletic footwear, and athletic shoe companies now make shoes for specific foot types, gait patterns, and training styles. With this increased specialization, it's really important to have a knowledgeable person help you choose running shoes, because wearing the wrong kind can hurt you.

Two terms you may encounter when shopping for running shoes are *pronate* and *supinate*. Both terms refer to the way in which the foot strikes the ground and rolls from the heel to the toe as body weight is transferred across the foot. People who pronate roll the foot inward as they go forward, whereas people who supinate roll the foot outward. A certain amount of pronation is considered normal. For those who pronate excessively or who supinate, some running shoes are made with wedges built into the heels to correct the problem. However, many more people think they need such correction than really do need it. So

don't be too hasty to assume you need special shoes or to accept a salesperson's diagnosis of a foot-strike problem, especially if you aren't having any running-related problems such as injuries.

Court sports. Court sports include basketball, volleyball, tennis, and other racquet sports. These sports require sprinting, jumping, stretching, and quick side-to-side movements. Court shoes need to provide a lot of stability to protect the foot, especially during those side-to-side movements. They should have a firm heel counter, and the shoe should be cut high enough to provide good support on the sides of the foot and at the ankle. High-tops, which cover the ankle, can be used for maximum ankle support. Court shoes have flatter soles than running or walking shoes and have a hard rubber outsole for traction.

Cross-training. If you're really going to get into running, you definitely want to have a good running shoe—and the same holds true for walking, tennis, basketball, and other sports. But if you're more likely to participate in a variety of activities in a more casual manner, then you probably want to buy a multiuse shoe called a cross-trainer. These shoes offer good support and shock absorption and work well for most sports. Cross-trainers are also great for people who work out at a health club or gym and use a variety of machines or do several activities.

Bicycling. Pressing down on the pedals of a bicycle can put a fair amount of pressure on the bottoms of the feet. When choosing shoes for cycling, therefore, it's important to look for a thick sole that will cushion and protect the foot where it contacts the pedal. For recreational cyclists, a sturdy pair of cross-trainers will usually do the trick. If your cycling hobby becomes more serious, however, you may want to look at the special cycling shoes sold at sporting goods stores and bike shops.

Swimming and water exercise. If you don't have any numbness or other problems with your feet, it's not absolutely necessary to wear protective footwear for swimming or water exercise. But wearing water shoes can help you avoid the types of scrapes and cuts that can easily occur around a pool or lake area. Wearing shoes is also a good way to protect against disease (such as athlete's foot) at a public pool or health club. Most water shoes have a soft rubber sole with a nylon mesh upper and offer simple coverage rather than support or stability.

Dress shoes

Finding dress shoes that are comfortable and good for your feet can be difficult, especially for women. The typical high-heeled pump has several problems. High heels place increased pressure on the vulnerable metatarsal heads. The insoles tend to have very little cushioning, and the outsoles tend to be made of leather or very hard rubber. The shoes tend not to be shaped like an actual foot; they often have pointed toes that cause rubbing and pressure and can eventually lead to deformity. And the lack of any vamp means that the shoes have trouble staying on your feet unless they are too small. Men's dress shoes can also have many of the same undesirable features such as low toe boxes, pointed toes, and very little shock absorption.

Fortunately, the workplace is becoming more casual, which means that a lot of people can avoid uncomfortable dress shoes at work and wear the comfort shoes we mentioned earlier. But if your workplace hasn't gone along with this trend, what can you do? Here are some ways to wear shoes that might not be the best for your feet while still trying to minimize foot problems:

■ Be aware of the condition of your feet. Examine your feet on a regular basis and look for any red spots, blisters, or ulcers. Also be aware of any numbness in your feet. Loss of sensation can happen very gradually, and big problems can develop before you know it. At the first sign of any foot problems, stop wearing the shoes that are causing them and see your doctor, who may recommend that you see a footwear specialist, such as a board-certified pedorthist, who can help you with special prescription footwear.

■ Minimize the amount of time spent in dress shoes. For example, wear your dress shoes *only* while at work; wear walking or comfort shoes to and from work and during your lunch hour or breaks. Also, take advantage of every opportunity to dress casually—such as the popular dress-down Fridays or days when you're not seeing clients.

■ Minimize the undesirable features on your dress shoes. Wear as low a heel as possible, and look for a more rounded toe, a higher toe box, and the fewest seams. Try to find shoes with some cushioning in the insole and softer, more shock-absorbing materials in the outsole. Some manufacturers make dress shoes with more attention to comfort. Rockport, for example, makes dressier shoes with high toe boxes, more shock absorption, and removable insoles. Although it has pointed toes, high heels, and no vamp, the Easy Spirit pump has additional padding in the insoles, making it better than most pumps.

For special occasions, such as weddings, even people with foot problems can wear shoes that may not be good for their feet, as long as these guidelines are followed—especially limiting the amount of time you actually wear the shoes.

Boots and sandals

If you live in a cold, snowy climate you're going to need some kind of boots or other winter footwear. It's especially important to protect your feet from the cold if you have any loss of feeling in your feet since you may not realize how cold your feet are getting. In looking for appropriate boots, you'll want to follow the same guidelines as you would for shoes. You may have more trouble finding a good fit because boots are generally not available in the same range of shapes and sizes as regular shoes.

There are a few alternatives to wearing boots. One is to wear regular walking or athletic shoes, possibly high-tops, that have been treated with a protective, water-proofing spray. They may not be as warm as winter boots, but if you're not going to be outside for long, they work fine.

Another alternative is to wear overshoes, so that you can wear your good, comfortable shoes but protect them from the weather. A new type of overshoe, called N.E.O.S. (a trademark of New England OverShoe Company), is made of a coated nylon fabric. It features a deep-lugged flat sole, and it is able to fit over any type of shoe.

In the warm weather, a lot of people like to wear sandals. Sandals can actually be good for people with diabetes because they allow the feet to be cooler and to breathe. However, you have to choose sandals carefully. Be sure to look for a good shape and the right size. Look for plenty of cushioning in the insole or even a removable liner that can be replaced with a specialized or custom-made orthosis. Many sandals are now made with a contoured insole with indentations to fit the contours of your foot. If you buy this type of sandal, be sure the contours match your foot. If they don't, areas of excess pressure can develop, eventually leading to skin breakdown.

Be sure the upper material is soft and doesn't rub or create pressure spots. Also, be sure there is enough strapping material to hold the sandal firmly on the foot, and look for buckles or Velcro to allow for adjustability. Never wear a thong-type sandal (with a strap between the toes); the rubbing between the toes can easily lead to skin breakdown. For women, sandals can often be an alternative to dress shoes, especially in the spring and summer. Manufacturers of good, comfortable sandals include Drew, SAS, Soft Spots, and Birkenstock.

Getting off on the right foot

Problems involving the feet are one of the most preventable complications for people living with diabetes. Wearing the right shoes can be a key factor in preventing future foot problems. And don't forget to practice other important foot-care basics, including washing, drying, and inspecting your feet daily and having your doctor examine your feet at every appointment. ❏

COPING WITH AMPUTATION

by James McGuire, P.T., D.P.M., C.Ped., W.C.S.

One of the most devastating complications of diabetes is amputation. Even with all the advances that science has made in the past 25 years, it has not succeeded in eliminating the necessity of amputation as a last resort for serious infection or gangrene. Each year in the United States, over 86,000 people with diabetes have an amputation of the foot or leg to preserve their life and halt the advance of serious infection. This number has not declined significantly in the past decade, even though serious infection and gangrene are mostly preventable.

This article is written to encourage anyone with diabetes to take the necessary steps to avoid ever having to face the choice to amputate. But it is also written to show each one of you who is facing the gut-wrenching decision to amputate your foot or leg that life doesn't have to end with an amputation. You can have as joyful and productive a life after an amputation as before. In fact, an amputation may eliminate many emotional and mobility problems, thus making your life even more fulfilling than before.

Why do an amputation?

An elective amputation is a choice to remove a body part because infection, loss of circulation, or deformity has rendered that part dysfunctional. It is both a terminal event and the first step toward improved health. The majority of amputations in the United States are caused by diabetes and its complications, including neuropathy (nerve damage), peripheral vascular disease (hardening or clogging of the arteries), and foot deformities such as hammertoes, bunions, or collapse of the arches. Having a combination of these complications significantly raises the risk of needing an amputation. Deformity alone may produce corns, calluses, and sore feet, but it doesn't necessarily lead to more serious problems. Ulcers and gangrene develop when foot deformities occur in combination with nerve and blood vessel disease.

Many studies have shown that the majority of amputations could have been prevented with good patient education and regular, preventive foot care by a podiatric physician. If you feel you could use more information about caring for your feet or more help doing it, speak to your doctor. A list of free foot-care resources is on page 231.

Diabetes complications

When you develop diabetes, it is not inevitable that you will have foot problems. A series of complications have to develop first that initially place you at risk and later may lead to more serious conditions and possibly amputation. You can intervene at any point, and the sooner the better. The road to fewer complications begins with accepting that you have diabetes and that you will have to take steps to control your blood sugar levels. For most people, those steps include changing well-established eating habits and behavior patterns.

It is essential that a person with diabetes develop an attitude of acceptance and a strong desire to learn all there is about it. Knowledge is power. It enables you to take control and to make sure you do everything you can to maximize the life you have now.

Most of the people with diabetes who I have seen go on to amputation had made a conscious or unconscious decision to deny the existence of their diabetes and resist the lifestyle changes that are necessary to avoid its complications. This same denial caused them to resist interventions that would have helped them to heal an ulcer or infection or cope with the decision to go forward with an amputation when other medical options had been exhausted.

Sometimes the large wounds created by rampant infection and loss of circulation just won't heal. It is important that people get straightforward, honest answers about their condition and the treatment options available to them. Physicians, wound-care specialists, therapists, and other health-care professionals counsel patients about treatment choices every day. As medical professionals dedicated to the treatment of people with diabetes, my colleagues and I are always willing to work with anyone who wants to avoid an amputation and go through the painstaking process of healing a wound. We try, however, to offer hope that is founded on expectations of success and not mere dreams that have little chance of fulfillment.

Preparing for the decision

The decision to amputate is usually not a rash or quick judgment. The complications that might necessitate an amputation take months to develop, and there are numerous opportunities to take steps to avoid them. There is also time for the person facing the possibility of an amputation to begin to prepare for it, practically and mentally. Many people squander this opportunity and refuse to address the problem. They then react emotionally and not rationally when the time arrives.

There are really only two choices when faced with the decision of whether to amputate: to give up and retreat from life or to face the situation with resolve and a positive attitude. Walking and the freedom of mobility are some of life's great joys. However, walking is not the essence of life, and a person can live a rich

TEAM PLAYERS

Whether you've had an amputation, are contemplating one, or are working to avoid the types of complications that sometimes lead to one, you may have occasion to work with some of the professionals listed here. This glossary may help to clarify everyone's role in your care.

AMPUTATION PREVENTION TEAM

Primary-care Physician	Physician primarily responsible for your medical care
Endocrinologist/ Diabetologist	Physician who specializes in the management of diabetes and related disorders
Podiatric Physician	Physician specializing in the medical and surgical management of problems of the foot and ankle
Vascular Surgeon	Physician specializing in the surgical management of blood vessel disorders
Certified Diabetes Educator	Medical professional with special training in diabetes care and education
Pedorthist	Certified footwear and orthotic (support and brace) specialist
Wound-care Specialist	Medical professional (such as a physician, nurse, physical therapist) with special training in wound care
Registered Dietitian	Credentialed food and nutrition expert

AMPUTATION REHABILITATION TEAM

Primary-care Physician/ Diabetologist	See "Amputation Prevention Team"
Physiatrist	Physician specializing in rehabilitation of people with physical disabilities
Psychologist/Psychiatrist	Mental health professional
Prosthetist	Certified artificial limb specialist
Physical/Occupational Therapist	Medical professional specializing in rehabilitation
Rehabilitation Nurse	Registered nurse with special training in rehabilitation
Social Worker	Licensed professional who helps people to obtain benefits and services from medical or government systems; some also provide psychotherapy
Wound-care Specialist	See "Amputation Prevention Team"
Podiatric Physician	See "Amputation Prevention Team"
Support Group	Peer group that provides encouragement, education, and social activities

and full life without it (although many amputees walk just fine). A sense of wholeness comes from an inner appreciation of who and what we are. Our spirit is more than just our physical bodies.

If we choose to see the loss of a limb or a portion of a limb as the loss of our spirit, our essential "whole," then an amputation may leave us with a sense of incompleteness and a profound depression that may be impossible for some to overcome. On the other hand, if we choose to see the loss of a diseased portion of our body as an attempt to prevent further damage and a step on the road to healing, then our essential "whole" remains intact and we can persevere and go on with a sense of hope and purpose.

It may sound simplistic, but the choice to give up or go forward is the choice each of us has every time a conflict or problem arises. It can be hard to pick yourself up and move on after a divorce, a business failure, or even a less profound setback. Likewise, it is very hard for some people to get on with life after an amputation. Although the physical success of the surgery itself is important, I have seen far too many people come through an amputation with a medically sound result, then lose hope and retreat into a world of depression and despair. More important than the physical outcome, then, is the spiritual outcome—how one copes with one's loss, adjusts to a changed body image and changed circumstances, and makes the most of the talents and capacity for life that one still has.

People almost always refuse the initial recommendation to get an amputation, even though it would likely be a relatively quick procedure, followed by rehabilitation, that would get them back to their lives with little delay. Instead, they go through numerous surgical procedures and spend months and months trying to save a toe, then the forefoot, and finally the heel. After months on crutches or in a wheelchair, hundreds of doctor visits, special shoes, wound treatments, and many different antibiotics, they generally end up with what was originally recommended to them: the amputation.

It is easy to understand why people fear amputation and to have great sympathy for them. Fear keeps all of us from being proactive in many areas of our lives. Rather than being a motivating force, fear tends to immobilize people, preventing them from seeing a way out. Fear also gives rise to a sense of hopelessness and despair. However, fear can often be assuaged with knowledge: of what it's really like to have an amputation, go through rehabilitation, and live with these changes to your body and your life. This type of knowledge is available to you, both from medical professionals and from the many people who have had amputations.

In addition to facing your fears, to cope with an amputation, you need to have a meaningful goal or purpose in your life. When working toward a goal, we are focused and hopeful, even if we don't eventually accomplish everything we had hoped to do. When we have no goal or purpose, it is easy to see life as pointless. As you contemplate your life after amputation, think about what's important to you and what you would like to accomplish in the coming months and years, even if you do not yet know all the steps you will need to get there.

Who to contact

There are many people who can help you prepare for an amputation and adjust to the changes in your life after the surgery and rehabilitation. A list of some of the professionals you may want to consult is displayed on page 229.

There are also a number of agencies and support groups available to amputees and their families. Most support groups would be more than happy to include you in one of their discussions to help you with your decision. A support group can also be invaluable to you later, during your rehabilitation.

If there is no support group in your area and you would like to start one, call Sabrina Kallies, R.N., at the Texas Diabetes Institute at (210) 358-7710 or e-mail her at skallies@university-health-sys.com. She can provide you with information about how to start a group.

Coping with new problems

There are numerous complications that an amputee may have to face. The most significant have to be the sense of loss and the natural grieving process that follow the removal of a body part. The depression, anger, and withdrawal that everyone experiences is a normal transition to healing and should not be denied. Unpleasant as it may seem, it is part of the recovery process. Good counseling—from your physician, a mental-health professional, or the therapist of your choice—can help you understand the stages of grief and recovery and guide you through the healing and rehabilitation process. Physical setbacks such as infection, phantom pain, or wound-healing problems can be tolerated more easily when a person is well informed and at peace with the recovery process.

Phantom pain, caused by nerves continuing to send signals after they have been cut, is particularly upsetting because it serves as a reminder of the missing body part. It also can be very painful and produce a great deal of anxiety. This was much more of a problem in the past. Recent advances in pain medication, therapeutic techniques, early prosthetic fitting, and a rapid return to activity greatly diminish the problems from phantom pain.

Tools of the trade

There have been so many advances in footwear and prostheses (artificial limbs) in recent years that you need not fear that you will appear odd or stand out because of your disability. Getting back to walking again is hard work, but with the help of such members of your rehabilitation team as your physical therapist, pedorthist (shoe specialist), prosthetist (artificial limb specialist), and podiatrist, it can be done.

Shoes for people with at-risk feet have improved in style and availability. Even custom-molded shoes that

FOR MORE INFORMATION

The organizations and Web sites listed here can provide information, support, and sometimes other services to people who have had an amputation.

AMERICAN ACADEMY OF ORTHOTISTS AND PROSTHETISTS
www.oandp.org
The professional society for orthotists and prosthetists.

AMPUTEE COALITION OF AMERICA
(888) AMP-KNOW (267-5669)
www.amputee-coalition.org
Call toll-free for information on support groups, prosthetic facilities, and rehabilitation centers in your area. Also home to the National Peer Network for peer counseling and *inMotion* magazine. The coalition operates the National Limb Loss Information Center, which offers fact sheets and answers to frequently asked questions, and is a partner in the Limb Loss Research and Statistics Program; you can link to both from the coalition's Web site.

AMPUTEE NET CENTER'S SUPPORT GROUP LIST
http://vandyke.digiweb.com/ampsup.htm
Names, addresses, and some phone numbers for support groups in the United States.

AMPUTEE ONLINE
www.amputee-online.com
News, information, and links on amputations. Also home to an e-mail newsletter.

AMPUTEE RESOURCE CENTER
www.usinter.net/wasa/arc.html
Information on how to start and maintain a peer support group, with descriptions of books and links to other resources.

AMPUTEE RESOURCE FOUNDATION OF AMERICA
www.amputeeresource.org
Information and articles from a certified prosthetist.

JONI AND FRIENDS AMPUTEE RESOURCE LIST
www.joniandfriends.org/helps/amputee.htm
Listing of agencies of interest to amputees.

UNITED AMPUTEE SERVICES ASSOCIATION
(407) 678-2920
www.oandp.com/resources/organizations/uasa
Support and education for people in south and central Florida.

PREVENTION RESOURCES
Call, write, or log on for these brochures on keeping your feet healthy and intact.

"Your Podiatric Physician Talks About Diabetes"
American Podiatric Medical Association
(800) FOOTCARE (366-8227)
www.apma.org
Click on "Foot Health Information," then click on "Diabetes."

"Diabetic Foot Problems and Treatments"
American College of Foot and Ankle Surgeons
(888) THE-FEET (843-3338)
www.acfas.org/patbrlist.html

"Foot Care"
American Diabetes Association
ATTN: Customer Service
1701 North Beauregard Street
Alexandria, VA 22311
(800) DIABETES (342-2383)
www.diabetes.org/ada/foot_care.asp

"Keep Your Feet and Skin Healthy"
National Diabetes Information Clearinghouse
1 Information Way
Bethesda, MD 20892-3560
(800) 860-8747
(301) 654-3327
www.niddk.nih.gov/health/diabetes/pubs/complications/index.htm

are made from casts of a person's feet are available in a wide variety of styles and colors. Modifications to the sole are less noticeable than in the past, and custom orthotic inserts (arch supports or insoles) are comfortable and more protective these days than they have ever been.

Artificial limbs are light, can be custom-colored to match your complexion, and can be made soft, so they even feel like your own skin. This is accomplished by using an internal skeleton or rigid frame (endoskeleton) made of a lightweight metal alloy covered with foam. One company can even make a painstaking copy of your remaining limb, adding body hair, toenails, and skin wrinkles to the prosthesis to produce a foot so lifelike that a casual observer can't tell the difference between the real foot and the prosthetic foot. Many amputee athletes, however, dispense with a cosmetic cover to save on weight and to cut wind resistance. Soft covers may also tear easily during athletic competition, making them impractical for these situations.

New technologies have improved to the point where amputees can run, hike, and even play tennis. These advances were evident at the Paralympics that followed the Olympic Games in Sydney, Australia, in 2000. There you even saw people with two artificial limbs running, jumping, and competing. These remarkable athletes exhibited a never-give-up spirit that was truly inspiring. Marlon Shirley, a below-knee amputee from the United States, came within 0.34 second of 2000 women's gold medalist Marion Jones' Olympic record time of 10.75 seconds in the 100-meter dash. The same technologies that allow these athletes to perform at such a high level are available to you to allow you to walk, run, and do other activities you enjoy.

For people with above-knee amputations, the challenges are greater, but the technologies are even more sophisticated. New knee joints almost think for themselves, using built-in mechanisms to provide a smooth, limp-free gait and to prevent buckling and falls. To see someone who has mastered gait with an above-knee prosthesis is always inspirational.

Although studies have shown that a significant number of people do not return to functional walking using their prosthetic limb, most of the people in these studies who had problems regaining mobility also had serious medical difficulties in addition to their amputation. It was these concurrent problems that prevented them from completing the rehabilitation process. Almost all amputees who are in reasonably good health prior to the amputation and are motivated to recover can walk again.

Leading by example

Although the technology is fascinating, the true miracles take place not on the workshop bench but in the hearts of people who overcome adversity and go on to live lives that are an inspiration to those around them. Your family needs you to succeed as much as you need it yourself. The vision of a mother, father, brother, or sister conquering fears to embrace and eventually overcome circumstances can be heartening for a family.

The opposite is also true. Hopelessness and despair can affect those around you. Families can lose hope along with the family member who retreats from life and refuses to face problems with dignity and resolve. You can unknowingly destroy the hope of the people who are dear to you when they watch your example and learn from you how to cope with their own future problems.

Elective amputation is one of life's most difficult challenges, but it is not one of life's greatest tragedies. There are far more devastating events in life that do not give you the opportunity to be proactive and make success out of what seems like failure. While the medical professionals involved in your care can advise you on how to avoid the complications that lead to amputation or, if necessary, cope with it when it occurs, the difference in final outcome is dependent on you and your attitude. ❏

EXERCISE

GETTING STARTED AND STAYING MOTIVATED

by Richard M. Weil, M.Ed., C.D.E., C.S.C.S.

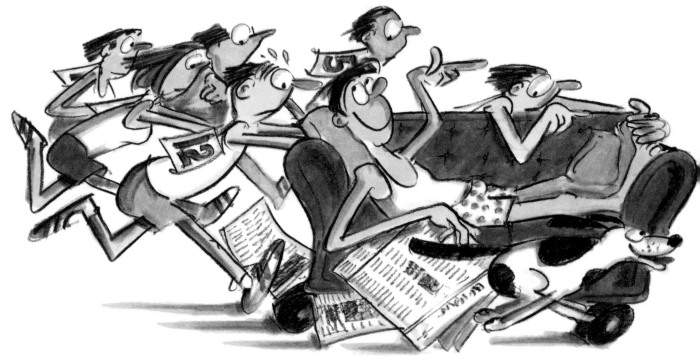

Y ou've heard it before: Exercise is good for you. You've heard it from your doctor, your diabetes educator, friends, magazines, and the evening news. But it's Sunday morning, you're relaxing at home, reading the paper, resting from a long, hard week, and the last thing on your mind is exercise. Even though you know it's a good idea, you just can't seem to do it.

You are not alone: According to data from the U.S. Centers for Disease Control and Prevention, only 27.7% of American adults are regularly active enough to achieve good health. So how *do* you get off the couch and start moving? And even more important, how do you stick with it?

Physical activity vs. exercise

Before we talk about getting motivated to exercise, let's define physical activity and exercise—because

there is a difference. Physical activity is any muscular activity that results in energy expenditure. Exercise is a subset of physical activity. Exercise is more vigorous (heart rate, breathing, and sweating all increase), sustained (it usually lasts 20 to 30 minutes), may require special clothing and a shower afterward, and usually involves a formal plan. It turns out that both are good for you, and here's why.

Recent guidelines from the U.S. Surgeon General are clear: You can be healthier and fitter if you accumulate 30 minutes of moderate-intensity physical activity on most, if not all, days of the week. The key words are "moderate-intensity" and "accumulate." Moderate intensity means walking at a speed of roughly 3 to 4 miles per hour, just fast enough to get a bit out of breath—but not gasping for breath—or engaging in any other activity that requires a similar level of exertion. Walking the dog, washing the car by hand, mowing the lawn, raking leaves, cleaning the house, and working in the garden can all qualify as moderate-intensity physical activity. It involves some effort, but not as much as you might think. And accumulating 30 minutes of activity means that you don't need to do it all at once. If you prefer, you can be active for, say, 10 minutes at a time, three times a day.

The recent activity guidelines from the Surgeon General are not intended to replace the old exercise guidelines (which were to exercise three to five times a week, 15 to 60 minutes per session, at 50% to 85% of your heart rate maximum). For those of you who go to the gym, take aerobics classes, or do more intense physical activity, there's no reason to stop what you're doing. You'll always get lots of benefits from working out. The Surgeon General's guidelines are simply intended to provide new options for those who are unwilling or unable to stick with formal exercise. Basically, you don't need to do Herculean amounts of exercise to lower your blood pressure and cholesterol, lose weight, reduce stress, feel better about yourself, become stronger, reduce your risk of heart disease, and help improve your blood sugar control.

The obstacle course

If exercise is so great, and you don't have to do as much as was once thought to get healthier, why aren't more of us doing it? Let's take a look at some of the common obstacles that keep us on the couch, and some ways to overcome inertia and get moving.

No time. Of course, some people barely have time to relax, much less exercise. People are busy with jobs, child care, volunteer work, social activities, and family responsibilities. Fitting in time to exercise can be difficult. There are two basic ways of approaching this problem. The first way is to simply schedule exercise into your life. Set a time for exercise and stick to it. Write it in your appointment book if you have to. Decide that you'll walk around your neighborhood for half an hour before dinner, or that you'll get on your stationary bike for 20 minutes before breakfast. Or sign up for a class that meets at a certain time, and block out that time on your calendar. When a distraction comes up—you're tired and don't feel like getting up early, for instance—look at your exercise as an appointment that you can't miss.

The other approach is to spread your physical activity throughout your day, to make your entire lifestyle more active. This is where the "accumulate 30 minutes of activity" part comes in. There are probably lots of small ways you could be more active. Do you take the elevator up to work? Try the stairs instead. Do you take the bus or subway regularly? Get off one stop earlier than usual and walk the rest of the way. If you have 30 minutes for a lunch break at work, go outside and walk around the block before eating. When you go shopping at the mall, try parking in the first space you see, rather than driving around and around for a space near the building. Rake your leaves by hand instead of using a leaf blower. These may all seem like little steps, but little steps add up, and that's the whole idea. After a while, small bouts of activity will seem normal to you. And the next time you're faced with a decision between the escalator and a flight of stairs, you'll choose the stairs without even thinking about it.

Both of these approaches work to improve health and well-being. To get started, you can think about which appeals to you more: getting your exercise over and done with in a single bound, or taking things in bits and pieces. Think about your own preferences and schedule and which method might work best for you.

It hurts. Exercise should not hurt. The "no pain, no gain" saying is no longer considered applicable to physical activity. This is not to say that exercise is always easy: You will have to push yourself sometimes. But pain should not be part of the equation. Listen to your body. If you get out of breath two minutes after you begin jogging, slow down, or walk instead. If climbing five flights of stairs is too difficult at first, start off with just one, and add the rest gradually. Your endurance will build up over time as your heart gets stronger. At the end of your exercise session, you should feel like you've moved your body (because you have), but there's no need to feel like you're about to collapse from exhaustion. You should walk away from your workout feeling like you could have done a little more.

If you're worried about soreness or stiffness, doing a few stretches for your major muscle groups before and after exercise can help prevent that achy feeling the next day. Sore muscles do sometimes occur if you've pushed yourself harder than usual, but the soreness usually fades within a few days. People who have higher fitness goals may encounter more frequent muscle soreness. If you're lifting weights at the gym to bulk up or running or biking long miles to prepare for a competition, you're probably going to be sore occasionally. But moderate daily activity should not hurt. Acute pain during exercise is always a signal to stop what you're doing immediately and seek help or apply proper first aid to the part of you that hurts.

It's boring. Boredom is a real problem for many people. Sitting on the stationary bike spinning the pedals, day after day, can get pretty dull. But there are ways to overcome this common problem. One is to try varying your routine, doing different activities on different days. Another is to experiment until you find an activity you like doing regularly. Walking, hiking, playing golf or tennis, riding a bicycle in the park, and swimming are all good choices.

Yet another approach to beating boredom is to find a way to distract yourself. Harold, for example, hates to exercise. Always has, always will. So to keep his mind off what he's doing and simultaneously reward himself for doing it, he tapes movies from cable TV and watches half an hour of a movie every time he's on his stationary bike. He only allows himself to watch the movie while he's biking; at the end of a half-hour workout, he turns the movie off. To see the next installment, he's got to start pedaling again. Harold found a clever solution: He combines something he likes to do with something he doesn't and ends up doing what he needs to do.

No equipment. It should be clear by now that you don't need any special equipment to get the type of physical activity recommended by the Surgeon General. Walking, the activity most people choose, requires no equipment other than a pair of sturdy, comfortable shoes. It's also convenient because you can do it just about anywhere. There's no need to join an expensive gym or health club.

Off on the right foot

When deciding what activity to try, there are several things to keep in mind. One is your current fitness level: If you've never run a step in your life, don't sign up for a marathon just yet. (But don't rule it out for the future, either!) Think about how far or for how many minutes you can comfortably walk now. Can you sustain a moderate or brisk pace for five minutes? Ten minutes? One of the most common mistakes new exercisers make is doing too much too soon, which inevitably leads to feeling sore and discouraged the next day. So start with what you can do easily. After all, your first goal is to make exercise a habit. Once you are doing it regularly, you can concentrate on increasing the duration and intensity of your exercise sessions.

A concern related to fitness level is any health problems you might have. For instance, if you have a bad knee, you might want to try a non-weight-bearing activity like swimming or bicycling rather than high-impact aerobics or jogging. If you aren't sure how a medical condition affects your ability to exercise, consult your doctor. Certain diabetes-related problems, including foot problems, heart disease, and retinopathy, often mean that it's better for you to pick a certain kind of physical activity over another. But don't let diabetic complications prevent you from exercising at all: No matter what the complication, there is some way you can work physical activity into your life.

Once you've assessed what your body can do, think about what you'd like to do and what's convenient. If you're not sure what you like or what fits into your

schedule best, test out different activities until one feels right.

How about exertion level? The easiest way to measure exertion is to use a "perceived exertion" scale. On a scale of 1 to 10, with 1 being very light activity and 10 very hard, your exercise should feel like a 5, somewhat hard. Pay attention to your breathing to rate how hard you're working.

Another way to measure how hard you're exerting yourself is to count your heartbeats. During exercise, your heart should beat at about 55% to 85% of its maximum rate. To calculate your *maximum heart rate*, subtract your age from 220. If you are 65 years old, for example, your maximum heart rate is about 155 beats per minute ($220 - 65 = 155$). Then figure out your range by multiplying 155 by 0.55 ($155 \times 0.55 = 85$) and then by 0.85 ($155 \times 0.85 = 132$). This means that your *target heart rate range* is 85 to 132 beats per minute. You can take your pulse during exercise to see where in the range your heart rate falls. (Make sure to consult your doctor if you've had any heart problems to make sure the 55% to 85% rule applies to you.)

The right frame of mind

So you've picked an activity to try, cleared it with your doctor, set aside time in your day to do it, and maybe even purchased a new pair of sneakers. But you're still sitting at home. Getting "psyched up" for exercising can be quite difficult. People have many different fears and concerns about exercise: Some people are afraid of looking silly or being embarrassed. Others feel they won't be able to exercise "right." And others suspect that exercise is futile and won't do any good no matter how hard they try. These are all legitimate concerns. Let's look at some ideas for overcoming a few common fears and frustrations.

Start small. One easy way to overwhelm yourself is to attempt too much at once. Exercise is a long-term project. Instead of being disappointed in yourself when you can't run 5 miles or do 50 sit-ups on your first try, set realistic goals and build up to them gradually.

Sometimes it helps to chart your progress in some way. Try keeping a calendar or journal where you write down what you've accomplished each day or week. That way, you can easily look back and see how far you've come. It's OK to start slowly. In fact, gradually increasing the amount and intensity of your activity puts less stress on your body. You don't have to be perfect at this for it to work.

Find a friend. Some people find that having company makes it a lot easier to stick with exercise. Make sure your workout partner is reliable, and make sure you have a contingency plan for when he or she doesn't show up.

Take a class. Taking a class is a good way to learn something new, and it can add the structure to your regimen that you might need, especially in the beginning. Make sure that you sign up for a class at your level, and if it will make you feel more comfortable, tell the instructor that you are a beginner and would appreciate a little bit more attention in the beginning. Most instructors are more than willing to help.

Think it out. If you just can't shake the feeling that you're out of your element in sneakers and sweatpants, try imagining your way out of the rut. Visualize yourself doing your activity, and "rehearse" it in your head. Just like a quarterback who reviews all the plays in his head over and over before the big game, you too can mentally prepare yourself for exercise.

Get some help. You may also want to consider turning to a professional for motivational and practical help. In addition to asking your doctor's advice, you could schedule a session with an exercise specialist such as an exercise physiologist or fitness trainer, who can help you choose an exercise program that's right for you. (Check to see whether your health insurance provides for such visits. If it doesn't, try petitioning your insurance company with a request to pay for one consultation visit.) Many gyms and YMCA's offer a free or low-cost orientation session at the beginning of your membership, where you can have a staff member show you how to use the equipment and give you recommendations for an exercise program.

Sticking with it

Getting started exercising is only half the battle. Here are some tips for sticking with exercise once you've started. Keep in mind that there is no end point to all of this. You can start now with one approach and change it later on.

■ Set aside special time for exercise by deciding at the beginning of each week which days you are going to exercise and when during the day you will do it. Goal setting and planning has been shown over and over again in research to help people adhere to an exercise plan.

■ Keep an exercise log or mark your calendar each time you exercise. At the end of the month, tally up the number of days you exercised and reward yourself. Sometimes, simply the satisfaction of knowing you did it is enough, but if you need more of a reward than that, do something like scheduling a massage or buying something special for yourself.

■ People who are experienced with sticking with exercise frequently report that it's better not to tell too many people that you're embarking on a lifestyle change. It seems that telling too many people only raises expectations and puts more pressure on you.

BENEFITS OF EXERCISE

Getting physical has numerous benefits for your body and your mind. Some of them take a while to kick in, but some will be evident after just one exercise session.

INSTANT GRATIFICATION

Elevated mood

Lower blood glucose

More energy during the day

Pride in your accomplishment

Sounder sleep

Stress relief

LONG-TERM RESULTS

Better feelings about yourself and your appearance

Change in body shape

Energy and ability to participate in recreational activities such as hiking and social dancing

Greater ease performing tasks of daily living, such as climbing stairs and carrying groceries

Improved blood sugar control

Improved cholesterol profile

Increased endurance

Lower blood pressure

Lower resting heart rate

Maintenance of weight

More self-confidence

Reduced insulin resistance

Reduced risk of heart disease and some types of cancer

Stronger bones

Stronger muscles, including heart

Instead, share your plans only with people very close to you.

■ If you're feeling stale, you can try varying your routine or even taking a short break (a few days at most). Sometimes your body needs the rest. If you're so inclined, take advantage of opportunities to try something new, perhaps an activity you've been thinking about for a long time. How about tennis lessons? Or swimming lessons? By participating in sports, you can put some of your fitness to good use, meet new people, and maybe even have a little fun.

■ If you've never thought about weight lifting (also called resistance training), now might be a good time to start. Contrary to popular belief, weight lifting isn't just for enormous men with bulging veins and biceps. In fact, resistance training is good for making just about anyone's muscles and bones stronger. It can help prevent osteoporosis and can make carrying groceries or lifting grandchildren easier. You don't need to belong to a gym to use weights, either: Many people use household items like soup cans or detergent bottles, or they use the weight of their own body for resistance by doing push-ups and sit-ups. A nice bonus to weight lifting is that you can often see and feel impressive results relatively quickly.

■ Don't get hung up trying to "make up" missed exercise sessions. In the long run, one or two missed sessions really make no difference. Just get back into your usual schedule as soon as possible.

■ A sure-fire way to discourage yourself is to compare yourself to what you used to be able to do or to focus on what you're not able to do at the moment. Instead, focus on what you've achieved, not what you haven't been able to do. Exercise is one of the best things you can do for your body, and you should take pride in knowing that you are doing it.

■ If you have had to take a break from exercise for whatever reason, take it slowly at first when you return. Sometimes it's necessary to cut back by as much as 50%, but rest assured that your fitness level will return within a couple of weeks.

Special considerations

Moderate physical activity is a good idea for almost everyone. However, there are a few circumstances that merit a little extra attention before you begin regular exercise or that make taking a day off the wiser decision.

It's been a while. So you haven't broken a sweat since high school football? If you haven't been exercising regularly, especially if you are over 40 or have a health concern such as high blood pressure or heart disease, it's a good idea to discuss your exercise plans with your doctor before you start.

Extreme weather. A little rain or cold need not keep you inside, but severe conditions should. Use common sense, and respect your limits. If you do go out, wear appropriate clothing, such as waterproof pants and a rain jacket and layers to keep warm. Always put your safety first.

Extremely hot weather raises the risk of heat exhaustion or heat stroke and must be taken seriously. If you live in an area that gets very hot or humid, avoid exercising during the middle of the day. Stick to the early mornings and evenings, when it's coolest outside, and be sure to drink lots of water, wear a hat with a brim, and dress in light, thin clothing. If you can't

ACTIVITY ASSESSMENT

This short questionnaire is meant to help you assess how much activity you already fit into your day and identify some ways in which you might become more active. It's not a test; its purpose is just to get you thinking about getting moving.

About how many city blocks do you walk on most days? _____

How many flights of stairs do you climb up or down on most days? _____

How many hours per week do you spend on housework or yard work? _____

How often do you engage in leisure-time activities such as bowling, gardening, golf, tennis, or dancing? _____

How often do you do planned exercise, such as walking, running, swimming, biking, or working out at a gym? _____

How many hours per week do you engage in active play with children or pets? _____

If you work, how many minutes or hours of your workday are not spent sitting or standing still? _____

Total _____

Tally up the number of minutes or hours you spend on physical activity each day or week. Use this as your starting point. If you currently spend a total of 20 minutes each day walking to and from the bus stop, try adding a short walk during your lunch break. If you don't perform any physical activity right now, start off with a small amount, and add more as you feel able.

avoid the heat outside, it may be better to do something inside or even take a break on some days.

Depression. Feeling depressed can sap your motivation to do much of anything: get out of bed in the morning, go to work, make social plans, and, certainly, exercise. Because exercise is often touted as a means of preventing and alleviating depression, you might think you should just force yourself to do it anyway. But that's not necessarily a good idea. Exercise can often boost your mood, but it is not a cure for severe depression, and putting pressure on yourself to exercise when you are very depressed can make things worse. Sometimes you just have to wait for the depression to pass. If it persists, however, you should speak with your physician, because treatment may be necessary.

Hypoglycemia. When you have diabetes, physical activity can lead to hypoglycemia (low blood sugar), especially in people who take insulin. So talk to your doctor or an exercise professional about strategies for avoiding it and treating it if it does develop. (For more information, see the article "Exercise and Blood Sugar" on this page.)

If this were easy

If physical activity were easy, more people would be doing it. Don't be too hard on yourself if you've had trouble starting or sticking with it. As you can see, there are many reasons it can be tough. But the benefits will be worth it. Physical inactivity is one of the leading causes of death in the United States, but it doesn't have to be. Even if you've never tried it before, exercise can help you turn your health around and get your diabetes under control. Good luck and good health. ❏

EXERCISE AND BLOOD SUGAR
Preventing Highs and Lows
by Richard M. Weil, M.Ed., C.D.E., C.S.C.S.

Physical activity has been proven to reverse and prevent heart disease, prevent osteoporosis, lower blood pressure, prevent certain types of cancer, reduce the risk of having a stroke, improve circulation, maintain weight, alleviate symptoms of depression, help control blood sugar and prevent Type 2 diabetes for some, improve self-esteem, and provide literally dozens of other benefits, including increased longevity. In short, we've all got lots of reasons to improve the quality of our lives through physical activity.

However, physical activity presents certain problems for people with diabetes, especially those who take insulin. The main problem is low blood sugar, or hypoglycemia, often defined as blood sugar below 60 mg/dl or, according to some authorities, 70 mg/dl. Hypoglycemia can happen during any type of physical activity: It can happen when you take a brisk walk or ride a bike or work out at the gym. So, as beneficial as physical activity is, the constant risk of low blood sugar can be a deterrent.

Nonetheless, people with diabetes can and do engage in regular physical activity, and some even perform vigorous exercise or participate in competitive sports. In this article, we help you learn how to manage your blood sugar during physical activity. There are no hard and fast rules, and every situation is just a bit different, so we present some real-world scenarios, talk about why blood sugar drops, and offer some guidelines for managing the situations you're likely to encounter.

Fueling your muscles

Whenever your body is in motion, it's your muscles that are making you go. Muscles are your engine and, like all engines, they need fuel. That fuel is carbohydrate and fat from the food you eat. But you don't use all the fuel from the food you eat immediately upon ingestion. Some carbohydrate and fat is stored for later use in liver, muscle, and fat cells. At any given time, a certain amount of fuel (glucose and fat) is circulating in your bloodstream, and a certain amount is in storage.

When you are sitting still, the fuel circulating in your bloodstream is enough to meet your needs. When you start to move, however, your muscles' fuel demands go up, and your body responds by releasing some of its stored fuel into the bloodstream. Once the fuel arrives at the muscles that need it, it leaves the bloodstream and enters the muscle cells.

When glucose arrives at the muscles that need it, insulin must also be present to allow the glucose to enter the cells. Insulin acts as a sort of key to unlock the cell. If insulin is not available, or if the receptors on our muscle cells do not respond properly to insulin (a situation known as insulin resistance), the glucose cannot enter the cells, and blood glucose levels go up. If insulin is available and the muscle cell receptors are working properly, blood glucose levels go down.

The good news for people with diabetes is that physical activity has an "insulin-like" effect: It increases the sensitivity of the cell receptors to insulin, so that whatever insulin is available works more efficiently. Physical activity thus reduces insulin resistance and allows more glucose to enter the muscle cell. During a bout of activity, when the demand for fuel is high, receptors become hypersensitive to insulin, so that more glucose can enter the muscle cells and meet the demand.

As more glucose enters the muscle cells, the drop in blood sugar levels can be rather dramatic. It's common for blood sugar to drop 30, 40, or even 50 points or more during activity, and it can happen rather quickly. The rate at which your blood sugar drops during activity and the amount it drops is dependent on many factors. These factors include the timing of your insulin injection or your last meal in relation to your activity, the type of insulin you take, the intensity of the activity (vigorous activity makes blood sugar drop more than low-intensity activity), and the duration of the activity (in most cases, 30 minutes of an activity will cause blood sugar to drop more than 10 minutes of the same activity).

Not only does blood sugar drop during activity, but it often continues to drop after activity. This is because your muscles continue to burn glucose at a higher rate as they cool down after activity and because they need to replenish the stored glucose that was burned during activity.

So, while the blood-glucose-lowering effect of physical activity is generally a good thing, it can also cause problems when blood glucose goes too low. To help you learn to prevent your blood glucose from dipping too low during and after activity, let's have a look at some people who were experiencing hypoglycemia with physical activity and what they did to solve their problems.

Low blood sugar: Case 1

Greta is 56 years old and has had diabetes for six years. She likes to take a brisk walk before dinner but finds that her blood sugar drops more than 60 points when she does. Because she is away from home when this happens, Greta gets nervous, so she normally treats her low blood sugar by drinking a 5-ounce container of orange juice and eating three glucose tablets.

Greta's hypoglycemia treatment contains about 30 grams of carbohydrate. However, a standard recommendation for treating blood sugar between 60 mg/dl and 70 mg/dl is to consume 15 to 20 grams of carbohydrate (the amount in three or four glucose tablets), wait 15 to 20 minutes, then do a blood sugar check to see if more carbohydrate is needed. If blood sugar is below 60 mg/dl, the standard recommendation is to consume 20 to 25 grams of carbohydrate, wait 15 to 20 minutes, then do a blood sugar check. Since Greta does not check her blood sugar level before taking her juice and glucose tablets, she does not really know how much carbohydrate she should consume, but most likely she is overtreating her hypoglycemia.

While Greta's treatment solves her immediate problem—low blood sugar—it creates another: high blood sugar at bedtime. Her doctor has told her that he would like her blood sugar to be below 160 mg/dl before bed, but when she has to treat hypoglycemia, her blood sugar at bedtime is often more than 210 mg/dl.

Why is Greta's blood sugar dropping so much during her walks? A look into her food diary reveals that at walk time, she usually has not eaten since lunch. Her long-acting insulin (she uses Lente) from the morning is still working just a bit, and, as mentioned earlier, physical activity makes her insulin receptors more sensitive to whatever insulin is available. Because she is walking, her muscles' demand for glucose is high, and her blood sugar drops.

What can Greta do to fix this situation? She could reduce the amount of Lente that she takes in the morning, but that might make her blood sugar high during the day. A better idea would be to have a snack 30 to 45 minutes before her walk. The snack should have some carbohydrate in it, so she might choose a few crackers, a slice of bread, or a small piece of fruit. Greta's dietitian can help her calculate how much to eat.

A simple rule to follow is that 15 grams of carbohydrate will raise your blood sugar approximately 30 mg/dl to 45 mg/dl in 15 to 20 minutes. Of course, this rule varies from person to person, but you can use it as a general guideline. The next time you have a snack, test your blood sugar immediately before you eat and 30 to 45 minutes later to see how much it rises. Then the next time you want to take a brisk walk, you can test 30 minutes beforehand and know whether or not you'll need a snack and how much to eat.

Low blood sugar: Case 2

Joel, age 61, likes to work out at the gym in the morning. He takes NPH and Regular insulin when he wakes up, has his breakfast, and then heads off for his workout. He normally does 35 minutes on a stationary bike and 20 minutes of weight lifting, in that order. Sometimes after the bike he starts to feel funny, and he knows his blood sugar is going low.

One morning he started to feel low after a particularly vigorous workout. He had not eaten all his breakfast (he wasn't hungry), and he did not have his meter with him so he couldn't check his blood sugar level. Recognizing the symptoms of low blood sugar, however, he bought a 16-ounce apple juice at the vending machine and drank all of it. Later that morning his blood sugar was over 300 mg/dl.

What caused Joel's problems? Well, he did not eat all of his breakfast, and that contributed to the low blood sugar during exercise. But he is, after all, only human, and he simply wasn't hungry enough to finish all his food that morning. He also did not have his meter at a time when he knew that he was at risk for hypoglycemia. Again, this is forgivable, but it meant that he could not check his blood sugar and see how much carbohydrate to consume to raise his blood sugar enough but not too much. As a result, he overtreated his hypoglycemia. He felt his blood sugar dropping and had more juice than he needed to raise his blood sugar. (Sixteen ounces of apple juice contains about 60 grams

GENERAL EXERCISE GUIDELINES

The guidelines that follow are just that: guidelines, not absolute rules. Each person's body works a little differently, so each person's food and insulin adjustments for exercise will also be a little different. There is one rule, however: Always review any adjustment in your insulin or meal plan with your doctor or diabetes educator. Here are some tips for keeping you safely on the move:

■ Plan on eating or drinking enough rapidly absorbed carbohydrate before activity to raise your blood sugar enough so that when it drops, it will be around 100 mg/dl after the activity. To know what's enough, keep in mind that 15 grams of easily absorbed carbohydrate, such as glucose tablets or gel, will raise blood sugar approximately 30 to 40 points in 15 to 20 minutes. Eating before activity will protect you against low blood sugar (hypoglycemia) during activity and compensate for any additional drop in blood sugar you may experience later on.

■ People tend to overtreat hypoglycemia. To avoid this, learn to trust your hypoglycemia guidelines. If you don't have guidelines, ask your diabetes educator or doctor.

■ The effect of activity on blood sugar can last for several hours after the activity. This is especially true for people with Type 1 diabetes, in whom the effect can last for 24 hours or more if the activity is long and intense.

■ It's OK to be physically active if your blood sugar is above 240 mg/dl, but you need to take some precautions: Check your blood sugar before physical activity. If it is higher than 240 mg/dl, perform your activity for 15 minutes and check again. If it decreases, it's OK to continue. If it rises, stop the activity and drink fluids. If it rises above 300 mg/dl and you have Type 1 diabetes, check for ketones. If you have ketones, call your doctor or diabetes educator.

■ Injecting insulin immediately before or after activity is OK, and decreasing insulin after activity can be a good strategy for controlling blood sugar.

■ Decreasing nighttime insulin before activity in the morning may be helpful in controlling morning low blood sugar.

■ Insulin decreases for physical activity can be as much as 10% to 90% of daily insulin requirements.

■ Blood glucose generally drops more in response to exercise later in the day (due to increased muscle activity and the possible availability of more insulin) than it does in the morning, when resistance to insulin tends to be higher.

■ Pay attention to when your insulin peaks. If it peaks during your physical activity, your blood sugar may drop more than you expect.

■ If you use insulin, it's a good idea to set up sliding scales for physical activity in addition to your standard meal scales.

■ The only way to learn how much your blood sugar will drop in response to physical activity is to check blood glucose before and after engaging in the activity.

of carbohydrate, three to four times the recommended amount for treating low blood sugar.)

Overtreating hypoglycemia is one of the most common mistakes that people with diabetes make. When you feel your blood sugar dropping, confirm your feeling by doing a blood sugar check with your meter, then trust your hypoglycemia guidelines. If you don't have guidelines, ask your diabetes educator or doctor. Every diabetologist and educator should have hypoglycemia guidelines in their offices. As scary and dangerous as hypoglycemia can be, learning to trust and follow the guidelines will help you treat hypoglycemia properly and safely. Not only that, but your blood sugar throughout the day will be easier to control.

Low blood sugar: Case 3

Dave is 68 years old and has been active for most of his life. On a typical day, he takes a brisk walk after lunch, and he plays tennis after dinner at least twice a week. He was diagnosed with diabetes when he was 64 and began taking insulin almost immediately. For the most part, his treatment plan has kept his blood sugar in his target range. However, his blood sugar levels often tend to be toward the lower end of his target range, so when he exercises, he frequently comes close to developing hypoglycemia.

Here's what happens to him on nights he plays tennis. He normally takes 7 to 11 units of Regular insulin before dinner on a sliding scale (meaning he adjusts his dose according to his blood sugar level before dinner and according to how much carbohydrate he plans to eat at dinner). His tennis game begins about 90 minutes after he's finished eating. At bedtime, his blood sugar tends to be low. He has had many episodes of waking in the middle of the night bathed in sweat, and this concerns him and his wife. When he checks his blood glucose level during those episodes, it is generally around 45 mg/dl.

What can Dave do to avoid these frightening occurrences of low blood sugar? Dave's nighttime hypoglycemia demonstrates that the effect of activity on blood sugar can last for several hours after the activity is complete. It also demonstrates that when a person engages in physical activity at the same time as his insulin is peaking (or is reaching peak effectiveness), the combination can have a potent blood-sugar-lowering effect. (Regular insulin peaks about two to three hours after it is injected, so Dave's tennis game is under way just as his dinnertime insulin is reaching maximum effectiveness.)

The best solution for Dave would be to reduce the amount of Regular insulin he takes before dinner on nights he plays tennis. Remember that activity has an insulin-like effect. In Dave's case, the activity combined with the insulin works together to lower his blood sugar more than normal, even hours after he's done playing.

With the assistance of his diabetes educator, Dave developed a sliding scale for tennis that was added to his normal dinner sliding scale. For example, his normal dinner sliding scale instructs him to take 7 units of Regular insulin before dinner when his blood sugar is between 100 mg/dl and 140 mg/dl. His tennis-night scale amends those 7 units to 4 units before a game. It's common to reduce an insulin dose by 50% or more before activity, but each person needs a slightly different adjustment. Your educator or doctor can help you devise a sliding scale just for you.

An alternative solution for Dave would be to eat more carbohydrate at dinner before his tennis games. But many people do not want to eat more, so for them, adjusting insulin is a better option.

Adjusting rapid-acting insulin

Rapid-acting insulin, such as insulin lispro (brand name Humalog) or insulin aspart (Novolog), has some obvious advantages when it comes to eating. Because rapid-acting insulin starts working within minutes of taking it, you can sit down to a meal, check your blood sugar, take your insulin, and eat; no more waiting 30 minutes before eating, as is generally necessary with Regular insulin. When it comes to physical activity, however, rapid-acting insulin raises management issues just like any other type of insulin. In short, the amount and timing of food, insulin, and activity all need to be taken into account in order to maintain blood glucose in the target range. And that can be quite a tall order. Let's have a look at the experience of one lispro user.

Renee, who has had Type 1 diabetes since she was a kid, is an editor and reporter for her small-town newspaper. She is 39 years old. Her job keeps her on the go, and she likes to take aerobics classes at lunchtime. She often wolfs down her lunch so she can get to class on time. The problem is that if she takes lispro right before eating, and the class starts just 15 minutes after she eats, her insulin is peaking just as class starts, and her blood sugar drops too much during the class. She ends up having to eat more to treat her low blood sugar. But she doesn't want to eat so much. She's concerned about her weight, and she finds it discouraging to have to eat every time she wants to exercise.

How can Renee adjust her diabetes-care plan so that she can exercise when she wants, eat what she wants, and avoid low blood sugar? Her first adjustment was to reduce the amount of lispro she took before lunch. Because Renee is very sensitive to the effects of lispro, as are many people, she and her doctor worked out a sliding scale for activity that lowered her dose of lispro by more than 50%, from 5 units to 2 units, before aerobics classes. She also added a half a piece of fruit to her lunch to keep her blood sugar from dropping too much.

But then another problem developed. When Renee followed her new scale, her blood sugar before dinner was often above 240 mg/dl. The reason was that the lunchtime lispro was gone from her system after two hours. But her liver continued to produce glucose between meals—the way it's supposed to. By dinnertime, even though she had some insulin working from her morning injection of Lente, it was not enough to keep her blood sugar level where she wanted it.

Renee considered increasing her morning dose of Lente to solve the problem, but because she is so active at her job, doing so would cause her blood sugar to be too low throughout the day. Instead, her doctor recommended switching to Regular insulin before lunch, because it works for a longer period than lispro. And indeed, Renee found that taking Regular before lunch worked better to "hold" her blood sugar from rising too much in the late afternoon on days she did aerobics.

Rapid-acting insulin can be a very helpful management tool for many people, but it isn't the best choice for every situation. If you use rapid-acting insulin and are having trouble keeping your blood sugar in your target range when you exercise, speak with your diabetes educator or doctor about making adjustments to your insulin regimen or using other forms of insulin some or all of the time.

High blood sugar

Every once in a while, your blood sugar may go up with activity. The reason is that your liver always produces glucose when you start activity. If you're not burning up as much glucose as your liver is producing, then it's possible for the level of glucose in your bloodstream to be higher after activity than it was before. This doesn't mean that the activity didn't contribute to your fitness, or that you didn't burn up glu-

STRATEGIC SNACKING

The following example shows how what you eat and when can make a big difference in your blood sugar control. Donald checked his blood sugar at 11:30 AM, right before he was ready to go jogging. It was within his target range, but since he knew it was going to drop during the jog, he ate some graham crackers and peanut butter. He jogged immediately after eating and, in spite of his snack, his blood sugar dropped. He treated the hypoglycemia with juice, and then had lunch. At 1:30 PM, his blood sugar was high.

TIME	BLOOD GLUCOSE	MEDICINE/ FOOD	ACTIVITY
7:45 AM	166 mg/dl	14 Lente, 10 Regular	
11:30 AM	124 mg/dl	graham crackers and peanut butter	
11:35 AM			30-minute jog
12:15 PM	51 mg/dl	8 ounces of juice and lunch	
1:30 PM	226 mg/dl		

What happened? Although Donald had the right idea to have a snack before exercise, the crackers and peanut butter he ate were not absorbed rapidly enough to prevent a drop during exercise. (Fat and protein slow digestion.) Then, after the workout, the crackers and peanut butter kicked in along with the juice and lunch, raising his blood sugar.

Donald tried again the next day. He was ready to jog at 3:45 PM and checked his blood sugar. It was 106 mg/dl, so he drank four ounces of juice, waited 15 minutes, tested again, and then jogged. This time, his blood glucose level was 137 mg/dl after his jog.

TIME	BLOOD GLUCOSE	MEDICINE/ FOOD	ACTIVITY
8:00 AM	138 mg/dl	14 Lente, 6 Regular	
Noon	161 mg/dl	4 Regular	
12:30 PM		lunch	
3:45 PM	106 mg/dl	4 ounces of juice	
4:00 PM	137 mg/dl		30-minute jog

The main difference between this day and the previous day is that Donald drank juice, a rapidly absorbed carbohydrate, and waited 15 minutes for his blood sugar to rise before jogging. This allowed him to jog safely without the risk of hypoglycemia.

In the future, he will allow himself 15 minutes before activity to raise his blood sugar if he needs to. When figuring out how much to eat, he will plan on having enough rapidly absorbed carbohydrate so that when his blood sugar drops during exercise, it will be around 100 mg/dl at the end of his jog. This will compensate for any additional drop he may experience later on.

cose. It just means that during that particular activity session, you had more glucose in your bloodstream than your muscles could burn.

Blood sugar also rises during activity when you have a low level of insulin in your system at the time you're active. Remember that physical activity has an insulin-like effect, but it's not insulin. It only works to lower your blood sugar when insulin is available. For this reason, people with Type 1 diabetes, whose pancreases do not produce any insulin, have a greater likelihood of blood sugar rising with activity.

In people with Type 1 diabetes, a blood sugar level above 300 mg/dl is dangerous because it raises the risk of ketoacidosis—a life-threatening complication. Whenever your blood sugar rises above this level, drink plenty of water and test your urine for ketones. If you have any ketones, contact your doctor or diabetes educator for advice.

STRIKING A BALANCE

Sometimes it's OK to change the time you eat and take insulin to accommodate your schedule and manage blood sugar. In the following sequence, you see how one person adjusted the timing of her insulin and meals in relation to activity.

Maritza took her insulin at 6:30 AM, waited half an hour, ate breakfast, and then biked for 35 minutes at 7:10. Because the Regular insulin was working but the food from breakfast had not had enough time to enter her bloodstream (it takes at least 15 to 20 minutes for glucose from food to be absorbed into the bloodstream), her blood sugar dropped to 47 mg/dl during her bike ride. At 7:50, therefore, she had to have more food, something she would have preferred not to do.

TIME	BLOOD GLUCOSE	MEDICINE/ FOOD	ACTIVITY
6:30 AM	112 mg/dl	9 NPH, 4 Regular	
7:00	104 mg/dl	breakfast	
7:10			35-minute bike ride
7:50	47 mg/dl	6 ounces of juice, raisins	
12:45 PM	162 mg/dl	lunch	

The next day, Maritza tried a new strategy. She took her insulin and then immediately hopped on her bike. After her workout, she had breakfast. You can see from her numbers (below) that this strategy helped keep her blood sugar from dropping. She was pleased because there was no need to eat any extra food as she had to do the day before. The reason this worked is that the insulin did not have time to start working, and typically in the morning, blood sugar does not drop as much as it does later in the day.

However, by 10:00 AM, Maritza's blood sugar was getting low. This is because exercise can continue to lower blood sugar hours after the activity has stopped.

TIME	BLOOD GLUCOSE	MEDICINE/ FOOD	ACTIVITY
6:45 AM	129 mg/dl	9 NPH, 4 Regular	30-minute bike ride
7:30	118 mg/dl	breakfast	
10:00	71 mg/dl		
12:30 PM	61 mg/dl	lunch	

Maritza tried a third strategy the following morning. She biked first, then took her insulin. She also reduced the amount of Regular insulin, from 4 units to 3. She did something else interesting: She ate 15 minutes after taking her insulin instead of 30 minutes after so that the food would get absorbed into her bloodstream before the insulin peaked. This prevented the mid-morning low she experienced the day before.

TIME	BLOOD GLUCOSE	MEDICINE/ FOOD	ACTIVITY
6:45 AM	99 mg/dl		30-minute bike ride
7:30	86 mg/dl	9 NPH, 3 Regular (normally 4)	
7:45		breakfast	
10:00	104 mg/dl		
12:30 PM	90 mg/dl	lunch	

One additional note: You should keep in mind that sometimes blood sugar will drop in the morning during activity because insulin from the night before is still in the bloodstream. For this reason, if you find that your blood sugar still drops in the morning after making interventions like the examples here, you may need to adjust the insulin from the night before.

Blood sugar above 240 mg/dl

For the longest time, people with diabetes have been told to restrict their physical activity when their blood sugar is above 240 mg/dl. The reason is that there is a risk of blood sugar rising higher. This is overly cautious advice that discourages many people from activity. One of the benefits of physical activity is that it improves your sensitivity to insulin. If you were to restrict your activity level every time your blood sugar was above 240 mg/dl, you'd never see the benefit.

Most people can be physically active when their blood sugar is above 240 mg/dl. In fact, people can be physically active even when their blood sugar is above 300 mg/dl. A recent study completed in Michigan showed that when more than 1,000 workout sessions were monitored among 76 people with Type 1 and Type 2 diabetes who started with blood sugar levels between 240 mg/dl and 300 mg/dl, during only four of the sessions did their blood sugar rise.

Here are some simple rules to follow. If your blood sugar is above 240 mg/dl, start your activity and after 15 minutes check your blood sugar again. If it decreases, continue your activity. If it rises, stop your activity. If you have Type 1 diabetes and your blood sugar rises above 300 mg/dl, test for ketones, drink plenty of water, and, if you have ketones, call your doctor or diabetes educator.

Even though exercising when your blood sugar is above 240 mg/dl is generally safe, it may not always be desirable. Some people don't feel well when their blood sugar is over 240 mg/dl, and that is certainly a good reason not to exercise at that particular time.

Oral pills

In general, the later-generation oral diabetes pills will not make you hypoglycemic with activity. However, many people feel symptoms of low blood sugar as their blood sugar drops during activity and assume they have hypoglycemia. If you treat yourself for hypoglycemia when you are not really hypoglycemic, you are likely to end up with higher blood sugar throughout the day. So it's important to check your blood glucose with your meter when you feel symptoms of low blood sugar. If you feel symptoms of hypoglycemia but your meter says your blood glucose is over 70 mg/dl, you may find it helpful to consume some tea, broth, or other no-calorie beverage.

Some oral pills, such as metformin (Glucophage), are frequently prescribed in combination with insulin. Because these drugs help make insulin work more effectively, hypoglycemia with physical activity is a real possibility with these combinations. If you are active and you take a combination of oral pills and insulin, you may need to lower your insulin dose to prevent hypoglycemia. Your doctor or diabetes educator can help you with that.

Anticipating your body's reaction

The key to managing blood sugar during and after physical activity is to anticipate whether your blood sugar will go up or down—and by how much—and learn what to do about it. The only way to learn to predict what your blood sugar will do is to regularly check and record your blood sugar levels immediately before and after activity. With the numbers in your logbook, you and your diabetes educator can come up with some creative ways to manage your blood sugar.

Once you have an idea how your body reacts to activity, you won't have to test every time. But doing it initially will give you some insight into how your body works, which in turn will give you a sense of control and satisfaction. With effective blood sugar management skills under your belt, you should be able to maintain a healthy, physically active lifestyle that you can feel good about. Good luck. ❏

GETTING STRONGER
Easier Than You Think
by Richard M. Weil, M.Ed., C.D.E., C.S.C.S.

Whether you're starting an exercise program for the first time or would like to augment your current plan of physical activity, resistance training has a lot to offer. One of the most obvious benefits is stronger muscles, which can make getting around, shopping, and other daily activities much easier to perform. Less obvious is resistance training's ability to help lower blood sugar levels, control body weight, improve coordination and balance, and maintain strong bones. Studies have shown that anyone, at any age, can do resistance training safely.

Resistance training is so named because it uses resistance to build muscles: The exerciser's muscles move or contract against some type of external resistance to develop or maintain strength. Resistance exercises can be done with weight machines, free weights (such as dumbbells or household objects), rubber surgical tubing, or rubber exercise bands. Calisthenics such as sit-ups and push-ups are also resistance exercises; in these exercises, your body acts as a weight.

Before you start

Resistance training is a safe pursuit, but check with your doctor or diabetes educator anyway before you start. Your doctor or educator can help you decide which exercises, if any, might not be safe for you.

If you have retinopathy, you *must* talk to your ophthalmologist before doing resistance exercise. This sort of exercise can cause a temporary rise in blood pressure, which can cause bleeding in your eyes if you have certain kinds of retinopathy. It's also important to avoid exercises that put your head below your heart if you have moderate or proliferative retinopathy. Your eye doctor should be able to advise you on what's safe and not safe for you.

A safety point for everyone to keep in mind is that resistance exercise will cause blood sugar to drop. So it's a good idea to check your blood sugar before and after exercising and to keep handy a food containing carbohydrate (such as glucose tablets, fruit juice, or raisins) in case your blood sugar level dips too much. Talk to your doctor or educator about making adjustments in your insulin regimen or food plan before and during exercise.

Getting started

When you start your resistance training program, work with a weight that you can lift (or push or pull) 12–15 times in a row without stopping. You may need to try out a few different weights to find a good starting weight for each exercise. You will most likely find that you need lighter weights for some exercises and can use heavier weights for others.

Whenever you perform resistance exercises, be sure to use proper form. This will prevent you from pulling a muscle or otherwise hurting yourself. Most health clubs and gyms have a fitness trainer who can show you proper form and observe you lifting to make sure you are maintaining it. If you are following diagrams and written instructions, read the exercise description carefully, and watch yourself in a mirror to make sure you are working the muscles for which the exercise is intended. Muscle awareness is important, so you should feel it in the muscle as well as see it in the mirror.

Here are some guidelines for safe lifting:
■ If you can't lift a weight 12–15 times with good form, it's too heavy, and you should try a lighter load.
■ If you have to arch your back or bend in an unfamiliar or awkward position to lift a weight (or pull a

rubber band or move your body), the resistance is too strong, and you should cut back.
■ Sometimes it takes a few sessions to feel the exercise in the muscle group for which the exercise is designed. Just remember to concentrate on the body part you're supposed to be working.
■ Holding your breath while lifting can temporarily raise your blood pressure to dangerous levels, so breathing properly is important when you do resistance exercise. You should exhale with effort. This means that when the weight feels heaviest (usually when you're pulling or pushing against gravity) you should exhale slowly. Inhale as you return to a resting position.

Once you have selected starting weights and know how to lift with good form, you're ready to get into a routine. The standard recommendation for anyone who wants to build strength is to work out three times a week, but even once or twice a week is better than nothing. Studies show that doing resistance exercise twice a week is enough to maintain strength. You can always increase the frequency of your lifting sessions when you're ready.

For general conditioning, you will want to do one to three sets of 12–15 repetitions of each exercise you choose to do. As the weeks go by, you'll notice that your weights get easier to lift. When this happens, it's time to increase the resistance. If you're using dumbbells, go up to the next weight. With rubber exercise bands, go up to the next resistance, or you can wrap the band around your hand to tighten it. Note that when you increase the weight or resistance, you need to drop the number of repetitions, at least initially. Start your higher weight with 12 (not 15) repetitions per set.

Training tools

Resistance training can be accomplished in many ways, so there's no need to invest in a fancy set of weights unless you want to. Here are some of the possibilities:

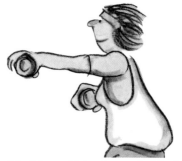

Household objects. Using household objects—preferably ones you can grip easily—is an easy and inexpensive way to start resistance training. Soup can exercises make a great routine for beginners. As you get stronger, you can increase the resistance by using bottles of water. (A 1-liter bottle filled with water weighs 2½ pounds.)

Soup Can Exercises

Use small, unopened soup cans, filled water bottles, or small dumbbells for these exercises. Repeat each movement 12 to 15 times.

FRONT RAISE
Start with your arms at your sides. With palms facing down, lift arms to the front until they are parallel to the floor. Return to starting position.

SIDE LATERAL RAISE
Start with your arms at your sides. With palms facing down, lift arms to sides until they are parallel to the floor. Return to starting position.

PUNCHES
Start with your elbows bent, hands at chest level. Extend one arm forward, pull it back, and extend the other arm, keeping your palms facing down.

KICKBACKS
Bend forward slightly from the hips and bend your knees slightly. Hold your weights at hip height, elbows pointing back. Straighten your elbows, extending your forearms and hands back. With arms extended, raise your weights as high as you can (another couple of inches). Return to starting position.

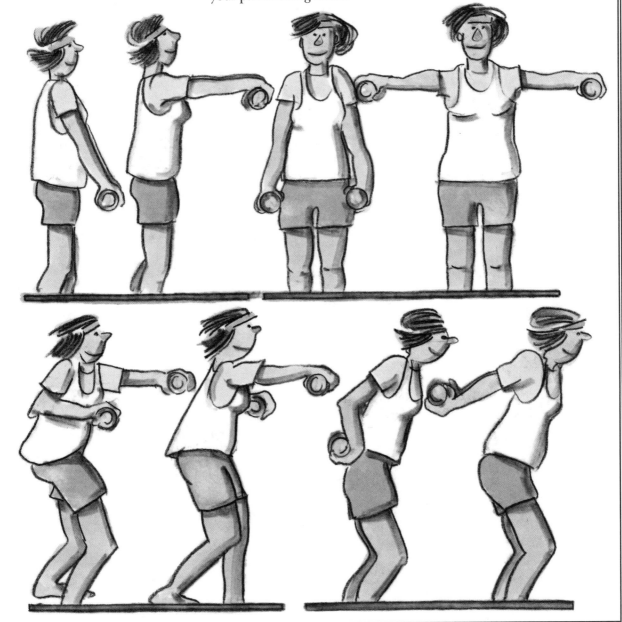

Calisthenics

These exercises use your body weight as the source of resistance. Repeat each 12 to 15 times.

WALL PUSH-UP

Stand 24 to 36 inches from a wall and extend your arms toward the wall, keeping your hands lower than your shoulders. Lean against the wall with your arms straight. Then bend your elbows and touch your nose to the wall, *keeping your back straight*. Push back to starting position.

CHAIR LIFT

Sit in a straight-back chair that has arms. Keeping your back straight, put your hands on the chair arms and push up so your buttocks and thighs lift off the chair. Hold for three seconds, then return to starting position.

TOE TOUCH

Stand with your feet shoulder width apart and your arms out to each side, parallel to the floor. Bend your knees, then bend forward from the hips and touch your left foot with your right hand. Return to starting position and repeat with your left hand and right foot.

Free Weights

Pick a weight you can lift or press 12–15 times without stopping to rest. For most beginners, a good starting weight is between 1 and 5 pounds.

If you have a history of frozen shoulder or other shoulder problems, start the overhead press, upright row, and overhead extension with a very light weight or no weight at all. If any of these exercises hurts, stop doing it and don't resume until you have talked to your doctor about it.

OVERHEAD PRESS
Start by holding your dumbbells to either side of your head, elbows at shoulder height. Extend your arms overhead, straightening your elbows. Return to starting position.

UPRIGHT ROW
Start by holding your dumbbells in front of your thighs. Pull the weights up to your armpits; your elbows should be slightly above shoulder height. Return to starting position.

BICEPS
Stand with your arms at your sides, knees bent slightly. Keeping your upper arm still, bring your hands toward your shoulders, bending only at the elbow. Lower your hands slowly to starting position.

OVERHEAD EXTENSION
Hold one dumbbell behind your head, elbow pointing to the side. Extend your arm upward by straightening your elbow; your arm will be at a slight angle, not perpendicular to the floor. Return to starting position. Repeat with your other arm.

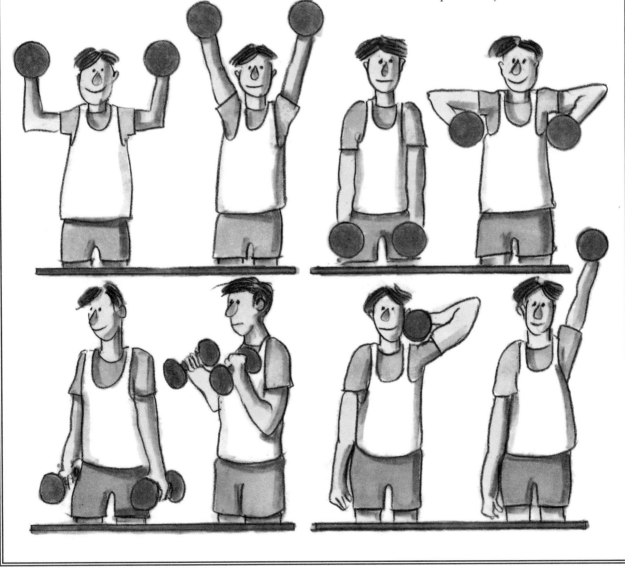

Rubber Band Exercises

Use a rubber exercise band or band of surgical tubing for these exercises. Select a resistance you can pull or push 12–15 times in a row, and be careful to always release the resistance in a slow, controlled manner. Allowing the band to "snap" your arm back to its starting position can injure your joints.

To maintain your balance while doing these exercises, stand with one foot ahead of the other (as if you were taking a step).

DOOR PULL

Place one end of a rubber band around the doorknob of an open door (or have a partner hold it), and hold the other end in your hand. Keeping your arm bent at a 90° angle, pull away from the door (or your partner), then return to your starting position, releasing the tension slowly. Repeat 12–15 times, then switch hands.

DOOR PUSH

Place one end of a rubber band around the doorknob of an open door, and hold the other end in your right hand. Standing with your right side to the door, hold your right hand at shoulder height in front of you, palm facing toward you. Push the band forward until you feel resistance. Return to your starting position, releasing the tension slowly. Repeat 12–15 times, then place your left side to the door and do the exercise with your left hand.

TWO-HAND STRETCH

Keeping your elbows at your sides, hold your hands in front of you and loop the rubber band around the backs of both hands. Keep your arms bent at a 90° angle. Slowly move your hands away from each other so that you feel resistance from the band. Return to your starting position, releasing the tension slowly. Repeat 12–15 times.

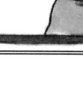

Your own body weight. Sit-ups, wall push-ups, and alternating toe touches are examples of exercises you can do at home that use your own body weight as a source of resistance. Using your own body weight can be difficult, so go slowly at first. If these moves prove to be too tough, try the soup can exercises first.

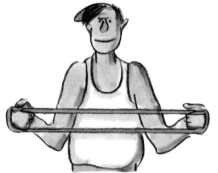

Rubber exercise bands. If you're feeling more ambitious, you can use rubber exercise bands or rubber surgical tubing. These bands are sold through some mail-order sources, at sporting good stores, and at surgical supply stores. You may even see them advertised on TV. Rubber exercise bands come in a variety of resistances, which are usually designated by color. Start with a band you can stretch 12–15 times.

Free weights. Many of the soup can exercises can be done with dumbbells, which may be easier to grip in your hands. Your local sporting goods shop should have everything you need. A good starting weight for dumbbells is from 1 to 5 pounds. Try the dumbbells in the store with some of the exercises illustrated here to determine what amount of weight is right for you.

The payoff

The best way to know if your training is working is to pay attention to how you feel as you go through your day. Do you have more energy? Is it easier to lift packages or carry bags of groceries? Can you get out of your chair or your car faster and with less effort? Do you simply *feel* stronger?

Feeling better and moving more easily may be all the motivation you need to continue your resistance exercise routine. But there are some other important benefits you may notice as you build your muscles, including the following:

Blood sugar control. Increasing the strength of your muscles causes them to burn more glucose. Conditioned muscles burn more glucose because they are more sensitive to insulin, and when insulin works better, your blood sugar level is typically lower. Research shows that resistance exercise is a good way to help keep your blood sugar level under control.

Weight control. Both men and women generally gain a pound of fat and lose a half pound of muscle every year between the ages of 25 and 55. Much of this fat gain, muscle loss, and overall weight gain may be the result of inactivity. As you lose muscle, your resting metabolic rate (the amount of calories your body burns at rest) slows down. If your resting metabolic rate is low, it becomes more difficult to burn calories.

Resistance training can help speed up your metabolism or prevent it from slowing down further. One study showed that if you do resistance training three days a week, the number of calories you need to maintain your weight increases by 15%.

People who are working on losing weight or planning to start a weight-loss plan can benefit a lot from doing resistance training. Typically, when people lose weight, 25% of their weight loss is muscle. Those who lose weight very quickly (more than 1% to 2% of body weight per week) lose even more muscle. Resistance exercise can both minimize the muscle loss and help maintain any weight loss by keeping the metabolic rate from slowing down.

Even if you are not overweight, doing resistance exercise is important because it can slow the rate of muscle loss that typically happens with age. Not only will your body look and feel more youthful, but you will lower your chances of experiencing the health risks associated with too much body fat and the poor balance, weakness, and frailty associated with low muscle mass.

Bone strength. More than 25 million Americans suffer from osteoporosis, a debilitating disease that causes the bones to deteriorate and weaken. Research shows that exercise, along with other measures such as calcium supplementation, is helpful in preventing and treating osteoporosis. Resistance exercise has been shown to be particularly helpful. Some studies show that lifting weights as little as two times a week can significantly increase bone health, sometimes making bones 3% thicker after just 12 weeks of lifting.

Studies have also shown that resistance exercise can reduce the risk of falling—a significant benefit for those at risk of bone fractures because of osteoporosis. People who participated in these studies developed better coordination and balance, so they walked more steadily.

Self-confidence. One of the greatest benefits of resistance exercise is that it will give you the strength and confidence to do the things you want to do independently. If you feel like you can do physical things, the quality of your life will be better. Most people who lift weights feel stronger, more in charge, and more self-reliant.

Whatever resistance routine you choose, the most important thing is that you keep it up. Start at a pace you're comfortable with, maintain consistency, and the results will follow. You really don't have anything to lose, do you? And your body will thank you. ❑

EXERCISES TO STRENGTHEN YOUR FEET

by Richard M. Weil, M.Ed., C.D.E., C.S.C.S.

Leonardo da Vinci said that the human foot is a work of art and a masterpiece of engineering. While some may quibble with da Vinci's aesthetic, it is indeed hard not to marvel at the construction of the foot: Each human foot is made up of 26 bones, 19 muscles, 107 ligaments, 33 joints, 250,000 sweat glands, and thousands of tiny nerve receptors. Your feet can bear four to five times your body weight and still bounce back quickly.

This resiliency is a good thing, too, considering the amount of use and stress your feet undergo. You march on them 8,000 to 10,000 times a day, smother them in socks and shoe leather, make them sweat, stub their appendages, and they still faithfully carry you everywhere you want to go. In your lifetime, your feet will lug you more than 115,000 miles—that's four times around the globe—yet you probably know more about how your car operates than how your feet do.

But it's never too late to learn, if not how your feet operate then at least to appreciate them for what they do. You've heard plenty about foot care—inspecting your feet, cutting your nails, and daily cleaning—so we decided it was time to pay homage to your feet with an article that will teach you how to exercise, stretch, and pamper them.

Exercising your feet. You've heard of strong biceps, pectorals, and even gluteals. But how about strong foot muscles—who ever talks about them? Feet are one of the most heavily used parts of the body, yet they are often taken for granted—at least until foot pain strikes. Over 70% of Americans will experience painful foot problems at least once. Exercises that strengthen the feet can often prevent or alleviate such problems. If your feet ache when you walk, hike, jog, or participate in other physical activities—and you and your podiatrist have ruled out anatomical foot problems or ill-fitting shoes as the cause—foot exercises may help. See pages 253 and 254 for some exercises that you can do to help you improve your foot strength and flexibility as well as the blood circulation in your feet.

RESOURCES

For the most part, strengthening and pampering your feet requires little equipment or outside help. However, if you are interested in buying exercise bands or a wobble board, reading up on specific foot problems, or finding a massage or reflexology professional in your area, the following addresses may be of help.

AMERICAN MASSAGE THERAPY ASSOCIATION
820 Davis Street, Suite 100
Evanston, IL 60201-4444
(847) 864-0123
www.amtamassage.org
Offers information about massage and provides referrals to licensed massage therapists.

AMERICAN PODIATRIC MEDICAL ASSOCIATION
9312 Old Georgetown Road
Bethesda, MD 20814
(800) FOOT-CARE
(366-8227)
www.apma.org
Publishes brochures about a variety of foot problems and provides referrals to podiatrists.

REFLEXOLOGY ASSOCIATION OF AMERICA
4012 South Rainbow,
Suite K-PMB# K55
Las Vegas, NV 89103-2059
www.reflexology-usa.org
Conducts and gathers research on reflexology. Provides research updates and referrals to reflexologists.

FOOT REFLEXOLOGY AWARENESS ASSOCIATION
P.O. Box 7622
Mission Hills, CA 91346
Publishes a newsletter on reflexology, offers information on groups and resources in your area, and provides referrals to reflexologists.

ORTHOPEDIC PHYSICAL THERAPY PRODUCTS
3700 Annapolis Lane,
Suite 175
P.O. Box 47009
Minneapolis, MN 55447-0009
(888) 819-0121
www.optp.com
Sells physical therapy products, including wobble boards and rubber exercise bands. Visit the Web site or call or write for a free catalog.

Exercising your ankles. Your ankles deserve some credit and attention, too. They're the hinge joints that allow your feet to flex and extend so you can walk, dance, and run. For some of us, however, ankle sprains are an all-too-familiar problem that may keep us from engaging in activities we enjoy. By exercising and strengthening your ankles, you can lower your chances of another sprain as well as increase your ankles' range of motion and degree of flexibility. You will also be improving circulation to your feet. A series of ankle-strengthening exercises is described beginning on page 254.

Finding your balance. Gymnasts and tightrope walkers are not the only ones who need to be concerned about balance. Many of us have difficulty with balance at one time or another, and some forms of diabetic nerve damage are known to disrupt physical coordination and balance. Fortunately, balance can be improved. With a fitness plan that consistently includes balancing exercises, you can gradually refine your sense of balance and coordination. To help get you started, we describe some balancing exercises on page 256.

Stretching it out. There's nothing like a good stretch. Even if you are too busy to do the foot and ankle exercises religiously, you probably won't mind just stretching out at the end of a long day. And that's not such a bad thing, because there's more packed into a simple stretch than you might realize: Stretching reduces muscular tension, increases range of motion and coordination, prevents injuries, and promotes circulation. In addition, it feels good. The stretches shown on pages 256 and 257 can be especially helpful if you have circulatory problems in your calves that cause you to experience cramping while you are walking or while you sleep.

Rubbing it out. Your poor neglected feet! They work for you all day long and never get a thank-you. Well, you can start thanking your feet today with a good foot rub. You may think of massage as a way to relieve neck and back tension. But if you think a back massage feels good, wait until you try a foot rub. Not only will your feet feel wonderful, but tension that's been building up all day will disappear from your whole body—including your lower back, shoulders, and neck—leaving you calm and relaxed. It's nice to have someone else rub your feet, but you can do a pretty good job yourself. One simple yet effective technique for a foot massage is shown on page 257.

You may also want to investigate a type of massage called reflexology that has been practiced in China for thousands of years. It is done by applying pressure to small areas, or "reflex points," on the feet. While some people believe that each reflex point corresponds to a particular area or organ in the body, others believe that reflexology just plain feels great. For information about contacting a reflexologist, you can call a local massage center, Y, or fitness center. Your doctor or diabetes educator might even be able to point you in the right direction. You can also contact the American Massage Therapy Association or the reflexology resources on page 252.

So there you have it. An article about feet without a mention of inspecting for sores or clipping your toenails. We hope you see your feet in a whole new light now and start to take care of them the way they've taken care of you for so long. ❏

STRONG FEET

Strength training for feet may sound funny, but it can make a big difference in how your feet feel at the end of the day. This is especially true if you walk a lot, dance, hike, or do other activities that keep you on your feet. For best results, do each exercise three times a week, leaving a day of rest in between each session.

TOE SPREADER

1. Remove your shoes and socks and sit in a chair with your back straight and your feet flat on the floor.
2. Spread your toes apart on your right foot, hold for three seconds, and then relax. Repeat 15 times.

3. Switch to your left foot and do the exercise 15 times.
4. Do two more sets of 15 on each foot.

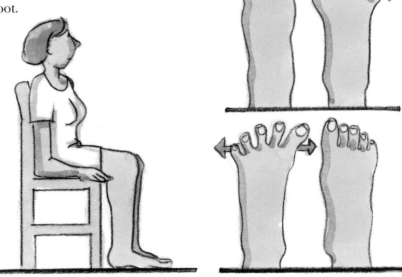

TOWEL PULLER

1. Remove your shoes and socks and sit in a chair with your back straight and your feet flat on the floor. (You can also try this one standing up.)
2. Place a medium-size hand towel on the floor with one edge under the toes of one foot. (If you like, you can use two towels and do both feet at once.) This exercise is easier on an uncarpeted floor.
3. Keeping your heel on the floor, drag and gather the towel under your foot by curling your toes. Do this until the entire towel is under your foot.
4. Repeat 10 times for each foot. If your toes or calves cramp during this exercise, do the calf stretch shown on page 256.

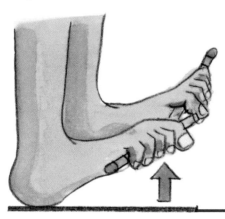

PENCIL GRABBER

1. Remove your shoes and socks and sit in a chair with your back straight and your feet flat on the floor.
2. Place two pencils on the floor, one under the toes of each foot.
3. Lift the pencils off the floor by curling your toes around them and either lifting your legs a few inches off the floor or flexing your feet so only your heels remain on the floor. Hold the pencils off the floor for five seconds. Hold on to the edge of the chair for support. If you have trouble grasping pencils, try thick, felt-tipped markers. You can also do this exercise with marbles, cord, or other small objects.
4. Return your feet to the floor, release the pencils, then lift them again.
5. Repeat the pencil lift 30 times, pausing between each set of 10.

STRONG ANKLES

These exercises strengthen the muscles that surround and support your ankles. They can be especially helpful if you're prone to ankle sprains.

ANKLE CIRCLES

1. Remove your shoes and socks and sit with your back straight in a chair or on a bed or sofa.
2. Extend one leg so your foot is a few inches above the floor, then rotate your foot in a clockwise direction 10 times. Next, rotate your foot in a counterclockwise direction 10 times.
3. Repeat the exercise with the other foot. Do three sets of 20 circles on each foot. This exercise also serves as an ankle stretch.

ANKLE CIRCLE VARIATIONS

1. Instead of rotating your foot, imagine that your toes are the tip of a pencil, then try writing your name in the air with the motion of your foot.
2. Grasp a pencil in your toes and try writing your name on a piece of paper on the floor.
3. Try these writing exercises standing as well as sitting. You may need to hold on to something for support while standing.

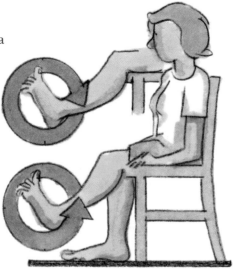

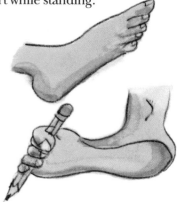

HEEL RAISES

1. Stand up straight, placing one hand on a wall or on the back of a chair for support if you need it.
2. Raise up onto your toes and hold for three seconds, trying to balance without the wall or chair if possible.
3. Lower your heels slowly to floor.
4. Repeat 30 times, with a brief pause after each 10 raises.

HEEL RAISE VARIATION

1. For a better stretch and increased range of motion, stand on the bottom step of a staircase, facing up the stairwell. Hold on to the railing or put one hand on the wall for support. Place your feet so that your toes and the balls of your feet are on the stair and your heels are suspended in air. Lower your heels below the level of the step.
2. Raise up onto your toes, then lower back to the starting position.
3. Repeat for three sets of 10 heel raises.

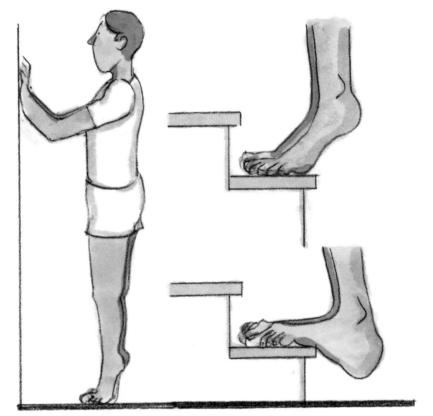

RUBBER BAND PULL

Exercise bands resembling large rubber bands can be used to condition many parts of the body, including the feet and ankles. They can be purchased at most sporting goods stores or through the mail, and they come in a variety of tensions, usually identified by color. Start with the lowest tension for these exercises.
1. Loop the rubber band around the leg of a sofa or heavy chair. Keeping your shoes on, sit on the floor facing the sofa or chair.
2. Slip the rubber band over your toe or tie it to the lowest part of your shoelace. Sit far enough from the sofa so the rubber band is extended but not stretched.
3. Lean back on your arms for support and flex your ankle. You should feel some resistance from the rubber band. Hold the flex for three seconds then slowly return to starting position.
4. Do three sets of 12 flexes for each foot.

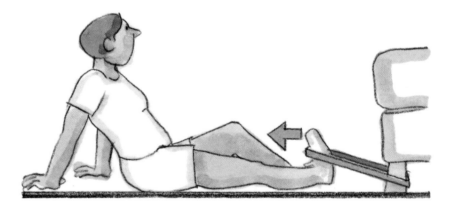

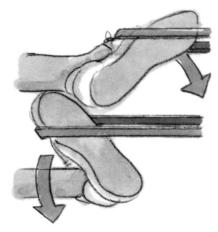

RUBBER BAND PULL VARIATION

1. Use the same starting position but flex and turn the ankle in. The big toe should lead. Hold for three seconds then slowly release.
2. Use the same starting position but flex and turn the ankle out. The little toe should lead. Hold for three seconds then slowly release.
3. Do three sets of 12 flexes for each foot.

BALANCING ACT

These exercises will improve your balance and strengthen your feet and ankles. If you have painful neuropathy or any loss of sensation in your feet, check with your doctor or diabetes educator before attempting any of the following exercises.

THE STORK

1. Stand with your back straight. You can leave your shoes and socks on if you like.
2. Lift one foot off the floor and balance. Try bending the knee of the raised leg and resting your foot on the inside of the opposite leg.

BALANCE TIPS

1. Most people try to "grab" the floor with their toes. Instead, relax your toes so your weight is evenly distributed over the entire foot, from heel to toe.
2. Relax your upper body, especially your shoulders. Breathe normally and don't shrug.

WOBBLE BOARD

The wobble board is a handy gizmo that helps strengthen feet and ankles and improve balance (see page 252 for purchasing information). Wobble board exercises are

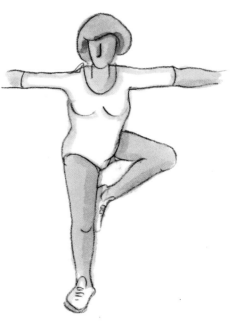

You may need to extend your arms out to your sides or hold one finger against a wall or on the back of a chair for support. (One finger is all you'll need.)
3. Hold the pose as long as you can, then lower your foot slowly to the floor.
4. Aim to balance for one minute. Most people can only do 5 to 10 seconds when they start. Spend 4 to 5 minutes on this exercise, trying to gradually increase your balance time. In addition to improving your balance, this exercise strengthens your feet and ankles.

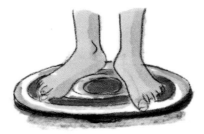

especially helpful for people with diabetes who have lost sensation in their feet and have problems with balance. As mentioned earlier, however, if you have painful neuropathy or have lost sensation in your feet, check with your doctor or educator before attempting the following.

1. Stand on the wobble board and try to keep it steady so the edges don't touch the floor.
2. Begin exercising on the board no more than three minutes a day, gradually building up to five to seven minutes over the first few weeks.
3. As your balance improves, try standing on the wobble board on one foot. If you need support, ask someone for assistance, or place one hand on a wall or the back of a chair.

STRETCHES

A few simple foot and ankle stretches first thing in the morning and right before you go to bed can start and end the day right. Hold all stretches at the point at which you feel a mild tension in the muscle you're stretching. Avoid bouncing, and maintain each stretch for 30 to 45 seconds or until the muscle feels loose. As it loosens, you can push the stretch a bit further until you feel more mild tension in the muscle.

CALF STRETCH

1. Stand a few feet from a wall or anything you can lean on for support.
2. Lean forward, placing your fore-

arms on the wall with your forehead on the backs of your hands.
3. Bring one leg forward, making sure to have both feet flat on the floor with toes pointing toward the wall.
4. Push your hips forward, keeping your back straight, until you feel a slight tension in the calf of the back leg.
5. Repeat 2 or 3 times for each calf.

CALF STRETCH VARIATIONS

1. Turn the back foot in; stretch gently.
2. Turn the back foot out; stretch gently.
3. Keep both feet facing forward, but elevate the toe of the back foot

by placing it on a stick, curb, or old shoe. Elevating the back toe will increase the angle of the stretch.

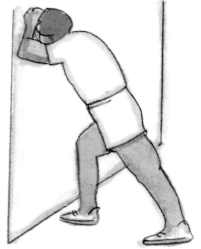

SOLEUS STRETCH

Do the basic calf stretch, but bend the back knee as well. You should feel the tension lower on the calf, near your Achilles tendon.

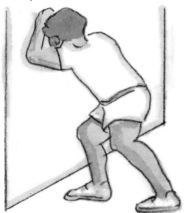

KNEELING TOE STRETCH

If you have Charcot joints, neuropathy, or circulatory problems, check with your doctor before attempting this stretch.

1. Get on all fours, then curl your toes under. You should feel a stretch on the undersides of your toes and in your arches.

2. For a more intense stretch, slowly raise your body to a kneeling position, so all your weight is on your knees and toes.

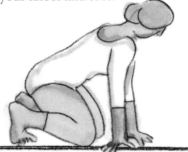

SITTING TOE STRETCH

This exercise stretches the toes in the opposite direction from the kneeling toe stretch. If you have Charcot joints, neuropathy, or circulatory problems, check with your doctor before doing this stretch.

1. Sit on the floor with your legs comfortably extended in front of you. Bend your right knee and grasp your right foot in both hands, allowing your right knee to sink as far as possible toward the floor.

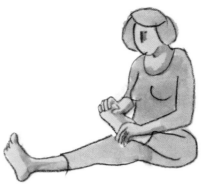

2. Point your right foot and gently pull your toes down, feeling the stretch on the top of your foot. Hold for several seconds then release your right foot, straighten your right leg, and rest your legs for about 30 seconds.

3. Repeat the stretch with your left foot.

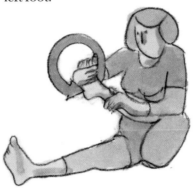

ANKLE STRETCH

Ankles are difficult to stretch, so take your time with this one. If it feels uncomfortable, discontinue it. If you have Charcot joints, neuropathy, or circulatory problems, check with your doctor before doing this stretch.

1. Sit on the floor or in a straight-back chair. If you choose the floor, you might want to lean against a wall for back support.

2. Bending your right leg at the knee, grasp just above the right ankle with your right hand and grasp the right toes with your left hand.

3. With your left hand, rotate your ankle in a clockwise fashion for 10 to 20 rotations. Then rotate your ankle in a counterclockwise fashion for 10 to 20 rotations.

4. Repeat stretch with your left foot.

MASSAGE

Here's the treat of all treats: a foot massage. If you're having trouble sleeping, try rubbing your feet. You'll be amazed how quickly you unwind. Try the following techniques by yourself or better yet, with someone else.

1. Sit on a bed or chair or on the floor with your back against a wall for support.

2. With both thumbs, massage up and down along the arch of your foot.

3. You can use a little moisturizer if you like; just be sure to clean it off when you're done, especially any that gets between your toes. (For people with foot ulcers or neuropathy, check with your educator before using a moisturizer.)

4. Massage with a pressure that feels good for at least two to three minutes. Do this before bed or while watching TV.

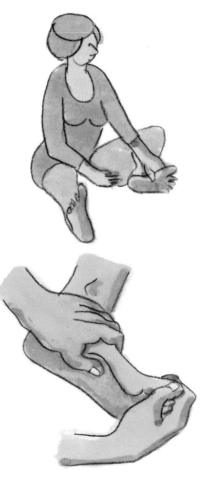

EXERCISING WITH COMPLICATIONS

by Richard M. Weil, M.Ed., C.D.E., C.S.C.S.

Complications from diabetes can be painful, inconvenient, and discouraging. If you're prone to not exercising in the first place, a complication might be all the reason you need to stay inactive. But complications don't have to put an end to exercise. In this article, we show you that there's an exercise for everyone, no matter what your condition, and that people with complications can enjoy the benefits of exercise just like everyone else.

About complications

At least 60% to 70% of all people with diabetes will experience one or more complications of diabetes in their lifetime. The onset and severity of a complication is frequently related to the degree of blood sugar control you maintain and the length of time you have had diabetes.

Exercise has a role in the management of complications. In some cases, exercise can reverse the complication. In others, it can slow down its development. And in still others, it can help a person manage the pain and discomfort of a complication or simply make daily functioning and activities easier.

Exercise helps by lowering blood sugar, improving blood flow to the blood vessels, strengthening the heart and bones, improving a person's range of motion, and elevating mood. Research shows that people who exercise regularly feel better and take better care of themselves.

Different complications affect different organs and systems of the body. Although exercise is encouraged in all cases, each complication presents its own particular precautions when it comes to exercise. For example, if you have moderate or proliferative retinopathy, which affects the eyes, exercises where your head is below your heart would not be advisable. We cover the major complications of diabetes in this article and tell you which exercises are safe and which are not.

Your ticker

Let's start with your heart. People with diabetes are two to 12 times as likely to develop heart disease as people who don't have diabetes. Exercise has been proven to reduce the risk of developing heart disease, sometimes by as much as 50%, and you don't necessarily have to do lots of it to get its benefits. One early study on heart disease and activity dates back to the 1950's. Researchers compared the health of London bus drivers with the health of the conductors who climbed the double-decker stairs collecting the tickets. They found that the conductors had a 30% lower chance of developing heart disease and had 50% fewer heart attacks than the drivers.

New research indicates that you only need to *accumulate* 30 minutes of activity throughout your day—climbing stairs, gardening, walking instead of taking the bus—to keep your ticker healthy. The message is that any activity is better than none, so the most important thing is to get started!

What activity or exercise will help you prevent heart disease? Walking, dancing, jogging, biking, hiking, weight lifting, and swimming are just a few of the activities that will strengthen your heart and prevent heart disease. You can also increase your activity level by participating in recreational sports you like. Activities such as tennis, badminton, volleyball, and skating will all give you some healthy heart benefits.

Always get your doctor's OK before you start an exercise program. If you're uncertain about what kind of exercise to do, ask your doctor for advice or for a referral to an exercise specialist who has experience with people with diabetes. No matter what exercise or activity you choose, always start out slowly and build up over time at a comfortable pace. One sure way to injure yourself or burn out is to try to make up for 20 or 30 years of inactivity in your first two weeks of exercise.

Silent ischemia. Sometimes, people who have had diabetes for a long time lose the warning signal of pain that is associated with spasms of the vessels in the heart or a heart attack. Such chest pain "without the pain" is called *silent ischemia*. The danger of silent ischemia is that you may not realize your heart isn't functioning properly. (Your doctor is the only one who can tell you if you have silent ischemia. He or she can detect it through fairly simple office tests.)

Having silent ischemia doesn't mean you shouldn't exercise. In fact, you need to exercise to keep your heart pumping strong. If you have silent ischemia, your doctor can prescribe drugs to prevent your heart from working too hard while you're exercising. He or she may also recommend that you have a stress test before you begin. You should ask your doctor for advice on getting started or ask for a referral to an exercise specialist, cardiac rehabilitation program, or local Y, hospital, senior center, or fitness center that has a special exercise program for people with cardiac problems.

Neuropathy

Neuropathy is a troubling chronic complication of diabetes that damages the nerves. It affects 60% to 70% of both people with Type 1 diabetes and Type 2 diabetes. Neuropathy can affect many different parts of the body. The most common type of neuropathy is *peripheral neuropathy,* which affects the feet, legs, and hands. Symptoms include pain, numbness, and tingling. The feet are usually affected first, and the pain is often worse when a person lies in bed at night. Although there are drugs to alleviate the symptoms of neuropathy, they don't work for everyone.

Exercise can't reverse neuropathy, but one study concluded that higher levels of physical activity are related to a lower risk of developing neuropathy. If you already have neuropathy, exercise can help you cope with it by increasing the blood flow to affected limbs, making your muscles stronger, and increasing your ability to perform the activities of daily living.

If you have peripheral neuropathy, exercises like walking, skiing, jogging, and aerobic dancing, where your feet support your body weight, may hurt. If they do, try non-weight-bearing activities such as stationary biking, recumbent biking, fan biking, rowing, and weight lifting. Chair exercise videos also provide a terrific workout. And you may want to try swimming or water aerobics, in which the water supports your body weight; you can also use flotation devices for more buoyancy.

Exercise will not make neuropathy worse, even if it hurts while you're doing it. However, some people have a high tolerance for pain while others don't. Exercise isn't supposed to hurt. If it does and you're uncomfortable, it's OK to stop and find an exercise that suits you better.

Be sure to inspect your feet after you exercise. If your feet are numb, you might not feel a blister or other sore develop. If you have trouble seeing the bottoms of your feet, have your doctor or someone else check them for you. If you choose to swim or do water aerobics, wear water socks while you are in the water or walking around the pool and locker room area. If you have an open wound, do not use the pool until it heals.

Loss of proprioception. Another problem related to peripheral neuropathy is the loss of *proprioception.* Proprioception is the reception of stimuli from receptors located throughout your body that let your brain know if you're moving or standing still and where your body is in relation to other objects. When you climb a flight of stairs or step off a curb, you have a good idea how high to lift your foot because you know where your feet are and how high the step is, even without looking. If you have a proprioceptor problem, your brain isn't getting the proper signal from the receptors responsible for this movement, and it's possible to lose your balance. The non-weight-bearing exercises listed above are good choices for people with this complication because they will help minimize your risk of falling.

Autonomic neuropathy. The other major type of neuropathy, called *autonomic neuropathy,* affects the nerves that control involuntary actions in your body. Silent ischemia is a form of autonomic neuropathy, and so is the loss of early warning signs of hypoglycemia, or *hypoglycemia unawareness.*

Hypoglycemia unawareness is a problem when you're exercising because you may not feel your blood sugar dropping. It's not uncommon for people with hypoglycemia unawareness to have a blood sugar level in the range of 30–40 mg/dl before they feel symptoms. The best solution to this problem is to prevent low blood sugar. That means you need to become familiar with how much your blood sugar drops during exercise by testing before, during (if the exercise lasts one hour or more), and after exercise and make adjustments in your insulin and/or snack beforehand. If you have questions about preventing and treating hypoglycemia during exercise, speak with your doctor or diabetes educator.

When autonomic neuropathy affects the cardiovascular system, it can cause a condition called *orthostatic hypotension.* This condition is characterized by a drop in blood pressure when a person stands up or sits up from a lying position. The drop in blood pressure can cause feelings of dizziness or weakness or can even cause a person to faint. If you experience orthostatic hypotension, you should be careful with exercises that require quick changes in body position or posture (such as standing up quickly) because of the risk of losing your balance or fainting.

Cooling down after exercise is a good idea for everyone, but for people with autonomic neuropathy, it is especially important. If you stop exercising abruptly without cooling down, blood can pool in your legs and feet rather than circulating back up to your heart. Such pooling can cause dizziness, fainting, and even a heart attack. Luckily, cooling down is easy: After your workout, simply continue the activity you've been doing at a lower intensity or walk around for five to 10 minutes, allowing your heart rate to return to normal.

Kidney disease

Nephropathy, or kidney disease, affects 20% to 30% of people with diabetes, and exercising with kidney disease can be tricky. That's because exercise naturally causes blood pressure to rise, but kidney disease and high blood pressure don't mix well. If you have kidney disease, it is important to take precautions to prevent your blood pressure from rising too high during exercise. Of course, one of the problems with blood pressure is that you can't feel it, so unless you have the opportunity to monitor your blood pressure during exercise, it's better to play it safe.

Playing it safe means doing exercises that involve large muscle groups, are low to moderate in intensity, and are rhythmic. Exercises with these characteristics are better choices for people with kidney disease than exercises that use smaller muscle groups or are highly intense. For example, swimming, dancing, walking, low-impact aerobics (without hand weights), yoga, and tai chi are better choices than high-intensity weight lifting (you can still tone and build strength with light

GET READY, GET SET

CHAIR EXERCISE VIDEOS

Sit and Be Fit Series
Arthritis
Chair Dancing
Feeling Good With Arthritis
Osteoporosis
Stroke
Sit and Be Fit videos are available through Collage Video, (800) 433-6769, www.collagevideo.com. You may also want to check for them at your local video store.

STRETCHING, YOGA, AND TAI CHI VIDEOS

Karen Voight's Pure and Simple Stretch
Stretching With Bob Anderson
Charlene Pricket's Home Stretch
Stretchin' to the Classics, Richard Simmons
Lilias, Alive With Yoga, Beginner
Richard Hittleman's Yoga Course, I
Tai Chi for Health
Tai Chi for Seniors
These videos are available through Collage Video, (800) 433-6769, www.collagevideo.com. You may also be able to find them at your local video store.

HELP FOR VISUALLY IMPAIRED ATHLETES

The Lighthouse, Inc.
111 East 59th Street
New York, NY 10022
(800) 829-0500
www.lighthouse.org
The Lighthouse offers recreational activities and exercise programs for people who are visually impaired or blind.

United States Association for Blind Athletes
33 North Institute
Colorado Springs, CO 80903
(719) 630-0422
www.usaba.org
The Association offers coaching in many sports. Contact it to inquire about programs that may be available in your area.

OTHER RESOURCES

Arthritis Foundation
(800) 283-7800
www.arthritis.org
Call, or check the Web site, for the phone number of your local chapter, which can tell you about exercise programs in your area.

Disabled Sports USA National Headquarters
451 Hungerford Drive, Suite 100
Rockville, MD 20850
(301) 217-0960
www.dsusa.org
Disabled Sports USA has community-based chapters across the United States that provide year-round sports, recreation, and social activities for people with orthopedic, spinal cord, neuromuscular, and visual impairments as well as other disabilities.

YMCA of the USA
(888) 333-YMCA (333-9622)
(312) 977-0031
www.ymca.net

YWCA of the USA
(212) 273-7800
www.ywca.org

weights), activities like basketball that involve jumping, and high-impact aerobics. Pedaling too hard on a stationary or outdoor bike can raise your blood pressure if you're out of shape or not accustomed to this type of activity, so start slowly if you choose to use these. Fan bikes used at a light intensity are a good alternative (if available) because they involve more muscle groups, which tends to keep blood pressure from rising very high.

If you do endurance aerobic sports like running, it's important to drink fluids before, during, and after the workout to avoid dehydration. To be on the safe side, drink 12 to 15 ounces 15 minutes before the workout, and 12 ounces every 15 minutes during the workout and immediately after.

Straining during an activity will raise your blood pressure, but sometimes straining is unavoidable. Remember this rule: Always exhale with effort. If you're lifting something heavy, breathe out during the lifting part. Another rule of thumb for safety: If the exercise feels too hard, it probably is, and if the veins in your neck are popping out and your face is red, it's definitely too hard.

Retinopathy and impaired vision

Retinopathy is damage to the small blood vessels in the back of the eye. In one study, researchers found that 97% of people with diabetes who use insulin and 80% of people with diabetes who do not use insulin have retinopathy 15 years after diabetes is diagnosed. There are several stages of retinopathy, ranging from mild background retinopathy to proliferative retinopathy. An ophthalmologist is best qualified to evaluate your particular case.

Despite the prevalence of retinopathy and the potentially serious consequences of exercising improperly, very little research has been done on safe exercise and eye disease. Thus, many of these exercise recommendations are based on common sense and the premise that one should avoid any activity that would raise blood pressure enough to risk rupturing blood vessels in the back of the eye. These would include exercises where the head is below the heart (such as sit-ups, especially on a slant board, toe touches, and yoga poses like the handstand or headstand), exercises where you risk significant rises in blood pressure (such as heavy weight lifting), high-altitude mountain climbing (above 14,000 feet), and activities like deep-sea diving where the effects of water pressure changes are unknown. (The safety of deep-sea diving remains controversial, however.)

If you have proliferative retinopathy (the most serious type), exercise could make things worse. Before you begin an exercise program, therefore, get treatment for your retinopathy. Once your eyes have

healed, ask your doctor when and how you can start activity again. Activities that require you to jump around, like high-impact aerobics, or contact sports, like football, should be avoided if you have later stages of retinopathy. On the other hand, exercises that involve the large muscle groups and that get your heart rate up with a minimal amount of strain or pressure are excellent if you have retinopathy. Such exercises include walking, either on a treadmill or outdoors, dancing, light jogging, and using a fan bike.

A word about weight lifting. It's true that weight lifting can raise your blood pressure, especially when heavy weights are used. However, that rise is momentary, and within seconds blood pressure returns to normal. Weight lifting is not off limits if you have retinopathy (or nephropathy for that matter) because the stronger you are, the less likely you are to strain doing activities of daily living or exercising. If you decide to lift weights, follow these precautions: Breathe properly (exhale with effort), keep the weight light enough so you don't strain (you should be able to lift it comfortably and with good form 12–15 times), and as always, get the OK from your doctor or ophthalmologist first. Remember, you can get stronger from lifting even light weights.

If you have low or poor vision, stationary biking or pedaling on a bicycle built for two can work nicely, as can water exercises. You can swim laps by guiding yourself along the wall of the pool or the lane ropes, and you can do water aerobics as well. (See "Get Ready, Get Set" on the opposite page for the addresses of organizations that help people with low vision stay active.)

Peripheral vascular disease

Peripheral vascular disease (or blood vessel disease) blocks blood from flowing freely through the blood vessels. The result is that the muscles are deprived of oxygen and other nutrients, which can lead to pain. Peripheral vascular disease usually affects the lower extremities first. About 10% of people with diabetes have it. Your doctor can prescribe drugs to help with the pain, but they don't work for everyone. In fact, exercise is the best intervention for peripheral vascular disease.

Probably the most common problem associated with peripheral vascular disease is *intermittent claudication,* a condition characterized by sharp pain in the calves or legs during exertion that usually subsides within a few moments of stopping the activity. It used to be that people with claudication were told to stop exercising whenever they felt pain, but new research shows that it's OK to just slow down and keep moving if you can tolerate the pain. Of course, you need to discuss this strategy with your physician.

If the pain from peripheral vascular disease is too great for weight-bearing activities like cross-country skiing, jogging, or even walking, then non-weight-bearing exercises would be a better choice. Recumbent bikes are very useful for people with claudication pain because your legs are out in front of you while you pedal, causing less pressure on the vessels in the feet and legs. Other helpful exercises include swimming, water aerobics, chair exercises, and weight lifting. When you have peripheral vascular disease, any exercise that gets blood flowing into your legs will help make the tasks of daily living easier, and in some cases, exercise can even reverse the disease.

Orthopedic problems

There is some evidence to show that arthritis is more common in people with diabetes, especially Type 1 diabetes. Exercise won't reverse arthritis, but it can help to manage the activities of daily living. In fact, the 1996 U.S. Surgeon General's Report on Physical Activity and Health emphasized that regular physical activity can help people with arthritis control pain and disability. If it's painful for you to reach into the cupboard, comb your hair, or walk down the street, then increasing the strength of your muscles and improving your range of motion will take some of the strain off your joints and increase your ability to move.

Good exercises for people with arthritis include biking, chair exercises, light weight lifting (where weights are lifted only as high or far as is comfortable for the individual), swimming (probably the best because the water keeps you from putting all your weight on the affected joint), and water aerobics. The Arthritis Foundation provides exercise and water aerobics programs in many areas of the United States and also has exercise video tapes. (See "Get Ready, Get Set" on page 260 for contact information.)

Charcot joints, which are bone or joint deformities in the foot, are a complication of diabetes that affects only a small percentage of the diabetes population. The immediate treatment of Charcot joint is no weight-bearing at all. Later, some people are able to resume activities with the help of an orthotic, or supportive device, that must be fitted by a podiatrist. Activities in almost every case are limited to non-weight-bearing exercises like swimming, recumbent biking (if OK'd by your doctor), and upper-body weight lifting.

An exercise for everyone?

With only a few exceptions, stretching, yoga, and tai chi would be helpful for almost anyone with complications from diabetes. These exercises improve range of motion, decrease the risk of injuries like muscle pulls, improve muscle tone, and help reduce stress with minimal amounts of risk. What's more, these are exercises you can do at home. In addition, many Y's, fitness centers, and city recreation departments now hold yoga and tai chi classes, and some cities have yoga or tai chi centers. Look in your local phone book or have a look at some of the videos that are widely available on these activities.

Get up and go

Complications don't make exercise easy, but many people with diabetic complications feel exercise is worth it. It can improve blood sugar levels, improve your sense of well-being, and help you feel more in control of your diabetes. In a nutshell, it can improve the quality of your life. I hope this article has shown you some ways that you can take care of yourself by exercising even if you do have complications. I encourage you to do the best you can. I think you'll be glad you did. Good luck. ❑

Nutrition and Meal Planning

You Are What You Eat
(AND HOW MUCH)

by Patti Bazel Geil, M.S., R.D., L.D., C.D.E.

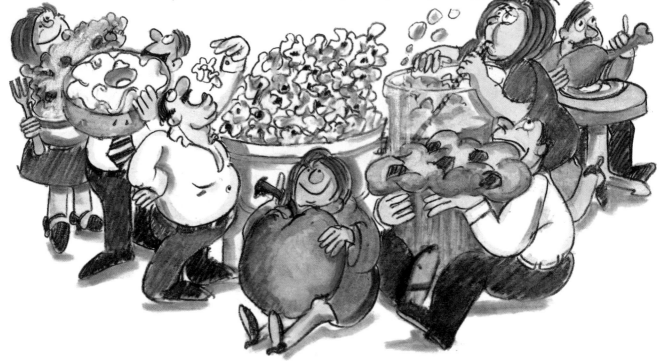

"To lengthen thy life, lessen thy meals." So said Benjamin Franklin, but even he would find it hard to follow this advice in today's "super-size" society. These days, instead of selling soft drinks in a customary 12-ounce cup, convenience stores sell 64-ounce barrels of beverage. Triple-decker burgers are common fast-food fare. And the size of the standard restaurant dinner plate has increased from 10½ inches to 12½ inches over the years.

As portion sizes swell, you may find your weight and blood sugar numbers creeping up, 1 pound and one fingerstick at a time, without an obvious explanation. If that's the case, beware: You may have fallen victim to the "bigger is better" mentality and become too nonchalant about the importance of portion control and accurate measurement of foods in the management of your diabetes. No matter what nutrition plan you follow—from carbohydrate counting to exchanges to the food guide pyramid—portion size is key in keeping your weight and blood sugar values in a healthy range.

Becoming "size-wise"

It's a frustrating feeling. You've been so good, sticking with your meal plan, eating only "healthy" foods. Your daily diet is a dietitian's dream: fruit juice, a bagel, and skim milk for breakfast; salad, soup, and a muffin for lunch; and for supper, grilled chicken breast, baked potato, carrots, and fresh fruit. Your evening snack? "Lite" microwave popcorn. You exercise regularly, take your diabetes medicines, and check your blood sugar as recommended. Yet at your recent clinic visit, you find your hemoglobin A_{1c} (HbA_{1c}) has risen, and you've gained 3 pounds in the past three months.

It's time for you to become "size-wise." Although only healthy foods may pass your lips, too much of a good thing does make a difference. Let's play detective with a sample diet recall to solve this mystery: How can a casual attitude to portion control lead to higher-than-expected blood sugar levels and steady weight gain over time?

Breakfast

Adding it up. Let's start with the liquids you report drinking for breakfast: fruit juice and skim milk. Are you using a measuring cup to find your recommended 4-ounce serving? Or are you just "guesstimating," using an old souvenir glass as a guide? Since 1 ounce of fruit juice has 15 calories and almost 4 grams of carbohydrate, and an ounce of skim milk has about 11 calories and 1½ grams of carbohydrate, being "off" by as little as 2 ounces per beverage adds 52 calories and 11 grams of carbohydrate to the day's total.

Bagels can be another source of hidden calories and carbohydrate. A 1-ounce bagel (or half of a 2-ounce bagel) is a starch exchange, containing about 80 calories and 15 grams of carbohydrate. However, a bakery bagel may weigh up to 4 ounces. Eating even ½ ounce more than you intended gives you an extra 40 calories and 7½ grams of carbohydrate over and above your starch exchange. And what about that "tiny" bit of cream cheese you spread on the bagel? Unfortunately, it's not a free food: A tablespoon of regular cream cheese adds 45 calories and 5 grams of fat to your day's total.

Bottom line. Measuring beverage and bagel portion sizes inaccurately and adding extras like cream cheese to your meal plan can lead to an extra 137 calories, 18½ grams of carbohydrate, and 5 grams of fat at breakfast alone.

Lessons to learn. Until you know exactly what your portion sizes should look like, use standard kitchen measuring spoons and measuring cups for liquids. Use a measuring cup for solids such as breakfast cereal. For measuring foods such as bagels in ounces, a food scale, which can be purchased for $5 or $10, is your best bet.

Lunch

Adding it up. Salad, soup, and a muffin for lunch—what could be healthier? Maybe you've always thought of salad as a free food, which it normally is, unless you eat more than 4 cups of salad greens. But is your salad a huge restaurant salad topped with bacon bits, eggs, and shredded cheese? A chef salad from a fast-food restaurant is far from free: You'll need to add 230 calories, 8 grams of carbohydrate, and 13 grams of fat. And don't forget to count the dressing! Even a tablespoon of reduced-calorie French dressing can con-

VISUALIZE PORTION SIZE

When you don't have your measuring cups and scale handy, these mental images may make it easier to eyeball your portion size.

A SERVING OF:	LOOKS LIKE:
1 cup of pasta or rice	a clenched fist
½ cup of vegetables	half of a tennis ball
1 cup of broccoli	a light bulb
3 ounces of meat, chicken, or fish	a deck of cards or the palm of your hand
1 ounce of cheese	two saltine crackers or a 1-inch square cube

tribute 40 calories, 5 grams of carbohydrate, and 2 grams of fat.

Soup may look thin and insubstantial, but it does contain calories, carbohydrate, and fat. Let's see how Grandma's cure-all for colds, chicken soup, affects your nutrition balance sheet. Broth-based chicken noodle soup generally has the fewest calories and least fat. By comparison, 1 cup of condensed cream of chicken soup prepared with water has 32 calories and 4 grams of fat more than 1 cup of chicken noodle soup, although their carbohydrate content is approximately equal. Preparing cream of chicken soup with whole milk rather than water adds 84 calories, 6 grams of carbohydrate, and 5 grams of fat to a 1-cup serving.

To keep tabs on what you're eating, measure your soup serving size in a liquid measuring cup occasionally. Consuming a mere extra 4 ounces (½ cup) of chicken noodle soup can amount to an extra 38 calories, 5 grams of carbohydrate, and 2 grams of fat. If you add a handful of oyster crackers to your soup, add another 80 calories, 15 grams of carbohydrate, and 1 gram of fat. Oyster crackers may be tiny but are not a free food; count 24 oyster crackers as a starch exchange.

Muffins are now mega-size, some weighing up to 3 or 4 ounces. Since you may be using a standard muffin (that is, a 1½-ounce muffin with 125 calories, 15 grams of carbohydrate, and 5 grams of fat) as the basis for a starch plus fat exchange, read your nutrition information carefully. A bakery muffin adds at least 150 calories, 15 grams of carbohydrate, and 10 grams of fat over and above a starch exchange.

Bottom line. Inattention to detail—having high-fat items in your salad, eating more soup than planned and adding oyster crackers, and eating a big muffin—

KEEPING IT DOWN TO SIZE

If you're not sure what a standard portion size is for the foods you want to eat, or you don't know how many calories or grams of fat and carbohydrate a portion contains, these books can help:

THE DIABETES CARBOHYDRATE AND FAT GRAM GUIDE
LeaAnn Holzmeister
American Diabetes Association
Alexandria, Virginia, 2000

BOWES & CHURCH'S FOOD VALUES OF PORTIONS COMMONLY USED
Jean A. T. Pennington
Lippincott-Raven Publishers
Philadelphia, 1997

THE COMPLETE BOOK OF FOOD COUNTS
Corrine T. Netzer
Dell Publishing Company
New York, 2000

can account for an extra 538 calories, 48 grams of carbohydrate, and 28 grams of fat from the lunch line.
Lessons to learn. Meet with a registered dietitian to learn more about which foods really are free. (By definition, a free food contains less than 20 calories or less than 5 grams of carbohydrate per serving.) Review your nutrition and meal plan information. Be aware that the term "reduced-fat" does not necessarily mean calorie-free. If in doubt, read food labels carefully, and weigh foods such as muffins to get a more accurate idea of their nutrition content.

Supper

Adding it up. Let's take a look at your typical supper: grilled chicken, baked potato, carrots, and fresh fruit. At first glance, this looks like a low-fat, low-calorie meal. But there may be some obstacles to good diabetes control hidden in your well-balanced plate. For example, it is easy to go overboard on portion size with meat because an extra ounce or so doesn't look like much. However, that extra ounce can add 50 calories and 1 gram of fat.

Baked potatoes range in size from 3 to 6 ounces; if you aren't careful, you can add an extra 80 calories and 15 grams of carbohydrate to your dinner total. To know what you're eating, weigh your potatoes before eating.

Carrots can be a wonderful source of vitamins, but are you really eating only ½ cup? Chances are you may

have been eating twice that amount, adding 25 calories and 5 grams of carbohydrate to the day. If you season the carrots with margarine, don't forget to account for the 45 calories and 5 grams of fat that a teaspoonful of it contains.

Fresh fruit is a great way to end your meal, but unless you know exactly what a 4-ounce apple looks like, you need to get out the food scale. A large red delicious apple can easily add an extra 60 calories and 15 grams of carbohydrate to an otherwise ideal diet record.
Bottom line. Even with minor additions, it's possible to pile on an extra 260 calories, 35 grams of carbohydrate, and 6 grams of fat, at supper.
Lessons to learn. Develop a visual image of the proper serving amount of meat: A 3-ounce portion is equal in size to a standard deck of playing cards or the palm of your hand. (Some other helpful comparisons are listed in "Visualize Portion Size" on page 265.) When you shop for fresh fruits and vegetables, weigh them individually in the produce section of the store. Buy only those that most closely match your perfect portion size—no more guesswork!

Snack

Adding it up. It's snack time! Your "lite" popcorn is just what the dietitian ordered. It has only 17 calories, 3 grams of carbohydrate, and less than 1 gram of fat per cup. But who eats just 1 cup? For most people, a typical serving size is closer to one bagful than one cupful. Let's say you rein yourself in at 3½ cups, leaving the rest of the bag for someone else. The extra 2½ cups still provide you with an extra 43 calories, 8 grams of carbohydrate, and 2 grams of fat.
Bottom line. Polishing off even more "lite" popcorn than you intended can lead to heavy changes in your blood sugar control as well as your weight. Add an extra 43 calories, 8 grams of carbohydrate, and 2 grams of fat to your records for the day.
Lessons to learn. Be sure the nutrition information you use from food labels is based on the serving sizes you normally eat. If you usually eat more than the serving size designated on the label, adjust your calories, carbohydrate, and fat count accordingly. "Lite" does not mean "free."

Crunching the numbers

Small changes and incidental extras such as those in the meal plan described above don't seem like much until you take a look at the bottom line: an extra 978 calories, 110 grams of carbohydrate, and 41 grams of fat in the day, all from "healthy" foods. If repeated daily over the course of a year, this can account for significant weight gain, resulting in major effects on blood sugar.

Theoretically, a person gains 1 pound for every 3,500 calories consumed above the normal intake. An extra

978 calories a day, therefore, could lead to weight gain of 1 pound every three or four days, totaling nearly 102 pounds by the end of one year! In reality, however, each person's metabolism is different, and a lot of extra calories are burned off as heat, so almost no one would actually gain the entire 102 pounds. What's more, most of us would change our eating habits if we started gain-ing weight that rapidly! Still, consuming extra calories each day or on most days will lead to gradual weight gain in anyone, and gaining even 10 or 20 pounds can have negative health consequences if you are currently at a healthy weight for your height or overweight.

The good news is that becoming aware of portion sizes and taking a closer look at what you really eat will

IT ALL ADDS UP

Many small extras can add up to big differences in the number of calories and grams of carbohydrate and fat you *intend* to eat in a day, compared to the amounts you really *do* eat.

What you *think* you're eating:

	CALORIES	CARBOHYDRATE (g)	FAT (g)
BREAKFAST			
4 ounces fruit juice	60	15	0
4 ounces skim milk	45	6	0
1-ounce bagel	80	15	0
LUNCH			
4-cup green salad	100	20	0
1 cup chicken noodle soup	75	9	3
1½-ounce muffin	125	15	5
17 grapes	60	15	0
4 ounces skim milk	45	6	0
SUPPER			
3 ounces grilled chicken breast	165	0	9
3-ounce baked potato	80	15	0
½ cup carrots	25	5	0
1 slice bread	80	15	0
4-ounce apple	60	15	0
SNACK			
1 cup "lite" popcorn	17	3	1
DAILY TOTAL	1,017	154	18

What you *really* may be eating:

	CALORIES	CARBOHYDRATE (g)	FAT (g)
BREAKFAST			
6 ounces fruit juice	90	23	0
6 ounces skim milk	68	9	0
3-ounce bagel	240	45	0
1 tablespoon cream cheese	45	0	5
LUNCH			
Chef salad with eggs, shredded cheese, and bacon bits	230	8	13
1 tablespoon low-calorie dressing	40	5	2
1½ cups chicken noodle soup	113	14	5
24 oyster crackers	80	15	1
4-ounce muffin	333	40	13
25 grapes	88	22	0
6 ounces skim milk	68	9	0
SUPPER			
4 ounces grilled chicken breast	220	0	12
6-ounce baked potato	160	30	0
1 cup carrots	50	10	0
1 teaspoon margarine	45	0	5
4-ounce piece cornbread	160	30	4
6-ounce apple	90	23	0
SNACK			
3½ cups "lite" popcorn	60	11	3
DAILY TOTAL	2,180	294	63

definitely lead to improvements in your health. So the next time a TV commercial for a fast-food burger chain has your mouth watering for a jumbo serving of fries, ask yourself: Is it wise to super-size? If you super-size your next serving of fast-food French fries, you add an extra 330 calories, 42 grams of carbohydrate, and 16 grams of fat to your meal. A super-size serving of fries alone has 540 calories, the same amount as in two hamburgers!

Measuring up

Even food professionals have a hard time accurately estimating the calorie and fat content of meals. A recent New York University study showed that when asked to estimate the nutrition content of a few typical restaurant meals, on average, dietitians underestimated calories by 30% to 50% and fat by 35% to 60%.

If trained nutrition professionals aren't always able to estimate accurately, does this mean you are doomed to a life of carrying around scales and measuring cups and spoons? Not at all. Take the time at home to train your eyes to help you judge correct portion sizes. Once you've weighed, measured, and become accustomed to seeing exactly what 1 cup of mashed potatoes or 4 ounces of fish look like at home, you'll be able to mentally carry these food pictures with you no matter where you go. When you are comfortable with your ability to eyeball, take a break from the scales and spoons. An occasional "refresher course" should keep your eyes sharp and your portion sizes in proper perspective.

An ounce here and a tablespoon there doesn't sound like much, but small changes do make a difference in the bottom line! ❑

CARBOHYDRATE COUNTING
Part 1: The Basics
by Patti Bazel Geil, M.S., R.D., L.D., C.D.E.

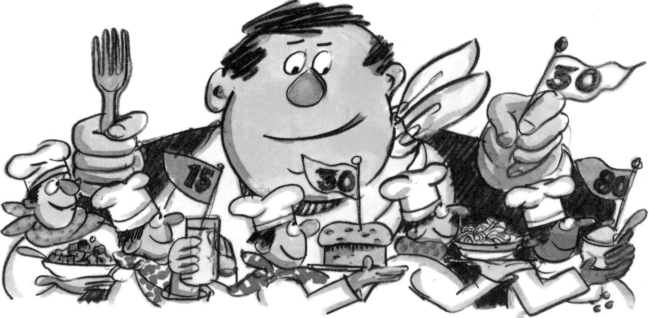

Freedom in food choices, flexibility in meal planning, an occasional sweet treat, and the bonus of improved blood sugar control. Sound too good to be true? Well, it doesn't have to be. These are some of the benefits of a meal-planning system called carbohydrate counting, and with a little time, effort, and motivation, you can make this system work for you.

If you are happy with your current meal plan, there's no need to change. But if you feel your current meal plan is too restrictive or too complicated, and you are willing to invest some time in record-keeping, blood-sugar monitoring, and learning more about food portions and nutrient content, then carbohydrate counting may be just the diabetes meal-planning approach you've been looking for.

The rising popularity of carbohydrate counting is the result of exciting changes in traditional diabetes diet dogma. As early as the 1970's, nutrition professionals questioned the conventional wisdom that simple sugars raise blood glucose levels higher than complex carbohydrates (starches) do. Scientific study ultimately proved that it is more important for people with diabetes to pay attention to the total amount of carbohydrate in their diet than to limit only concentrated sources of carbohydrate such as table sugar, honey, and regular soft drinks. As a result, diabetes professionals no longer consider sugar a "forbidden food," but rather just one source of carbohydrate that can be enjoyed in moderation if blood sugar levels remain in a person's target range.

The results of the Diabetes Control and Complications Trial (DCCT), published in 1993, proved conclusively what many already knew intuitively: Better blood sugar control reduces the risk of complications from diabetes, including nerve damage, damage to the eyes, and kidney disease. The DCCT also shed some new light on the role of diet in controlling blood sugar levels. The 1,441 people who participated in the DCCT used a variety of meal-planning approaches based on individualized assessments by registered dietitians. Researchers found that no single diet approach worked better than the rest. Health professionals now realize that just as there is no one drug regimen that is right for everyone with diabetes, there is also no single meal-planning approach that meets everyone's needs.

The 1994 American Diabetes Association Nutrition Recommendations and Principles for People with Diabetes Mellitus tied these findings together and endorsed an individualized approach to meal planning. Of the many meal-planning options that are now available, carbohydrate counting has become one of the most popular. This article explains the basic method of carbohydrate counting, which involves keeping carbohydrate intake consistent from day to day. This approach may be especially useful for people with Type 2 diabetes. In Part 2 of this article, we will cover more advanced carbohydrate-counting techniques, including adjusting your diet to special situations and balancing insulin to grams of carbohydrate.

About carbohydrates

Foods that contain carbohydrate, such as grains, vegetables, fruit, milk, and sugar, have the most immediate impact on blood sugar level. Almost 90% of the starches and sugars we eat appear in the blood as glucose (blood sugar) within two hours after eating. Eating small amounts of carbohydrate raises blood sugar somewhat; eating larger amounts of carbohydrate raises blood sugar more. For example, eating two large bowls of cereal raises your blood sugar more than eating ½ cup of cereal. Exactly how much a certain amount of a certain food raises blood glucose varies from person to person.

Learning which foods contain carbohydrate is essential for carbohydrate counting. Carbohydrate is found in any food containing starches or sugars, including breads, crackers, cereals, pasta, rice and other grains, dried beans, vegetables, milk and yogurt, fruit and fruit juice, and table sugar, honey, syrup, and molasses, as well as foods sweetened with these items. Other foods such as cake, ice cream, candy, snack foods, pizza, casseroles, and soups contain a combination of carbohydrate, protein, and fat.

Certain foods such as meat, fish, eggs, oils, cheese, bacon, butter, and margarine contain little or no carbohydrate; the calories in these foods come from fat and protein. Foods that don't contain carbohydrate do not need to be accounted for in the carbohydrate-counting approach because they don't raise blood sugar levels as much as carbohydrate-containing foods do. Of course, these foods cannot be ignored altogether since they do contain calories and eating too many calories and too much fat and protein can have negative health consequences other than raising blood glucose levels.

Even though all carbohydrates, whether they are from chocolate chip cookies or mashed potatoes, theoretically affect blood sugar the same way, the carbohydrate-counting approach should not be regarded as an invitation to a nutrition free-for-all. Foods high in sugar are often high in fat and calories and low in vitamins and minerals. Ignoring the principles of good nutrition can lead to weight gain and high blood lipid levels (high cholesterol and high triglycerides). Choosing healthful foods should always remain your

FIND THE CARBOHYDRATES

Seven of the 12 foods listed below contain carbohydrate. Can you find them?

Olive oil	Oat bran cereal
Skim milk	Sausage pizza
Grapes	Bacon
Poached egg	Black-eyed peas
Whole wheat bagel	Sour cream
Carrots	Ground beef

The seven foods that contain carbohydrate are skim milk, oat bran cereal, grapes, sausage pizza, whole wheat bagel, black-eyed peas, and carrots.

TWO VIEWS OF 1800 CALORIES

Many people with diabetes are familiar with using exchanges for meal planning. Here's how a day's menu would be analyzed using the exchange system and using carbohydrate counting.

Menu	Exchanges	Carbohydrate (g)
BREAKFAST		
1 cup skim milk	1 milk	12
1 cup bran cereal	2 starch	30
1 medium fresh peach	1 fruit	15
LUNCH		
2 ounces turkey	2 lean meat	0
2 slices whole wheat bread	2 starch	30
2 teaspoons mayonnaise	2 fat	0
1 cup carrot sticks	1 vegetable	15
1 ounce potato chips	1 starch, 2 fat	15
1 large apple	2 fruit	30
DINNER		
3 ounces grilled chicken	3 lean meat	0
⅔ cup baked beans	2 starch	30
½ cup corn	1 vegetable	15
2-inch cube cornbread	1 starch, 1 fat	15
1 small frosted cupcake	2 starch, 1 fat	30
SNACK		
3 graham cracker squares	1 starch	15
1 cup skim milk	1 milk	12
TOTAL	1,811 calories	264 g

main consideration, no matter which meal-planning approach you use.

Measuring up

Carbohydrate in foods is measured in grams, but you don't need to be a metric whiz to give carbohydrate counting a try. What you do need to know is that 15 grams of carbohydrate equal one carbohydrate choice. To find out how many grams of carbohydrate one serving of a particular food contains, you must either read the Nutrition Facts label or use a reference book that lists the amount of carbohydrate in the food. (Although a gram is a measure of weight, you cannot determine how many grams of carbohydrate a food contains simply by weighing it.) For a list of some reference books that can help you determine carbohydrate content, see "Resources" on page 271.

Even though you cannot directly weigh grams of carbohydrate, you will do a fair amount of weighing and measuring as you get started counting carbohydrates. That's because carbohydrate counting is based on portion sizes, and to make sure your portion size is accurate, you will need to use a food scale, measuring cups, and measuring spoons. Lest you think these tools are unnecessary, note the difference in the amount of carbohydrate when you measure a food exactly and when you estimate portion sizes:

■ 1 measured cup of cooked macaroni = 30 grams of carbohydrate
■ 1 typical plate of cooked macaroni = 120 grams of carbohydrate
■ ½ frozen bagel (1 ounce) = 15 grams of carbohydrate
■ 1 bakery bagel = 45 grams of carbohydrate

Start on the right track by measuring foods accurately for the most effective blood sugar control. When your eye gets accustomed to proper portion sizes, you can take a break from measuring, but it is helpful to take a refresher course periodically.

When using food labels to determine the carbohydrate content of a food, use the number for the total grams of carbohydrate per serving. Pay special attention to the serving size listed on the label. If the serving size is different from the one you normally eat, you will need to adjust the carbohydrate information. For example, if the serving size specified on the package is four cookies, containing 40 grams of carbohydrate, and you eat six cookies, you will have consumed 60 grams of carbohydrate, not 40.

Consistency counts

The goal of carbohydrate counting is to improve your blood sugar control by matching the amount of carbohydrate you eat with the amount of insulin available to metabolize it. Those people who inject insulin have some control over how much insulin is available. But whether or not you inject insulin, when you first begin carbohydrate counting, you will need to test your blood sugar 1½ to 2 hours after eating to see how it reacts to different carbohydrate-containing foods and different amounts of food. You will learn through experimentation and blood-glucose testing how much carbohydrate you can eat at each meal without your blood sugar level going too high.

The basic approach to carbohydrate counting involves setting a target carbohydrate goal for each of your meals and snacks. If you do not currently follow a specific meal plan, use your typical carbohydrate intake as a starting point. Write down your usual food intake, noting exact portion sizes, and calculate your carbohydrate intake. Test your blood glucose 1½ to 2 hours after each meal. A test result in the range recommended for you suggests that the amount of carbohydrate you ate is right for you. A test result higher than the recommended range suggests that you may need to eat less carbohydrate to achieve your blood glucose goals. A session with a registered dietitian can be particularly helpful to provide information and support in this new way of meal planning.

If you currently use the exchange system, you can convert from exchanges to carbohydrate counting by noting the amount of carbohydrate in each of the food exchanges in your meal plan. (As a quick review: One starch, fruit, or other carbohydrate exchange contains 15 grams of carbohydrate; one milk exchange contains 12 grams of carbohydrate; one vegetable exchange contains 5 grams of carbohydrate; and one meat and meat substitute or fat exchange contains 0 grams of carbohydrate.)

Once you know how many grams of carbohydrate you want to eat at a meal, you can decide which carbohydrate-containing foods you feel like eating and adjust portion sizes accordingly so that you meet but don't surpass your goal. For example, if your carbohydrate goal for breakfast is 60 grams, you might eat either of the two breakfasts below, each of which contains about 60 grams of carbohydrate:

BREAKFAST 1	Amount	Carbohydrate (g)
Orange juice	½ cup	15
Scrambled egg	1	under 1
Toast	2 slices	30
Margarine	1 teaspoon	0
Jelly	1 tablespoon	15
Coffee	1 cup	0
Total grams		60

BREAKFAST 2	Amount	Carbohydrate (g)
Shredded wheat	½ cup	15
Skim milk	1 cup	12
Bagel	2 ounces	30
Cream cheese	1 tablespoon	0
Coffee	1 cup	0
Total grams		57

A blood sugar test 1½ to 2 hours after breakfast should confirm that it doesn't matter what the source of carbohydrate is; it's the total amount that counts. In this way, carbohydrate counting helps you keep blood glucose levels consistent from day to day, but frees you from eating the same thing every day.

RESOURCES

Looking for guidance on carbohydrate counting? These books and booklets can help get you started with information, advice, and recipes.

The following three booklets, published by The American Dietetic Association and the American Diabetes Association, explain carbohydrate counting at three levels of complexity:

"Getting Started" teaches consistent carbohydrate intake.

"Moving On" is a guide to recognizing and managing patterns of blood glucose, food, medication, and exercise.

"Using Carbohydrate/Insulin Ratios" offers instructions in intensive management of blood glucose.

The booklets can be ordered by calling The American Dietetic Association, at (800) 877-1600, extension 5000. You can also order online, via the Association's Web site, by going to www.eatright. org/catalog/diabetes.html

THE DIABETES CARBOHYDRATE AND FAT GRAM GUIDE
Lea Ann Holzmeister
The American Dietetic Association and the American Diabetes Association, 2000
This handy reference book shows how to count carbohydrate and fat grams and includes dozens of charts listing foods, serving sizes, and nutrient data for all types of foods.

Order by calling The American Dietetic Association, at (800) 877-1600, extension 5000. You can also order online, via the Association's Web site, at www.eatright.org/catalog/diabetes.html

THE CARBOHYDRATE COUNTING COOKBOOK
Tami Ross and Patti Geil
John Wiley & Sons
New York, New York, 1998
This cookbook has instructions for carbohydrate counting as well as 125 recipes, each of which lists the number of carbohydrate choices and grams of carbohydrate per serving. A unique index lists recipes according to carbohydrate content, making it easy to keep intake consistent from day to day.

Order by calling John Wiley & Sons at (800) 225-5945.

The amount of work involved in even the most basic form of carbohydrate counting may seem overwhelming at first, but good diabetes control is worth it. During the first few weeks you try carbohydrate counting, you will need to spend time weighing and measuring foods and calculating your actual intake. After a few weeks, however, you will begin to accumulate a customized list of your favorite foods with their carbohydrate content, saving yourself the time of recalculating whenever you want to eat a favorite food or snack. Keep records of the amount of carbohydrate you eat, the amount of insulin you use and/or the amount of oral medicine you take, and your blood sugar results. You will learn to make adjustments with the help of your health-care team to achieve improved blood sugar control. ❏

CARBOHYDRATE COUNTING
Part 2: Beyond the Basics

by Patti Bazel Geil, M.S., R.D., L.D., C.D.E.

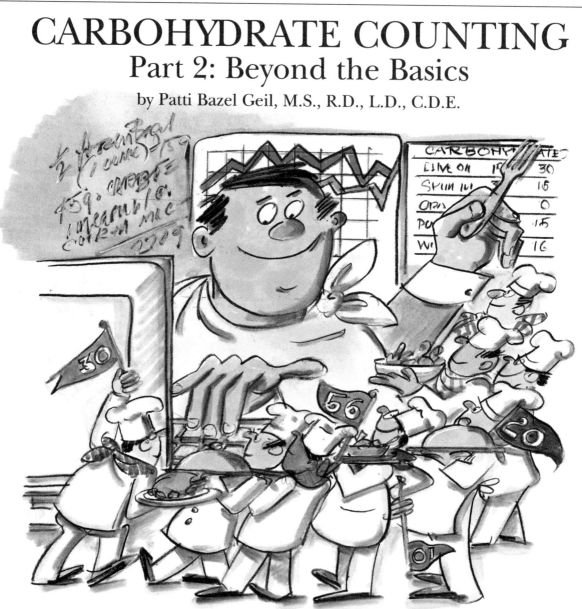

Carbohydrate counting is a very precise method of diabetes meal planning that can help you improve your blood sugar control. Part 1 of this article (page 268) covered the fundamentals of carbohydrate counting: identifying sources of carbohydrate, measuring the amount of carbohydrate in foods, and setting goals to eat consistent amounts of carbohydrate at each meal and snack. Underlying it all is the importance of keeping food and blood sugar monitoring records to enable you to see exactly how the amount of carbohydrate you eat affects your blood sugar.

Are you ready to move beyond the basics? Advanced carbohydrate counting gives you even greater flexibility in your lifestyle, along with improved blood sugar control. As you become more skilled in carbohydrate counting, you may be ready to take on the challenges of advanced forms of carbohydrate counting: pattern management and carbohydrate-to-insulin ratio. Advanced carbohydrate counting requires special skills and considerations. Pattern management involves working with your health-care team to find patterns in your blood sugar levels that are related to the foods you eat, the diabetes medicines you use, and your day's physical activity. It can be used by people with either Type 1 or Type 2 diabetes. If you have Type 1 diabetes and are taking multiple daily injections of insulin or using an insulin pump, learning about your carbohydrate-to-insulin ratio will allow you to make adjustments in your insulin dose based on the amount of carbohydrate you choose to eat.

Research has proven that it is more important for people with diabetes to monitor the total amount of carbohydrate in their diet than the source of the carbohydrate. You can enjoy formerly forbidden sweet treats in moderation if you know how to keep blood sugar levels in control using advanced carbohydrate counting.

Pattern management

If you enjoy playing detective, then pattern management will certainly appeal to you. Successful pattern management involves three steps: studying records of food, medication, physical activity, and blood sugar levels; interpreting the patterns you find in the records; and determining the steps to take to achieve your blood sugar goals.

Knowing your target blood sugar goals is the first step in pattern management. For example, you and your health-care team may decide that your blood sugar level should stay between 70 mg/dl and 150 mg/dl before meals and below 180 mg/dl one to two hours after meals. These levels are the goals you'll attempt to meet. Detailed records of factors that affect your blood sugar are the tools you'll use to meet your goals. Ideally, you should keep track of the following information:
■ Times and results of your blood sugar readings.
■ Times of meals and snacks, plus the foods eaten and the grams of carbohydrate consumed.
■ Times, type, and dose of insulin or other diabetes medicines.
■ Times, duration, and intensity of physical activity.
■ Other factors such as stress or illness that can influence blood sugar control.

Keep this very valuable information in a logbook. Review it daily, and bring it to all your clinic visits. You and your health-care team will study it and note blood

sugar levels outside your target range. You may find it helpful to use different colored highlighter pens to draw attention to levels above or below your target range.

Look for patterns in your blood sugar levels and note how often they occur. Your notes and records will help you find explanations for levels outside your target range. For example, if your blood sugar levels are too low several times a week, ask yourself the following questions:
■ Did I delay or skip meals or snacks?
■ Did I eat less carbohydrate than usual at the meal or snack just before my blood sugar tested low?
■ Does my diabetes medication need to be adjusted? Did I take the correct dose?
■ Did I participate in more physical activity than usual?

If you find blood sugar levels running too high, ask yourself these questions:
■ Did I eat more carbohydrate than usual at the meal or snack just before my blood sugar tested high?
■ Does my diabetes medication need to be adjusted? Did I take the correct dose?
■ Did I participate in less physical activity than usual?
■ Was I ill or under stress?

The final step in pattern management is to determine the action you need to take to bring your blood sugar level back into your target range. Some possible strategies include the following:
■ Changing the amount or timing of the carbohydrate you eat.
■ Changing the dose of your insulin or oral medicine or the timing.
■ Increasing or decreasing the amount of physical activity you perform or changing the time of day you exercise.

Pattern management requires more work on your part, but better blood sugar control reduces your risk of complications from diabetes, including nerve damage, damage to the eyes, and kidney disease. Better blood sugar control is worth the effort!

To see an example of the type of detective work involved in successful pattern management, take a look at "The Case of the Elevated Blood Sugar Levels" on page 275.

Carbohydrate-to-insulin ratio

If you are using intensive insulin therapy or an insulin pump, you may want to learn how to adjust your dose of short-acting or rapid-acting insulin (such as Regular or lispro) so it matches the amount of carbohydrate you decide to eat. To do this, you need to know your carbohydrate-to-insulin ratio. Most people need 1 unit of fast-acting insulin for each 10–15 grams of carbohydrate consumed. Your personal ratio can be calculated by your registered dietitian and health-care team based on your records of food intake, physical activity, insulin dose, and blood sugar readings.

For example, if you generally eat 50 grams of carbohydrate at breakfast and need 5 units of Regular insulin to achieve target blood sugar levels, your ratio is 10 grams of carbohydrate to 1 unit of insulin. If you know you'll be eating an extra biscuit at breakfast, you'll be able to add an extra unit of Regular insulin to your usual prebreakfast dose to cover the additional grams of carbohydrate. Remember, individual needs vary and may change over time. In addition, your ratio at breakfast may be different from your ratio for the remainder of the day, based on your degree of insulin resistance, or how efficiently your body uses insulin, and level of physical activity. Careful blood sugar testing and follow-up will keep you within your target range.

Before you try the carbohydrate-to-insulin ratio method of carbohydrate counting, your blood sugar levels must be in good control. You must be skilled in record-keeping, and you must be able to adjust your insulin to bring blood sugar levels that are outside your target range back into control. Instructions and support from your health-care team are essential.

Special situations

Advanced carbohydrate counting requires skills and considerations that may be new to your diabetes regimen. The following food factors are important, whatever level of carbohydrate counting you choose to try:

Fiber. Because fiber is a carbohydrate that is not digested and absorbed in the same way as sugar and starches, it has much less effect on blood sugar. Therefore, a high-fiber meal won't raise blood sugar as much as a lower-fiber meal, even if both have the same amount of carbohydrate. Keep this rule of thumb in mind: If a serving of food contains 5 or more grams of fiber, subtract them from the total grams of carbohydrate in the serving to find how much carbohydrate to count toward your meal total. For example, if you eat a bowl of cereal with 8 grams of fiber per serving, subtract 8 grams from the total grams of carbohydrate in the serving and only count what's left toward the meal total.

Combination foods. If you read Part 1 of this article, which deals with basic carbohydrate counting, you learned how to use exchange lists, labels, and food value books to calculate the amount of carbohydrate in your food. What about foods that aren't found in these references? You won't have to give up your grandmother's special potato salad if you take the time to separate the recipe ingredients, weigh or measure them, and calculate the approximate grams of carbohydrate in a serving. Here's an example of

how to calculate the carbohydrate choices in a recipe:

GRANDMA'S POTATO SALAD

Ingredient	Amount	Carbohydrate (g)
Potatoes	1 pound	80
Hard-boiled eggs, chopped	2	0
Chopped onion	⅓ cup	2
Chopped celery	1 cup	5
Mayonnaise	1 cup	0
Vinegar	2 tablespoons	0
Salt	1 teaspoon	0
Sugar	1 teaspoon	3
White pepper	¼ teaspoon	0
	TOTAL GRAMS	90

If you know that this recipe makes five servings, you can divide 90 by 5 to calculate that a serving will contain approximately 18 grams of carbohydrate. Once you've calculated the amount of carbohydrate in several of your favorite dishes, you'll find it's much easier to keep track of your carbohydrate intake.

Free and fat-free. You may be including fat-free foods in your meal plan and assuming that they are also low in carbohydrate. If so, take a closer look at the nutrition information for these foods. Some fat-free foods are high enough in calories and carbohydrate to affect your blood sugar control. Here are some foods whose carbohydrate content may surprise you:

Food	Carbohydrate (g)
Fat-free ranch salad dressing (2 tablespoons)	11
Fat-free cream cheese (2 tablespoons)	1
Fat-free fig cookies (2)	22
Fat-free vanilla ice cream (½ cup)	20

You may also be surprised at the amount of carbohydrate in foods traditionally considered "free" foods such as salads. A large salad with lettuce, tomatoes, carrots, peppers, celery, and croutons may contain as much as 12 grams of carbohydrate, or almost as much as one carbohydrate choice.

Eating out. Does carbohydrate counting mean the end of eating out? No one wants to go into a restaurant with food scales in hand, but you can take this meal-planning method on the road with a bit of preparation. Try practicing at home. After you've learned to estimate portion sizes accurately, you'll be able to know at a glance the amount of carbohydrate in your restaurant meal.

THE CASE OF THE ELEVATED BLOOD SUGAR LEVELS

This simple case study illustrates the basic steps of pattern management: studying the data, identifying patterns, interpreting the data, and determining possible actions or strategies.

PATIENT INFORMATION

TIMOTHY MITFORD
Type 2 diabetes, treated with diet and oral
  diabetes medicine every morning
Elevated presupper blood sugar levels

BLOOD SUGAR TARGETS
70–150 mg/dl before meals
Less than 180 mg/dl one to two hours after meals

CARBOHYDRATE GOALS
40 grams at breakfast
40 grams at lunch
60 grams at supper

RECORDS
Timothy's blood sugar records for three consecutive days were as follows:

Day	Activity	Time	Blood sugar (mg/dl)	Lunch	Carbohydrate (g)
Thursday	Office work	11:30 AM	146	Double cheeseburger	31
				Medium French fries	49
				Diet soft drink	0
				TOTAL GRAMS	80
		6:00 PM	242		
Friday	Office work	12:00 PM	151	Pepperoni pizza, 2 slices	45
				Garden salad with fat-free dressing	5
				Diet soft drink	0
				TOTAL GRAMS	50
		5:30 PM	212		
Saturday	Gardening	11:30 AM	133	Grilled chicken breast, 3 ounces	0
				Rice pilaf, ½ cup	30
				Watermelon, 1 cup	12
				Sugar-free iced tea, 12 ounces	0
				TOTAL GRAMS	42
		6:00 PM	101		

THE INVESTIGATION: Timothy and his dietitian studied his records, circled blood sugar levels outside of the target range, and identified a pattern of elevated sugar levels, particularly before supper.

They also noted that these elevated levels occurred most often during the work week, when Timothy ate a fast-food lunch and spent the afternoon in his office doing paperwork. He ate more carbohydrate at lunch than his established goal. His weekend routine was considerably different, allowing for more physical activity and better blood sugar levels.

TAKING ACTION: Timothy and his health-care team considered several strategies for improving his evening blood sugar levels. Their possible solutions included the following:

ADJUST FOOD. Timothy could try to stay within his lunch carbohydrate goal of 40 grams. He may need to decrease his portion sizes or bring lunch from home during the workweek.

ADJUST PHYSICAL ACTIVITY. Timothy could increase his afternoon physical activity by taking a brisk walk during his lunch hour. Depending on his office location, he may be able to walk to and from his lunch location instead of taking a cab or driving.

ADJUST MEDICATION. Timothy may need to increase the dose of his oral diabetes medicine or add a second drug.

It also helps to scout out the menu ahead of time. If you know what's on the menu, you can estimate the carbohydrate content of the foods you are most likely to order. If possible, order takeout portions of your favorite restaurant foods so you can bring them home to weigh and measure.

If you eat in fast-food restaurants often, don't focus on carbohydrate content alone and ignore the protein and fat content of your meals. The main focus of your meal plan should be healthy eating. Fortunately, nutrition information is yours for the asking at most fast-food restaurant chains. Keep this information handy so you'll know the carbohydrate content of your usual fast-food fare.

Thinking for your pancreas

Carbohydrate counting enables you to think like a pancreas and achieve good blood sugar control. However, several factors in addition to carbohydrate can influence your thinking.

A high-fat meal can slow down the time your stomach takes to empty, delaying the after-meal rise in your blood sugar levels. If you eat a very high-fat supper, your bedtime blood sugar may be higher than usual. The same thing may occur if you happen to eat more protein than usual.

And seemingly small differences in cooking methods may have surprising effects on your blood sugar. For example, pasta absorbs more water the longer it cooks, so pasta cooked al dente can contain significantly more carbohydrate than the same amount of tender-cooked pasta.

What about alcohol? Alcohol generally lowers blood sugar, so extra insulin isn't required unless a mixed drink contains sugar-sweetened beverages or fruit juices. As always, use alcohol with caution. Speak with your health-care team to learn how to handle these special situations.

Lifestyle flexibility and good diabetes control are the biggest advantages of carbohydrate counting. However, tight control may lead to low blood sugar and/or weight gain. Weight gain can occur for several reasons, including the following:
■ As blood sugar control improves, you lose fewer calories as sugar in the urine.
■ You may be so focused on carbohydrate that you forget about the calories from protein and fat.
■ You may be using high-calorie foods such as candy bars and ice cream to treat low blood sugar instead of the more effective 15 grams of pure carbohydrate from glucose tablets or fruit juice.
■ You may be enjoying the flexibility of carbohydrate counting a bit too much by indulging yourself in high-calorie sweet treats or larger portion sizes that you may not have eaten in the past.

Your registered dietitian and health-care team are available to help you learn about carbohydrate counting and encourage you as you face the challenges of living with this effective method of meal planning. Carbohydrate counts in good blood sugar control! ❏

HEALTHY EATING FOR OLDER ADULTS

by Linnea Hagberg, R.D.

Who is the most likely to be nutritionally at risk: a 45-year-old woman, her 20-year-old daughter, or her 70-year-old mother? If you guessed the 70-year-old, you're correct. Good nutrition is important to good health at any stage in life. Aging, however, brings many changes, including a number that can affect nutritional well-being. For those in or approaching the later years of life, a bit of extra dietary vigilance can help maximize the opportunity for an active, healthy future.

For starters, older adults require and generally consume fewer calories than their younger counterparts, yet they need about the same amount of vitamins and minerals, and in some cases, they need more. To meet their nutrition needs, then, older people must obtain a lot of nutrients from a relatively small amount of food—no simple feat. Spending calories on foods that contain a high proportion of vitamins and minerals—that is, choosing nutrient-dense foods—is the best way to accomplish this task. This doesn't mean a steady diet of skinless chicken and broccoli (although those *are* healthful foods). It means paying a bit more attention to food choices and making small changes where necessary. For example, switching from corn flakes to higher-fiber bran flakes at breakfast, eating a sweet potato instead of white rice at dinner, and choosing a calcium-rich dietetic pudding rather than a cookie are all changes that result in a better nutrient intake for about the same number of calories.

In addition to a reduction in calorie needs, aging can be accompanied by numerous changes, many of which affect how or what people eat. Of course, no two people age in just the same way. Some persons may find they feel about the same in their 70's as they did in their 60's or even their 50's, while others may experience serious medical problems or find they suddenly have to cope with a major change in lifestyle. Still others may find they are simply slowing down a bit and have less interest in food shopping, cooking, or even eating. Some change is an inevitable part of aging, however, and being aware of potential nutrition trouble spots can help avert problems.

Nutrient needs

Many older adults have a problem absorbing vitamin B_{12}, even if they eat plenty of foods that contain the vitamin. This is because an estimated 20% to 30% of people in their 60's and almost 40% of those over 80 have a condition known as *atrophic gastritis*. This condition causes a reduction in stomach acid, which makes it difficult for the body to separate vitamin B_{12} from the proteins it is bound to in food and hinders its absorption into the body. A lack of vitamin B_{12} can lead to neurological problems, mental confusion, and dementia. Since there aren't obvious symptoms of atrophic gastritis, older adults may want to choose a breakfast cereal fortified with vitamin B_{12} (a form that can be absorbed regardless of stomach acid production) or discuss taking a B_{12} supplement with their doctor.

Getting enough vitamin D and calcium to maintain healthy bones and stave off osteoporosis—a disease characterized by thinning, fragile bones that affects 10 million Americans—is another area of concern for older adults. Aging hampers the body's ability to absorb vitamin D from food. And while vitamin D is also manufactured by the body via a reaction of substances in the skin after exposure to sunlight, the aging body is less efficient in this process.

Vitamin D is not well distributed in the food supply. The major source of vitamin D in the American diet is fortified milk. Other dairy products such as yogurt and cheese do not contain the vitamin. Some breakfast cereals are also fortified with a small amount of vitamin D. Goals for vitamin D vitamin intake by a healthy individual in the absence of adequate exposure to sunlight have been established by the Food and Nutrition Board of the U.S. Institute of Medicine: 10 micrograms a day for ages 51 to 70, which is equivalent to 400 International Units (IU's) a day, and 15 micrograms (600 IU's) a day for ages above 70; these

TIPS FOR THE SOLO COOK

If you're used to shopping or cooking for a crowd (or if you're not used to shopping or cooking at all) planning and preparing meals for just yourself can be a challenge. But everyone needs and deserves good, nutritious food, so it's worth the effort to learn to feed yourself well. Here are some tips to make the process easier:

■ Plan ahead. Sketch out menus and shopping lists for a few days at a time.

■ Assume you'll have leftovers. Plan combination dishes like soups, casseroles, salads, and pasta preparations to use them up.

■ Use the same ingredient in more than one way. For example, a head of cabbage can be sautéed, layered in a casserole with ground meat or rice, and turned into cole slaw.

■ To cut down on the number of times you need to cook each week, try occasionally making large dishes that can be divided into several individual servings, frozen, and used later in the week or month. Or cook extra food one night to be used the next.

■ Set up your kitchen for one person. You may need to buy smaller cooking pans and storage containers. Consider buying a microwave oven if you don't already own one.

■ For inspiration, look for cookbooks written specifically for solo diners at your local library or bookstore.

■ Supplement fresh produce with canned and frozen varieties. Buy frozen fruits and vegetables in plastic bags. That way, you can use as much as you want and pop the rest back into the freezer.

■ If necessary, ask your butcher to repackage meat or poultry into smaller packages.

■ Buy one new food item each week to add variety to your meals.

are "Adequate Intake" figures, which the Institute uses when there is not enough scientific data to develop an official Recommended Dietary Allowance. Older adults who fall short of these goals may wish to discuss taking a supplement with their doctor. Those who do take supplements, however, should be careful not to take more than their doctor recommends, since too much vitamin D can be harmful.

Older adults may also be shortchanging themselves on calcium. Dietary recommendations call for those age 51 and older to take in 1200 milligrams of calcium (the National Institutes of Health recommends 1500 milligrams a day for those 65 and older). Many Americans, however, consume only half that amount.

One of the best sources of both calcium and vitamin D is milk; one cup contains 300 milligrams of calcium and 100 IU's of vitamin D, plus protein, vitamin B_{12}, and a number of other nutrients. (People limiting calories or fat in their diet should drink nonfat or low-fat milk.) A greater proportion of older people, however, may have trouble breaking down lactose, the sugar in milk. Many of those who do have difficulty digesting milk can tolerate small daily amounts (one or two cups a day in ½-cup to 1-cup portions) or find they can eat yogurt or aged cheese. A number of reduced-lactose dairy products are also widely available, as are calcium-fortified soy milk and orange juice. Calcium is also contained in leafy, dark greens like collards and kale and in canned salmon and sardines eaten with their bones. As with vitamin D, those unable to get enough calcium from their diet should consider making up shortfalls with a supplement.

Although often overlooked as a nutrient, water is vital to the health of older adults. Water serves many roles in the body, from controlling temperature to dispersing medicines to helping the kidneys function properly. Fluid needs don't go up with age; like younger adults, healthy older adults need eight glasses or more a day. What does change, however, is the ability to feel thirst, which is reduced in many older people. To meet their fluid needs, then, older adults need to use cues other than thirst as reminders to drink. For example, it can be helpful to make it a regular habit to drink a full glass of water in addition to any other beverage with every meal and snack, or to drink a glass of water every two hours. Getting plenty of fluids and adequate amounts of fiber (discussed below) will also help relieve constipation, a common problem in older adults.

Water is not the only choice for fluids. Other beverages, including fruit juice, milk, and herbal and decaffeinated teas also count. However, water contains no calories, sugar, or other unwanted extras, so it remains the best first choice.

Fiber facts

Fiber is another nutrient worth considering when discussing the well-being of older adults. Getting enough fiber has health benefits for young and old alike, but aging increases the likelihood of two conditions—diverticulosis and constipation—that respond well to a high-fiber diet.

According to the National Institute of Diabetes and Digestive and Kidney Diseases, a branch of the U.S. National Institutes of Health, nearly half of Americans aged 60 to 80, and almost everyone over the age of 80,

has a condition known as *diverticulosis*, in which small pouches called diverticula bulge outward through weak spots in the colon. These pouches can be formed when pressure, usually from constipation, builds in the colon. Although many people with diverticulosis have no symptoms, the pouches can become infected or inflamed, causing abdominal pain and fever, a condition known as diverticulitis.

Constipation is another common condition for older adults. In the 1991 National Health Survey, more than 4 million people reported they are constipated most or all of the time, and adults age 65 and over were among those who reported the complaint the most. Diets rich in fiber help relieve constipation. However, while current recommendations call for Americans to consume 20 to 35 grams of fiber a day, the average older adult takes in only about 15 grams per day.

One good way to start adding fiber to your diet is to choose a breakfast cereal with at least 5 grams of fiber per serving. Other fiber-rich foods include fruits and vegetables, especially those with edible peels and skins; whole wheat bread and whole grains such as oatmeal and brown rice; and dried beans and peas. Adding cooked beans to other dishes is a great way to boost the fiber content of a meal. For example, try adding black beans to cooked rice, white beans to tuna fish, and kidney beans or chick peas to tossed salads.

Sensory changes

In addition to having an increased need for specific nutrients, older adults are also more likely to be affected by a number of factors, including sensory changes, that can affect overall food intake.

Aging can bring about a decrease in the acuity of some senses. About half of adults over age 65, for example, experience some impairment in their ability to smell food. Taste buds may also lose their sensitivity. As a result, older adults may feel that their food lacks flavor, find they have decreased pleasure or interest in eating, or begin reaching for the salt shaker or sugar bowl to compensate. Alterations in taste and smell can sometimes be related to underlying medical conditions such as an inflammation of the mucous membranes or sinuses. They can also be caused by certain drugs, so it's worth talking over any changes in taste or smell with a doctor before chalking them up to old age.

If the source of taste changes can't be located, however, there are other steps to take. Research indicates that enhancing food with herbs and flavoring agents such as lemon or lime juice, flavored vinegars, artificially sweetened maple syrup, or butter flavor granules results in greater food intake. Those with a greater loss of smell show the most gains in food intake. Combin-

FOOD PYRAMID FOR ADULTS 70+

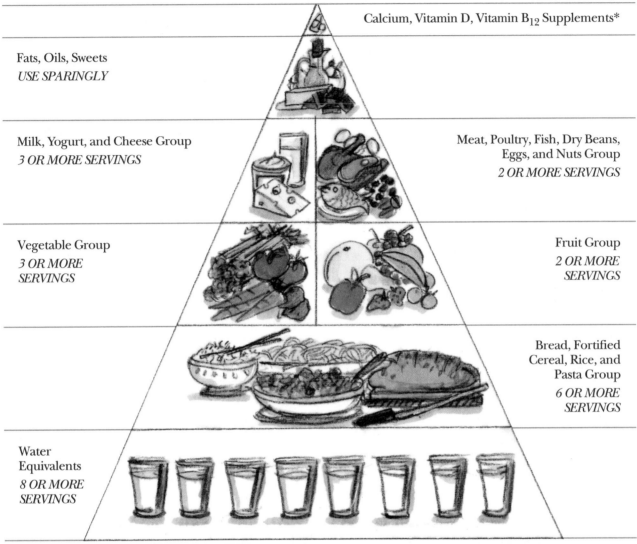

Calcium, Vitamin D, Vitamin B_{12} Supplements*

Fats, Oils, Sweets
USE SPARINGLY

Milk, Yogurt, and Cheese Group
3 OR MORE SERVINGS

Meat, Poultry, Fish, Dry Beans,
Eggs, and Nuts Group
2 OR MORE SERVINGS

Vegetable Group
*3 OR MORE
SERVINGS*

Fruit Group
*2 OR MORE
SERVINGS*

Bread, Fortified
Cereal, Rice, and
Pasta Group
*6 OR MORE
SERVINGS*

Water
Equivalents
*8 OR MORE
SERVINGS*

*Not all individuals need supplements; consult your health-care provider.   © Copyright 1999 Tufts University

A DAY IN THE LIFE OF THE PYRAMID

The following menu represents a one-day meal plan based on the minimum recommendations of the
70+ Food Pyramid. This menu contains approximately 1,760 calories and 30 grams of fiber.

BREAKFAST
1 cup water
1 serving (1 ounce) bran flakes
½ cup skim milk
½ red grapefruit
1 slice whole wheat toast with
  1 teaspoon margarine
Coffee or tea

MID-MORNING
1 cup water
1 cup split pea soup

LUNCH
Tuna fish sandwich with
  lettuce on two slices whole
  wheat bread
1 cup skim milk
1 piece fresh fruit
1 cup water

AFTERNOON
1 cup water
1 ounce low-fat whole wheat
  crackers

DINNER
1 piece baked or broiled
  chicken
1 small baked sweet potato
½ cup steamed spinach
1 cup water
½ cup artificially sweetened
  pudding made with skim milk

EVENING
1 cup skim milk
1 ounce graham crackers

ing different textures—for example adding chewy raisins to oatmeal or crispy lettuce to a sandwich—is also helpful, as is alternating bites of different foods during a meal and making meals with a variety of tastes, textures, and colors.

Bear in mind, too, that smoking, drinking coffee, and eating very hot or very cold food decrease the ability to taste and smell.

Aging and health problems

Increasing age brings an increasing likelihood of being affected by one or more medical conditions, such as Type 2 diabetes or high blood pressure, that necessitate making dietary changes. For many, this may be the first time they have to pay significant attention to what they eat. Some people may be faced with more than one problem requiring dietary changes, a situation that can make meal planning a real juggling act. Working with a professional such as a certified diabetes educator or a registered dietitian can be helpful.

As a result of the increase in medical conditions, older people are more likely to be taking prescription or over-the-counter drugs. Some drugs may affect specific nutrients—for example some diuretics cause the body to lose potassium. Other drugs can have side effects such as stomach distress or appetite suppression, or they can affect the way food tastes, which in turn can affect food intake. People who suspect that a particular drug is causing such side effects may wish to check with their doctor to see if another drug could be substituted. Even if switching drugs is not a possibility, other measures such as changing the timing or dose of a drug may be.

Other medical conditions can affect diet indirectly, by interfering with a person's ability to shop for or prepare food. Arthritis, for example, can make it hard to cook, while vision problems can make driving and shopping, as well as preparing food, difficult. So can a medical problem that saps strength and makes it difficult to find the energy to prepare food.

While physical limitations can sometimes cause overwhelming and obvious changes, subtler changes can also take place. For example, a person who cannot get out to shop frequently may find it hard to keep fresh fruits and vegetables on hand. Someone who has trouble cooking may grow to rely on frozen meals, many of which lack vitamins, minerals, and fiber and contain too much fat and sodium. Modern food-processing techniques and a growing consumer interest in healthful foods have made these particular problems relatively easy to remedy. For example, frozen and canned fruits and vegetables, which last much longer than fresh varieties, are nutritious choices if they aren't packed in syrup or processed with added salt. And there are a variety of low-fat and low-sodium frozen dinners on the market that can be nutritionally enhanced by a glass of milk, an extra vegetable or salad, and a piece of fresh fruit for dessert. (Read the Nutrition Facts label to find out how many calories and how much carbohydrate, fat, protein, fiber, and sodium a product contains.) The key is to recognize that changes have occurred so that they can be addressed.

Changes in family structure

Older people may also find themselves alone after many years of living with a loved one, or they may find that due to the death or disability of a spouse, they are newly faced with the role of shopping and cooking. Some people may find it difficult to motivate themselves to cook when it is "only" for themselves. Others may lack the necessary skills. Additional challenges to the solo cook and diner include difficulty eating a varied diet or trouble with eating regular meals, an issue of particular importance to those with diabetes.

Inviting friends or neighbors for meals or having a standing date to share meals with others can help motivate the single cook. If regular meals are a problem, changing to six smaller meals and snacks a day may be helpful. (Check with your diabetes-care team before making big changes in your meal plan.) More tips for the single cook are on page 277.

The 70+ food pyramid

Even given the many changes that can occur with age, for the most part, a healthful diet for older adults is much the same as that for everyone else. It is a diet that emphasizes whole grains, fruits, and vegetables with judicious amounts of dairy products, meat, fish, poultry, and eggs. To reflect some of the special needs of older adults, however, researchers at Tufts University developed a Modified Food Pyramid for 70+ Adults (see page 279), based on the familiar USDA Food Guide Pyramid. The 70+ Pyramid is intended as a guide for relatively healthy and active older adults who live independently.

While the 70+ Pyramid looks much the same as the USDA Pyramid, a level has been added to the base of the Pyramid to reflect the need for fluid intake, and the top carries a reminder of the potential need for some supplements. Except for dairy products, where the recommendation is for three servings a day, the number of servings in the 70+ Pyramid is the lowest number of servings from the USDA Pyramid. This pattern reflects the lower food intake characteristic of older adults.

Again, to maximize the intake of necessary vitamins, minerals, and fiber while eating less food, the researchers recommend selecting nutrient-dense foods. This means choosing whole grains (for example, eating whole wheat bread instead of, say, rye or white) and dark green, red, orange, or yellow fruits and vegetables (for example, eating broccoli in place of celery or a red grapefruit rather than a pear) as often as possible. The Tufts researchers also recommend choosing cruciferous vegetables (such as broccoli, cabbage, and Brussels sprouts) often and substituting legumes (dried peas, beans, or lentils) for meat twice a week.

It's never too late to make healthful changes in eating. Considering that the 80+ group is slated to be one of the fastest-growing populations, a little dietary care in your late 60's or early 70's might well be paving the way for a healthier age 90. ❏

HOW TO CUT BACK ON SATURATED FAT

by Ann M. Coulston, M.S., R.D., and Patricia M. Schaaf, M.S., R.D.

You may have heard you should cut back on saturated fat in your diet. Or maybe you've heard you should cut back on *all* fats. But you also know that, for good blood glucose control, people with diabetes need to keep careful track of the amount of carbohydrate they eat. So how do you sort out all the dietary advice you hear? And how do you go about adding, subtracting, or limiting various nutrients in your diet and still end up with meals you enjoy?

When you have diabetes, good places to turn to for dietary advice are the American Diabetes Association and The American Dietetic Association. The joint Associations have developed nutrition recommendations aimed at helping people with diabetes meet their total nutrient needs while striving for good blood glucose and blood lipid (cholesterol and triglyceride) control. The recommendations address calorie intake to achieve and maintain a healthful body weight, as well as the percentage of total calorie intake that should come from a combination of animal and vegetable proteins (10% to 20%). The remaining 80% to 90% of calories should come from carbohydrate and fat, but the American Diabetes and Dietetic Associations do not recommend a specific percentage of total calories from either carbohydrate or fat. Those percentages must be worked out on an individual basis. This is where working with a registered dietitian can be especially helpful.

The Associations do recommend that a person's intake of saturated fat be no more than 10% of calories, and that dietary cholesterol intake be less than 300 milligrams per day. (For some individuals, lower ceilings, such as 7% and 200 milligrams, respectively, are advised.) That's because eating too much saturated fat and cholesterol can contribute to the development of cardiovascular disease, and people with diabetes are already at increased risk. To help you meet these guidelines, this article focuses on ways to limit saturated fat and cholesterol in your diet.

Fats are triglycerides

The fats found in foods such as oil, butter, nuts, meat, fish, and poultry are called *triglycerides*. Each triglyceride molecule is made up of three *fatty acids* (fats, to the layperson). Fatty acids are classified as saturated fats, polyunsaturated fats, or monounsaturated fats according to their chemical composition. Triglycerides made mostly of saturated fatty acids tend to be solid at room temperature; coconut oil and butter are examples of foods containing mostly saturated fats. By contrast, triglycerides that contain mostly polyunsaturated or monounsaturated fats tend to be liquid at room temperature; canola oil, olive oil, and safflower oil fall into this category. After a person eats a food containing fat, the triglyceride molecules break down and release the fatty acids to be used by the body.

Most of the triglycerides found in foods are a combination of all three types of fatty acids. However, many fats and oils have more of one type of fatty acid than the other two types. Therefore, your food choices can affect the overall fatty acid composition of your diet.

FINDING THE FAT

FOOD	CALORIES	TOTAL FAT (g)	SATURATED FAT (g)	MONO-UNSATURATED FAT (g)	POLY-UNSATURATED FAT (g)	CHOLESTEROL (mg)
BEEF						
Serving size = 3 ounces cooked						
Round eye	149	4.9	1.8	2.1	0.2	59
Top round steak	153	4.2	1.4	1.6	0.2	71
Round tip sirloin roast	157	5.9	2.1	2.3	0.2	69
Top sirloin	166	6.1	2.4	2.6	0.2	76
Flank steak	176	8.6	3.7	3.5	0.3	57
Tenderloin steak	179	8.5	3.2	3.2	0.3	71
PORK						
Serving size = 3 ounces cooked						
Tenderloin	159	5.4	1.9	2.2	0.5	80
Sirloin chop	184	8.8	3.1	3.8	0.7	73
Loin chop	206	11.8	4.5	5.3	1.0	68
Rib chop	217	13.0	5.0	5.9	1.1	62
Canadian bacon	157	7.2	2.4	3.4	0.7	49
Ham	134	4.7	1.6	2.2	0.5	47
POULTRY						
Serving size = 3 ounces cooked						
Skinless chicken breast	140	3.0	0.9	1.1	0.7	72
Chicken breast with skin	168	6.6	1.9	2.6	1.4	71
Skinless chicken thigh	178	9.3	2.6	3.5	2.1	81
Chicken thigh with skin	210	13.2	3.7	5.2	2.9	79
Skinless turkey breast	115	0.6	0.2	0.1	0.2	71
Skinless turkey leg	175	8.2	2.6	2.4	2.3	77
SEAFOOD						
Serving size = 3 ounces cooked						
Orange roughy	76	0.8	0.0	0.5	0.0	22
Prawns/Large shrimp	84	0.9	0.3	0.2	0.4	166
Cod	89	0.7	0.1	0.1	0.3	40
Sole/Flounder	100	1.3	0.3	0.3	0.4	58
Halibut	119	2.5	0.4	0.8	0.8	35
Salmon	127	3.8	0.6	1.0	1.5	57
Light tuna (in oil)	168	7.0	1.3	2.5	2.5	15
Light tuna (in water)	99	0.7	0.2	0.1	0.3	26
Sardines (in oil)	177	9.8	1.3	3.3	4.4	121
Clams	126	1.7	0.2	0.2	0.5	57
DAIRY						
Whole milk (8 ounces)	139	7.5	4.9	2.0	0.3	31
2% milk (8 ounces)	113	4.4	2.9	1.1	0.2	17
1% milk (8 ounces)	95	2.4	1.6	0.6	0.1	9
Soy milk (8 ounces)	75	4.4	0.5	0.7	1.9	0

Nutrition and Meal Planning

DAIRY (continued)	CALORIES	TOTAL FAT (g)	SATURATED FAT (g)	MONO-UNSATURATED FAT (g)	POLY-UNSATURATED FAT (g)	CHOLESTEROL (mg)
2% yogurt (¾ cup)	116	2.6	1.9	0.7	0.1	11
2% cottage cheese (¼ cup)	51	1.1	0.7	0.3	0.0	5
American cheese (1 ounce)	106	8.9	5.9	2.2	0.4	27
Mozzarella cheese (1 ounce)	79	4.9	3.1	1.4	0.1	15
Feta cheese (1 ounce)	81	6.1	5.1	—	—	25
Cheddar cheese (1 ounce)	114	9.4	7.7	2.1	0.4	30
Swiss cheese (1 ounce)	107	7.8	5.1	2.1	0.3	26
Jack cheese (1 ounce)	106	8.6	5.4	2.5	0.3	25
Parmesan cheese (2 tablespoons)	57	3.8	2.4	1.1	0.1	10

EGGS

	CALORIES	TOTAL FAT (g)	SATURATED FAT (g)	MONO-UNSATURATED FAT (g)	POLY-UNSATURATED FAT (g)	CHOLESTEROL (mg)
Egg (medium, raw)	78	5.3	1.6	2.0	0.7	212
Egg Beaters (¼ cup)	69	4.8	0.8	1.1	2.7	1

NUTS
Serving size = 1 ounce

	CALORIES	TOTAL FAT (g)	SATURATED FAT (g)	MONO-UNSATURATED FAT (g)	POLY-UNSATURATED FAT (g)	CHOLESTEROL (mg)
Peanuts	165	14.0	1.9	7.0	4.4	0
Almonds	166	14.6	1.4	9.5	3.1	0
Walnuts	172	16.1	1.0	3.6	10.6	0
Pecans	189	19.2	1.5	12.0	4.7	0
Cashews	163	13.2	2.6	7.7	2.2	0
Macadamias	204	21.7	3.3	17.1	0.4	0
Pistachios	164	13.7	1.7	9.3	2.1	0
Sunflower seeds	165	14.1	1.5	2.7	9.3	0

FATS/OILS
Serving size = 1 teaspoon

	CALORIES	TOTAL FAT (g)	SATURATED FAT (g)	MONO-UNSATURATED FAT (g)	POLY-UNSATURATED FAT (g)	CHOLESTEROL (mg)
Canola oil	40	4.5	0.3	2.8	1.2	0
Olive oil	40	4.5	0.6	3.3	0.4	0
Safflower oil	40	4.5	0.4	0.6	3.4	0
Corn oil	40	4.5	0.6	1.1	2.7	0
Sunflower oil	40	4.5	0.6	0.7	3.1	0
Shortening	38	4.3	1.1	1.9	1.1	0
Mayonnaise	33	3.7	0.5	1.1	1.9	3
Butter	34	3.8	2.4	1.2	0.1	10
Margarine (tub)	34	3.8	0.7	1.5	1.5	0
Margarine (stick)	34	3.8	0.6	2.2	0.9	0

OTHER

	CALORIES	TOTAL FAT (g)	SATURATED FAT (g)	MONO-UNSATURATED FAT (g)	POLY-UNSATURATED FAT (g)	CHOLESTEROL (mg)
Olives, black (8)	41	3.9	0.5	2.8	0.3	0
Avocado (1 ounce, or ⅛)	50	4.9	0.7	3.2	0.6	0
Chocolate (1 ounce)	145	8.7	4.7	3.2	0.3	6
Tofu, regular (4 ounces)	86	5.4	0.8	1.2	3.1	0
Peanut butter (2 tablespoons)	188	16.0	3.1	7.6	4.6	0
Sour cream (2 tablespoons)	62	6.0	3.7	1.7	0.2	13
Cream cheese (1 tablespoon)	50	5.0	3.5	—	—	15
Bacon (2 slices, 13 grams)	75	6.4	2.3	3.1	0.8	11

SAMPLE MEAL PLAN

This sample one-day menu provides about 2,000 calories and is
low in saturated fat and high in monounsaturated fat.

FOOD	AMOUNT	CALORIES	TOTAL FAT (g)	SATURATED FAT (g)	MONO-UNSATURATED FAT (g)	POLY-UNSATURATED FAT (g)	CHOLESTEROL (mg)
BREAKFAST							
English muffin	1 whole	134	1.0	0.2	0.3	0.4	0
Natural peanut butter	2 tablespoons	187	16.0	2.2	7.9	5.0	0
2% milk	1 cup	121	4.7	3.1	1.2	0.2	18
SNACK							
Orange	1 medium	62	*	—	—	—	—
LUNCH							
Whole wheat bread	2 slices	172	2.9	0.7	1.3	0.7	0
Light tuna in water	2 ounces	66	0.5	0.1	0.1	0.2	17
Mayonnaise	1 tablespoon	99	11.3	1.6	3.2	5.8	8
Lettuce	2 leaves	5	*	—	—	—	—
Avocado	4 slices	65	6.1	1.0	3.8	0.8	0
Apple	1 medium	81	*	—	—	—	—
SNACK							
Almonds	¼ cup	209	18.5	1.8	12.0	3.9	0
Dried apricots	6 whole	100	*	—	—	—	—
DINNER							
Beef round, cooked	3 ounces	149	4.9	1.8	2.1	0.2	59
Baked potato	1 medium	145	*	—	—	—	—
Sour cream	1 tablespoon	31	3.0	1.9	0.9	0.1	6
Green string beans	1 cup	44	*	—	—	—	—
Salad:							
Shredded lettuce	1 cup	9	*	—	—	—	—
Cherry tomatoes	3	11	*	—	—	—	—
Ripe olives	5 large	26	2.4	0.3	1.8	0.2	0
Black beans, cooked	¼ cup	57	*	—	—	—	—
Parmesan cheese	1 tablespoon	29	1.9	1.2	0.6	0	5
Salad dressing:							
Olive oil	1 tablespoon	119	14.0	1.9	10.0	1.1	0
Balsamic vinegar	1 tablespoon	14	*	—	—	—	—
SNACK							
Pretzel sticks	1 ounce	108	1.0	0.2	0.4	0.4	0
Totals:		**2,043**	**88.2**	**18.0**	**45.6**	**19.0**	**113**

Note: The grams of the three fatty acids do not add up to the total fat because trace amounts of fatty acids are not accounted for.
Asterisk indicates food items with less than 0.5 gram total fat.

Recent clinical studies have shown beneficial effects of a diet low in saturated fat and high in monounsaturated fat. The data from these studies not only show that this type of diet lowers blood cholesterol and blood lipids, but they show that it improves blood glucose control in people with Type 2 diabetes. So even though a diet high in monounsaturated fat may increase the total fat in your diet, it may also have a number of beneficial effects on your diabetes control.

The table "Finding the Fat" beginning on page 282 lists how much of each of the three types of fatty acids is found in everyday foods. Dairy products, especially those made from whole milk, tend to have a greater percentage of saturated fat than unsaturated fats. Choosing low-fat or nonfat dairy products over the whole milk type will therefore lower your saturated fat intake. Many of the items in the meat, poultry, and seafood lists have more monounsaturated fat than saturated fat per serving. And several plant foods, including olives and avocados, are very rich sources of monounsaturated fat. Identifying foods you enjoy that are good sources of monounsaturated fat is an important step toward controlling the amounts of saturated fat and cholesterol you eat.

Fat versus carbohydrate

"But wait a minute," you may be thinking. "Are you actually encouraging me to eat fat?" Dietitians and researchers have posed a similar question: "As people with diabetes follow the nutrition recommendations to consume less than 10% of calories from saturated fat, should they replace foods high in saturated fat with monounsaturated fat or with carbohydrate?"

To answer this question, let's review the history of diet therapy for diabetes. The classic problem of diabetes is high blood glucose. Before the discovery of insulin and, more recently, oral medicines, diet therapy focused on severely restricting dietary carbohydrate. With the introduction of effective drug therapy, restrictions on carbohydrate were eased. By 1986, the American Diabetes Association recommendations for dietary carbohydrate were set at 55% to 60% of the total calories a person consumed. However, this recommendation came about not because of scientific evidence to support a high carbohydrate intake but because of data that showed that a low fat intake reduces the risk factors associated with heart disease. Since people with diabetes are at increased risk for heart disease, medical scientists felt that the low-fat, high-carbohydrate recommendations made some 30 years ago by the American Heart Association *for the general public* seemed appropriate for people with diabetes.

However, clinical research and experience since 1986 have shown that high-carbohydrate diets tend to increase plasma triglycerides, lower high-density lipoprotein (HDL) cholesterol (the "good" cholesterol), and have no favorable impact on low-density lipoprotein (LDL) cholesterol (the "bad" cholesterol), particularly in people with Type 2 diabetes. These findings created a carbohydrate-versus-fat dilemma and encouraged scientists to further investigate the effects of diet on people with diabetes.

Today, evidence suggests that diets that contain no more than 30% to 35% of total calories from fat, in which the composition of fat has been modified to reduce saturated fat and dietary cholesterol, offer the best overall control of blood glucose and blood lipid metabolism in people with diabetes.

Calculating fat intake

"Finding the Fat" on pages 282 and 283 illustrates that no food contains only one type of fat. For each item, this table provides the total fat (triglycerides) and its respective composition of fatty acids. For example, the first food listed in the table is beef, round eye. The total fat for a 3-ounce serving (a piece about the size of a deck of playing cards) is 4.9 grams. The fatty acid distribution shows that there are more grams of monounsaturated fat (2.1 grams) than saturated fat (1.8 grams). If you compare round eye with an equal portion of skinless chicken breast, you can

REFERENCE MATERIALS

For more about meal planning, we recommend the following:

"Exchange Lists for Meal Planning"
American Diabetes Association

"The First Step in Diabetes Meal Planning"
American Diabetes Association

Publications of the American Diabetes Association can be ordered from the Association's Web site at http://store.diabetes.org or by calling (800) ADA-ORDER (232-6733)

The following is a software package, used by many professionals, that automates dietary intake analysis, fitness and weight management, recipe development, and menu planning:

THE FOOD PROCESSOR
Nutrition Analysis and Fitness Software

Available from ESHA Research, P.O. Box 13028, Salem, OR 97309. Phone (800) 659-3742, extension 100.

see that the total fat and saturated fat content in chicken breast is slightly less than in the beef. However, a serving of chicken breast has slightly more cholesterol than a serving of beef. Now compare beef, top round steak with skinless chicken thigh. The total fat, saturated fat, and cholesterol content are higher in the chicken thigh.

These comparisons illustrate that it is possible to target the saturated fats in your food choices. It is also important to remember that because foods are mixtures of all fatty acids, it is difficult to eliminate an individual fatty acid from your diet. And finally, some food choices are low in saturated fat but higher in cholesterol. So how do you figure out what to eat?

For starters, you need to determine how many grams of saturated fat and cholesterol you usually eat per day by keeping a food diary in which you list all the foods and beverages you eat and drink each day. Then use "Finding the Fat" and the Nutrition Facts label found on all food packages to count the number of grams of saturated fat and the number of milligrams of cholesterol in the foods you eat. Information on monounsaturated and polyunsaturated fat content is not provided on all Nutrition Facts labels, but there are reference books that provide this information. You should be able to find these books in a public library or well-stocked bookstore. Many restaurants provide nutrition information for the items they serve, but you may have to ask for it.

Portion control is a key factor. Remember, if you eat portions of food that are larger than those specified in your meal plan, you are also eating larger amounts of saturated fat and cholesterol. Three ounces of skinless chicken breast contains 0.9 gram of saturated fat and 72 milligrams of cholesterol, but only if the serving of chicken you eat is really 3 ounces!

Your daily saturated fat limit depends on your recommended intake of calories (the number of calories you need to achieve or maintain a healthy weight). Here's how to figure out your daily saturated fat limit, assuming it represents 10% of total calories: First, find 10% of your recommended calorie intake by multiplying the number of calories by 0.1. For example, 0.1 × 2,000 calories = 200 calories. To convert calories into grams of fat, divide your result by 9 (because there are 9 calories per gram of fat). Following our example, 200 calories ÷ 9 calories per gram = 22 grams. So in a 2,000-calorie diet, saturated fat should be limited to no more than 22 grams per day. "Sample Meal Plan" on page 284 contains only 18 grams of saturated fat and is a good guide for planning.

The current diabetes nutrition recommendations say you should limit your daily intake of polyunsaturated fat to about 10% of calories (the same as for saturated fat). The amount of monounsaturated fat (sometimes referred to as the "good fat") in your diet should be greater than this amount. How much greater depends on individual blood glucose and blood lipid goals. If you need to decrease the amount of carbohydrate in your diet to meet optimal blood glucose control, you can substitute monounsaturated fat for carbohydrate (while maintaining the same calorie intake). For example, you might omit a serving of fruit or bread at lunch and substitute the same number of calories in nuts, seeds, olives, or avocado.

Nutrition experts recommend eating a variety of foods from each food group—meat, dairy, fruits and vegetables, and grains—to make sure your diet includes a variety of nutrients, while still controlling the amounts of saturated fat and cholesterol. The meat group (meat, fish, and poultry) gives you protein, iron, and the B vitamins niacin, riboflavin, and thiamin; fruits and vegetables are rich sources of vitamins A and C and many other antioxidant nutrients; and dairy products are a good source of calcium. But no one food group contains all the essential nutrients.

Food records and monitoring

A daily food record is essential to determine what and how much you are eating. If this is done in a stepwise fashion, it will not be an overwhelming task. Start by recording all foods and beverages you consumed after each meal. At the end of each day, count the grams of saturated fat and cholesterol you've eaten. If you are at a healthy weight and your daily intake for saturated fat and cholesterol are within the recommended range, but your blood lipids (total cholesterol, HDL cholesterol, LDL cholesterol, and triglycerides) are outside the recommended range, you may need to decrease the amount of saturated fat, cholesterol, or total carbohydrate in your diet. But you can only learn to adjust your diet by knowing how much of these your current food and beverage intake contains.

Keeping daily blood glucose levels in the optimal range set by your health-care team will encourage favorable blood lipid levels. Testing your blood glucose regularly and keeping records will help you determine which nutrients in meals you need to alter. If a high-carbohydrate meal plan routinely leads to high blood glucose after you eat, try decreasing the total carbohydrate and replacing it with monounsaturated fat. The percentage of carbohydrate needed to maintain optimal blood glucose and blood lipid goals will vary from person to person. The ideal amount depends on the individual.

It is also important for you to take your daily blood glucose and food records to your regular diabetes clinic appointments. Your records will help your health-care team help you become more independent in your diabetes management. ❏

Nutrition and Meal Planning

EATING YOUR WAY TO LOWER CHOLESTEROL

by Linnea Hagberg, R.D.

A beating heart is the motor that keeps our bodies running. The heart is responsible for pumping blood, oxygen, and nutrients to all our organs and muscles. But to be able to pump blood, the heart also needs its own blood supply. If blood flow to the heart should happen to be impeded, the motor can't get enough gas, and it breaks down.

Impeded blood flow to the heart is a serious and common problem. It is most often caused by coronary artery disease (often called heart disease), a condition in which fatty deposits accumulate in the cells lining the walls of the coronary arteries (the arteries supplying the heart muscle with blood). The major complications of heart disease are angina (chest pain) and heart attack.

In the United States, coronary artery disease is the leading cause of cardiovascular disease, and cardiovascular disease is the leading cause of death among both sexes. Unfortunately, people with diabetes are at high risk of developing heart disease. The good news is that many of the factors contributing to heart disease can be controlled.

Many factors affect a person's risk of developing heart disease. Some of them, including age, sex, family history, and the fact of having diabetes, cannot be changed. But several significant risk factors, namely, cigarette smoking, obesity, inactivity, and high blood pressure, can be changed by actions you take. Another major risk factor that you can help control is your cholesterol level.

High levels of total cholesterol and low-density lipoprotein (LDL) cholesterol in the blood, a condition that affects almost 20% of American adults, greatly raise the risk of developing heart disease. Lowering levels of total and LDL cholesterol decreases that risk. In fact, studies show that reducing blood cholesterol by 1% reduces the risk of a heart attack by 2%. This means that a drop in total cholesterol from, say, 230 mg/dl to 200 mg/dl can reduce the risk of a heart attack by approximately 30%.

How can you go about lowering your cholesterol? Just like high blood sugar, high cholesterol often responds to dietary changes, weight loss, if necessary, and increased physical activity. And, just like high blood sugar, it tends to respond best when dietary changes and increased activity are put into place simultaneously. A recent study in *The New England Journal of Medicine* looked at men and women who had high cholesterol levels. The researchers found that a low-fat, low-cholesterol diet reduced cholesterol somewhat, but it took regular exercise in combination with diet to cause significant declines.

For many people, drugs are also necessary to lower cholesterol to healthy levels. But diet, weight control, and exercise remain important components of a cholesterol-lowering program, even when drugs are used. This article looks at adjustments you can make to your diet to help reduce your cholesterol level.

Comprehending cholesterol

Before investigating strategies to lower cholesterol or prevent it from becoming elevated in the first place, it's helpful for us to step back and review just what cholesterol is all about.

Cholesterol is a waxy, fatlike material that is present in all cells. Although cholesterol is often portrayed as a villainous substance, the body actually requires it in moderate amounts for a variety of purposes, including digesting fat, making cell membranes, and manufacturing certain hormones. But too much cholesterol causes serious damage.

Cholesterol in the body comes from two sources. Most (about 80%) is made by the body, primarily in the liver. The remainder comes from the food we eat. All cholesterol, regardless of where it comes from,

BOOSTING HDL CHOLESTEROL

It is possible to increase your HDL (good) cholesterol. Try the following steps:

■ Replace saturated and polyunsaturated fats with monounsaturated fats, but don't go above 30% of calories from fat, unless your doctor or dietitian specifically advises you to do so.

■ Exercise. Regular aerobic exercise has been shown to help increase HDL cholesterol (and reduce LDL cholesterol). Aim for at least 30–45 minutes of exercise, four times a week.

■ If you are overweight, try to reduce. Obesity lowers HDL cholesterol (and raises triglycerides).

■ If you smoke, stop. Among the hazards it causes, smoking lowers HDL cholesterol.

travels through the body in the bloodstream. Cholesterol is transported by protein-covered packages called *lipoproteins*. There are several different kinds of lipoproteins; the most commonly discussed are high-density, low-density, and very-low-density.

Low-density lipoproteins (LDL's) carry most of the cholesterol. If there is a real villain in the world of cholesterol, LDL cholesterol is it. When present in high levels, LDL cholesterol can mix with other substances in the blood and form buildups on the walls of the blood vessels leading to the heart and brain. These buildups, known as plaques, cause the normally flexible arteries to become harder and thicker and are the hallmark of the condition known as atherosclerosis. This hardening of the arteries results in a diminished blood flow to the heart. Plaques can also break off and form clots, causing a heart attack or stroke. Because of its potential to do damage, LDL cholesterol is sometimes referred to as "bad" cholesterol. There is evidence that people with diabetes may produce more of a type of LDL cholesterol—in which the particles are smaller and denser—that is particularly likely to cause atherosclerosis.

If LDL cholesterol is the villain, then high-density lipoprotein (HDL) cholesterol can be considered the hero. HDL cholesterol gets its name because it is carried by high-density lipoproteins. It earns hero status because it carries cholesterol away from the arteries to the liver, where it can be removed from the body. Thus, HDL's can help prevent damaging cholesterol from building up in blood vessels. HDL cholesterol is often referred to as "good" cholesterol. Because HDL choles-

terol is good for your heart, having low levels of it is considered by experts to be a separate risk factor for heart disease.

Although not a form of cholesterol, a type of fat called triglycerides also circulates in the blood, in VLDL's, or very-low-density lipoproteins. The exact role that triglycerides play in determining heart disease risk is still being studied, but elevated levels are gaining in importance as yet another risk factor for heart disease.

Cholesterol by the numbers

Cholesterol levels are measured through a blood sample. All adults should have their cholesterol levels checked regularly. The frequency of testing is based on past levels and the presence of other risk factors for heart disease.

In its position statement on Management of Dyslipidemia in Adults with Diabetes, the American Diabetes Association established guidelines for determining the risk of heart disease. (See "Cholesterol Guidelines" on page 290.)

These guidelines are used to decide when steps to lower cholesterol should be taken and what those steps should be. Keep in mind, however, that cholesterol is only one piece of the heart disease picture. A health-care professional can help you get a better idea of your individual risk profile and what you can do to help yourself.

The fat factor

You might think that high blood cholesterol is the result of eating too many foods that are high in cholesterol. Although dietary cholesterol does contribute to high blood cholesterol, the single greatest dietary influence on blood cholesterol is actually fat, in particular, saturated fat. To bring down high cholesterol, the first step is to limit total fat in the diet to 30% or less of total calories. Even people who are at a healthy weight and who have normal cholesterol values would be well-advised to observe this 30% limit in order to help prevent future problems.

For a person eating 1,500 calories a day, applying the 30% rule means that no more than 450 calories (1,500 × 0.30) should come from fat. Since each gram of fat contains 9 calories, this translates to a daily goal of not more than 50 grams of fat (450 ÷ 9) a day. A person eating 2,000 calories a day should observe an upper limit of 65 grams of fat per day.

Limiting fat to 30% of calories or less is in line with the general dietary guidelines of virtually every major health organization, including the American Diabetes Association. If you're currently following a diabetes meal plan designed especially for you by a registered dietitian, your diet is probably already in line with this recommendation. (Some people who have high triglycerides may be advised to reduce the amount of carbohydrate they eat and to replace those calories with monounsaturated fat, which may necessitate pushing the percent of calories from fat in their diet closer to 35%. Such dietary changes, of course, should certainly be discussed with a doctor or dietitian before being adopted.)

Most Americans, however, take in about 34% of their calories from fat, which leaves some room for improvement. However, for many people, drastic change isn't necessary because small substitutions and changes can add up. For example, people eating 1,500 calories a day would need to cut about 7 grams of fat from their daily intake to drop from 34% of calories from fat to the 30% goal. Here are some ways this could be accomplished:

■ Substituting jelly for margarine on a piece of toast or opting to use low-fat salad dressing instead of regular dressing.

■ Choosing a plain fast-food hamburger instead of a deluxe version.

■ Spreading a sandwich with mustard instead of mayonnaise.

■ Regularly cutting out a nutritionally empty, high-fat snack such as potato chips.

All fats are not equal

If cutting back on total fat is the first step toward lowering blood cholesterol, considering what type of fat you're eating is the second. Not all fats are the same, and different kinds of fat have different effects on your blood.

All fats contain 9 calories per gram, but the resemblance stops there. Fats are composed of individual building blocks called fatty acids. The major fatty acids in food are saturated, polyunsaturated, and monounsaturated. Food is composed of a mixture of these fatty acids in various proportions.

Saturated fatty acids are usually solid at room temperature. The bulk of saturated fat in the diet comes from animal foods such as meat, poultry skin, egg yolks, butter, whole milk, and dairy products made from whole milk. A few vegetable oils such as palm, palm kernel, and coconut oil are also very high in saturated fat. Eating too much saturated fat can raise blood cholesterol levels.

Polyunsaturated fatty acids are usually liquid at room temperature. Vegetable oils, such as safflower, corn, soybean, and sunflower oil, and seafood are the major dietary sources of these fatty acids. Fish, particularly some cold-water species like Atlantic salmon, mackerel, herring, and halibut, are good sources of omega-3 fatty acids, a particular kind of polyunsaturated fat. Soybeans and nuts are also high in this type

of fat. While the link is still being investigated, there is evidence that diets rich in omega-3's may have benefits that include reducing triglyceride levels and reducing the risk of forming blood clots. In general, though, polyunsaturated fats can lower blood cholesterol levels.

Monounsaturated fatty acids are also liquid at room temperature; primary dietary sources are olive and canola oils and nuts. Not only can monounsaturated fats lower blood cholesterol, but there is evidence that monounsaturated fat lowers LDL cholesterol without affecting HDL (good) cholesterol, a distinct advantage.

Within the overall limit of 30% of calories from fat, then, to control cholesterol, foods high in monounsaturated and polyunsaturated fats should be emphasized, while saturated fat should be held to a minimum. For example, have tuna fish in place of a hamburger, or substitute a vegetarian meal for one based on meat. Choosing foods low in saturated fat will also automatically help reduce intake of dietary cholesterol since these substances are frequently bundled together in food.

Some people, however, may benefit from consuming a diet with a slightly higher percentage of calories from fat (up to 35%) provided monounsaturated fats are emphasized and body weight goals can be met. Saturated fat should be limited to 7% of calories or less while calories from polyunsaturated fat should be kept to 10% of calories or less. A doctor or registered dietician can help devise appropriate diets to meet individual circumstances.

Lowering saturated fat

Keeping saturated fat intake below 7% was one of the recommendations contained in guidelines issued in 2001 by the U.S. National Cholesterol Education Program for individuals whose LDL cholesterol is above optimal levels; other guidelines included low consumption of *trans* fatty acids. The limitation of saturated fatty acid intake to no more than 7% of calories in persons with elevated blood cholesterol levels is also recommended by the American Diabetes Association.

This 7% ceiling amounts to 12 grams of saturated fat for a 1,500-calorie intake and 16 grams for a 2,000-calorie diet. Because the recommendations for saturated fats are relatively low, even a few grams either way can make a difference.

Since saturated fatty acids come primarily from foods of animal origin, choosing the leanest versions of animal foods whenever possible is a good way to cut back. This means choosing very lean cuts of meat and poultry, removing skin from poultry, and choosing only skim or 1% milk and other low-fat dairy products.

CHOLESTEROL GUIDELINES

The American Diabetes Association has set out the following guidelines for determining a person's risk of heart disease.

RISK	LDL CHOLESTEROL	HDL CHOLESTEROL (for men)	(for women)	TRIGLYCERIDES
High	130 or more	under 35	under 45	400 or more
Borderline	100–129	35–45	45–55	200–399
Low	under 100	over 45	over 55	under 200*

*Triglyceride levels under 150 are desirable.

Switching from 2 cups of 2% milk to 2 cups of skim milk cuts out more than 5 grams of saturated fat (and 9 total grams of fat). Eating half a skinless chicken breast instead of two skinless thighs can save 2 to 3 more grams. (Dark meat has more fat than light meat.) Fish is one of the leanest sources of dietary protein and, as mentioned above, it is also rich in omega-3 fatty acids. Replacing other meats and poultry with small portions of fish two or three times a week can accordingly be a helpful step.

Portion size is also important when limiting saturated fat intake. Stick to a total of 5 to 7 ounces of lean protein a day.

The Nutrition Facts panel on food labels is a helpful tool for determining the amount of saturated fat in a packaged product. Use it to compare the saturated fat content of packaged foods and then choose products with lower amounts. For example, the Nutrition Facts panel on one brand of frozen cheese ravioli may show that the product contains 4 grams of saturated fat per serving, while an equivalent portion of frozen cheese tortellini contains only 2 grams. At first glance, saving 2 grams of saturated fat may sound modest, but you should bear in mind that it's actually close to 15% of a 12-gram goal.

Trans fats

Although they occur naturally in only a few foods, *trans* fatty acids are also worthy of mention. *Trans* fatty acids are formed when liquid oils are chemically hardened, a process known as hydrogenation. This occurs when oil is turned into margarine or vegetable shortening. Recent studies indicate that *trans* fats act similarly to saturated fats to raise cholesterol. *Trans* fats tend to be less of a problem than saturated fats simply because we eat less of them. Still, it makes sense to limit *trans* fatty acids.

The harder the fat, the more *trans* fatty acids it contains, thus stick margarine or vegetable shortening contains more *trans* fatty acids than does tub or liquid margarine. Commercial baked goods, such as packaged cakes, cookies, and pastries, and other high-fat processed foods, such as French fries and restaurant foods fried in partially hydrogenated vegetable shortening, are major dietary contributors of *trans* fatty acids. Unfortunately, at the present time, *trans* fatty acids are usually not listed on food labels or in the nutrient information obtained from restaurants. To limit intake of *trans* fats, avoid products that list hydrogenated or partially hydrogenated oils high in the list of ingredients, as well as commercially fried foods.

When choosing fats to use in cooking and eating, the best route for avoiding both *trans* and saturated fatty acids is to use liquid oils, when you use fats at all. For example, sauté food in a bit of olive or canola oil rather than cooking it in butter or margarine. Invest in high-quality nonstick skillets, and get an oil mister that allows you to spray small quantities of oil on pans and food instead of pouring directly from the bottle. On bread, try skipping fat altogether and eating it plain. This may be easier when the bread has plenty of its own flavor and texture, as with a crusty whole wheat sourdough loaf. When you do use spreads, whenever possible go with soft tub or liquid varieties that are expressly labeled "*trans* fatty acid free."

Limiting dietary cholesterol

As well as limiting the total amount of fat you eat and the amount of saturated fat in your diet, it helps to limit specific foods that are known to have a high cholesterol content. (Many high-fat foods are also high in cholesterol, so it's easy to cut out both at once.)

Guidelines issued by the American Diabetes Association call for keeping dietary cholesterol at no more than 300 milligrams a day for most individuals and under 200 milligrams a day if your LDL cholesterol level is a concern.

Eggs are especially high in cholesterol: A single large egg yolk contains 274 milligrams of cholesterol. While a recent study published in *The Journal of the American Medical Association* found that eating an egg a day did not raise the likelihood of having a heart attack or stroke for the general population, this did not hold true when researchers looked only at study participants with diabetes. The researchers pointed out that more study is necessary before conclusions can be drawn, but in the meantime, it makes sense to adhere to the American Heart Association's reminder to limit consumption of egg yolks (all the cholesterol is contained in the yolk), making sure that you stay within your daily cholesterol limit. Organ meats, such as liver, are also very high in cholesterol.

What's left to eat?

Once you've cut back on fatty meats, egg yolks, butter, cheese, and other high-fat dairy products, fried foods, stick margarine, and cookies, donuts, muffins, pastries, and other bakery items, what can you eat to fill the gaps? First, remember that there is no need to entirely eliminate any one food from your diet. Just use higher-fat foods less frequently, and, when you do eat them, keep a sharp eye on your portion size. For example, rather than eating a grilled cheese sandwich, make an open-face sandwich using a piece of bread, sliced tomato, and a tablespoon or two of grated sharp Cheddar. Think of using meat or poultry as an accompaniment instead of the main event by using it in stews, casseroles, pasta, or other mixed dishes. And make substitutions wherever you can. For example, substitute mushrooms for some of the beef in stew, add chopped tart apples and celery to tuna or chicken in a salad, use egg whites or egg substitutes in place of whole eggs, use ground turkey breast instead of regular ground meat, or try a mix of extra lean ground beef and imitation ground beef made from soy.

Almost all plain fruits, vegetables, grains, legumes, and beans fit easily into a cholesterol-lowering diet. Exceptions include some packaged rice or other grain mixes and creamed vegetables or those with added sauces which may be higher in fat. To add flavor without fat, try lemon juice, herbs, and spices. Or chop a clove of fresh garlic and heat it in a nonstick skillet with a teaspoon or less of olive oil and toss in lightly cooked vegetables. Top salads with low-fat salad dressings, or try balsamic vinegar with just a dash of extra-virgin olive oil.

Legumes (dried beans and peas) contain soluble fiber, a form of fiber that can help lower cholesterol if eaten regularly, so they make a good addition to the diet. Other plant foods that contain soluble fiber include oat bran and oatmeal and some fruits like apples and grapes. To introduce more legumes and beans into your diet, try a bowl of lentil soup as a main dish, or make vegetarian chili using beans instead of ground beef for protein. Bear in mind that, unlike other protein foods, beans are high in carbohydrate, so adjustments to your meal plan may be necessary.

Soy foods are also gaining in prominence in diets meant to lower cholesterol. In a review of 38 studies looking at the relationship between soy intake and blood cholesterol and triglyceride levels, researchers found that when people with high cholesterol levels replaced animal protein with soy protein, their triglyceride, total cholesterol, and LDL cholesterol levels dropped, while HDL cholesterol remained about the same. The cholesterol-lowering effect of soy protein was strongest in those who had higher levels of blood cholesterol to begin with.

The U.S. Food and Drug Administration has approved a label claim stating that 25 milligrams of soy protein a day can help lower cholesterol when consumed in conjunction with a diet low in total and saturated fat. This is the equivalent of about 1 cup of tofu.

Substituting soy-based foods for meat and poultry products can provide benefits even if consumption doesn't reach 25 milligrams of soy protein a day. For example, soy foods are low in saturated fat. A serving of 100 grams (about 3 ounces) of tofu contains a little more than 1 gram of saturated fat while the same amount of extra-lean ground beef contains about 6 grams of saturated fat.

All-around good health

Cutting down on fat while eating plenty of grains, beans, fruits, vegetables, and low-fat dairy products has benefits beyond lowering your cholesterol. This type of diet can help you bring down high blood pressure, keep blood sugar in control, lose extra weight, and get the nutrients you need to stay healthy and energetic. ❏

THE FACTS ON FATS

by Nancy Cooper, R.D., C.D.E.

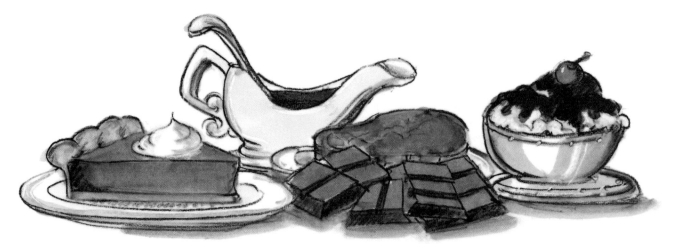

Think about some of the foods that might be considered favorites among many Americans: a bowl of rich ice cream, a piece of melt-in-your-mouth chocolate, a slice of succulent prime rib, homemade gravy made from the turkey pan drippings on Thanksgiving, and that light and flaky crust on the pumpkin pie. All of these foods share a common trait—they contain fat. And fat is what provides the great flavor and texture associated with these and many other foods.

Of all the nutrients in the diet, fat probably receives the most attention from consumers and health professionals alike. In the world of health promotion and chronic disease management, fat generally has a bad reputation. But as nutritionists know, a certain amount of fat is vital for good health. In this article, we examine the different types of fat found in foods, the roles they play in the body, and their impact on health. We also provide you with some guidelines for selecting fats—including butter, margarine, shortening, and oils—you can add to your food at the table or use in cooking. On page 295, we provide a chart of some fat products available in grocery stores today and their nutrition facts.

Like carbohydrate and protein, fat is an important nutrient in the diet. It provides energy (9 calories per gram, compared with 4 calories per gram for carbohydrate and protein) and fatty acids necessary for good health. Fat also plays a role in maintaining healthy skin, regulating cholesterol metabolism, and contributing to substances in the body (called prostaglandins) that regulate other body processes. Fat carries fat-soluble vitamins A, D, E, and K and aids in their absorption from the intestine.

The body uses dietary fat as a calorie source for energy. Whatever is not needed immediately for energy is stored by the body in fat (adipose) cells. These body fat deposits not only store energy for future use but also play a role in insulating the body from cold temperatures and in supporting and protecting the body's internal organs. Fat helps to satisfy the appetite by making you feel full after eating. This happens because fat slows down the rate at which food leaves the stomach. (This explains why it is common to feel hungry soon after eating a low-fat meal.)

Despite all the important functions of fat, evidence is clear that a diet with *too much* fat can lead to many health problems, including heart disease, some types of cancer, diabetes, and obesity. More and more consumers and health professionals are recognizing that moderating fat intake is good advice for people of all ages, and while Americans have lowered the proportion of fat in their diets somewhat in recent years, we still have a way to go. On average, Americans currently consume about 34% of their calories from fat; most health authorities recommend we reduce our fat intake to 30% or less of our total calories. (Fat consumption in children under the age of two should not be restricted, however.)

The different types of fat

All fats are a mixture of saturated, monounsaturated, and polyunsaturated fatty acids. Fatty acids, the building blocks of fats, differ primarily in the amount of hydrogen they contain. Saturated fatty acids contain the most hydrogen (they are saturated with hydrogen), and unsaturated fatty acids (including monounsaturated and polyunsaturated fatty acids) contain the smallest amount of hydrogen. Fats with a higher level of saturated fatty acids are firmer at room temperature and need more heat to melt or burn; examples include butter and lard. Fats with a higher amount of unsaturated fatty acids (such as vegetable oils) tend to be liquid at room temperature.

The amounts and proportions of these types of fats in the diet affect levels of blood cholesterol in the body. High blood cholesterol levels are a risk factor for heart disease. Studies have shown that a diet high in some saturated fatty acids tends to raise blood cholesterol levels, while a diet high in unsaturated fatty acids tends to lower cholesterol levels. Saturated fats occur typically in animal products such as meat, egg yolks, whole milk, and whole milk products—including butter, cream, and cheese. Higher amounts of unsaturated fats are found in liquid vegetable oils and nuts.

Although they are made from liquid vegetable oils, shortening and margarine are solid at room temperature because the oils have been partially hydrogenated to increase their firmness and melting point. Hydrogenation also increases the stability of the fat or oil, which lengthens a product's shelf life. During this process, however, the fats become more saturated—and less desirable to consume in a heart-healthy diet.

Remember that national dietary guidelines suggest we reduce our total fat intake to 30% or less of our total daily calories. Because saturated fats tend to raise blood cholesterol levels, it is also recommended that we limit our saturated fat intake to one-third of the total fat calories we consume (or 10% or less of total calories). For example, if you eat 2,000 calories per day, your fat intake should be around 65 grams of total fat, and those 65 grams should include no more than approximately 20 grams of saturated fat. (When converting grams of fat into calories, remember that each gram of fat contains 9 calories. So 65 grams of fat × 9 calories per gram = 585 calories from fat.) As one way to reduce saturated fat intake, the American Heart Association recommends using soft (tub) margarine and spreads and vegetable oils instead of butter and other solid fats like shortening.

Specific fatty acids in food that you might hear about or see listed or discussed on food labels include not only polyunsaturated fatty acids and monounsaturated fatty acids but also omega-3 fatty acids and *trans* fatty acids. Polyunsaturated fatty acids are part of the larger category of unsaturated fatty acids, which tend to lower blood cholesterol levels. Sources of polyunsaturated fat in the diet include corn, safflower, soybean, and sunflower oils. The fat found in seafood is mainly polyunsaturated.

Monounsaturated fatty acids have an advantage over polyunsaturated fatty acids. Research suggests that while both of these types of fatty acids lower cholesterol levels, the monounsaturated ones lower the "bad" cholesterol (LDL cholesterol) without lowering the "good" cholesterol (HDL cholesterol). This is desirable because studies suggest that HDL cholesterol has a protective effect against heart disease. Sources of monounsaturated fatty acids include canola oil, olive oil, some nuts, and olives.

Omega-3 fatty acids are polyunsaturated fatty acids with a slightly different structure. They are found primarily in seafood, especially higher-fat and cold-water fish such as mackerel, salmon, sardines, albacore tuna, and lake trout. Their benefit comes from their ability to lower the risk of heart attacks by preventing blood platelets from clotting and sticking to artery walls. Omega-3 fatty acids may also help reduce hardening of the arteries.

The best way to obtain omega-3 fatty acids is to consume fish two or three times a week as part of a healthy diet. Supplements of omega-3's are available in capsule form, but they are not thought to be as effective as the fatty acids obtained by eating fish itself. In addition, the safety and proper dose of the supplements have not been determined.

Trans fatty acids have been labeled a culprit in the fight against high cholesterol and heart disease. *Trans* fatty acids are produced when unsaturated fats and oils are hydrogenated. Commercially prepared high-fat baked goods, partially hydrogenated stick margarine, solid cooking fats like shortening, and French fries are all high in *trans* fatty acids. (Stick margarine contains more *trans* fatty acids than soft tub margarine and spreads.) *Trans* fatty acids also occur naturally in some foods such as beef, butter, and milk fat.

Some clinical studies have shown that when consumed in large quantities, *trans* fatty acids may raise levels of LDL cholesterol (the so-called "bad" cholesterol), but not as much as saturated fats do. In addition, high levels of *trans* fatty acids in the diet (twice the amount typically consumed by the average person) may reduce levels of HDL cholesterol (the so-called "good" cholesterol). However, at average levels of intake, *trans* fatty acids do not appear to reduce HDL cholesterol levels significantly.

Much more research is needed on the issue of *trans* fats in the diet to determine what level of intake can be considered a health risk. So far, research has shown that *trans* fatty acids resemble saturated fats in some but not all ways. Reducing the intake of saturated fat continues to be the major priority in fat-modified diets. Following a healthy diet and sticking to the recommended levels of total fat and saturated fat intake will likely keep levels of *trans* fat in an appropriate range. In the future, as we learn more about the role of these fats in the diet, we may see levels of *trans* fat listed on the Nutrition Facts panel of food labels.

Fats and cholesterol

Two new spreads have appeared in the margarine and butter section of the grocery store that specifically address the issue of *trans* fats and blood cholesterol levels. They are called Benecol and Take Control. Both of these products contain plant sterols—substances derived from plant sources such as vegetable oils, soybeans, and corn. These plant compounds are thought to be effective in reducing blood cholesterol levels by blocking the absorption of cholesterol in the digestive tract, thereby lowering the level of bad LDL cholesterol while maintaining the good HDL cholesterol.

Benecol and Take Control also contain ingredients found in other margarine spreads, including liquid vegetable oils, water, and salt. Both have zero or negligible amounts of *trans* fatty acids. The products can be used as you would butter, margarine, or other spreads—on toast, vegetables, crackers, muffins, or any other food. Benecol can be used in cooking, but Benecol Light—a reduced-fat, reduced-calorie version of the product—is not recommended for this purpose. The makers of Take Control do not suggest using it in cooking. Because of their high price, these products do not easily lend themselves to baking.

Benecol and Take Control have been tested in Europe and the United States. Participants in research studies were instructed to eat a specific number of servings per day of Benecol or Take Control as part of a diet low in saturated fat and cholesterol. With this regimen, LDL cholesterol levels were reduced by up to 14%, with no significant change in HDL levels. Benecol has been used in Europe for several years, and there are no known reports of adverse effects at this time. Still, it is important to remember that these products are intended for people with moderate to high cholesterol levels, and they are not intended to be a substitute for cholesterol-lowering drugs. In fact, if you are taking medicine for high cholesterol, it would be a good idea to check with your doctor before including the new cholesterol-lowering margarines in your treatment plan. The American Heart Association also warns that people with normal cholesterol levels should not use such products as a preventive measure since they do not prevent the underlying cause of elevated LDL cholesterol levels.

If you decide to try one of these new spreads, be prepared to spend a few more dollars when you go shopping.

Another factor related to nutrition and blood cholesterol levels is dietary cholesterol. About 70% of your circulating cholesterol is manufactured by your liver; the rest you get from what you eat. Dietary cholesterol is a fatlike substance found only in animal products such as meats, poultry, fish and shellfish, organ meats, dairy products, butter, and egg yolks. It is never found in vegetable oils, margarine, egg whites, or plant foods such as grains, fruits, and vegetables.

Cholesterol is a part of all body cells and plays a key role in the formation of body hormones and brain and nerve tissues. Whether it comes from food or is made by the body, cholesterol circulates in the bloodstream and is known as "serum cholesterol" or "blood cholesterol." Many factors affect blood cholesterol levels, including heredity. Recommended levels of dietary cholesterol for most people are about 300 milligrams or less per day.

Keep in mind that cutting back on dietary cholesterol is just part of keeping blood cholesterol under control. Though the effect of dietary cholesterol on blood cholesterol is not clearly understood, saturated fat intake appears to have an even greater impact on blood cholesterol levels than cholesterol obtained from food.

Figuring out fats

In the chart beginning on the opposite page, we list several types of commonly used fats. They are grouped into the following categories: table spreads, shortening, and oils. We also include nonstick cooking sprays, which can be used in place of regular fats to coat cooking utensils and pans, and butter-flavored sprinkles, a substitute that can be used at the table. Within each product category, the items are arranged alphabetically by brand name. We have included only a selection of products available in grocery stores. This list does not include everything on the market today, and there may be products in our list that you cannot find in your area.

For each product entry you will find nutrition information per serving, including total calories, total fat, saturated fat, polyunsaturated fat, monounsaturated fat, cholesterol, and sodium. Since these types of products have zero or negligible amounts of carbohydrate and protein, these two nutrients are not included in the chart. In addition, some products do not provide information on polyunsaturated or monounsaturated fat on the label, so this information is missing for some entries.

You can use this chart to compare the nutrition profile of various fats you might use in your diet. In the table spreads category, there are many options available:

Butter. If you are trying to follow a heart-healthy diet, limit your use of butter because most of its calories come from saturated fat, and it also contains a fair amount of cholesterol. If you keep your fat intake to the recommended 30% or less of total calories per day, a daily pat of butter probably won't hurt you, but

FATS BY THE GRAM

BUTTER, MARGARINE, AND SPREADS

	SERVING SIZE	CALORIES	TOTAL FAT (g)	SATURATED FAT (g)	POLYUNSATURATED FAT (g)	MONOUNSATURATED FAT (g)	CHOLESTEROL (mg)	SODIUM (mg)
Benecol								
Light	1 tablespoon	30	3	0	1	1	0	65
Regular	1 tablespoon	45	5	0	1	2	0	65
Blue Bonnet								
Light Stick	1 tablespoon	50	6	1	1	1	0	75
Stick	1 tablespoon	70	7	1	2	1	0	100
Tub	1 tablespoon	60	7	1	3	1	0	110
Brummel & Brown Tub	1 tablespoon	45	5	1	2	1	0	90
Canola Harvest Tub	1 tablespoon	100	11	1	0	6	0	110
Crystal Farms								
Butter Blend Margarine Stick	1 tablespoon	100	11	5	—	—	3	90
Corn Oil Margarine Stick	1 tablespoon	100	11	2	4	5	0	130
Unsalted Butter Stick	1 tablespoon	100	11	7	0	3	30	0
Fleischmann's								
Fat Free Squeeze Spread Butter Original	1 tablespoon	5	0	0	0	0	0	130
Lower Fat Margarine Stick	1 tablespoon	50	6	1	2	1	0	75
Lower Fat Margarine Tub	1 tablespoon	40	4	0	1	2	0	90
Margarine Stick	1 tablespoon	100	11	2	3	3	0	115
Margarine Unsalted Stick	1 tablespoon	100	11	2	3	3	0	0
Original Light Tub	1 tablespoon	40	4	0	1	2	0	90
Original Margarine Tub	1 tablespoon	80	9	1	4	3	0	90
Original Unsalted Tub	1 tablespoon	80	9	1	4	2	0	0
Hain Margarine Stick	1 tablespoon	100	11	2	5	2	0	140
I Can't Believe It's Not Butter								
Easy Squeeze	1 tablespoon	80	8	1	5	2	0	95
Light Stick	1 tablespoon	50	6	1	1	1	0	90
Light Tub	1 tablespoon	50	5	1	2	1	0	90
Nonfat Spread Tub	1 tablespoon	5	0	0	0	0	0	90
Regular Stick	1 tablespoon	90	10	2	2	2	0	95
Regular Tub	1 tablespoon	90	10	2	4	1	0	95
Spray	1 spray	0	0	0	0	0	0	0
Italian Rose Garlic Spread Tub	1 tablespoon	100	10	2	—	—	0	140
Land O Lakes								
Butter Stick	1 tablespoon	100	11	8	2	0	30	85
Country Morning Blend Light Stick	1 tablespoon	50	6	3	1	1	10	110
Country Morning Blend Margarine Stick	1 tablespoon	100	11	2	3	3	0	90
Country Morning Blend Margarine Tub	1 tablespoon	100	11	2	4	3	0	80
Honey Butter Tub	1 tablespoon	90	8	4	2	2	15	35
Light Butter Stick	1 tablespoon	50	6	4	0	2	20	70
Light Unsalted Butter Stick	1 tablespoon	50	6	4	0	2	20	0

Note: To ensure readability, all values represented in the table have been rounded to the nearest whole number.
There is no Carbohydrate column because most of these products contain very little carbohydrate.

BUTTER, MARGARINE, AND SPREADS
(continued)

	SERVING SIZE	CALORIES	TOTAL FAT (g)	SATURATED FAT (g)	POLYUNSATURATED FAT (g)	MONOUNSATURATED FAT (g)	CHOLESTEROL (mg)	SODIUM (mg)
Land O Lakes *(continued)*								
Light Whipped Butter Tub	1 tablespoon	35	3	2	0	1	10	45
Roasted Garlic Butter								
With Olive Oil Tub	1 tablespoon	100	11	5	1	5	20	95
Spread With Sweet Cream								
Tub	1 tablespoon	80	8	2	3	2	0	70
Unsalted Butter Stick	1 tablespoon	100	11	8	2	0	30	0
Whipped Butter Tub	1 tablespoon	70	7	5	1	0	20	50
Move Over Butter Whipped	1 tablespoon	60	6	1	2	1	0	70
Organic Valley Butter Stick	1 tablespoon	100	11	8	0	3	30	75
Parkay								
Buttery Spray	1 spray	0	0	0	0	0	0	5
Light Stick	1 tablespoon	50	6	1	1	1	0	75
Stick	1 tablespoon	90	10	2	3	2	0	105
Tub	1 tablespoon	80	8	1	4	3	0	100
Promise								
Buttery Light Stick	1 tablespoon	50	6	1	1	1	0	50
Buttery Light Tub	1 tablespoon	50	5	1	3	1	0	55
Regular Stick	1 tablespoon	90	10	2	4	2	0	90
Regular Tub	1 tablespoon	90	10	1	4	1	0	95
Ultra Fat Free	1 tablespoon	5	0	0	0	0	0	90
Ultra Tub	1 tablespoon	30	3	0	1	2	0	55
Shedd's Spread								
Country Crock Stick	1 tablespoon	70	7	1	2	1	0	110
Country Crock Tub	1 tablespoon	70	7	1	2	1	0	110
Smart Balance								
Buttery Spread Tub	1 tablespoon	80	9	2	2	3	0	90
Light Spread Tub	1 tablespoon	45	5	1	1	2	0	100
Smart Beat								
Fat Free Smart Squeeze	1 tablespoon	5	0	0	0	0	0	100
Super Light Margarine Tub	1 tablespoon	20	2	0	1	1	0	105
Spectrum Naturals Tub	1 tablespoon	80	10	0	3	6	0	55
Take Control Tub	1 tablespoon	50	6	0	2	2	<5	110

SHORTENING

	SERVING SIZE	CALORIES	TOTAL FAT (g)	SATURATED FAT (g)	POLYUNSATURATED FAT (g)	MONOUNSATURATED FAT (g)	CHOLESTEROL (mg)	SODIUM (mg)
Alessi Olive	1 tablespoon	120	14	2	1	10	0	0
Bella Cucina Olive	1 tablespoon	120	14	1	1	11	0	0

OILS

	SERVING SIZE	CALORIES	TOTAL FAT (g)	SATURATED FAT (g)	POLYUNSATURATED FAT (g)	MONOUNSATURATED FAT (g)	CHOLESTEROL (mg)	SODIUM (mg)
Bertolli								
Extra Light Olive	1 tablespoon	120	14	2	2	10	0	0
Olive	1 tablespoon	120	14	2	2	10	0	0
Canola Harvest Regular	1 tablespoon	130	14	1	5	8	0	0
Colavita								
Canola and Olive	1 tablespoon	120	14	1	4	9	0	0
Olive	1 tablespoon	120	14	2	1	10	0	0

	SERVING SIZE	CALORIES	TOTAL FAT (g)	SATURATED FAT (g)	POLYUNSATURATED FAT (g)	MONOUNSATURATED FAT (g)	CHOLESTEROL (mg)	SODIUM (mg)
Crisco Vegetable	1 tablespoon	120	14	2	6	6	0	0
Cuisine Perel Chili Grapeseed	1 tablespoon	80	14	1	11	2	0	0
Hain Canola	1 tablespoon	120	14	1	4	8	0	0
Hollywood								
Canola	1 tablespoon	120	14	1	4	8	0	0
Peanut	1 tablespoon	120	14	2	5	7	0	0
Safflower	1 tablespoon	120	14	1	11	2	0	0
Jacques Pepin's Kitchen								
Herbes De Provence								
Flavored Olive Oil	1 tablespoon	120	14	2	1	10	0	0
Three Peppercorn								
Flavored Olive Oil	1 tablespoon	120	14	2	1	10	0	0
Loriva								
California Walnut	1 tablespoon	120	14	2	9	3	0	0
Rice Bran	1 tablespoon	120	14	2	6	6	0	0
Roasted Peanut	1 tablespoon	120	14	2	5	7	0	0
Toasted Sesame	1 tablespoon	120	14	2	6	6	0	0
Mazola								
Canola	1 tablespoon	120	14	1	4	8	0	0
Corn	1 tablespoon	120	14	2	8	3	0	0
Right Blend	1 tablespoon	120	14	1	4	7	0	0
Olitalia Grapeseed	1 tablespoon	120	14	1	9	2	0	0
Planters Peanut	1 tablespoon	120	14	2	4	6	0	0
Sunera Canola	1 tablespoon	130	14	1	4	9	0	0
The International Collection								
Garlic Flavored	1 tablespoon	120	14	1	2	11	0	0
Hazelnut	1 tablespoon	120	14	1	2	11	0	0
Sweet Almond	1 tablespoon	120	14	1	4	9	0	0
Toasted Sesame	1 tablespoon	120	14	2	6	6	0	0
Walnut	1 tablespoon	120	14	1	10	3	0	0
Wesson Vegetable	1 tablespoon	120	14	2	8	3	0	0

NONSTICK COOKING SPRAYS

	SERVING SIZE	CALORIES	TOTAL FAT (g)	SATURATED FAT (g)	POLYUNSATURATED FAT (g)	MONOUNSATURATED FAT (g)	CHOLESTEROL (mg)	SODIUM (mg)
All Brands								
(Canola Harvest, Pam,								
Mazola, Weight Watchers, etc.)	⅓-second spray	0	0	0	0	0	0	0

BUTTER FLAVOR SPRINKLES

	SERVING SIZE	CALORIES	TOTAL FAT (g)	SATURATED FAT (g)	POLYUNSATURATED FAT (g)	MONOUNSATURATED FAT (g)	CHOLESTEROL (mg)	SODIUM (mg)
Butter Buds								
Butter Flavor	1 teaspoon dry	5	0	0	0	0	0	75
Sprinkles	1 teaspoon	5	0	0	0	0	0	120
Molly McButter								
Cheese Flavor Sprinkles	1 teaspoon	5	0	0	0	0	0	125
Roasted Garlic Sprinkles	1 teaspoon	5	0	0	0	0	0	125

Note: To ensure readability, all values represented in the table have been rounded to the nearest whole number.
There is no Carbohydrate column because most of these products contain very little carbohydrate.

if you like a lot of butter, you might consider using margarine or a butter blend instead.

Margarine. As in butter, 100% of the calories in margarine come from fat, but the fat is mostly unsaturated with no cholesterol.

Vegetable oil spreads. These contain less than 80% fat by weight (the amount required in margarine), but the calories and total fat vary greatly between brands.

Diet, light, or reduced-calorie margarine. All of the calories in these products come from fat, but the percent fat by weight is reduced to about 45% because water has been added (and is sometimes the first ingredient listed on the label). Per serving, these products generally have half the fat of regular margarine.

Butter-margarine blends. These may be anywhere from 15% to 40% butter. In addition to its taste, they contain some of butter's cholesterol and saturated fat.

The amount of saturated fat contained in a margarine or spread depends on which oil it is made from and how it was made. When shopping, read the label for ingredients and nutrition facts to guide your selection. Here are some tips to keep in mind:

■ Look for a margarine or spread with at least twice as much unsaturated fat (polyunsaturated and monounsaturated fat combined) as saturated fat. If a brand does not give you a breakdown of types of fat, you might want to choose another one.

■ Although the oils used in margarine are usually low in saturated fat, they do vary. Those lowest in saturated fat are canola, safflower, and corn oil, in that order.

■ Avoid margarine with hydrogenated or partially hydrogenated oil listed first on the ingredients list because these products are likely to be more saturated. Look for margarine or spreads with liquid oil listed as the first ingredient.

■ The softer or more fluid a margarine, the less saturated it is. For this reason, choose liquid or tub margarine over stick margarine. You will also get fewer *trans* fatty acids with softer margarines.

■ If you are watching sodium in your diet, consider using unsalted varieties of margarine or spreads.

When shopping for vegetable oils, there are many choices available today, including flavored oils to add zest and adventure to your recipes. All oils have roughly 120 calories per tablespoon, with all the calories coming from fat, and no cholesterol. Don't be fooled by "light" oils—they are simply lighter in taste and/or color, not in calories or fat. Most oils are low in saturated fat (no more than 2 grams per tablespoon). Olive and canola oils are the highest in heart-healthy monounsaturated fats.

One easy way to reduce your fat intake is to use a nonstick cooking spray. All fats have 9 calories per gram, and it is easy to add a lot of fat when cooking with oil. Nonstick cooking sprays come in handy for coating pans, and they contain no fat and negligible amounts of calories per serving. Many brands are available in several different flavors.

Sprinkle-on butter substitutes, such as Butter Buds and Molly McButter, are powders that are typically made from carbohydrate and are virtually fat-free and cholesterol-free. They can be used on hot, moist foods such as baked potatoes or cooked vegetables. But they won't do for spreading on toast or in recipes, nor can they be used in cooking. One teaspoon has about 5 calories, 1 gram of carbohydrate, and up to 125 milligrams of sodium.

Fat plays a vital role in the taste, appearance, and texture of foods you enjoy. While you may want to trim the amount of fat you eat, you need not try to cut it out altogether. Moderation, balance, and variety are still the best principles of a healthy diet, and the Nutrition Facts panel of the food label can assist you in evaluating the amount and type of fat in the foods you eat. By balancing high-fat items with lower-fat choices— along with appropriate amounts of grains, fruits, vegetables, dairy products, and meat and meat substitutes—you can enjoy a diet with a wide variety of foods and still meet your personal health goals. ❏

FRESH MEAT

by Nancy Cooper, R.D., C.D.E.

Americans have always loved meat. From colonial times, when wild game was the most plentiful form of meat, to modern times, when raising animals for meat has become an industry, meat has been the focus of the American meal. So great is our hunger for meat that the United States has become one of the world's largest meat-producing and meat-consuming nations.

In recent years, however, the role of meat in the American diet has been questioned amid nutrition recommendations to eat less fat, especially saturated fat, and cholesterol. Vegetarian diets have become more common, and many consumers now consider red meat an unhealthy food. Poultry, on the other hand, has gained popularity because it is lower in fat than many types of meat. So, while Americans are eating more meat and poultry than ever before (about 180 pounds per person in 1998), our choices have changed. Total beef and pork consumption has declined since 1975, and intake of chicken and turkey has risen. According to the U.S. Department of Agriculture (USDA), today we eat about the same amount of poultry as beef—about 65 pounds per person in 1998.

As many people are aware, red meat is one of the major sources of fat in the American diet, and eating too much fat has been linked to an increased risk for several diseases, including heart disease and some cancers. In addition, a high-fat diet can promote obesity, which is a risk factor for heart disease, cancer, and diabetes.

But this is not to say meat is a "bad" food. Through advances in breeding, feeding, and management techniques, the beef cattle and hogs of today are leaner than ever. Meat packers and processors have also helped lower the fat content of meat by trimming the fat surrounding cuts of meat to between ⅛ inch and 1/16 inch, rather than to ¼ inch, as done in the past. As in anything else, moderation is the key when it comes to eating meat. It is overconsumption of meat that can put health at risk.

Meat and poultry provide many valuable nutrients, including iron, zinc, vitamins B_6 and B_{12}, protein, phosphorus, riboflavin, and niacin. Meat can easily be part of a healthy, low-fat diet, especially if you follow these tips:
■ Eat small portions of meat, about 3 to 4 ounces at a meal (about the size of a deck of cards). Four to 5 ounces of raw meat cook down to about 3 to 4 ounces.
■ Choose lean cuts of meat.
■ Substitute chicken and turkey for some of the red meat in your diet.
■ Treat meat as a side dish that complements the vegetables, grains, breads, and fruits at a meal.
■ Limit fattier cuts of meat, such as prime beef, bacon, sausage, and ribs, to special occasions.
■ Trim visible fat from meat and remove the skin from poultry before eating.
■ Choose low-fat cooking methods such as grilling, broiling, roasting, poaching, or stir-frying with little added fat.

Safety tips

We've all heard horror stories about food poisoning caused by improperly prepared meat. Luckily, the risks of food poisoning from meat and poultry are virtually eliminated by storing, handling, and cooking them properly. As you handle raw meat or poultry and prepare your dish, keep in mind these guidelines:
■ Keep your refrigerator below 40°F and your freezer at or below 0°F.

■ Thoroughly wash your hands, including under your fingernails and between your fingers, with soap and warm water before and after handling raw meat.
■ Use a clean dish towel every time you prepare meat.
■ Defrost frozen meats in the refrigerator or microwave or in cold water. If you use cold water, change the water frequently or put it in the refrigerator to ensure that the water stays cold. Never thaw meat at room temperature. If you do, the outside will thaw before the inside does, leaving the outside susceptible to bacterial growth while the inside is still frozen.
■ Wash knives, utensils, kitchen counters, and cutting boards thoroughly in hot, soapy water after preparing raw meat and before preparing other foods.
■ Marinate meats and poultry in the refrigerator. Keep cooked meat away from the marinade, and do not serve the marinade as a sauce unless it has been boiled for several minutes.
■ Use a clean plate for serving cooked meat. Do not put cooked meat on the same plate that previously held the raw meat. Likewise, use clean utensils for serving.
■ Keep meat refrigerated until cooking time, and refrigerate leftover cooked meat within an hour of cooking.
■ Avoid eating raw meat. Steak tartare may be considered a delicacy, but it is dangerous to eat.

Beef

Today's beef is 27% leaner than it was 25 years ago, thanks to leaner animals and closer trimming of the fat. To choose a low-fat piece of beef, you will need to consider both grade and cut.

Grading is a voluntary process established by the USDA. For a fee, government graders evaluate beef quality by looking at the amount of marbling (flecks of fat within the lean tissue), the texture of the meat, and its color and appearance. Marbling gives beef juiciness, tenderness, and flavor, so the grading system rewards fatty beef by giving it the highest grade—prime—followed by choice and select. Beef graded below select is not usually found in grocery stores; it is used in processed meat products. (Note: Grading is not the same as inspection. The USDA inspects all meat to ensure that it is clean and safe.)

Select grade beef has 5% to 20% less fat than choice beef of the same cut, and 40% less fat than prime. It is generally less juicy, tender, and flavorful as a result, but with moist methods of cooking and proper carving (against the grain) these cuts can be very tasty. Unlike the amount of fat, the amount of nutrients does not vary from one grade to the next. Because grading is voluntary and costs the meat packer money, some of the beef in supermarkets is ungraded. Ungraded beef is not necessarily lower quality than graded beef. In fact, ungraded beef found in supermarkets would typically be graded choice or select had the meat packer decided to grade the beef.

The cut indicates the part of the animal from which a piece of meat comes, and some parts are fattier than others. Select grade beef of one cut may have more fat than choice beef of a different cut. For example, 3½ ounces of select chuck roast has about 14 grams of fat, while the same amount of choice top round has only 6 grams of fat.

Slaughtered beef cattle are first divided into primal cuts, which include chuck, sirloin, round, brisket and flank. Primal cuts are further divided into retail cuts, which are what you find in the store. There are at least 300 different retail cuts of beef, and a meat counter may display 50 or more of them. (Meat labels will always list both the primal and retail cut names.)

The following lean cuts of beef have about 9 grams of fat per 3½-ounce portion: top round, eye of round, round tip, sirloin, tenderloin, top loin, and flank steak. Fattier cuts of beef include most chuck cuts and cuts from the short plate, including skirt steak (the preferred meat for fajitas) and short ribs. Look for cuts with little marbling and external fat. If your store has a butcher, you can have him or her trim away the excess fat.

Most ground beef comes from the chuck, sirloin, or round. Packages are labeled by cut, fat content, or both. Ground beef labeled 75% lean is 25% fat by weight, not by calories. Because fat has more than two times the calories of protein, a patty made from this beef would derive 64% of its calories from fat when cooked. Lean ground beef is 21% fat by weight when raw and gets 61% of its calories from fat when cooked. Extra-lean ground beef is 17% fat by weight when raw and gets 57% of its calories from fat when cooked.

To get the leanest ground beef, buy a lean cut of sirloin or round and have the butcher trim it of all external fat and grind it for you. You can also grind it yourself using a meat grinder or food processor. When buying packaged ground beef, look for the highest percent lean label on the package.

Cut and grade are good indicators of fat content, but they don't help you recognize fresh meat. Check the freshness date on the label, and choose meat with the latest "sell by" date. Fresh beef has creamy white fat, not yellow fat, and feels springy to the touch. Fresh beef is typically a bright red color; older beef will have a browner color.

Beef is very perishable and should be stored in the coldest part of your refrigerator. Keep the meat in its original wrapping and use within a few days. To keep it longer, wrap it in freezer paper or freezer wrap, date it, label it, and freeze it. Roasts and steaks will keep for six to 12 months, and ground beef for two to three months.

Veal

Veal comes from young calves. Considered a specialty food in the Unites States, it has a delicate flavor and light texture. Americans eat less than 1 pound of veal per person per year, but in parts of Europe, veal is eaten as often as beef is eaten in the United States.

Veal is similar in fat content to some of the leanest cuts of beef—3½ ounces of trimmed roasted veal sirloin, for example, has around 6 grams of fat. A lean leg of veal has only 3 grams of fat per 3½ ounces—about the same as a skinless chicken breast. Although the cuts of veal are similar to those of beef, there are fewer of them. The top round, leg cutlet, arm steak, sirloin steak, loin chop, rib chop, and scallops made from the leg are the leanest cuts. Ground veal is a lean alternative to ground beef, especially if the meat is from the leg or shoulder.

When buying veal, look for light pink, fine-grained meat with little marbling. Any fat should be firm and white. Store veal as you would beef; when frozen and wrapped in a moisture-proof freezer paper or wrap, it will keep up to six to nine months.

Pork

Pork has had an unfavorable reputation for many years because so many pork products, including bacon, sausage, spareribs, and hot dogs, are high in fat. According to the USDA, Americans' consumption of pork has increased only slightly, if at all, over the past 25 years; in 1998 we ate an average of about 49 pounds per person per year, roughly one-quarter less than our beef intake. Yet recent research has shown that fresh pork is 31% leaner than it was in 1983. With selective breeding, pork producers have changed the fat and muscle composition of hogs, producing leaner animals over the past decades. Modern ways of feeding and raising have also contributed to the pig's leaner form.

Pork is an excellent source of protein, B vitamins, iron, and zinc. In addition, pork has slightly less saturated fat than beef. Guidelines for including pork in the diet are similar to those for beef: Choose lean cuts, eat small portions, and trim visible fat. As with beef, there are leaner cuts and higher-fat cuts to choose from, but don't look for grades on pork to give you a clue about the fat content. Because pork is more consistent in quality than beef, it is not graded.

Like beef, pork is divided into primal wholesale cuts, which are named for the part of the animal they come from, and is further divided into the retail cuts that you find in your supermarket. For fresh pork, the

MEATY MEASURES

Serving size = 3½ ounces cooked, unless otherwise noted.	CALORIES	CALORIES FROM FAT	FAT (g)	SATURATED FAT (g)	SODIUM (mg)	PROTEIN (g)
Beef						
Chuck, arm pot roast, choice, braised	219	81	9	3	66	33
Flank steak, choice, broiled	207	90	10	4	83	27
Ground, extra lean, broiled	256	144	16	6	70	25
Ground, regular, broiled	289	189	21	8	83	24
Round, eye of, choice, roasted	175	72	8	2	62	29
Tenderloin, prime, broiled	232	108	12	5	63	28
Tenderloin, select, broiled	199	81	9	3	63	28
Top sirloin, choice, broiled	200	72	8	3	66	30
Chicken						
Broiler/fryer						
Dark meat, without skin, roasted	205	90	10	3	93	27
Dark meat, with skin, roasted	253	144	16	4	87	26
Light meat, without skin, roasted	173	45	5	1	77	31
Light meat, with skin, roasted	222	99	11	3	75	29
Roaster						
Dark meat, without skin, roasted	178	81	9	2	95	23
Light meat, without skin, roasted	153	36	4	1	51	27
Rock Cornish hen, without skin, roasted (½ of a 1½-pound bird)	147	36	4	1	69	26
Lamb						
Foreshank, choice, braised	187	54	6	2	74	31
Ground, broiled	283	171	19	8	81	25
Leg, sirloin, choice, roasted	204	81	9	3	71	28
Leg and shoulder, cubed, broiled	186	63	7	3	76	28
Shoulder, arm, choice, roasted	192	81	9	4	67	26
Pork						
Center loin, chops/roasts, broiled	202	72	8	3	60	30
Center rib, chops/roasts, broiled	216	90	10	3	65	30
Ham, fully cooked, lean, roasted	145	54	6	2	1,203	21
Ham, fully cooked, regular, canned, roasted	226	135	15	5	941	21
Ham, fully cooked, whole, roasted	159	54	6	2	1,327	25
Leg, roasted	211	81	9	3	64	29
Loin, broiled	210	90	10	4	64	29
Tenderloin, broiled	164	45	5	2	56	28
Top loin, chops/roasts, broiled	203	72	8	3	65	31
Turkey						
Dark meat, without skin, roasted	187	63	7	2	79	29
Dark meat, with skin, roasted	221	108	12	4	76	28
Light meat, without skin, roasted	157	27	3	1	64	30
Light meat, with skin, roasted	197	72	8	2	63	29
Veal						
Ground, broiled	172	72	8	3	83	24
Loin, roasted	175	63	7	3	96	26
Shoulder, arm, roasted	164	54	6	2	91	26
Sirloin, roasted	168	54	6	2	85	26
Top round, leg, roasted	150	27	3	1	68	28

Note: To ensure readability, all values represented in the table have been rounded to the nearest whole number. Nutrient information is based on *Bowes & Church's Food Values of Portions Commonly Used,* 17th edition. We have omitted the columns for carbohydrate and fiber because meat contains no carbohydrate and no fiber.

cut determines the fat content. Cuts that provide less than 9 grams of fat per 3-ounce cooked portion include pork tenderloin (the leanest cut of pork), sirloin chop, loin roast, loin chop, sirloin roast, rib chop, and rib roast.

Only one-third of the pork produced in the United States each year is sold fresh; the remainder is cured, smoked, or processed. Historically, curing was used to preserve meat so it would last through the winter. Today, pork is cured for flavor. Because two of the main ingredients used in curing are salt and sodium nitrite (which has been linked to cancer development), cured pork products can be high in sodium. Bacon, Canadian bacon, and ham are popular forms of cured pork, with Canadian bacon and ham being leaner than bacon.

When shopping for fresh pork, look for cuts that are well trimmed of fat and meat that is pinkish to gray-pink in color (An exception to this rule is pork tenderloin, which is deep red in color.) The fat should be creamy white, and any bones should be red and spongy at the ends. (The whiter the bone end, the older the animal was when it was slaughtered and the less tender the meat will be.) When choosing cured pork products, be sure to read the label for nutrition information as well as cooking and storage tips.

Refrigerate fresh pork in the original wrapper and use within two to three days. Frozen pork chops and roasts will last four to six months. Cured pork products will last up to a week in the refrigerator once they are opened or cut. Frozen, fully cooked hams will keep one to two months.

Lamb

While lamb is the principal meat eaten in parts of Europe, North Africa, the Middle East, and India, Americans consume only about 1 pound per person per year. As with beef and pork, modern breeding and feeding methods have improved lamb's taste and texture, and the meat is also leaner due to close trimming of the external fat. Lamb is graded prime, choice, or good. Most of the lamb in supermarkets is choice, which is comparable to choice beef in its content of fat, protein, iron, zinc, and vitamin B_{12}. However, the grading of lamb is not based on marbling. High-grade lamb has thick, well-shaped muscles in the loin and rib cuts.

Lamb has fewer retail cuts than beef. Leaner cuts, such as the foreshank and parts of the leg, are generally less tender than cuts from areas where the muscles are used very little, such as the loin and rib. However, because lambs are smaller, younger animals than beef cattle, even lean cuts are more tender than corresponding cuts of beef. Lean cuts of lamb (with less than 10 grams of fat in a 3½-ounce cooked portion) include the shank half leg roast or hind shank, loin chops, arm chops, and foreshank.

Prepackaged lamb is usually dated for freshness, so check the label. Other signs of freshness include firm, pinkish-red meat (lamb darkens with age), bones that are moist and reddish at the joint, and creamy white fat. As with other meats, store lamb in the coldest part of the refrigerator in its original wrapping. As a rule, the larger the cut, the longer it keeps. Whole roasts will stay fresh up to five days; chops and steaks, for two to four days; and ground or cubed lamb, one to two days. If frozen, larger cuts will last six to nine months, and smaller cuts can be frozen for three to four months.

Chicken

In the United States, chicken consumption has risen since the 1940's, when changes in breeding and marketing made it more affordable. The price of chicken today, when adjusted for inflation, is only one-third of its price in the early 1960's.

But price is not the only reason we consume so much chicken. To reduce fat in their diets, many Americans have decided to eat less red meat and more poultry. Cooked skinless light chicken meat is 33% to 80% leaner than cooked beef, depending on the beef's cut and grade. Yet chicken is comparable to beef in quantity of protein, vitamins, and minerals (except that beef has slightly more iron and zinc). Still, not all chicken is created equal: A 3½-ounce cooked portion of white meat without skin contains about 4 grams of fat, while the same size portion of skinless dark meat has close to 10 grams of fat. Skinless dark chicken meat supplies the same amount of fat as light meat with skin. Dark meat with the skin is the fattiest combination of all, with about 16 grams of fat per 3½-ounce roasted portion.

As with beef, chicken is graded for quality by the USDA only if the processor requests it and pays a fee. As a result, you often find ungraded chicken on the market. Graded chicken is most likely to be grade A; lower-quality chicken is grade B or C and is usually sold for use in packaged and processed products. The fat content is not the criteria for grading chicken. Instead, chicken is graded based on characteristics such as shape, presence of feathers, and unbroken skin.

Over 50% of the chicken sold in the United States is purchased in parts (breasts, drumsticks, wings, and thighs). Whole chickens can also be purchased and come in several varieties. Broilers or fryers are all-purpose birds that weigh 2½ to 5 pounds; roasters are slightly older and larger than broilers or fryers, weighing 3½ to 6 pounds; capons are male chickens weighing 9½ to 10½ pounds; Rock Cornish hens weigh ¾ to 2 pounds and are perfect for one or two servings; stewing chickens are mature hens weighing 4 to 6 pounds with flavorful but tough meat; and free-range chickens are chickens that have been allowed outside instead of being raised entirely indoors.

To buy fresh chicken, check the "sell by" date on the package. This date is the last recommended date of sale, but the meat may remain fresh for two to three days more if properly refrigerated. If the "sell by" date is near, don't buy the chicken unless you're sure you'll use it soon. If the chicken has a peculiar smell, don't buy it no matter when the "sell by" date is. Whole chickens should have a plump, rounded breast, and chicken parts should be moist and plump. The color of the skin will vary from white to yellow, depending on the breed of chicken and its diet. (Skin color is not related to quality.) Frozen chicken should be rock-hard and show no ice crystals or freezer burn.

Fresh chicken is highly perishable and should be refrigerated immediately. Store it in the original wrapper and be sure any juices that leak from the package do not leak onto other foods. If you purchase a whole chicken, store the giblets separately because they will spoil before the meat. Fresh chicken keeps for two to three days; frozen chicken can be kept for nine to twelve months.

Trim the fat off chicken before cooking, but leave the skin on to keep the meat moist. (An insignificant amount of fat is transferred to the meat from the skin during cooking.)

Turkey

Long the favorite meat for holiday feasts, turkey is becoming a regular part of the diet for more and more people. Skinless turkey breast is one of the leanest of all meats, supplying just a few grams of fat per 3½-ounce cooked serving. These days, you don't have to buy a whole bird. Consumers can purchase the parts they prefer, such as breasts, cutlets, thighs, and drumsticks. Convenience and nutrition have contributed to a 133% increase in U.S. turkey consumption over the past 20 years.

As with chicken, almost all of turkey's fat is found in the skin. However, eating cooked turkey breast with the skin would still only furnish about 8 grams of fat per 3½ ounces because the meat is so lean. Dark meat without skin has about 7 grams of fat per 3½-ounce serving, and with the skin, it has about 12 grams of fat per 3½ ounces. Turkey is high in nutrients such as protein, the B vitamins, iron, and zinc.

Most turkeys found in the supermarket are either fryer/roasters (the youngest and most tender, weighing 5 to 9 pounds), hens (female turkeys weighing 8 to 18 pounds), or toms (male turkeys weighing up to 24 pounds). Ground turkey, especially if it is made from light meat, is a tasty, leaner alternative to ground beef. (The same is true of ground chicken.) Packaged ground turkey may also contain dark meat and be higher in fat; check the ingredients label to see which parts are used.

Like other meats, turkey is graded by the USDA only if the processor requests it and pays a fee. Like grade A chicken, grade A turkey is well-shaped, free of feathers, and has a layer of fat with unbroken outer skin. When buying fresh turkey, check the "sell by" date and do not buy turkey with a date that is too near. When buying a whole bird, be sure to select one that will fit in your oven. And beware of self-basting birds—many basting solutions contain large amounts of oil or butter in addition to seasonings and broth.

Fresh turkey should be stored in the same manner as other meats—in the coldest part of the refrigerator in the original wrapping—and used within two days. Store the giblets separately, and make sure the turkey juices do not leak onto other foods. Frozen turkey parts can be kept six to nine months; a whole frozen bird will keep up to a year, but remember that you do not know how long it stayed in the store's freezer before you bought it.

The table on page 301 lists information on calories, calories from fat, fat, saturated fat, sodium, and protein for various cuts of meat and poultry. To make sure the nutrients in your meat match what's listed in the table, trim all meat of visible fat and use the cooking method indicated. ❑

ALCOHOL AND MIXERS

by Nancy Cooper, R.D., C.D.E.

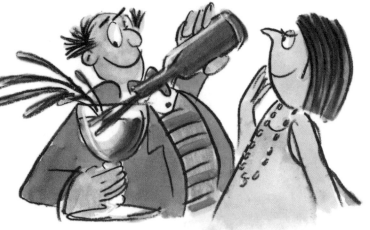

For centuries, people have enjoyed wine, beer, and ale. Many people find that moderate amounts of alcohol enhance their appetite and add pleasure to eating. Now it appears that alcoholic beverages may contribute not only to good meals but to good health. Evidence suggests that moderate alcohol consumption may lower the risk for certain chronic diseases such as heart disease and possibly diabetes in some people.

Where alcohol is concerned, if a little might be good, a lot is not necessarily better. The U.S. federal government's *Dietary Guidelines for Americans, 2000* state, "If you drink alcoholic beverages, do so in moderation." Health experts suggest that women have no more than one drink a day and that men have no more than two drinks a day. One drink is defined as 12 ounces of regular beer, 5 ounces of wine, or 1½ ounces of 80-proof distilled spirits. Drinking more than the recommended amount raises the risks of numerous, serious health concerns.

The decision of whether or not to drink alcohol is an individual one. There are many people who choose not to drink for personal or health reasons. There are also those who should avoid drinking for health and safety reasons, including women who are pregnant or trying to get pregnant (drinking while pregnant can cause birth defects), individuals taking drugs that interact with alcohol (check with your doctor or pharmacist about using prescribed or over-the-counter drugs with alcohol), people who are unable to moderate their drinking or have a history of alcohol abuse, and teenagers and children. Even among those who can drink safely, there are times when it is inappropriate to drink, such as before driving or using heavy machinery.

For people with diabetes, it is important to know how alcohol affects blood glucose levels and the rest of the body and how to drink safely. This article discusses the effects of alcohol in people with diabetes and offers guidelines for safe use. We have also included a table of nutrition information for some common alcoholic beverages.

Alcohol metabolism

Unlike carbohydrate, protein, and fat, alcohol is not broken down through the process of digestion. It is absorbed directly into the bloodstream through the lining of the stomach and wall of the small intestine. If there is no food in the stomach, alcohol is absorbed quickly into the bloodstream, usually within about 20 minutes. The presence of food in the stomach slows down alcohol absorption slightly.

From the bloodstream, alcohol travels to virtually every cell in the body, and it has a special affinity for the cells of the brain. Although alcohol is a depressant, it initially produces feelings of euphoria and a release of inhibitions. Over time, however, alcohol dulls various brain activities, including concentration, coordination, and response time. Alcohol can also cause drowsiness, sleep disturbances, slurred speech, and blurred vision.

Because alcohol has a diuretic effect, it can promote water loss from the body, making people feel thirsty after drinking a lot. (The feeling of thirst often occurs the morning after a night of heavy drinking.)

Normally, the liver metabolizes most of the alcohol consumed. (A small percentage of alcohol is eliminated via the kidneys in the urine or via the lungs in exhaled air.) The liver breaks down alcohol slowly, at a rate of about one-half ounce per hour. So the average man will require about two hours to metabolize 1 ounce of alcohol—the amount in about 12 ounces of beer or 1½ ounces of whiskey.

Alcohol affects women differently than men due in part to body size and composition. Alcohol is carried in body fluids, and since women have a smaller volume of fluid in the body, the same amount of alcohol is more concentrated in the bloodstream of a woman than it is in a man. In addition, an enzyme that helps break down alcohol in the body is less active in women, so the same amount of alcohol will affect the average woman more than it does the average man.

Diabetes and alcohol

In a person with diabetes, one of the main risks associated with drinking alcohol is hypoglycemia, or low blood sugar. The body does not require insulin to metabolize alcohol. In fact, alcohol tends to increase the blood-glucose-lowering ability of insulin. It does not cause the pancreas to release more insulin; it simply makes the insulin or other glucose-lowering drugs "work" harder at lowering blood glucose. This is one of the ways in which drinking alcohol can increase the risk of hypoglycemia.

If a person whose diabetes is under control has a drink, blood glucose levels are unlikely to be significantly affected by the alcohol as long as it is consumed with food. However, drinking on an empty stomach can cause hypoglycemia, especially if it has been a long time since a person's last meal. As little as 2 ounces of alcohol (one to two drinks) taken on an empty stomach can have this effect. Since the symptoms of low blood sugar mimic drunkenness, a person may not realize he or she is experiencing hypoglycemia. If hypoglycemia goes unrecognized, appropriate treatment is delayed and sometimes not given at all. It's important to know that the hypoglycemic effects of alcohol can last for many hours after you have stopped drinking.

Occasionally, alcohol can cause blood glucose levels to go up. This may be because alcohol is an appetite stimulant, and it is easy to overeat while drinking. Another reason is that large amounts of alcohol can interfere with the way glucose is used and stored by the body. The increase in blood glucose is usually temporary, and it can be followed (sometimes several hours later) by a drop in blood glucose levels.

In spite of the dangers of excessive alcohol intake for people with diabetes (including difficulty controlling blood glucose, increased levels of blood fats called triglycerides, and worsened painful neuropathy), some evidence suggests that light to moderate alcohol consumption by people with diabetes may be associated with less insulin resistance in the body and a lower risk for cardiovascular disease. But this does not mean that all people with diabetes (or anyone else for that matter) should start to drink if they don't currently do so.

The risks

People who abstain from drinking alcohol usually do so for a reason, such as a family or personal history of alcohol abuse or intolerance, medical concerns, or taking medicines that interact with alcohol. It would not be prudent for people in any of these situations to start drinking in an effort to lower their risk of heart disease.

For long-term heavy drinkers, excessive alcohol use can lead to many additional health concerns, including an increased risk for high blood pressure and stroke, heart disease, certain cancers, liver disease, and pancreas damage. Heavy drinking can also put women at greater risk for osteoporosis.

As discussed earlier, drinking can cause hypoglycemia in people with diabetes. And heavy drinking may worsen neuropathy, produce or worsen insulin resistance, and raise triglyceride levels, especially in people who already have elevated triglycerides.

Each individual should weigh the potential benefit of drinking alcohol against the spectrum of health concerns related to its use or overuse, including increased risk of cancer, liver disease, drug interactions, depression, and unintentional injuries and accidents. Light to moderate alcohol use may be of benefit for people with diabetes or those at risk for cardiovascular disease, but it is not recommended for anyone who, for whatever reason, cannot restrict his or her drinking to these levels.

Guidelines for safe use

Following are guidelines for including alcoholic beverages occasionally in your diet. Occasional use is defined here as one or two drinks or ounces of alcohol, once or twice a week. If you drink alcohol on a daily basis, you should limit the amount, and you may need to adjust your food plan to account for the calories in the alcohol.

■ Use alcohol only when your diabetes is in control. Drinking when your blood glucose is out of control will only make matters worse. Check with your diabetes health-care team for advice on controlling your diabetes through diet, exercise, and medicine. Be aware of the effect alcohol can have on your blood glucose levels, and test your blood glucose regularly and record the results so you can discuss them with your health-care team.

■ Use alcohol in moderation. Most major health organizations recommend limiting your alcohol intake to no more than one or two servings each time you drink. A drink is 1½ ounces of distilled spirits (whiskey, scotch, vodka, gin, rum, etc.), 4 to 5 ounces of wine, 2 ounces of sherry, or 12 ounces of beer.

■ Remember (particularly if weight control is a concern) that alcohol can add a lot of calories to the diet. Alcohol contains 7 calories per gram. In comparison, protein and carbohydrate contain 4 calories per gram, and fat contains 9 calories per gram. It can be very easy to forget that what we drink can give us so many extra calories!

■ If you take insulin, you can occasionally add up to two drinks to your meal plan. Because alcohol can cause hypoglycemia, no food should be omitted from your usual eating plan when you drink.

■ If you do not take insulin, the calories from alcohol can be substituted for fat exchanges in an exchange meal plan, because alcohol is metabolized in a manner similar to fat. Each drink is equal to two fat exchanges.

■ Avoid drinking on an empty stomach or after vigorous exercise. These situations make you more prone to hypoglycemia, as does alcohol itself. The best time to have a drink is with a meal or just after you have eaten.

■ If you find it hard to stick to just one or two drinks, drink slowly and make one drink last a long time. Put your glass down frequently and focus on socializing instead. Or alternate an alcoholic drink with a nonalcoholic one, such as diet soda or mineral water. When you do this, you consume less alcohol and give your body a chance to metabolize the alcohol you have already had. You can also dilute beverages with ice, water, club soda, or a little fruit juice to increase their volume.

■ When you are drinking to quench your thirst, choose a nonalcoholic drink, since alcohol has a dehydrating effect.

■ To keep your calorie intake lower, choose light beer or light wine, which have fewer calories and less carbohydrate and alcohol than regular versions.

■ If you love the taste and ritual of drinking but can't limit yourself to just one or two servings, you may want to try nonalcoholic beer or alcohol-free wine as an alternative. For every 15 grams of carbohydrate in a nonalcoholic beer or wine, you can count one carbohydrate choice in your food plan.

■ Measure liquor for mixed drinks with a jigger to help control the amount you use. If you pour straight from the bottle, you are likely to use a larger quantity.

■ Be wary of mixing alcohol with medicines. Alcohol can block the effects of some drugs and amplify the effects of others. Certain medicines can also intensify the effects of alcohol on your body. If you take the diabetes pill metformin, limit your use of alcohol as a precaution against developing liver problems. Check with your health-care team to see if you should avoid alcohol when taking any of your prescribed or over-the-counter medicines.

■ Drinking too much can make you forgetful, which can interfere with your schedules and plans. Try not to get careless with your diabetes management goals of eating meals and snacks on time, following your meal plan, and testing your blood glucose regularly.

■ Carry visible identification. This is a good idea all the time, and especially when you are drinking away from home. Don't take any chances that possible symptoms of hypoglycemia will be confused with drunkenness.

Following is a table that lists the average calorie, carbohydrate, and alcohol content of alcoholic (and a few nonalcoholic) beverages. Items listed are general types of beverages, not brand specific, since there is little variation between most brands. Use this chart along with our safe sipping tips above to guide you in consuming alcohol safely and without disrupting your diabetes control.

Because alcoholic beverage labels do not typically list nutrition information, we include the titles of several books currently on the market that provide nutrition information for a wide variety of foods and beverages: *The Corinne T. Netzer Encyclopedia of Food Values,* by Corinne T. Netzer, Dell Books, New York, New York, 1992; *The Diabetes Carbohydrate and Fat Gram Guide,* by Lea Ann Holzmeister, The American Diabetes Association, Alexandria, Virginia, 2000; and *The Joslin Guide to Diabetes,* by Richard S. Beaser with Joan V. C. Hill, Simon & Schuster Books, New York, New York, 1995. ❏

MEASURING OUT THE DRINKS

ALCOHOLIC BEVERAGES	SERVING SIZE	CALORIES	CARBOHYDRATE (g)	ALCOHOL (g)
Beer				
Regular	12 ounces	150	13	13
Light	12 ounces	100	5	11
Nonalcoholic	12 ounces	70	13	1
Cocktails				
Bloody Mary	5 ounces	115	5	14
(tomato juice, vodka, lemon juice)				
Bourbon and soda	4 ounces	105	0	15
Daiquiri (rum, lime juice, sugar)	2 ounces	110	4	14
Gin and tonic (tonic water, gin, lime juice)	7.5 ounces	170	16	16

ALCOHOLIC BEVERAGES
(continued)

	SERVING SIZE	CALORIES	CARBOHYDRATE (g)	ALCOHOL (g)
Manhattan (whiskey & vermouth)	2 ounces	130	2	17
Martini (gin & vermouth)	2.5 ounces	155	< 1	22
Piña colada (pineapple juice, rum, sugar, coconut cream)	4.5 ounces	260	40	14
Screwdriver (orange juice, vodka)	7 ounces	175	18	14
Tequila sunrise (orange juice, tequila, lime juice, grenadine)	5.5 ounces	190	15	19
Tom Collins (club soda, gin, lemon juice, sugar)	7.5 ounces	120	3	16
Whiskey sour (lemon juice, whiskey, sugar)	3 ounces	120	5	15
Distilled Spirits				
All types, 80 proof	1.5 ounces	100	0	14
Gin, 90 proof	1.5 ounces	110	0	16
Brandy, cognac	1 ounce	75	0	11
Liqueur				
Coffee, 53 proof	1.5 ounces	175	24	11
Coffee with cream, 34 proof	1.5 ounces	155	10	7
Creme de menthe	1.5 ounces	185	21	15
Wine				
Dry	4 ounces	80	1	11
Dessert, dry	2 ounces	45	1	9
Dessert, sweet	2 ounces	90	7	9
Champagne	4 ounces	100	4	12
Wine cooler	12 ounces	220	30	10–17
Nonalcoholic wine	8 ounces	66	17	—

DRINK MIXERS

	SERVING SIZE	CALORIES	CARBOHYDRATE (g)	ALCOHOL (g)
Plain water, mineral water, club soda	any	0	0	—
Soft drink, regular	4 ounces	50	14	—
Soft drink, sugar-free	any	0	0	—
Tonic water	4 ounces	45	12	—
Tonic water, sugar-free	any	0	0	—
Tomato juice	4 ounces	25	5	—
Fruit juice	4 ounces	60	15	—
Margarita mix	4 ounces	130	29	—
Bloody Mary mix	8 ounces	40	9	—
Piña Colada mix	4.5 ounces	180	43	—
Mai Tai mix	4.5 ounces	140	33	—
Sweet & Sour mix	5.8 ounces	200	51	—
Rum Runner mix	3.5 ounces	160	39	—
Strawberry Daiquiri mix	3.5 ounces	150	35	—

Note: To ensure easy readability, all nutrient values in the table have been rounded to the nearest whole number. The numbers in our Carbohydrate column represent the total number of grams of carbohydrate (including simple sugars, starches, and other carbohydrates). We do not list simple sugars separately because they affect blood glucose no differently than starches and have the same number of calories per gram.

A QUICK GUIDE TO VEGETARIAN EATING

by Karmeen Kulkarni, M.S., R.D., C.D.E.

Ask people to name an essential nutrient that they don't get enough of, and most will answer "protein." Not only is this not true, but it is a misperception that can have unfortunate health consequences. In fact, most of us eat a lot more protein than we need, up to twice as much more. There's nothing wrong with that exactly; only certain people—such as those with kidney disease—need to watch how much protein they consume. The problem is that we get most of our protein from animal sources; approximately 70% comes from meat, poultry, fish, and dairy products. And animal protein almost always brings along an uninvited guest: fat. Anybody going to suggest that we don't get enough of that in our diet?

We've grown so accustomed to associating red meat with protein that we often overlook another, perhaps even better, way to get the protein we need. Animal products may be the primary protein source in the United States, but they're not the only source. Almost everything we eat contains some. Beans, lentils, legumes, potatoes and other vegetables, and breads and cereals all contain a fair amount. These foods are rich in vitamins and minerals as well and—here's the best part—*they are all low in fat.* So it's nutritionally savvy to take advantage of these alternative protein sources.

The fact is you can get all the protein you need from a well-balanced vegetarian meal plan. And that's not all you get. Studies have shown that a vegetarian diet promotes weight loss and provides effective weight management. It also appears to decrease the risk of hypertension, coronary artery disease, and some forms of cancer. And it *may* reduce the incidence of Type 2 diabetes and lower insulin requirements in people who have diabetes.

At one time, people who turned to vegetarianism did so for religious or ethical reasons. Clearly, there are now legitimate health reasons for choosing this dietary path as well.

A veggie by any other name

There's no one "correct" way to be vegetarian. But obviously, plant foods are the centerpiece of any vegetarian diet. That's not only fruits, vegetables, and beans, but also grains, seeds, and nuts. Any truly vegetarian diet excludes meat, fish, and fowl, but the hardest-core practitioners known as *vegans* shun dairy products, eggs, and even egg substitutes as well. More commonly, people will include dairy products (*lacto-vegetarians*) or dairy products and eggs (*lacto-ovo-vegetarians*). Even fish and poultry make it on to some menus. Unless you are making a political or religious statement, how strict you choose to be is up to you. But each of these diets is preferable, from a health standpoint, to the (heavy on the) meat-and-potatoes diet so many of us are used to.

The pros of plant foods

Simply put, vegetarians have a lower incidence of chronic disease than nonvegetarians. More than anything else, this can be attributed to a large reduction in the amount of fat provided by a vegetarian diet. Typically, animal products are responsible for the bulk of the fat we eat every day, so cutting out animal products can drastically cut down on your fat intake. And that's a plus for many reasons.

Less fat means fewer calories, and fewer calories means weight loss. (Vegetarian diets are extremely heavy with carbohydrates. Carbohydrates offer only 4 calories per gram while fat has 9 calories per gram, so you'd have to really stuff yourself on a vegetarian diet to get anywhere near the total calories of a higher-fat diet.) Of course, weight loss is important because people who carry additional pounds are at greater risk for diseases like hypertension, coronary artery disease, stroke, and diabetes. Vegetarians, specifically vegans, manage to stay closer to their ideal body weight than nonvegetarians.

Perhaps even more important, most animal fat is saturated fat. In addition, cholesterol is only found in animal products, so vegetarian diets offer another plus in this regard. Saturated fat and cholesterol can clog blood vessels with fatty deposits, leading to coronary artery disease. Needless to say, the incidence of heart and blood vessel trouble is much lower in vegetarians.

Studies show that vegetarians also have lower levels of low-density lipoprotein cholesterol—the "bad" cholesterol—and total cholesterol. (Levels of high-density lipoprotein cholesterol and triglycerides vary, depending on the type of vegetarian diet.) According to one study, a very-low-fat vegetarian diet, which got less than 10% of its total daily calories from fat, in combination with a healthy lifestyle of no smoking, moderate exercise, and stress management actually reversed severe coronary artery disease. For people with diabetes, who

VEGETARIAN FOR A DAY

Here is a sample meal plan that provides 1250 calories and adequate protein for an adult man or woman. It also fulfills a typical day's other nutritional requirements for some groups of people. (Since different persons have different nutritional needs, meal plans need to be individualized.)

	EXCHANGES	PROTEIN
BREAKFAST		
¾ cup dry cereal	1 starch/bread	3 grams
1 slice whole wheat toast	1 starch/bread	3 grams
1 teaspoon margarine	1 fat	0 grams
1 cup raspberries	1 fruit	0 grams
8 ounces skim milk	1 milk	8 grams
LUNCH		
2-ounce whole grain roll	2 starch/bread	6 grams
2 ounces string cheese	2 meat	14 grams
1 cup green salad	1 vegetable	2 grams
6 ounces V8 juice	1 vegetable	2 grams
8 ounces fruit yogurt	1 skim milk	8 grams
DINNER		
1 small baked potato	1 starch/bread	3 grams
½ cup corn	1 starch/bread	3 grams
4 ounces tofu (stir-fry)	1 meat	7 grams
2 cups stir-fry vegetables	2 vegetable	4 grams
1 orange	1 fruit	0 grams
8 ounces skim milk	1 skim milk	8 grams
Total grams of protein		**71 grams**

often have high cholesterol levels, this is very good news.

And that's not all. Although vegetarian diets offer adequate protein, the amount is still often less than that provided by animal-based diets. And that's good. Lower-protein diets may improve kidney function in people with kidney disease. In addition, studies seem to suggest that vegetarian protein is better than animal protein for these people. Although these studies are not conclusive, the results have been encouraging enough to suggest a switch to a vegetarian meal plan.

In addition, lower protein intake may improve the body's absorption and retention of calcium. New studies have shown that animal fat and protein erode the skeleton over time. Protein breaks down into acid in the blood, and the body counters with antacids, which unfortunately, can strip away calcium as well. So less animal protein can mean less trouble for people who have osteoporosis.

Less protein can also benefit people with Parkinson disease because extra protein has been shown to inhibit the effectiveness of some drugs prescribed for this condition.

Finally, because plants provide us with so much fiber while animal sources provide none, a move to vegetarianism means lots more of this important nutritional component in your diet. Fiber promotes intestinal regularity, and soluble fiber helps to lower blood cholesterol levels.

Answering the naysayers

Not everyone believes that vegetarian diets are as healthy as supporters make them out to be. In fact, some people worry that a diet that excludes animal products has to come up short in offering some essential nutrients needed by the body. Let's put these doubts to rest:

Protein. Protein is made up of building blocks called *amino acids*. Our bodies need a full complement of these amino acids, 20 in all, to function properly. Most of them can be produced internally, but we have to get nine "essential" amino acids from our diet. Animal protein offers all these essential amino acids, but most plant protein does not. (Soy products are a major exception.)

Don't consider this a major drawback. All it means is that you have to vary the plant foods your eat. Different plant sources offer different essential amino acids, so by mixing and matching them you can get all the protein your body needs.

Keep this simple equation in mind: legumes plus grains equals complete protein. Legumes have low levels of some essential amino acids and high amounts of others. Cereals have a complementary makeup; they have plenty of the amino acids that legumes lack and not enough of the other types. Together, they mesh nicely to provide a complete protein that offers the full plate of amino acids.

In truth, you don't really have to make a calculated effort to combine complementary plant foods at each meal. Rather, it makes more sense to prepare a diverse vegetarian menu that can add up to complete proteins over the course of the day. It's actually a lot less complicated than it sounds. And if you need help, don't hesitate to check in with your dietitian.

Iron. The traditional American diet gets most of its iron from red meat. This iron is known as *heme iron*. Plants provide a different type of iron called *nonheme iron*. Although nonheme iron isn't absorbed as well as heme iron, generally, most plant products offer enough to keep vegetarians at no risk of iron deficiency. Dark green leafy vegetables such as spinach, potatoes, whole grains, dried fruits, nuts, and egg yolks are your best bets for iron. A tip: Nonheme iron is absorbed more efficiently when it is consumed along with vitamin C.

Vitamin B$_{12}$. Vitamin B$_{12}$, which plays a vital role in growth and development, is found primarily in meat, milk, and dairy products. So although nonvegans do not have to worry, total vegetarians may be at increased risk for vitamin B$_{12}$ deficiency. Fortified breakfast cereals, some nutritional yeast, and soy beverages all can provide vegans with sufficient amounts of vitamin B$_{12}$. But as a precaution, you can take vitamin supplements as well.

Calcium. Similarly, you may expect vegans to experience a calcium shortage, since so much of it comes from milk and meat. In fact, vegetarians usually absorb and retain more calcium from foods than nonvegetarians. Soybeans, leafy vegetables, and dried beans are good calcium sources.

Zinc. Zinc, which is essential for growth, cell development, and wound healing, also comes primarily from protein-rich foods, such as liver and other meats and eggs. However, you can get plenty of zinc from legumes, whole grains, and nuts.

Total calories. Not only are vegetarian diets low in fat, but their fiber content makes them particularly filling, so you may very well be satisfied on fewer calories than you are used to. Many people would consider that an advantage. But for some—specifically, infants, children and teenagers, pregnant women, and other individuals—getting sufficient calories each day is a nutritional priority. Not to worry; a well-planned vegetarian diet can give anyone more than enough calories.

So our answer is "yes" to all the detractors that ask "is there enough?" However, some people with diabetes may have a different concern—not "is there enough?" but in the case of carbohydrate "is there *too much*?" Inevitably, a vegetarian diet will give you more carbohydrates than a more traditional meal plan. When a diet is low in fat and lower in protein, what's left to offer sufficient calories but carbohydrates? But the only concession you may have to make is in your insulin dosing. You and your doctor can figure out a new regimen over time. However, if you want to lower the carbohydrate content of your new diet a little, you can increase your fat content by eating foods high in monounsaturated fats, such as avocados, and by cooking with olive oil and canola oil.

Recipe for success

That truth is that it's not difficult at all to devise a diet that gives you the protein, vitamins, minerals, and calories required by the Recommended Dietary Allowances. However, there's more to a vegetarian diet than simply avoiding meat. After all, you can eat cheese and potato chips all day and call yourself a vegetarian, but you won't be a very healthy one. The key is variety.

A wide range of foods can go a long way toward ensuring a well-balanced diet that gives you all the nutrients you need. If you decide to go veggie, we suggest that you talk over the particulars with your dietitian. But here are some basic guidelines to help you get started:

■ Choose a variety of fruits and vegetables high in vitamin C. Vitamin C may have some anticancer properties and it helps you to absorb iron. The recommended minimum amount of five servings of fruits and vegetables per day should give you more than enough vitamin C (and vitamin A as well). Foods that provide vitamin C include oranges and orange juice, grapefruit and grapefruit juice, strawberries, cantaloupe, sweet red peppers, Brussels sprouts, broccoli, cauliflower, and potatoes.

■ Opt for fortified, enriched cereals and whole-grain or unrefined breads and pastas. There's more fiber and vitamins in these products than in their refined counterparts such as white bread.

■ Dairy products are an excellent source of protein, B$_{12}$, and calcium, but if you include them in your diet, be sure to select low-fat or nonfat versions. Whole-fat products will undermine many of the benefits associated with an otherwise low-fat vegetarian diet.

■ Similarly, don't forget other good sources of vitamin B$_{12}$ such as fortified breakfast cereals and soy beverages.

■ If you include eggs in your meal plan (they are excellent iron sources) try to eat no more than three or four yolks per week. Egg yolks are very high in cholesterol.

■ Consult the Exchange Lists for Meal Planning (published by the American Diabetes Association and The American Dietetic Association) or another nutrition resource book to help you figure out how much protein you're getting from your new food choices. Each starch/bread exchange—for instance, 1 bread slice, 1 small baked potato, ½ cup corn or black beans, or ⅓ cup rice, pasta, or lentils—provides 3 grams of protein. Each vegetable exchange—½ cup cooked or 1 cup raw of most kinds—gives you 2 grams of protein. Each milk exchange—1 cup of milk or yogurt—provides 8 grams of protein. One egg or an ounce of most types of cheese provides 7 grams of protein. Fruit, however, has no protein.

The recommended daily allowance for protein for adult men and women is between 50 and 63 grams a day. The numbers are slightly less for teenagers and young adults. Clearly, there are a lot of ways to get to your total allotment without too much trouble. For one way to accomplish this goal, see the sample meal plan on page 309.

Of course, you don't have to switch over all at once. In fact, it may be better to go slow. Give your taste buds time to get used to the idea. Start by substituting pasta and vegetables for a hamburger at dinner, or a lentil salad instead of a ham sandwich for lunch. Each step brings you closer to your goal.

Vegging out

You never have to go totally vegetarian to receive many of the health benefits described in this article. But whatever meal planning path you choose, keep in mind that although a little meat never hurt anyone, you really don't need any to maintain your health. Even the more nutritionally vulnerable among us can thrive on a balanced vegetarian diet.

One of the best parts of moving toward a vegetarian diet is having the opportunity to expand your culinary horizons. For too long and for too many people, vegetables have been nothing more than peas and carrots and tomato and lettuce salads. But there are many more exotic choices just waiting for you to try them. Oh, there's one more thing: Eating vegetarian is usually a whole lot easier on the pocketbook than a traditional meat-filled diet.

Most of the world's population is already primarily vegetarian. You have to think that they're on to something. ❑

DIABETES SNACK BARS
WHAT CAN THEY DO FOR YOU?
by Belinda O'Connell, M.S., R.D., L.D.

A carbohydrate is a carbohydrate is a carbohydrate. Ever since 1994—when the American Diabetes Association began advising people with diabetes to count *all* carbohydrates in the diet rather than just limiting sugar and sweets—dietitians have been chanting this mantra to their clients with diabetes. (Carbohydrate is the type of nutrient that affects blood sugar levels the most; fat and protein have much less of an effect.)

What the dietitians mean when they recite their catchy slogan is that all foods that contain carbohydrate—from fruit, to oatmeal, to common table sugar—have similar effects on blood glucose levels when consumed in equivalent portions. And this is true—most of the time. So when doesn't a carbohydrate act the way we expect a carbohydrate to act?

Several new snack bars that have come on the market within the past several years contain special forms of carbohydrate that do not cause the rapid increase in blood glucose levels typically seen when carbohydrate-containing foods are eaten. These snack bars, which include Gluc-O-Bar, Choice DM bar, Extend Bar, Ensure Glucerna bar, and NiteBite bar, were created specifically for the management of diabetes and are considered "functional" or "medical" foods. Functional or medical foods are defined as foods that may provide benefits beyond basic nutrition. Some are intended to treat or prevent disease; others are designed for the dietary management of a disease.

The labels of the new "diabetes" snack bars bear such nutrition claims as "Slow release glucose bar," "Long acting carbohydrate snack," "Improves blood glucose control," "Blood sugar stabilization," and "Reduces risk of hypoglycemia." Can these bars really do all that they claim to do? If so, how do they work? To answer these questions, we need to look at what carbohydrates are and how they are digested.

What is a carbohydrate?

The word *carbohydrate* is a general term that refers to any of several compounds found in foods. These compounds are very similar and share many characteristics but do have subtle differences in their chemical form. Much as there are different types of gasoline for automobiles, there are different types of carbohydrate, all of which work in roughly the same way.

All carbohydrates are built from single units of sugar. These sugar units can exist alone or be combined with others, forming either small groups with just a few sugar molecules, or long chains with hundreds of sugar molecules. The longer chains of carbohydrate are often referred to as "complex carbohydrates" (and sometimes as starches) and the smaller units as "simple sugars." The most common sugar found in carbohydrates is called glucose.

When foods with carbohydrate are eaten, digestive enzymes break the long chains of sugar into single units of sugar, usually glucose, that the body can absorb. After it is absorbed, glucose is transported in the bloodstream to other cells in the body. The increase in blood glucose levels seen after eating is referred to as the *postprandial,* or after-meal, blood glucose level. Under normal circumstances—in both people who have diabetes and those who don't—digestion and absorption of carbohydrate occur quite quickly, with a maximum increase in blood glucose levels by 30 minutes after eating and a return to normal levels within two hours, as long as insulin levels are adequate.

In the past, it was assumed that smaller carbohydrate molecules (the simple sugars) were broken down and absorbed more quickly than the longer carbohydrate chains (the complex carbohydrates). We now know that this assumption is not correct and that other factors are more important than the size of the carbohydrate molecule in determining how quickly it is digested and how it affects blood glucose levels. This understanding is what led to the dietary guidelines issued in 1994, which recommend controlling the total amount of carbohydrate consumed rather than just limiting sugar and sweets. Some of the factors that alter the rate at which a carbohydrate-containing food is digested and absorbed into the bloodstream as glucose include the specific form of carbohydrate in the food, the presence of other nutrients such as protein, fat, and fiber, and the type of processing the food has undergone.

The snack bars designed for people with diabetes are made with forms of starch that are either naturally digested more slowly or have been chemically processed to slow the rate of their digestion. This type of starch is referred to as "resistant starch" because it is resistant to (or less easily broken down by) digestive enzymes. Because these snack bars are digested more slowly and over a longer time period, they cause a lower peak blood glucose level immediately after being eaten, and they continue to enter the bloodstream over several hours, helping to keep blood glucose levels stable.

What makes starch resistant?

Starch contains two main forms of carbohydrate: amylose and amylopectin. Both are made up of hundreds of glucose molecules linked together, but the arrangement of the glucose molecules differs significantly. Amylopectin contains many separate chains of glucose that branch off a common stem, much like a tree trunk with many individual branches. Amylose, on the other hand, is a long, straight chain of glucose molecules without any branches.

In food, amylose and amylopectin molecules are found clustered in bunches. The size and three-dimensional shape of these clusters affect the rate at which they are digested. Amylose molecules are able to form very tight groups with very little space between them because the glucose chains are so straight and orderly. Amylopectin molecules form very loose bunches that have lots of gaps between molecules because the branches stick out in all directions, holding the molecules apart. Picture amylose as straight branches stacked very tightly together and

amylopectin as a pile of brush with many gaps and spaces between branches.

These structural differences cause the two types of starch to be digested differently. The gaps and spaces in the amylopectin bunches let digestive enzymes easily attack the starch and chop apart, or digest, the glucose molecules rapidly. With amylose, the closeness of the molecules makes it difficult for digestive enzymes to find a place to start, so it is digested more slowly. Because of this, amylose starch is considered to be more "resistant" to digestion. Foods that contain very high amounts of amylose starch cause a smaller increase in blood glucose levels than foods containing mostly amylopectin.

The way a food is processed can also alter the rate of starch digestion. For example, cooking generally causes the starch molecules to move further apart, increasing ease of digestion. Food manufacturers use other processing methods to increase the amount of resistant starch in a product. These methods make the molecules of amylose associate even more closely than they do in their unprocessed form, decreasing the rate of digestion.

NiteBite, Gluc-O-Bar, and Extend are made with uncooked cornstarch, a natural form of resistant starch. The manufacturers of the NiteBite bar also claim that the proportion of sucrose to protein to uncooked cornstarch in their snack bar extends the rate of blood glucose release.

The Choice DM bar is made with a specially processed form of resistant starch called CrystaLean, which is produced by Opta Food Ingredients, Inc. Because CrystaLean is incompletely digested, it has a lower caloric content than standard carbohydrates. Opta estimates that CrystaLean provides 2.4 calories per gram of carbohydrate, compared with 4 calories per gram of fully digestible carbohydrate.

The Ensure Glucerna bar does not use resistant starch but instead contains soluble fiber, which forms a viscous gel in the small intestine and slows the absorption of glucose.

Benefits of resistant starch

Including resistant starch in the diet has several potential benefits for people with diabetes. Some of those benefits include lower blood glucose levels after meals and a lower risk of low blood sugar during the night.

Decreased blood glucose levels after meals. Good blood glucose control is the single most important factor in preventing the chronic health complications associated with diabetes, and current research suggests that controlling blood glucose levels after meals is an important component of overall blood glucose management. The most common method used to minimize blood glucose levels after meals is to limit

SNACK BAR PROFILES

Listed below are examples of snack bars formulated to meet the needs of people with diabetes. They are available at many pharmacies and grocery stores, by mail order, or via the World Wide Web. We list nutrition information (provided by the manufacturer) for one flavor of each brand. Nutrition information may be slightly different for other flavors. Abbreviations used: g is grams, and mg is milligrams.

CHOICE DM
Mead Johnson Nutritionals
(800) 247-7893
www.choicedm.com

PEANUTTY CHOCOLATE
Calories: 140
Carbohydrate: 19 g
Protein: 6 g
Fat: 4.5 g
Saturated fat: 2.5 g
Cholesterol: <5 mg
Sodium: 80 mg
Fiber: 3 g

ENSURE GLUCERNA
Ross Products Division
Abbott Laboratories
(800) 227-5767
www.ensureglucerna.com

CHOCOLATE GRAHAM
Calories: 140
Carbohydrate: 24 g
Protein: 6 g
Fat: 4 g

Saturated fat: 1 g
Cholesterol: <5 mg
Sodium: 75 mg
Fiber: 4 g

EXTEND BAR
Clinical Products, Ltd.
(877) 3-EXTEND (339-8363)
www.extendbar.com

PEANUT BUTTER CRUNCH
Calories: 160
Carbohydrate: 30 g
Protein: 4 g
Fat: 2.5 g
Saturated fat: 0 g
Cholesterol: 0 mg
Sodium: 85 mg
Fiber: 0 g

GLUC-O-BAR
APIC USA, Inc.
(877) 458-2622

CHOCOLATE
Calories: 130
Carbohydrate: 22 g

Protein: 6 g
Fat: 2 g
Saturated fat: 1 g
Cholesterol: 0 mg
Sodium: 95 mg
Fiber: 1 g

NITEBITE
ICN Pharmaceuticals, Inc.
(800) 795-1880
www.nitebite.com

CHOCOLATE FUDGE
Calories: 100
Carbohydrate: 15 g
Protein: 3 g
Fat: 3.5 g
Saturated fat: 1.5 g
Cholesterol: 5 mg
Sodium: 40 mg
Fiber: 0 g

the amount of carbohydrate consumed at meals and snacks and to match the amount of carbohydrate eaten with a person's medication and activity level. For many people, however, limiting the amount of carbohydrate in the diet can be difficult. This is where foods made with resistant starch may be helpful.

In research studies, resistant starch has been shown to decrease blood glucose levels after meals in people with either Type 1 or Type 2 diabetes. For people with Type 2 diabetes, this means their bodies do not have to produce as much insulin to metabolize the carbohydrate. The blood glucose response to resistant starch can vary from person to person, from meal to meal, and from one type of resistant starch to another. Generally, however, it is 15% to 25% lower than that seen with equivalent portions of nonresistant starches. Because resistant starch results in a lower peak blood glucose level after consumption, some people may be able to have increased quantities of carbohydrate at a

meal without having a corresponding increase in blood glucose level.

Lowered risk of low blood sugar. Snack bars made with resistant starch may also be helpful in preventing low blood sugar during the night when they are eaten as part of a bedtime snack. Because resistant starch is digested more slowly, it may provide a source of glucose for an extended time period after being eaten. This "slow release" of glucose over the nighttime hours, when people are sleeping and not eating, may provide enough carbohydrate to prevent the drop in blood glucose some people experience overnight. It has also been hypothesized that resistant starch could prevent exercise-related low blood sugar when eaten as a snack before exercise.

Other benefits. Because resistant starch is incompletely digested and absorbed in the small intestine, the portion that is undigested proceeds to the large intestine. In the large intestine, it undergoes bacterial fermentation. The resulting fermentation products are believed to be beneficial in maintaining healthy colon cells.

Since resistant starch provides fewer calories than fully digestible starch, it may be beneficial in promoting weight loss. However, the effect of resistant starch on weight and weight loss is largely unknown at present.

In addition to improving blood glucose levels, some research suggests that resistant starch may have a positive effect on blood cholesterol and blood triglyceride levels. (Triglycerides are a type of blood fat that, when present at high levels, is associated with heart disease.) These studies are still preliminary, and more research is needed to clarify these effects.

Do the snack bars deliver?

Several studies have been done on the "diabetes" snack bars. Companies' nutritional claims are based on tests in people with diabetes, on general research, or on research conducted with other food products. In general, the snack bars appear to have positive effects on diabetes management, with some bars having a clinically significant impact on blood glucose levels. But the limited number of research studies does not provide enough information to make definitive conclusions yet.

The effects of Ensure Glucerna were tested in people with Type 2 diabetes. Each subject consumed three different snack bars, each containing 50 grams of carbohydrate but differing quantities of dietary fiber and guar gum, in a random order on three separate occasions. (Guar gum is a soluble fiber that forms a viscous gel in the intestinal tract and is believed to decrease the absorption of glucose.) The subjects' peak blood glucose level after eating, total blood glucose level over time, and insulin level were significantly lower for the bar with the highest concentration of guar gum. In addition, four hours after eating, the blood glucose level for the guar gum bar remained significantly higher than for the other bars, suggesting slowed glucose absorption. (Researchers look at both the peak or maximum blood glucose level after a food is eaten and the length of time a person's blood glucose level stays elevated above normal after eating to test the effect of a food.)

In a test of Choice DM, which is made with resistant starch, subjects with Type 2 diabetes also consumed three different snack bars with similar carbohydrate levels (just under 50 grams) in a random order on three different days. Peak blood glucose and total blood glucose levels over time were significantly lower for the Choice DM bar, compared to the two other bars. Insulin levels over time were also lower for the Choice DM bar than for one of the other snack bars.

The effect of including uncooked cornstarch in the bedtime snack of adolescents with Type 1 diabetes has been tested in several clinical trials. (NiteBite, Gluc-O-Bar, and Extend Bar, as noted above, all contain uncooked cornstarch.) In one study, the uncooked cornstarch was provided in the form of the discontinued Zbar. In this trial, adolescents at a diabetes camp consumed either the Zbar or a standard snack bar as a bedtime snack for five consecutive nights each. The incidence of early morning and nighttime low blood sugar was significantly lower for the bar containing uncooked cornstarch than for the standard snack bar.

Extend Bar is a revamped—reportedly tastier—version of the Zbar. Tested under similar conditions, Extend Bar also prevented nighttime low blood sugar without increasing the incidence of high blood sugar.

Investigators have also evaluated the effect of NiteBite on the incidence of low blood sugar during exercise in people with Type 1 diabetes. Subjects in this study followed their usual exercise regimen and consumed either the NiteBite bar or a "usual" snack before exercise on two consecutive days. Subjects in both groups had similar rates of low blood sugar during and two hours after exercise, but total calorie consumption and the incidence of high blood sugar after exercise were significantly lower with the NiteBite bar.

Are snack bars for you?

Given the apparent benefits of "diabetes" snack bars, should you give them a try? For people who like eating energy bars or granola bars for a quick breakfast or snack, bars containing resistant starch may prove helpful in preventing low blood sugar and minimizing blood glucose levels after meals. They may also allow some people to eat more carbohydrate at a meal since they raise blood glucose less than other carbohydrates. For example, if you normally have 4 carbohydrate choices for lunch—say, a sandwich (2 choices), an apple (1 choice), and a cup of milk (1 choice)—you may be able to add a resistant starch snack bar (containing 15 grams of carbohydrate) to your lunch without an undue rise in blood sugar. Another benefit of some snack bars is that they are fortified with nutrients such as calcium, folate, vitamin E, and vitamin C. However, while snack bars may be helpful for controlling blood glucose levels after meals, they have no proven benefit over restricting the amount of carbohydrate you eat, and they need to be used as part of a comprehensive diabetes management plan.

If you are interested in trying a diabetes snack bar, work with your dietitian or doctor to determine how to fit it into your meal plan. The bars discussed in this article contain 15 to 30 grams of carbohydrate, so they are technically one to two carbohydrate choices, but they may require less injected insulin than a typical carbohydrate choice. You will need to check your blood sugar levels more frequently to determine their effect on you. If you use insulin, you will need to check your blood sugar to determine how much insulin, if any, you need to take with them.

People trying a snack bar between meals should check their blood glucose before eating the bar, one hour afterward, and two to four hours after eating the snack bar on several occasions. Keeping records of the amount of carbohydrate you eat at meals, your medication, and your activity level will help you determine the effect of the snack bar on your blood glucose level.

If you are trying a snack bar as part of your bedtime snack to prevent low blood sugar overnight, be sure to keep detailed daily records of food, medication, and activity. Keeping carbohydrate intake and activity levels as consistent as possible will also help you determine the effect of the snack bar on your blood glucose level. You should also check your blood glucose level before your snack, at bedtime if this is more than half an hour later, and in the morning when you first wake

up. For people who frequently have low blood sugar during the night, checking your blood glucose in the early morning (around 3 AM) is also helpful.

Since snack bars containing resistant starch do not cause a rapid increase in blood glucose levels, they are *not* appropriate for treating low blood sugar. You still need to carry another source of carbohydrate (such as glucose tablets) for this purpose.

Snack bars may be helpful in certain instances as part of a good diabetes management plan, but they cannot improve blood sugar levels on their own. Other strategies for keeping blood sugar in target range—such as appropriate meal spacing, taking insulin or pills according to a schedule, and counting carbohydrates or following a meal plan—are still the cornerstones of your diabetes-care plan.

The bars discussed in this article tend to be expensive—often costing more than a dollar a bar—so keep in mind that they are not necessary for good control but are simply another tool that can increase the flexibility of your diabetes treatment plan. ❑

MEETING FOR BETTER EATING
TEAMING UP WITH A DIETITIAN
by Patti Bazel Geil, M.S., R.D., L.D., C.D.E., and Tami Ross, R.D., L.D., C.D.E.

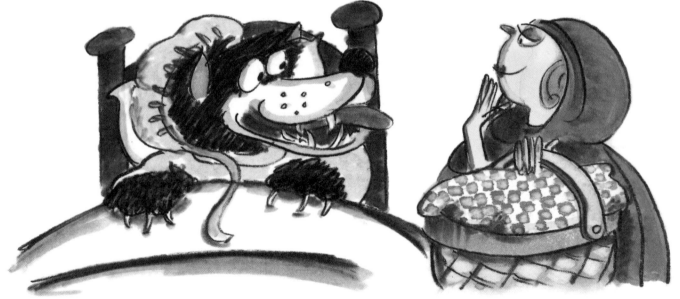

When Ted, 52, went for his yearly checkup, he was shocked when his doctor diagnosed him with diabetes. Ted knew that he was about 30 pounds overweight and that he had high blood pressure, but he assumed the fatigue he'd been feeling lately could be

blamed on his stressful job as a mutual funds manager and the fact that he was past 50. He never dreamed he could have a serious chronic disease.

At the checkup, his physician prescribed an oral diabetes drug and advised Ted to begin checking his blood glucose at home. The doctor also told Ted that

TOP TEN REASONS TO SEE AN R.D.

1. You want to improve your diabetes control.

2. Your lifestyle or schedule has changed (new job, moving, marriage).

3. Your nutrition needs are changing rapidly (growing children, pregnancy, breast-feeding).

4. You've begun an exercise program or your diabetes medication has changed.

5. You feel bored or frustrated with your meal plan.

6. You have unexplained high and low blood sugar levels.

7. You're concerned about your weight or blood fat levels (cholesterol or triglycerides).

8. You've developed nutrition-related complications such as high blood pressure or kidney disease.

9. You'd like an update on what's new in diabetes nutrition.

10. You'd like a routine review of your meal plan. Diabetes experts suggest visiting your dietitian at least twice a year for follow-up.

taking a pill is only one part of a diabetes management plan. He said Ted also needed to make some changes in his diet and increase his physical activity to control his blood glucose level.

Ted's only physical activity was a little gardening in the summer, and he was willing to give exercise a try. But the idea of changing his diet made him uneasy. His job required him to have frequent business lunches with clients, and he didn't want to be distracted by having to search the menu for special foods. In addition, Ted can't tolerate milk products, which was a big enough problem by itself. He wanted to take care of his health, but he worried that his diabetes would interfere with his job, and he was uncertain about whether he could handle all the responsibilities that seem to come with diabetes.

To help him with the nutrition side of diabetes, Ted's doctor referred him to a registered dietitian (R.D.). Ted wasn't sure what to expect from this meeting. Although he could use some help figuring out what to eat to improve his blood sugar control, he dreaded the idea of being put on a strict weight-loss diet or being told to give up his favorite foods and instead eat things he doesn't like or doesn't know how to prepare. He also suspected the R.D. would scold him for his eating habits, which include occasionally eating at fast-food restaurants and having dessert.

Many people with diabetes can probably relate to how Ted was feeling. It's not uncommon to be apprehensive about meeting with a dietitian, particularly if a doctor has told you to change your diet. After all, food is one of life's great pleasures. If you are in Ted's situation, and you feel nervous or uncertain, remember that visiting an R.D. is not like a trip to the principal's office. Although the registered dietitian is the nutrition expert on the diabetes team, that doesn't mean he or she will act as the "food police" and forbid you to ever enjoy food again. Instead, a visit to the R.D. means you will receive nutrition education that is individualized for you. Ideally, your R.D. will help you understand the role that food plays in your blood sugar control and offer you ideas and resources to manage your diet and your blood sugar.

What's a dietitian?

These days, many people consider themselves nutrition experts, or "nutritionists," whether it's the cafeteria cook, nutraceutical salesperson, or TV infomercial host. As someone with diabetes, you must make sure the person you are consulting for nutrition information is truly a credentialed health professional. You can't afford to follow the advice of an untrained person or take to heart the latest fad diet.

In your search for reliable nutrition information, you need to consult a registered dietitian (R.D.), registered with the Commission on Dietetic Registration of The American Dietetic Association (ADA). An R.D. must earn a bachelor's degree in nutrition (or a related field) from an accredited college or university, complete an ADA-approved internship, and pass an extensive registration exam. In order to maintain registration, all R.D.'s are required to complete at least 75 hours of continuing education every five years. In addition, some states now also require R.D.'s to be licensed by their state. (Dietitians with a state license will have an "L.D." following their name.)

While all R.D.'s should have a good understanding of the nutrition recommendations for diabetes, some go on to gain further experience and knowledge. They specialize in diabetes management and can become Certified Diabetes Educators (C.D.E.), certified by the National Certification Board for Diabetes Educators.

Registered dietitians work in a variety of settings. You might link up with an R.D. at a local hospital, clinic, or health department; in private practice; or through your county extension office or health maintenance organization. Your doctor may be able to refer you to a dietitian. If not, the list on page 317 entitled "Finding the Food Experts" suggests several good avenues for finding an R.D. who specializes in diabetes management.

Like most professionals, registered dietitians charge a fee, either by the hour or by the session, based on their experience and other factors. Fees for nutrition counseling can vary widely. Some R.D.'s are a part of a hospital or physician's staff, and their fees are included in the cost of your visit. Others are paid directly by their clients. Before you meet with a registered dietitian, find out the fee schedule, number of expected visits, and preferred method of payment. If your health-care plan or insurance carrier covers the cost of nutrition counseling, find out how many visits are covered and what referral forms or other paperwork your plan requires for reimbursement.

If your health-care plan initially rejects your claim to cover the cost of nutrition therapy, don't take no for an answer! Your health-care team may be willing to write a letter of appeal, highlighting the fact that nutrition counseling can actually save health-care dollars. For example, if you have Type 2 diabetes, the weight loss and improved blood glucose control that result from successful nutrition counseling may enable you to reduce or eliminate expensive diabetes medicines, as well as avoid future complications and health problems.

Expect your initial visit with the R.D. to last anywhere from half an hour to two hours. While realistically you may have only one visit with a dietitian because of insurance limitations or other restraints, education is best accomplished through a series of visits scheduled every two to four weeks for two to four months, with each visit ranging from 15 to 45 minutes. Follow-up visits to assess progress are scheduled as needed. Children can benefit from a visit every three to six months, to make sure their meal plan is providing adequate nutrition for normal growth and development. For adults, a visit every six to 12 months can help keep a person on track and allow changes to be made in one's meal plan as one's lifestyle changes.

Getting to know you

The dietitian's job is to help you develop an individual nutrition plan that will enable you to manage your blood sugar and meet your other goals and that will be satisfying to you. To do this, he or she will need to learn about you, your diabetes, and the way you eat. Information may be gathered through a questionnaire, simply by talking with you, or both. So when you visit a dietitian for the first time, be prepared to answer questions—lots of questions! Being open and honest with your answers will enable the R.D. to formulate the best nutrition approach for you.

At your appointment, expect to have your height and weight measured, followed by a review of your weight history, medical history, and level of physical activity. Your lab values, blood glucose results, and

FINDING THE FOOD EXPERTS

To find a registered dietitian near you, try contacting the following organizations. You may want to request information specifically about R.D.'s who specialize in diabetes nutrition:

THE AMERICAN ASSOCIATION OF DIABETES EDUCATORS
www.aadenet.org
(800) 832-6874

THE AMERICAN DIABETES ASSOCIATION
(800) 342-2383
www.diabetes.org

THE AMERICAN DIETETIC ASSOCIATION
(800) 366-1655
www.eatright.org

MEAL-PLANNING RESOURCES

If you'd like more information about the diabetes meal planning approaches mentioned in this article, try the following:

For a copy of "Exchange Lists for Meal Planning," contact the American Diabetes Association at (800) ADA-ORDER (232-6733) or order via the World Wide Web, at http://store.diabetes.org.

To order a set of three booklets that explain carbohydrate counting, from the basics to more advanced techniques, call The American Dietetic Association at (800) 877-1600, extension 5000. You can also order online, via the Association's Web site, www.eatright.org/catalog/diabetes.html.

To get a single, free copy of "The First Step in Diabetes Meal Planning," call the American Diabetes Association at (800) 342-2383 or e-mail customerservice@diabetes.org.

medicines will be evaluated to help determine the best meal plan for you. The dietitian will probably ask about any nutrition education you've received in the past and will almost certainly ask about your current eating habits. The idea is to base your new meal plan as closely as possible on the eating habits and preferences you already have. At this point, having a food journal—in which you have noted everything you ate over a period of three to seven days—can be very helpful. Be sure to mention any food allergies, intolerances, preferences, and dislikes. In Ted's case, he needs to make sure the dietitian knows that he frequently eats in restaurants and cannot tolerate dairy products.

To make the most of your initial visit, it's a good idea to bring along information on paper for the R.D. to review. A checklist of what to bring with you includes the following:

■ The consult/referral form from your doctor's office.
■ A copy of the findings from your most recent medical checkup. (You will need to get this from your doctor's office.)
■ Recent medical test and lab results, such as your hemoglobin A_{1c}, 24-hour urine, and lipids (cholesterol and triglycerides). (You will also need to get this from your doctor's office.)
■ Your blood glucose meter. (Not all R.D.'s will ask you to bring your meter, but an R.D. who is also a C.D.E. can review your blood glucose testing technique, go over any test results stored in the meter with you, and show you how to clean and calibrate the meter, if necessary.)
■ Your blood glucose logbook.
■ A list of all medicines and supplements you take, along with the doses.
■ Any diet information you have received in the past or are currently following.
■ A food journal listing everything you ate or drank during the past three to seven days. Be sure to include serving sizes and how the food was prepared (fried, baked, grilled, boiled, etc.).
■ Food labels or products you have questions about.
■ A list of goals that you hope to accomplish.
■ A list of questions you want answered.

You might also want to consider bringing along a family member or support person to help provide information (especially if he or she does most of the cooking in your home) and to lend an extra set of ears.

Because you'll be sharing a lot of personal information, it's important to feel comfortable with the dietitian. After all, it can be embarrassing to admit to your habit of raiding the refrigerator at midnight! Remember that the R.D. is not there to judge you on your weaknesses but rather to help you work toward your goals by applying professional knowledge of nutrition to your dietary needs.

Setting goals

After the dietitian gets to know you and your needs, it's time to discuss setting goals. The general goal of everyone with diabetes is to keep his or her blood sugar in the target range as much as possible, and the right diet can help you do that. The American Diabetes Association recommends keeping your blood sugar between 80 mg/dl and 120 mg/dl before meals, and having it go no higher than 180 mg/dl after

meals. Ask your doctor if these numbers are good targets for you, or if your range should be different.

Some other common goals include attaining or maintaining optimal blood cholesterol and triglyceride levels, attaining or maintaining a reasonable weight, preventing diabetes-related complications, and improving overall health through good nutrition. Whether you adopt these goals as your personal goals and how you decide to achieve them is an individual matter. There's no one correct diabetes management plan; your R.D. can help you develop a plan that's tailored just for you.

When you discuss goals with your dietitian, be sure to mention the things you are willing to do—and those you are not. Ted's doctor had told him to lose 30 pounds, but Ted felt overwhelmed just thinking about losing weight. He had tried following weight-loss diets in the past, and he always felt deprived while he was dieting and depressed when the weight didn't come off. Besides, he didn't see how it was possible to cut back on his food intake, since he already ate only three meals a day and never snacked.

You may decide you are not willing to give up a particular food. For example, to cut down on your fat intake, your dietitian might suggest that you switch from regular salad dressing to fat-free salad dressing. But if you look forward every day to creamy ranch dressing on your salad, say so. It probably can be incorporated into your meal plan, although perhaps in smaller amounts than you usually eat, and fat can be trimmed from a different area of your diet. There's no point in constructing a plan that will be too difficult or unpleasant for you to follow.

A dietitian should explain why certain changes in your eating habits and lifestyle are needed. If yours doesn't, and you don't understand the recommendations, be sure to ask about them. Likewise, if your dietitian uses terms you don't understand, ask for clarification.

Working toward your goals

You and your dietitian may discuss a number of goals that you'd like to work on, but success is more likely if you choose just two or three to work on at a time. While general goals are helpful, the best goals are specific and measurable. Ted and his dietitian decided together that he would initially focus on two goals: getting a true sense of how much he ate each day and incorporating more physical activity into his life, as recommended by his doctor. Ted scheduled a follow-up visit with the dietitian in two weeks to assess how things were going.

To accomplish the first goal, Ted agreed to keep a food diary for one week. He would write down everything he ate each day, including portion sizes and how

GOING FOR THE GOALS

The best diabetes nutrition goals are measurable and attainable. The following list shows how a general goal can be individualized to make it more specific and achievable.

GENERAL GOAL	PERSONALIZATION
Eat a variety of foods.	I will eat at least three servings of fruits and vegetables each day.
Control portion sizes.	I will weigh and measure my foods three days next week.
Eat less fat.	I will substitute a small salad for an order of French fries at lunch twice this week.
Get some physical activity on a regular basis.	I will walk for 15 minutes during my lunch hour four days a week.
Check blood glucose on a regular basis.	I will check my blood glucose twice a day for the next week.
Don't skip meals.	I will eat breakfast five days a week.
Reach and maintain a healthy weight.	I will eat three cups of popcorn instead of the entire bag for my evening snack.

the food was cooked. At home, he would measure his portion sizes with measuring cups and spoons; at restaurants, he would estimate, noting the size of the plates on which the food was served.

For the second goal, Ted decided to begin walking for exercise 20 minutes per day, five days per week. Many people with diabetes benefit from working with an exercise specialist such as a physical therapist or an exercise physiologist when starting a physical activity program. Since Ted had no foot problems or other medical conditions that might limit his ability to exercise, and Ted's doctor had given him the OK to start walking several times a week, Ted sought only the support of his dietitian as he increased his physical activity.

Keep in mind that the goals you agree on are not set in stone; they can always be revised as needed. In fact, it's often easier and more effective to begin with intermediate goals, or small steps, that get you closer to your ultimate goals. Instead of jumping right in and promising yourself you'll lose 20 pounds by your cousin's wedding next month, start with a more modest—and more realistic—plan to gradually reduce the amount of calories you eat each day. Learning to manage your diabetes doesn't happen in one session of nutrition instruction; it is a lifetime process. Periodically reviewing your progress with your dietitian gives you the opportunity to update your goals—and your meal plan—as your needs change. How will you know if you're on the right track? Changes in your blood glucose levels, hemoglobin A_{1c} values, lipid levels, body weight, blood pressure, and simply how you feel show you how your treatment plan is working.

Find time to follow-up

Follow-up visits can contribute greatly to the continued success of your diabetes nutrition management. Ideally, a follow-up visit with the R.D. should be scheduled one to two weeks after your first visit. When Ted and his R.D. reviewed his food diary at the follow-up visit, he admitted to being surprised at how much food he had been eating. Restaurants, where Ted often has business lunches, tend to serve large portions, causing him to eat far more calories than he thought he was.

Once Ted had accomplished the goal of raising his awareness of his portion sizes, he and his R.D. replaced it with a new goal: When eating out, Ted would try to make his meals a little smaller by leaving some of the steak on his plate or taking home the leftover pasta to have for dinner that night. They also talked about choosing foods with less fat. For example, Ted could choose chicken or fish that had been broiled rather than fried, or pasta with tomato sauce rather than a cream sauce.

In the area of physical activity, Ted found that he had only been able to walk two days a week, primarily because he was too tired to exercise after a long day at work. He and his R.D. decided to try a different schedule: Ted would walk three days a week before work and both days on the weekend. He hopes this adjustment will make walking for exercise more compatible with his lifestyle.

The follow-up visit also gave Ted the opportunity to ask questions he'd thought of in the past two weeks. He brought in menus from his favorite business-dining restaurants so he and his dietitian could design strategies for ordering. And he asked the R.D. to help him learn about carbohydrates, so that he could avoid having high blood sugar after meals.

Learning about meal planning

To help people with diabetes control their blood glucose levels, dietitians have developed a number of meal-planning approaches. (The days when everyone with diabetes received a 1500-calorie exchange diet sheet are long gone!) But while any number of people might use the same approach, each person should have an individualized meal plan that takes into consideration his food preferences and the number of calories and nutrients he needs to maintain good health and blood sugar levels in his target range.

Since carbohydrate is the nutrient that affects blood glucose levels the most, one of the key steps in developing a meal plan is determining how much carbohydrate (how many servings or how many grams of carbohydrate) a person can eat at each meal or snack without causing blood sugar levels to go too high. Your dietitian can suggest ballpark amounts to start with, based on experience with other people who have diabetes as well as on your current eating habits. Fine-tuning your meal plan, however, requires checking your blood glucose 1½ to 2 hours after eating to see how your meal affected you. (This is one of the many reasons keeping a blood glucose log is important!)

Ted decided to start with a simple meal-planning approach called "The First Step in Diabetes Meal Planning," which is based on the Diabetes Food Guide Pyramid. The Pyramid divides foods into six categories and suggests how many servings of each to eat each day for good nutrition. The food groups and recommended number of daily servings are grains, beans, and starchy vegetables (6 or more servings), vegetables (3–5 servings), fruits (3–4 servings), milk (2–3 servings), meat and meat equivalents (2–3 servings), and fats, sweets, and alcohol (eat sparingly).

Ted's dietitian explained which foods contain carbohydrate (grains, beans, and starchy vegetables; fruits; vegetables; milk; and most sweets) and told him that spreading his servings of those foods over the day would help keep his blood glucose levels stable. Ted and his dietitian then decided on the number of servings of carbohydrate-containing foods he would eat at each meal. Because Ted does not consume milk products, his dietitian told him about other food sources of calcium. And Ted decided to aim for three servings of vegetables per day, which was considerably more than he had been eating. Ted agreed to check his blood glucose 1½ to 2 hours after meals for a week to see how his chosen amount of carbohydrate affected his blood glucose. Then he and his dietitian would discuss any changes that needed to be made.

"The First Step in Diabetes Meal Planning" is just one of many meal-planning approaches. Two other popular approaches are the "exchange" system and the "carbohydrate-counting" system. People who like structure often like to follow an exchange meal plan. Like the Diabetes Food Guide Pyramid, the exchange system also divides foods into categories (or lists), in this case, starches, fruit, milk, other carbohydrates, vegetables, meat and meat substitutes, and fats. A booklet called "Exchange Lists for Meal Planning" shows which foods belong to which category. A meal plan based on the exchange system specifies how many exchanges (or choices) from each list a person should eat at each meal or snack. A dietitian can help you determine how many exchanges from each list are right for you.

People who want more flexibility may prefer the carbohydrate-counting approach. Their meal plans generally specify only how much carbohydrate to eat at each meal, but not the source of carbohydrate nor the amount of protein or fat. To know how much carbohydrate is in a serving of food, a person must either read the Nutrition Facts label (on packaged food) or consult a reference guide that contains nutrition information. As with all meal plans, determining how much carbohydrate to eat at each meal and snack depends largely on your blood glucose readings following meals.

Knowledge is power

If your diabetes was diagnosed recently, the very thought of changing your lifelong eating habits isn't easy to digest. Meal planning may be one of the most challenging aspects of diabetes care, but consulting with a dietitian right from the start can be a great help, particularly since many people with Type 2 diabetes can successfully manage their diabetes through diet and exercise alone.

However, if you've had diabetes for some time and haven't talked with a dietitian recently, it's not too late! You can still benefit from a nutrition refresher, even if you've read and learned a lot on your own. Maybe you've unconsciously slipped into some "not-so-good" eating habits. A visit with a dietitian might be just what you need to get back on track. Nutrition and meal planning can improve blood glucose control and have positive effects on blood pressure and cholesterol. Just a few small changes in food choices can make a big difference. Since the nutrition recommendations for people with diabetes are constantly evolving, periodic "checkups" help guarantee that your nutrition plan is up-to-date. ❏

MIDNIGHT MUNCHING
HOW TO OVERCOME "WEREWOLF SYNDROME"
by William H. Polonsky, Ph.D., C.D.E.

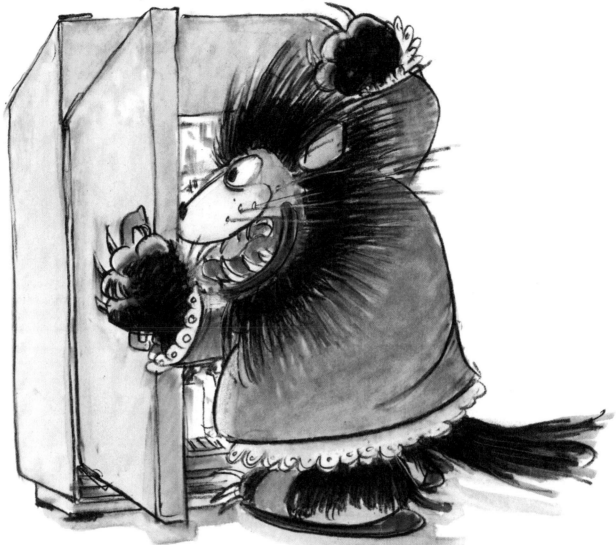

It always happens at night. After a good day of eating balanced meals, exercising, and testing, a low grumble awakens deep down inside. The kitchen beckons, tempting you with its treasures, and soon you find yourself transported there, seemingly against your will. Like the legendary werewolf, who sprouts hair, claws, and an uncontrollable urge to feast when the moon rises, people with werewolf syndrome lose control when the sun goes down. Their eyes grow large and their thoughts turn to food, food, and more food! Soon, they are on the prowl, and God help any goodies in their path.

Simply put, werewolf syndrome is a common form of problematic nighttime eating. It can lead to frus-

trating, uncontrollable behavior and anxious, guilty feelings. And if you have diabetes, in which case you have probably been encouraged to watch your weight and manage your eating carefully, you can see how werewolf eating can lead to a breakdown in diabetes control. Is all this beginning to sound a little familiar to you?

Let's meet Dana, a 43-year-old married woman with two young children and a successful career in advertising. She has been living with diabetes for the past two years and has worked hard to follow her health-care team's recommendations, but she is very frustrated with herself. Although she exercises regularly, tests her blood sugar level several times a day, and eats three small, nutritious meals each day, her blood sugar levels remains elevated. For example, her morning blood sugar level is typically over 200 mg/dl. Given these numbers, her doctor has told her that it may be time to begin insulin soon.

Dana knows that her problem kicks in during the evening hours. On a typical night, shortly after dinner, she starts to feel anxious and uncomfortable. As though drawn by a powerful magnet, she steals into the kitchen, where she nibbles at whatever little goodies she can find (usually pie, cake, and cookies). After her snack, she gets angry with herself and retreats to the living room. Throughout the evening, however, she returns to the kitchen again and again, consuming ever larger and larger amounts. And once this dance begins, she finds herself unable to stop it.

By the end of the evening, Dana is angry with herself and angry with her diabetes. And strangely, as delicious as she imagines that her cakes and cookies will taste, she doesn't really find them that satisfying anymore. By the next morning, she has committed herself to redoubling her willpower and never letting another nighttime eating episode occur. Still, she is as powerless as is the werewolf in the grip of a full moon. Despite her very best efforts, including a recent meal-planning session with a registered dietitian, her nighttime overeating episodes have been occurring more frequently.

Identifying a werewolf

Like Dana, all victims of werewolf syndrome share three common characteristics.

First, they tend to eat reasonably well during daylight hours. Unfortunately, they sometimes eat too well. In other words, they restrict their daytime eating so severely that that their meals are often too small, too unsatisfying, or too boring.

Second, people who have this problem tend to lose control during the evening hours. During their nighttime forays, they commonly eat large amounts of food, especially tasty "forbidden foods" that are certain to drive up blood sugar levels. They feel powerless to stop, even though they may not be hungry at all.

Overeating episodes are usually not organized snacks or meals. Rather, people often eat while standing in front of the refrigerator or at the kitchen counter. Or, like Dana, werewolf eaters may sneak in and out of the kitchen, pausing only for nibbles and returning again and again for little snacks that can add up to quite a bit. Remarkably, many werewolf eaters are never sure what they really want to eat; they wander from one food to the next, but nothing ever hits the spot.

Third, people with werewolf syndrome tend to drive themselves crazy in the process! Rather than enjoying this plunge into an eating frenzy, they end up tormenting themselves. Not only is their eating rarely pleasurable, they are also likely to be furious with themselves afterward and feel guilty or depressed about what they have done. Because of these feelings, they tend to feast alone. Unfortunately, no matter how much they punish themselves and no matter how strong their self-discipline may be, they are usually unable to prevent further bouts of werewolf eating.

When you are trying to manage a tough challenge like diabetes, living with werewolf syndrome is even more of a problem. Frequent nighttime eating can lead to significant weight gain as well as chronically elevated blood sugar levels. In either case, diabetes can become more and more difficult to control, so understanding the problem and taking action to solve it are essential. If you are a victim of werewolf syndrome, take heart; despite its sharp claws and scary appearance, the werewolf can be tamed.

What brings out the werewolf?

In contrast to the classic werewolf tales, werewolf eating is not really caused by magical spells, the bite of another werewolf, or the rising of the full moon. The real triggers are, unfortunately, a bit more mundane.

Stomach hunger. If your daytime meals are typically small, it's likely that you'll become hungry in the evening. Perhaps you've been on a diet and are eating as little as possible. Perhaps you're feeling so bad about *last* night's binge that you've decided to punish yourself and eat only popcorn today. Or maybe you're trying to follow a diabetes meal plan that is just too limited and restrictive for you. In any of these cases, your stomach growls at you louder and louder throughout the day. And by evening, even though your willpower may be incredibly strong, the biological urge to eat becomes irresistible. Unfortunately, when in a state of overwhelming hunger, you are unlikely to eat just a small amount. The mind and body overreact and become voracious. Thus, werewolf eating can actually be caused by dieting and other major food restrictions.

Eyeball hunger. What if you eat plenty of food during the day, but still feel hungry at night? Your stomach may be full, but your eyes, mouth, and brain may actually be starving for food. This can occur when you are not satisfied with your food choices at mealtimes.

Dana, for example, ate a sufficient amount of food during the day to ward off stomach hunger in the evening, and yet she couldn't control her eating at night. As it turned out, Dana's daytime meals were completely uninteresting to her. Being a perfectionist, she had strictly followed the food choices her dietitian had selected for her (to make sure that her carbohydrate intake was balanced during the day, to avoid

Nutrition and Meal Planning

weight gain, and to provide good nutrition), without considering her own personal tastes and desires. In the end, she treated her meals as if they were merely fuel for her machine. She admitted that nothing she ate hit the spot and that she felt she was eating "nothing but birdseed" all day. And so, not surprisingly, during the quiet and unstructured hours of the evening, a part of her brain would revolt and seek relief from this feeling of deprivation. Then she would search out the truly satisfying foods that she never allowed herself to eat during the day.

When your diabetes management plan or your weight-loss plan is too restrictive (in terms of food *types*, not just food *amounts*), you may be depriving yourself of the joys of eating: the sensory stimulation and satisfaction that your mind and body crave. Eventually, you may rebel and try to satisfy in one evening all those cravings you have so carefully repressed during the day.

Boredom. If your evenings just aren't very exciting, it's normal to look for ways to spice them up. Many people report that werewolf eating begins when they feel understimulated, dissatisfied, or lonely at night. They may be watching television, but they aren't really interested in what they are watching. They may wish they had someone to talk to or to do something with, but there is no one at hand. At times like these, even though they're not hungry at all, a trip to the kitchen may feel like the only pleasure or distraction available. In the end, however, most people discover that overeating rarely relieves boredom.

Unconscious eating. Many werewolf eaters have reported that they will innocently sit down to watch television with a box of cookies, crackers, or chips by their side. The next thing they know, the box of cookies is empty and there are crumbs all over their shirts. What happened? Did someone break into the house, knock them unconscious, eat all the cookies, and then sprinkle crumbs all over them? Well, probably not. Werewolf eating may occur when you are preoccupied with another activity that has become linked, by habit, to eating. Such activities commonly include reading, doing household chores, or watching television.

For example, one werewolf eater noted that, without ever thinking about it, he ate a quart of ice cream each night as he read the newspaper. The mere act of picking up the newspaper was an unconscious trigger to start eating. This was such an automatic behavior for him that he tended to ignore all the subtle but important body cues that might have prevented him from overeating. When he finally paid attention, he realized that he wasn't that hungry and that he really didn't like the taste of ice cream as much as he thought he did.

Anger and anxiety. Negative emotions are a common trigger for werewolf syndrome. If you're feeling angry, nervous, sad, frustrated, or lonely, you may try to comfort yourself through eating. For example, Dana was rarely aware of why she felt anxious in the evening, but reaching out for her favorite foods was a very familiar way for her to soothe herself.

For most of us, eating has been used as a strategy for emotional calming since childhood. In fact, we often regard certain familiar foods as "comfort foods" simply out of habit or because they evoke soothing feelings or memories. Unfortunately, eating is not a very effective means of stress management. No matter what we eat, the bad feelings don't recede for very long. And after a serious bout of werewolf eating, there is even more to feel bad about!

To make matters worse, once a werewolf eating episode has begun, it is almost impossible to stop. A common reaction is, "Well, I've blown it now, so I might as well just keep eating, and I'll start fresh tomorrow." With permission now granted, the floodgates for eating are opened. The werewolf may emerge night after night, in part because of people's typical responses to these episodes: To compensate for overeating the night before, many people will start the new day by restricting their eating even more severely. This can lead to more hunger and even stronger feelings of deprivation, which results in the reemergence of the werewolf that evening.

Seven steps to control

To defeat the werewolf, something greater than willpower is necessary. Take the case of Margaret, a 67-year-old widow who has had diabetes for 11 years. For the past decade, she had been struggling with obesity and chronically high blood sugar levels. As an example of her daily battle, Margaret reported that she placed a bowl of M&M's, her favorite food, on her coffee table each and every evening "just in case guests arrived." The truth was, however, she almost never had guests. Each evening, she would sit down to watch TV (with her bowl of candy always within arm's reach) and within a few hours, the bowl was empty. She berated herself for her lack of willpower. But Margaret did not really need more willpower. Instead, she needed to use common sense and think more clearly about what exactly was triggering her overeating. This way she could, with help, devise strategies for overcoming those problems. Here are seven of the most useful strategies.

1. Alternative nighttime activities. If you think that your nighttime overeating may be caused by boredom, it's time to find some other ways to enliven your evenings. During the hours when the werewolf starts to prowl, add some structure to your life by trying a new activity. For example, you might take a walk, call a friend, take a bath, or write that letter you've been meaning to write. It is especially important to pick an activity that is not passive (such as watching TV), not related to food, and that might even be fun. Actively doing something can help to interrupt your normal habits (such as eating a box of cookies while reading the newspaper), help to take you away from the temptations of your kitchen, and stimulate your mind and body. Many a werewolf has been halted in his tracks by such a strategy, so give it a try!

2. Make your environment work for you. Like Margaret, your most important strategy may be to alter your "eating geography." If you tend to eat unconsciously while reading or watching TV, consider ways to *physically* reduce those temptations. For instance, if you have a soft spot for candy, make it less accessible. Put sweets away in the cupboards, or don't buy them at all. If you tend to eat while watching TV, experiment with some alternative evening activities, such as reading, walking, knitting, or making phone calls.

3. Change your daytime eating. If your daytime eating is too restricted, leaving you hungry or dissatisfied by evening, consider adjusting your meal plan. This is best done in consultation with a dietitian. Together, you can experiment with ways to reduce feelings of stomach hunger, perhaps by increasing your intake of fruits and vegetables, which could raise the amount of food you eat without adding too many calories. You can also work to limit eyeball hunger, perhaps by incorporating small amounts of "forbidden foods" like chocolate into your daily meal plan. By evening, you will then feel more satisfied and less deprived.

4. Regular nighttime snacking. For some people, the more they try to avoid nighttime eating, the more insistent the werewolf becomes. If this sounds like you, the solution may be to incorporate a regular snack into your evening routine. In other words, if the werewolf continues to visit you each night, despite all of your best efforts, it may be necessary to make a compromise. Try this experiment for a week (one night won't be enough): Schedule an enjoyable, satisfying snack each night, at a time shortly before you might start overeating. To be on the safe side, you might want to talk to a dietitian about adjusting your other meals accordingly.

Dana tried this approach and chose to schedule a time for a small plate of cookies every night. By giving herself permission to enjoy such forbidden foods every evening, she found herself less hungry, more satisfied, and less anxious during the remainder of the evening. Thus, she was able to avoid her typical nightly binge of *many* cookies, pie, and cake.

5. Alternative strategies for resolving negative feelings. If your werewolf syndrome is typically triggered by negative emotions like anger, sadness, or anxiety, it is important to take time to identify those feelings and to explore the stresses that lie behind those emotions. This way, you are more likely to discover an effective way to resolve those feelings, rather than drowning them in food.

Dana was able to do this by talking about her feelings with a close friend. She realized that her evening anxiety would build each night, shortly after her husband sat down to watch TV. For the rest of the evening, he would completely ignore her, and she would start wondering where the love had gone in their marriage and whether their relationship would survive. Soon thereafter, she would begin her forays into the kitchen. Once Dana realized the source of her anxiety, she courageously chose to confront the situation. By talking to her husband about her feelings and needs (and by listening to his, as well), the quality of their evenings together improved dramatically, her feelings of anxiety were alleviated, and her werewolf syndrome was greatly eased.

6. Make use of your friends and family. Werewolf syndrome is usually a solitary and lonely experience. Overcoming this torturous habit is difficult, especially when it involves new actions like taking a walk, changing your eating patterns, or redesigning your eating geography. Consider how your friends and family can help you out. Maybe you would be more willing to take a nighttime stroll if you had some company. Perhaps it would be easier to reduce your TV snacking if your spouse agreed to cut back as well. Or maybe if you didn't feel obligated to keep the house stocked with cookies for the kids, you'd have an easier time dodging them yourself. Take a risk and ask your loved ones for specific help and support. Remember, most of the actions you would like them to share with you will be good for *their* health as well.

7. Increasing your eating awareness. While this idea may seem odd, learning how to heighten your enjoyment of food can be a powerful way to weaken the werewolf within. Because werewolf eating is often so rapid, unconscious, and full of anxiety, victims rarely have a deep awareness of what they are eating. For example, when she was watching TV, Margaret could munch through several bowls of M&M's without even realizing it. The reason was that her attention was usually focused on the television, not on her candy consumption. When she began to limit her indulgences to times when the television was off, and then focused her full attention on eating her candies, she found that she enjoyed them much more. However, she also found—to her great surprise—that she became full after only a few handfuls. In other words, by paying close attention to what she was eating, she began to notice and respond to the subtle cues of satiety.

Try this experiment on your own. Bring your favorite werewolf food to a quiet, restful place. (On your first go, you might fare better if you don't do this in the evening.) Sit down and make sure there are no other distractions. Focus all of your attention on the sensory experience of what you are eating. You might even want to close your eyes with each bite. You don't have to try to enjoy it or hate it; just taste it as deeply and fully as you can.

Try this "eating awareness" exercise for at least 10 minutes, five days in a row, and see what happens. It may sound odd to recommend eating a food like candy or cookies that can raise your blood sugar. However, as a victim of werewolf syndrome, you are likely to eat these foods anyway (and we know that trying to use willpower to deprive yourself of these foods usually doesn't work). Why not experiment with eating these goodies in a healthier, more controlled manner? To be safe, consider talking to your health-care provider about adjusting your medicines and meals accordingly.

Defeating the werewolf

By following these seven strategies, Dana was able to conquer her werewolf eating. Most important, she adjusted her food choices and meal plan so that her meals were more personally enjoyable (while still quite nutritious), she incorporated a tasty snack into her evenings, and she resolved her nighttime feelings of anxiety by confronting her husband about her frustrations. As her nighttime overeating ceased, her blood sugar dropped to near-normal levels, her anger with her diabetes disappeared, and her mood improved significantly.

Margaret, too, was successful. She was able to remove her M&M's from the coffee table, practiced the "eating awareness" exercise with all of her most tempting foods, and asked a neighbor to start an evening walking program with her. With a significant reduction in her nighttime overeating, her blood sugar level and weight began to drop slowly, and her energy level and mood began to climb.

While battling werewolf syndrome is not easy, it can be done. By recognizing and understanding your situation, carefully considering your triggers to overeating, refusing to blame yourself any longer, and taking thoughtful action, you can successfully begin this process of change. ❏

THE LOWDOWN ON LOW-CARB DIETS

by Patti Bazel Geil, M.S., R.D., L.D., C.D.E.

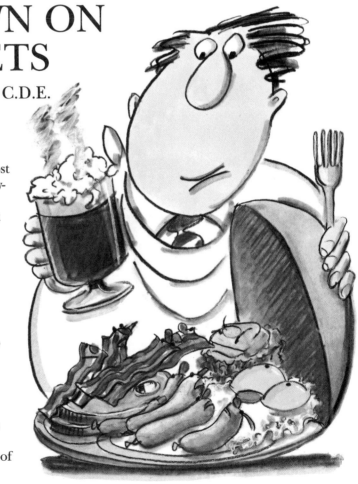

Counting carbohydrate grams has replaced counting fat grams as Americans' newest nutrition obsession. Almost everyone knows someone who is following a high-protein, low-carbohydrate diet in an attempt to lose weight. Anecdotes abound about overweight people eating bacon and eggs for breakfast, double cheeseburgers for lunch, and steak and lobster platters for dinner—all while watching the pounds melt away.

The low-carb diet craze has been responsible for several best-selling books, in addition to numerous Web sites and TV infomercials. *Sugar Busters, Protein Power, The Zone,* and *Dr. Atkins' New Diet Revolution* generated great debate among nutrition professionals. A few low-carb books, including *Dr. Bernstein's Diabetes Solution* and *The Insulin Control Diet: Your Fat Can Make You Thin,* have been promoted to people with diabetes as a way of achieving normal blood glucose levels.

If you have diabetes, you are no doubt aware of the importance of healthy eating and well-

WHAT'S FOR BREAKFAST?

Here's how three different diet plans set the table for breakfast, the "most important meal of the day." (These menus are only samples.)

AMERICAN DIABETES ASSOCIATION/
AMERICAN DIETETIC ASSOCIATION
½ small banana
1 slice toast
1 teaspoon margarine
1 egg
4 ounces skim milk
Coffee

TOTAL: 14 grams protein, 10 grams fat, 29 grams carbohydrate, 275 calories

DR. BERNSTEIN'S DIABETES SOLUTION
2 hard-cooked eggs
3 meatless sausage breakfast links
1 tablespoon cream
Coffee

TOTAL: 26 grams protein, 16 grams fat, 5 grams carbohydrate, 271 calories

DR. ATKINS' NEW DIET REVOLUTION
2-egg western omelet
3 ounces V-8 juice
½ slice bran crispbread
1 tablespoon cream
Coffee

TOTAL: 14 grams protein, 16 grams fat, 8 grams carbohydrate, 243 calories

controlled blood glucose levels, as well as the importance of maintaining a reasonable body weight. Is turning the food pyramid upside down by eating less carbohydrate and more protein and fat beneficial if you have diabetes?

If you are interested in improving your eating habits and health, congratulations! But before you leap onto the low-carb diet bandwagon, you owe it to yourself to take a careful look at the pros and cons of this way of eating.

Promises, promises...

Carbohydrate, protein, and fat are the three basic sources of calories, or energy, in foods. Carbohydrates (commonly known as sugars and starches) are our body's main source of energy. The carbohydrate content of a food—almost all of which is broken down into glucose—is what affects blood glucose levels the most. Protein has much less of an effect on blood glucose levels. (Research is ongoing to determine exactly how much of an effect it has.) And fat (from foods such as bacon, nuts, and mayonnaise) slows the digestion process, so eating a high-fat meal raises the blood sugar slowly.

When glucose from food enters the bloodstream, the pancreas releases insulin, a hormone that helps the cells in our body use the glucose as a source of energy. Insulin also helps the body store extra calories as fat.

The most popular low-carb diets promise rapid weight loss without limiting calories from protein and fat. The basic premise behind their claims is that carbohydrates are harmful because they increase insulin levels. And excess insulin, they claim, causes weight gain, elevated blood lipids, high blood pressure, increased appetite, and mood changes, as well as diabetes. In fact, high insulin levels and insulin resistance (a condition in which the body produces plenty of insulin but the cells can't use it properly) are fingered as the culprits that make Americans the heaviest people on earth. Many diet promoters also claim that "fat doesn't make you fat." In their meal plans, therefore, pasta, breads, cereals, fruits, and vegetables are severely limited and are replaced by high-fat foods such as sausage, cream, and butter. (See "What's for Breakfast?" on this page.)

Enjoying your favorite high-fat foods without a side dish of guilt sounds wonderful, but the truth is that there is very little science to support the low-carb diet approach. It is technically true that fat does not make you fat, but insulin does not make you fat either. The *calories* in fat—and in any other type of food—are what cause people to put on pounds. The simplistic approach touted by low-carb diet proponents ignores the fact that Americans are eating more total calories (100 to 300 extra per day) and exercising less than ever before, leading to weight gain.

People who have insulin resistance do tend to have large quantities of insulin in their blood, but it is not simply a result of eating a high percentage of calories as carbohydrate, nor is there evidence that insulin resistance causes obesity. In fact, research indicates that the opposite is true: Obesity causes insulin resistance.

Insulin resistance is cause for concern. (To read more about it, see the article "Insulin Resistance" on page 25.) People who have high insulin levels (with or without diabetes) and who also have obesity, high triglycerides, low HDL ("good") cholesterol, and high blood pressure may have "Syndrome X," which raises the risk of heart disease. Weight loss, physical activity, and a lower-carbohydrate diet, which substitutes unsaturated fat (nuts, peanut butter, margarine, mayonnaise, and olive oil) for some carbohydrate may prove helpful in this case. But for people who don't have Syndrome X and are concerned about their weight, calorie control is more important than carbohydrate control.

The untold story behind the weight loss

A low-carbohydrate diet can lead to an immediate weight loss, but because of the makeup of the diet, it is difficult to keep the pounds off and promote good health over the long term. When a person severely restricts carbohydrate intake, the body immediately turns to stored glucose (called *glycogen*) for energy. The glycogen has water attached to it that is released when it is used. Much of the quick weight loss on a low-carb diet is caused by the loss of water as the body uses its glycogen stores.

If a carbohydrate deficit continues, the body begins to break down lean body mass (muscle protein) in an effort to provide glucose to crucial organs. The waste products from this breakdown of protein are processed by the kidneys and flushed from the body along with large amounts of water. The initial exciting weight loss that has people singing the praises of low-carb diets is mainly an unhealthy loss of muscle tissue and water. When carbohydrate is included in the diet again, the water will reaccumulate, and the scales will reflect this as pounds regained.

Although low-carb diet promoters tout a particular combination of fat, protein, and carbohydrate as the reason that pounds disappear, it's a fact that people lose weight on these diets because they are eating fewer calories than they usually do. An analysis of a day's sample menu from four popular low-carb diet books reveals that they range from 1,000 calories to 1,400 calories daily initially, with long-term maintenance menus providing no more than 1,800 calories per day. This is well below the number of calories overweight Americans eat on a daily basis. The calorie restriction alone will promote weight loss in most people.

Low calorie intake will inevitably lead to a loss of body fat if a negative calorie balance is maintained—that is, if you consistently burn more calories than you take in. When you haven't eaten enough carbohydrate to supply your body with energy, the body begins to break down fat instead, to slow the loss of muscle protein or lean body mass. When this fat breakdown occurs, by-products called *ketones* appear in the blood. Having an abnormal amount of ketones is called ketosis. One of the most rigid low-carb diets promotes ketosis as "the dieter's best friend" and encourages daily ketone testing to assure that the dieter stay in the ketotic state. People with diabetes, however, should be aware that if ketones form faster than their body can get rid of them in the urine, they build up in the

POTENTIAL SIDE EFFECTS

The potential physical consequences of low-carbohydrate diets range from mild to serious to life-threatening. Here is a list of short-term and long-term side effects.

Constipation
Dehydration
Dizziness
Fainting
Fatigue
Gout
Increased risk of heart disease
Increased risk of some cancers
Increased workload on kidneys
Keto-breath
Kidney stones
Low blood pressure
Nausea
Short-term weight loss
Vitamin and mineral deficiencies, including osteoporosis

blood, making it acidic. This is a potentially life-threatening situation. In addition, further water loss occurs as the kidneys work harder to remove the ketones from the body.

Sizing up the side effects

Side effects from low-carb diets range from unpleasant to downright dangerous. (See "Potential Side Effects" on this page.) Low-carb dieters who are in ketosis often have "keto-breath," which is described as smelling like a cross between nail polish and overripe pineapple. Constipation can occur when fruits, vegetables, and grains are eliminated from the diet during severe carbohydrate restriction. Fatigue and nausea are associated with the ketotic state. Dehydration and low blood pressure result from water loss; people on a low-carb diet may complain of dizziness or even fainting after standing up quickly. Kidney stones and gout are more likely to occur on a high-protein, ketosis-inducing diet than on a higher-carbohydrate diet with more fruits and vegetables. Vitamin and mineral deficiencies, including calcium depletion and osteoporosis, are far more likely when entire food groups are eliminated from a meal plan.

Even more serious are the long-term effects of the low-carb way of eating. High protein intake places an

TOO GOOD
TO BE TRUE?

Although we all sometimes hope for a quick and easy solution to our problems, as often as not, that miracle cure just doesn't exist. Be wary of any offer that promises too much too soon. Here are some guidelines for what to watch out for. Be skeptical of diets that:

■ Claim to be quick, painless and effortless
■ Claim to have special, secret, foreign, ancient, or natural ingredients
■ Claim to be effective for a wide variety of conditions
■ Rely on personal success stories rather than scientific data for documentation
■ Claim that the medical community or government agencies refuse to acknowledge their effectiveness

increased workload on the kidneys. This should be of concern to people with diabetes, who are at increased risk of kidney disease. If you already have damage to your kidneys, the low-carb diet is not for you. The risk of many cancers is likely to be increased when most fruits, vegetables, whole grains, and beans are eliminated from the diet. Risk of heart disease is higher on a low-carb, low-fiber diet that is high in animal protein, cholesterol, and saturated fat. These three components raise serum cholesterol, particularly the LDL or "bad" cholesterol. Because people with diabetes are already two to four more times likely to get heart disease, this is not a risk to be taken lightly.

Finally, weight control by carbohydrate restriction alone isn't likely to work over the long term. Short-term loss of water weight appears to be a dieter's dream and is the basis of many word-of-mouth success stories surrounding low-carb diets. However, permanent weight control is still a matter of calorie balance: To lose weight, you need to take in fewer calories than you burn. There is no scientifically proven "metabolic magic" in a lifestyle that eliminates entire food groups. If you have diabetes, your focus should be on controlling blood glucose levels, engaging in regular physical activity, taking medicine as needed, and following a healthy eating plan for life.

Will cutting carbs control diabetes?

Controlling blood glucose by controlling carbohydrate intake is an approach that has been used since the discovery of insulin. In 1922, Leonard Thompson became the first person with diabetes to receive insulin. He was also prescribed a diet that was 10% protein, 70% fat, and 20% carbohydrate. The scientific rationale at that time was that curtailing carbohydrate would keep blood glucose in control. (Thompson reportedly followed this diet for 13 years before dying of bronchial pneumonia.)

This is quite a contrast to the current, mainstream diabetes diet recommendations of approximately 10%–20% protein, with the remainder of calories to be divided between carbohydrate and fat, depending on eating habits and blood glucose and blood lipid goals. The effect carbohydrate has on an individual's blood sugar depends on many factors, including the amount of carbohydrate eaten at a meal, the way in which the food is prepared, how quickly the carbohydrate breaks down into glucose in the bloodstream, and the combination of protein, fat, carbohydrate, and calories eaten at a particular sitting.

The American Diabetes Association Nutrition Recommendations stress that it's the total amount of carbohydrate you eat, rather than the source of carbohydrate, that is most important. Your blood sugar will be affected similarly whether you eat 45 grams of carbohydrate from cookies or 45 grams of carbohydrate from a baked potato. The carbohydrate counting meal-planning approach advises people with Type 1 diabetes to match their insulin dose to the amount of carbohydrate they plan to eat. For people with Type 2 diabetes, consistent carbohydrate intake to keep blood glucose in the target range is advocated. (To learn more about carbohydrate counting, call The American Dietetic Association, (800) 877-1600, extension 5000, to order a set of three booklets on the subject; the Association's Web site, www.eatright.com, is also helpful.)

There are still those whose approach to diabetes control is extreme carbohydrate limitation, as outlined in *Dr. Bernstein's Diabetes Solution*. Dr. Bernstein's plan limits carbohydrate to 30 grams daily (the amount found in two slices of bread), which is divided into 6 grams at breakfast, 12 grams at lunch, and 12 grams at supper. He advocates eating very small amounts of "slow-acting" carbohydrate plus 3 ounces or more of protein at each meal. His book gives no specific restrictions for the amount of fat. He also recommends multiple daily injections of small amounts of insulin for Type 1 diabetes and weight loss, exercise, and medication as needed for Type 2 diabetes. The goal is blood glucose levels within the normal range of 85 mg/dl to 90 mg/dl.

Dr. Bernstein's approach requires meticulous attention to detail and doing without foods on his list of "No-No's in a Nutshell," which includes all fruits, many vegetables, milk, and most grains and grain products. Potential pitfalls of this approach include vitamin and mineral deficiencies, as well as constipation from lack of fiber. In addition, it can lead to the development of a very real sense of deprivation from eliminating entire food groups.

Carbohydrate clashes: Coming to conclusions

The debate over the effects of low-carb diets will no doubt continue, as long as there are best-selling diet books on the market. People with diabetes should be especially alert for results from scientific studies on carbohydrate that are published in peer-reviewed journals. Nutrition is such an important part of diabetes care that you must be able to distinguish trustworthy information from book-promoting publicity, which should be viewed with a skeptical eye. (See "Too Good to Be True?" on the opposite page.)

Just as there is no single medicine that works perfectly for all people with diabetes, there is no single dietary approach that fits all. The effect of carbohydrate on weight loss and diabetes is obviously an area that requires much more research. Until more evidence accumulates, it is best to continue with a balanced meal plan, limited in fat and saturated fat, that contains enough carbohydrate to provide energy but not so much that it disrupts blood sugar control.

If you have insulin resistance, you may do well on an eating plan that substitutes unsaturated fats for some carbohydrates. Your health-care team should always evaluate your individual condition before you decide on the nutrition approach for you. The bottom line isn't which diet plan allows you the most omelets for breakfast, but rather which healthy eating approach gives you the best control of your blood glucose while protecting your long-term health and letting you enjoy your food! ❑

NUTRITION RESEARCH
WHY IT CHANGES AND HOW TO UNDERSTAND IT
by Belinda O'Connell, M.S., R.D., L.D.

It's a typical morning all across America. Thousands of health-conscious people get up and eat a nutritious, high-fiber breakfast (skipping the eggs, bacon, and butter). Then they open the morning paper to read that according to the latest study, fiber may not prevent colon cancer after all. Or maybe eggs aren't as bad as health experts thought. Or it's now believed that salt affects the blood pressure of only a select few, not everybody, as was previously declared. You see it in the news all the time: another nutrition "flip-flop." On Monday, margarine is good for you; on Tuesday, it's not. Researchers in California say eat more fiber to prevent cancer; researchers in Boston say fiber isn't protective after all. For people trying to eat a healthy diet, it can be pretty frustrating. Who do you believe? Why all the conflicting information? And how is a person supposed to know what to eat?

Research results can and should vary

As frustrating as it may be, results of research studies can and should vary. The scientific method is based on disproving your assumption or hypothesis. Good scientists start out with a theory or idea that they want to test. For example, they may start with the theory that dietary fiber prevents colon cancer or that eggs increase cholesterol levels. Then they design a study to try to disprove that theory.

If a hypothesis withstands rigorous tests, we assume it is true—until the next study comes along with new information or better tests, perhaps supporting the earlier research, but just as likely contradicting it. Contradictory results show that scientists are doing their job—testing new theories rigorously, under new and varied conditions, and building on the information obtained from earlier studies.

This is especially true for health and nutrition questions. Health questions are very complex and difficult to answer because many different factors influence the occurrence of disease, and each study can only look at one small part of that relationship. Scientists look at each individual study as part of a bigger picture, one of many pieces of information that together answer a question such as, "Do eggs increase cholesterol levels?" No one study is seen as a definitive answer.

The story about the three scientists and the elephant illustrates this point. Three scientists are blindfolded and put in a room with an elephant. Each is allowed to examine the elephant and then is asked to describe what an elephant looks like. The first scientist, who started at the trunk, says, "Oh, I know exactly what an elephant looks like. It is a long, skinny, muscular animal with no bones. It is very flexible and can wriggle and slide around quite freely." The second scientist, who was placed by the elephant's foot, says, "Oh, no, you are quite mistaken. An elephant has bones, huge bones, and is not at all flexible. My measurements show that an elephant is very heavy and hardly moves at all." The third scientist, who was placed behind the elephant at its tail, says, "You are both wrong. Elephants are very skinny and wave around high in the air. They move quite quickly and have a furry patch on one end."

Different types of studies ask different questions and therefore often give slightly different answers. Because of this, many separate studies are needed to answer a single question. Scientists expect that each study will have some results that support previous research and some results that are contradictory or totally new and will, over time, help us to build a better picture of what the truth is. There are also times when scientists simply differ on the best way to interpret a study's results. Much like analyzing art or the nuances of language, the task of analyzing information from a study is somewhat subjective: There is often more than one way to look at study results.

As readers of health information, we need to learn to accept that there will be a certain amount of variability in "cutting edge," or new, health research. It's just that: new and generally still a little unclear. Fact-finding is a process that takes time. It's much like getting to know a person: When you first meet, you have a set of initial impressions. After you have had many contacts, under different conditions and in different settings, you have greater knowledge and understanding of the person, and your feelings about the individual may change considerably over time.

Unfortunately, the media often fail to present a research study as part of a larger picture. Often when they publish results of a new study, they make it seem as though scientists are constantly contradicting each other. To better interpret what you read or hear in the news, it helps to understand the different types of research and what they can and can't prove.

Epidemiological studies

There are two main types of health studies: epidemiological studies and experimental studies. The studies you most often see reported in the news with splashy headlines are epidemiological studies. This type of study looks at the distribution of disease in a population and attempts to identify factors that are associated with that disease. Epidemiological studies are used to identify potential protective factors and potential risk factors for disease. For example, a study might find that dietary fiber appears to protect against getting Type 2 diabetes; another might find that increased body weight appears to be a risk factor for developing Type 2 diabetes. However, this type of study can only suggest relationships; it cannot prove cause and effect.

Epidemiological studies measure associations or relationships between factors. But the fact that two things often occur together does not necessarily mean that one causes the other. (For example, Christmas always occurs in December, but December does not cause Christmas.) This type of research is helpful in identifying factors that potentially influence disease. Scientists can then conduct other kinds of studies to determine whether the identified factors really do have any effect. Many of these initial associations turn out to be mere coincidence.

Ecological studies. There are several types of epidemiological studies. One, the ecological study, looks at the incidence of disease in large groups of people and does not collect specific information on individuals. This type of study looks at general trends in a country overall. Because of this, ecological studies are more likely than other types of studies to have spurious results not supported by later research. But this type of study is often used as a starting point for identifying an interesting question that researchers can then explore further using other styles of research.

For example, an ecological study looking at eating patterns in different countries found a correlation between early cow's milk consumption (before three months of age) and the incidence of Type 1 diabetes. In this study, the United States and the Scandinavian countries had the highest intake of cow's milk products and the greatest incidence of Type 1 diabetes. Incidence of diabetes was found to be lower in countries such as Japan and Korea, where infants are breast-fed and cow's milk consumption is much lower.

Intriguing as this observation is, it does not come close to proving that cow's milk can cause Type 1 diabetes. There are many factors that differ between these two population groups, including genetics, average weight, and other dietary and cultural factors that are likely to have a greater influence on the incidence of diabetes. But it does raise an interesting question that researchers are currently exploring further. (At this time, the American Academy of Pediatrics encourages breast-feeding if possible and using only breast milk or formula for the first year of life to delay the introduction of regular cow's milk for health reasons *unrelated* to diabetes.)

Retrospective studies. Another type of epidemiological study is the retrospective study, in which a questionnaire is generally used to collect information about the diet and health of individuals. Retrospective studies sort out specific protective and disease-causing factors better than ecological studies do.

As the name implies, retrospective studies look into the past. Researchers contact people who have a disease, such as cancer, and ask them questions about what they ate or what their health habits were before they had cancer. The researchers also pose the same questions to a group of people who are similar but who do not have cancer. They then compare the information from the two groups to see if there are any differences. They may find, for example, that the people who developed cancer had a much lower intake of fruits and vegetables than the people who did not develop cancer.

Retrospective studies are generally the first step a researcher takes to investigate a relationship between diet and disease. They are quicker and less expensive than many other types of research, because it's relatively easy to target those people who have the disease of interest. Unfortunately, this type of research has some serious limitations, including recall bias, accuracy in measuring diet, confounders, and appropriateness of the control group. Let's take a look at each of these limitations.

Sometimes, when you know that you have a disease, it may affect the way you remember or answer questions about your diet in the past. This is called *recall bias.* People who have a disease such as cancer who believe that diet plays a role in cancer development or who have heard reports in the news about diet and cancer may assume that they had less of a potentially protective nutrient such as fiber or more of a potential risk factor such as fat. Or they may feel uncomfortable reporting their true dietary intakes because they believe they "caused" their cancer by eating in a particular way.

Even if recall bias weren't a problem, there are other reasons it can be difficult to accurately measure what a person ate in the past. Dietary questionnaires typically ask questions such as, "How often in the past month did you eat orange squash, carrots, and sweet potatoes?" or "How many cola beverages did you drink per month as an adolescent?" It is to be expected when you are asking people to remember how often and how much they ate of specific foods up to 20 or 30 years ago that there will be a certain amount of inaccuracy in what they recall. Most of us have trouble remembering what we had for dinner two nights ago—forget about 20 years ago.

Confounding refers to hidden variables that can confuse results. For instance, a study may find that high-fat diets are a risk factor for heart disease, but other factors that are commonly associated with a high-fat diet—such as a low intake of fruits and vegetables or a high intake of meat—may actually be responsible for the effect, not fat. Or a study may find that a vegetarian diet protects against heart disease, but vegetarians may exercise more or smoke less than nonvegetarians.

Confounders are important to consider and adjust for in nutrition research, because people who tend to have healthier diets often have healthier lifestyles. But in many cases, researchers do not know all the factors they may have to adjust for, and that can lead to differences in results.

Selection of the comparison or control group for a study is important because that is the group you are using to determine what is "normal." A control group should be randomly selected and unbiased so that it accurately represents the population in general. That way, the study's results can be applied to everyone.

But this can be difficult to do. A study may be biased because people who have time to participate in a study may be different (older, younger, less apt to be employed) than the general population. Or a study may be biased toward a higher income and education level if the questionnaire requires a great deal of reading. It may be biased toward one sex (for example, if phone numbers are picked from the phone book at random and called during the day, more women may be home at that time), or toward one ethnic group (a study conducted in rural Minnesota would have primarily Caucasian subjects).

Prospective studies. Prospective, or forward-looking, studies use methods of collecting information that are similar to those used in retrospective studies. The difference is that they collect information over an extended period of time, starting in the present.

Prospective studies select a large group (called a *cohort*) of healthy people to study and use questionnaires to collect information on their current diet and health. The cohort is then followed over time, with additional information collected at regular intervals. As people in the cohort develop diseases, researchers can look back at the information that was collected to see if there are differences in diet, exercise, etc., in those who got sick, compared to those who did not.

A drawback of prospective studies is that it can take many, many years for a disease such as cancer to develop. This can make it very expensive and logistically difficult to continue a study long enough to get meaningful results. But because this type of study collects information as it goes, it is less likely to be affected by recall bias and memory issues. The data collected tend to be more accurate than that obtained from retrospective studies. But there are still plenty of difficulties with accurately measuring diet and nutrient intakes. These difficulties are discussed later in the article.

Epidemiological research is more likely than other types of research to provide contradictory results because it is conducted in the "real world," not under controlled or laboratory conditions. Because of this and the other issues discussed, epidemiological studies are best at picking up strong associations, such as the association between smoking and lung cancer, rather than more subtle associations. The degree to which a study can identify when two factors are associated is referred to as *sensitivity*.

When two factors are strongly associated with one another, different studies are more likely to get similar results, making it easier to make definitive conclusions. But even if every epidemiological study conducted clearly showed that two factors, such as dietary fat and heart disease, are associated with one another, it would still not prove that dietary fat causes heart disease. Epidemiological studies cannot prove cause and effect.

Experimental studies

To prove that one factor (such as dietary fat) causes another (such as heart disease), you need to specifically test that hypothesis under experimental conditions. Many theories are initially tested in animals or in simulated environments such as a cell culture or a test tube. Researchers may feed mice a high-fat diet and then look to see if they develop heart blockages. These types of experiments are helpful in determining if an association discovered in an epidemiological trial has a possibility of acting as believed in people (plausibility) and in determining how two factors may interact (mechanism of action).

But animal models, even the best, are just that: models. Finding that a factor is protective or causes disease in an animal proves nothing for humans, because animals have different metabolism, anatomy, and life spans. Animals are also commonly given much higher doses of an experimental compound than would be given to humans, which can lead to differing results. Animal studies are useful for identifying factors that are likely to be important, disease-causing agents in humans, so that experiments conducted with human subjects can be safely planned. But in the end, only studies conducted with humans, called *clinical trials,* can actually prove something about disease in people.

Clinical trials are also called *intervention trials,* because one "intervention" (change) is made in the normal environment, and the effect of this change is then monitored. Clinical trials are used to show a cause-and-effect relationship between two factors. It has been said that clinical trials are the only way to go from questions and hypotheses to answers.

The gold standard for clinical trials is the randomized, double-blind clinical trial. In this type of study, one group receives a treatment (the experimental or intervention group), and a second group receives no treatment (the control group). In the best-designed studies, all participants are similar and are assigned on a random basis to either the experimental group or the control group. (This ensures that any confounding factors, which may skew the results of the study, are evenly distributed between the two groups and are therefore less likely to cause problems.) The experimental group is given the active treatment, and the control group is given a placebo or "dummy treatment."

Ideally, neither the researchers nor the subjects know who is receiving the active treatment until after the study is completed. This is called *blinding.* Blinding is important because it ensures that the beliefs of the researchers and the subjects do not influence the collection of data. For instance, if people knew they were getting a dietary supplement that might improve their energy level, they might perceive and report that they feel better, have more energy, or need less sleep. Or a scientist who is testing whether a pill helps with weight loss might unintentionally measure hip and waist circumferences differently on the subjects getting the experimental pill.

Blinding is an important way to help maintain objectivity in a study. Unfortunately, it is difficult or impossible to do for many nutrition studies. People know if they are following a low-fat diet or eating 10 high-fiber oat bran muffins a day—you can't conceal it!

Clinical trials avoid many of the pitfalls of epidemiological research. There are no problems of recall bias due to memory inaccuracies. There are fewer problems related to diet measurement, because researchers are providing an exact amount of the test substance. And there are fewer problems due to confounding if subjects are randomly assigned to control and experimental groups.

Clinical trials provide clearer results when they have the expected, beneficial (or positive) effect. For instance, if a study found that subjects with diabetes who followed a regular exercise routine had significantly lower blood glucose levels than a control group of subjects, who had the same diet and the same average weight but did not exercise, it could be reasonably assumed that the exercise caused the improvement.

Like all research studies, however, clinical trials have their own, unique problems. For one, they are expensive and often cannot be conducted for long enough periods, and with enough people, to measure certain diseases like cancer that take a long time to develop. Clinical trials can also only be used to answer certain types of questions, because scientists cannot ethically conduct experiments that could harm study subjects. For this reason, few nutrition studies are conducted in children, because the removal or addition of a nutrient could affect a child's growth and development. In addition, clinical trials can only look at common diseases, because it is difficult to find enough subjects with unusual diseases, and it would take too long for enough people to come down with an unusual disease in a long-term trial.

Clinical trials have some other limitations. To ensure that there are few differences between the control and experimental groups that might bias the research study, clinical trials often set up narrow selection criteria for study subjects. For instance, a study looking at the effects of following a low-fat diet on heart disease rates may enroll only older Caucasian men. But while this may make the study results clearer in some respects, it also makes it more difficult to say whether the results can be applied to other groups, such as women, younger men, or men of different ethnicities.

It is difficult to interpret results from a clinical trial when no association is found or when the results are not what the researchers had expected. Any number of things can cause such "negative" results: Researchers could have used a dose that was too high or too low to cause an effect or included subjects who

RED FLAGS OF JUNK SCIENCE

Most people realize that some studies are better than others, but it can be hard to know which is which. The following "red flags" should raise your suspicions that what you're reading is bad science:

■ Recommendations that promise a quick fix

■ Dire warnings of danger from a single product or regimen

■ Claims that sound too good to be true

■ Simplistic conclusions drawn from a complex study

■ Recommendations based on a single study

■ Dramatic statements that are refuted by reputable scientific organizations

■ Lists of "good" and "bad" foods

■ Recommendations made to help sell a product

■ Recommendations based on studies published without peer review

■ Recommendations from studies that ignore differences among individuals or groups

The Red Flags were compiled by FANSA, the Food and Nutrition Science Alliance, a coalition of four professional organizations—The American Dietetic Association, the American Society of Nutritional Sciences, the American Society of Clinical Nutrition, and the Institute of Food Technologists.

were unable to respond to the intervention. They might have conducted the study for too short a time to see an effect, enrolled too few people to measure an effect, or simply tested the wrong thing. Nutrition studies are more likely than many studies to run into these and other problems.

Problems unique to nutrition studies

The field of nutrition is notorious for having contradictory studies. We had the oat bran craze, we were told that margarine would prevent heart disease, and at one time, it seemed that beta-carotene could protect us from almost anything. Why does nutrition research seem so prone to mistakes? Why so many about-faces and upsets?

Well, first of all, there aren't as many true nutrition flip-flops as the media would have you think. Headlines change much more often than experts' recommendations do. But good nutrition studies are difficult to conduct, and even the best are likely to run into some problems due to the nature of the questions asked.

Problems with measuring diets

All methods for collecting information about the way people eat have weaknesses. Nutrition studies often rely heavily on questionnaires that ask people to accurately remember very small details about their typical diet. This is very difficult to do. Can you remember if you salted the green beans you ate for dinner last Tuesday? Can you accurately estimate the amount of peanut butter you spread on your toast this morning? Was it 1 teaspoon or 1 tablespoon? Do you know if the restaurant you ate at used vegetable oil or lard to fry your fish? Do you know if your spouse used canned vegetables at dinner? Were they regular or low-sodium? And were they green beans, wax beans, or actually peas? Or harder yet, how often did you eat citrus fruit or drink citrus juices in the past month? How about the past 20 years?

There is a lot of room for inaccuracies to creep into the data, even when people are doing their best to ask good questions or answer questions honestly. And we all know that some questions about what we eat are embarrassing to answer honestly. Who wants to reveal they ate the whole carton—yes, a half-gallon carton—of ice cream? It is well known among researchers that people inaccurately recall portions of the foods they eat and that underreporting is especially common among people who are trying to lose weight or are on a diet. In addition, the databases used to calculate the nutrient content of a diet from the actual foods eaten are of variable accuracy and quality. For some nutrients, such as fiber, phytochemicals (protective compounds found in plants such as lycopene and beta-carotene), and trace minerals, this can affect study results.

Problems such as these can lead to what we call *misclassification errors*. Many epidemiological nutrition studies group subjects according to their level of nutrient intake and then compare disease rates in people with "high" nutrient levels with those in people with "low" nutrient levels. The cutoff points between high and low levels are set arbitrarily, and they are different for every study. Because of this, different researchers may come to slightly different conclusions about the healthfulness of a nutrient. In addition, difficulties in accurately measuring diets can mean that some study subjects are placed into the wrong group of nutrient intake (high when they are really low, or low when they are really high). This type of misclassification error can confuse results, making it look as though a nutrient has a smaller effect on

disease than it actually has, or no effect when it really has some effect. This can contribute to variable results and differences between two research studies.

One way around these problems is to have study subjects eat a certain diet or provide them with the food they eat during the study. But this is expensive and means that a study needs to be fairly short-term, limiting the types of questions the study can answer. Some of the most important questions—such as "Does diet impact cancer or heart disease?"—take a long time to answer. Nutrition studies that ask subjects to follow a certain diet can also run into problems with compliance. Let's face it: Not everyone is going to eat exactly what they are supposed to every day, especially if what they are supposed to eat is unpleasant or extremely different from the way they normally eat.

Because it is impossible to measure what a person actually eats every day for a long period of time, many long-term studies assume that a person's diet remains relatively constant over time. Yet we know this isn't true: Diets change over time and with the seasons. This means that even if subjects can accurately recall what they ate over the past month, the study may inaccurately estimate their intake of a particular nutrient over the past year. Nutrients like beta-carotene that are found primarily in seasonal vegetables are most likely to have this problem. Other studies may measure how someone currently eats and assume that the person's diet has always been the same. But, as you have probably noticed, diets can change greatly with life events such as starting college, retiring, getting married, or experiencing changes in health status.

Nutrition requirements

The impact of a change in diet, such as taking a vitamin or mineral supplement, is often dependent on the study subject. For example, supplements are more likely to have a beneficial impact on people who have low levels of nutrients in their body. You see no effect when you give an extra dose of something that wasn't needed in the first place. (It's like trying to pump extra gasoline into an already full tank: The extra gasoline isn't used; it just spills out onto the ground.)

Under ideal conditions, a study would be able to select the people who have nutrient deficiencies and are most likely to respond to the treatment. But we do not have reliable methods for measuring body levels of many nutrients. So in most cases, the people included in a study have varying likelihoods of responding to the treatment. This explains some of the contradictory results we see in nutrition studies.

This is exactly the situation we see with chromium supplementation in people with diabetes. We know that chromium plays a role in glucose metabolism, because if we remove it completely from the diet, diabetes-like symptoms occur. But most studies conducted in the United States show little benefit from chromium supplements. One reason for this is that most people in the United States are believed to have adequate amounts of chromium in their body to start with. When studies have focused on people who were more likely to have nutrient deficiencies—such as older people, people with chronic high blood glucose (which can lead to increased urinary loses of many nutrients), and people from developing countries—chromium supplementation has been found to be more effective.

Scientists would like to be able to choose people who have low chromium levels for studies, but at this time there are no accurate tests to measure body chromium stores. So most studies probably end up including people who have both lower and higher body levels of chromium. Those with low chromium levels may respond to the chromium supplement, and those with adequate levels probably do not. In a sense, the group of people who show no response cancels out the group that shows a positive response, and the study shows no effect overall from providing a chromium supplement.

Picking the right dose

It is important to pick the right amount of a nutrient to provide in a study. Give too little, and you might not see an effect; give too much, and you might cause negative side effects. This seems straightforward enough, but it is actually quite difficult to pick the right amount. This is because nutrient requirements vary between individuals, with age, sex, body size, activity level, and many other characteristics. In addition, nutrients can interact with one another, changing the levels needed. In some cases, taking very high amounts of one will decrease the absorption of the others. This effect is most common with minerals such as iron, zinc, chromium, and copper. This is why many nutritionists recommend taking a general multivitamin rather than separate, high-dose supplements of individual nutrients.

Picking the right form of a supplement can also affect whether a study shows a positive effect or not. Different forms of nutrients are absorbed and function differently. Some are more effective than others. If two studies use different forms of the same nutrient, they may get very different results. For instance, studies that have used a form of chromium that is eas-

SEEKING NUTRITION INFORMATION

A few reliable sources of nutrition and diabetes information include the following:

THE AMERICAN DIETETIC ASSOCIATION
www.eatright.org
(800) 366-1655
Offers referrals to registered dietitians and information about nutrition, including free fact sheets and booklets.

THE DEPARTMENT OF HEALTH AND HUMAN SERVICES
www.healthfinder.gov
Provides links to numerous health information Web sites. (This resource is only available through the Internet.)

NUTRITION ACTION HEALTH LETTER
(Published by the Center for Science in the Public Interest)
www.cspinet.org
Suite 300
1875 Connecticut Ave. NW
Washington, DC 20009
A newsletter about nutrition and health that is published 10 times a year. The Web site contains articles from the newsletter in addition to lots of other nutrition information.

THE NATIONAL INSTITUTE OF DIABETES AND DIGESTIVE AND KIDNEY DISEASES
www.niddk.nih.gov
(301) 654-3327
Three booklets—"I Have Diabetes: What Should I Eat?"; "I Have Diabetes: How Much Should I Eat?"; and "I Have Diabetes: When Should I Eat?"—are available for free in English and Spanish. They are also posted on the Web site.

TUFTS UNIVERSITY NUTRITION NAVIGATOR
www.navigator.tufts.edu
A Web site that evaluates other nutrition Web sites and provides links to reliable information. (This resource is only available online.)

TUFTS UNIVERSITY HEALTH & NUTRITION LETTER
www.healthletter.tufts.edu
(800) 274-7581
Sample articles from this monthly newsletter are posted on the Web site.

THE AMERICAN DIABETES ASSOCIATION
www.diabetes.org
(800) DIABETES (342-2383)
Call to request a free information kit about nutrition and diabetes.

ily absorbed (called chromium picolinate) have shown more positive effects than studies conducted using other forms of chromium.

Another source of variability is the amount of nutrients in a study subject's usual diet. Because most studies cannot afford to provide the food eaten by study subjects, researchers ask that subjects continue to eat their usual diet. This means that each person in the study is getting a slightly different amount of the nutrient being studied: the amount found in their usual diet, whatever that happens to be, plus what they are given in the study.

Study design

Nutrition studies also run into problems with study design. When planning a study, you try to keep all factors (variables) the same, except the one you are testing. So if your question is, "Do high-carbohydrate diets increase blood glucose levels?" you would give one group of people a high-carbohydrate diet and a second group of similar people a low-carbohydrate diet. Then you would measure the differences in their blood glucose levels.

But when you increase or decrease the amount of carbohydrate in the diet (without changing anything else), you are also changing the number of calories people are consuming. That makes it difficult to tell if any effects you measure are due to the change in carbohydrate percent or the change in calorie level. If you try to keep the calorie intake of the groups the same, which most studies do, then you need to give more calories as fat or protein when you decrease carbohydrate to make up the difference. But this still raises the question whether the differences measured are due to the change in carbohydrate or something else.

How nutrients affect disease

It can be difficult to sort out exactly how a nutrient affects the development of a disease. This is perhaps the most significant reason that the results of nutrition studies are often contradictory. The effects of many individual nutrients on the disease process are relatively small, and studies may not be sensitive enough to measure their effects, leading to negative results. In some cases, it has been helpful to change the amount of several nutrients in the diet simultaneously, because the nutrients interact with one another and together have measurably significant results.

Diet studies are also difficult to do because foods are complex. They have many beneficial compounds in them, so it can be hard to determine just what it is that may be healthful. We have many studies that show that diets high in fruits and vegetables are helpful in preventing chronic diseases such as cancer. Scientists hypothesized that it was the amount of beta-carotene (an antioxidant nutrient) in these foods that made them healthful. But when they tested this theory by giving study subjects beta-carotene supplements, they were surprised to find that beta-carotene wasn't protective. In fact, the supplements actually increased the risk of cancer in certain subjects (men who smoked).

Role of the media

We remember best the clinical trials that fail because these are the studies that the media emphasize the most. The media often hype a story or inflate a controversy to sell papers and magazines or encourage you to watch a particular TV news show. It isn't very exciting to report that there is a new study that suggests that earlier research told only part of the picture, but that overall, if you look at the total body of research on the topic, there are no significant changes in the scientific community's opinion. Boring! (But truthful.) It is much more interesting and profitable to have head-turning headlines such as "Butter is Back" or "Carbs Make You Fat." Often, however, the headlines are more misleading and controversial than the article that follows, which may do a good job of explaining the research—but that is not always the case.

Even when a writer isn't trying to hype a study or make it seem more exciting or controversial than it is, the story may not be completely accurate or take into account all the studies that came before the most recent one. Many newspaper and magazine writers cover all areas of science, not just health, and many do not have the educational background to understand all the scientific issues of the topic they are reporting on. Writers also tend to work on short deadlines and often have to rely on summaries and press releases for their information—rather than reading and analyzing the research study themselves. So it is helpful to remember that you need to read with a critical eye and not assume that someone else's conclusions are correct. (For tips on finding reliable nutrition news, see "Seeking Nutrition Information" on page 335.)

In many cases, new studies are reported without being placed in a historical context, and too much emphasis is placed on just one study. Keep in mind the metaphor of the elephant and the three scientists: No one study provides all the answers. Research results of multiple studies need to be evaluated together to create the most accurate picture. If you ask your dietitian's opinion of the latest nutrition flip-flop you saw in the news, you will probably be told that this is an overblown presentation of the facts and that the recommendations of the actual experts, not the news media, are still more or less the same and will stay that way until we have more studies and a better understanding of the facts.

Getting accurate information

When looking for information on a particular nutrition topic, look for studies that have been reported in peer-reviewed journals. Studies published in peer-reviewed journals have been rigorously reviewed before publication by experts working in the field of the research. This ensures that the studies are valid and accurately represent the facts. (If you aren't sure whether a journal is peer-reviewed, try calling the publisher, whose phone number should be printed near the front of the journal.) Health newsletters from well-established health and educational institutions can also be a reliable source of information.

Be wary of the health information you read in popular, general-interest magazines; the American Council on Health and Science has found them to have varying accuracy. (The ACHS has researchers and health professionals evaluate the accuracy of nutrition information in popular magazines.)

Evaluate information you find on the World Wide Web very carefully. Most of the health information on the Web is not reviewed by experts, and when evaluations have been conducted, even the best sites have had less than perfect accuracy. Web sites maintained by a health organization, the government, or an academic institution are more likely to provide appropriate, unbiased information than commercial organizations (typically with Web site addresses that end in .com), which are often selling advertising or a product and have a vested interest in promoting one opinion over others.

Picking out a "good" study

When reading a report on a new nutrition research study, there are a few key factors you should be looking for:

Study type. Look for studies involving human subjects rather than test tube or animal studies. The most conclusive research answers generally come from clinical trials, and the cream of the crop is the double-blind, randomized clinical trial.

Study design. Important factors are selection of an appropriate control group, the number of people included in the study (larger studies are generally but not always more sensitive), the length of the study, and a discussion of the way scientists controlled for variables that could affect the study's outcome, such as other health habits, income, weight, etc. Consider also whether the food was provided by the study and whether the study was conducted in a controlled environment or in the "real world."

Statistical issues. A discussion of statistical issues such as confounding or the sensitivity of a study are beyond the scope of many magazine articles. But they are important issues and can lead different scientists to come to different conclusions about the merits of a study. Ideally, a writer will consult with several experts in the field—not just the scientist reporting the new study—before interpreting the results.

The results of a study are considered significant if there is only a very small chance that those results could have occurred purely by chance. Statistics is a mathematical way of assessing that chance or "probability." Most studies use what are called "P values" with a P value less than or equal to 5% ($P=0.05$) considered significant. This means that the results of the study would occur less than 5% of the time by chance and not because of a true association or effect. A P value of 1% ($P=0.01$) or lower is considered an even more stringent test of a study's results.

Relevance. It is important to evaluate how meaningful the results of a study are in the real world. In some cases, a study may show that a treatment has a statistically significant effect, but it is not what we would call clinically significant. For example a researcher may find that herb X causes a "significant" decrease in blood glucose levels, in statistical terms, when blood glucose levels in real numbers dropped from an average of 110 mg/dl to 100 mg/dl. Ten points lower, though nice, is not a big enough decrease to warrant the expense and side effects of a new treatment.

Applying research results to yourself

When evaluating new research, use common sense. Most health experts agree that the basics of a healthy lifestyle include regular exercise, not smoking, and eating a balanced diet that includes a variety of foods and emphasizes fruits, vegetables, and whole grains. There haven't been many changes on this front over the years, and it's unlikely there will be.

Avoid looking for the one magic factor that will improve your health and keep you from needing to do the hard work it takes to eat well and exercise. Don't try to revamp your entire diet every time a new study comes along; this is frustrating and counterproductive. Take new research for what it is—some new, interesting ideas that might be helpful in adjusting your basic, healthy eating plan.

Finally, evaluate the relevance of a new research study to your life. Check with your health-care team to get their opinion of the study's merits and of whether it could be helpful for you. These people should know you and your personal health history. They should know the steps you've already taken to improve your health and can help you figure out which changes will help you the most. We all have a finite amount of time and energy to spend on health-related issues, and focusing our energies where we will get the biggest bang for our buck, so to speak, is important. ❑

WEIGHT-LOSS SUPPORT GROUPS

by Linnea Hagberg, R.D.

Consider the statistics: Over 60% of American adults are now classified as either overweight or obese, and about a quarter of American adults are currently on a diet. With numbers like these, it's no wonder that weight loss has become an industry in itself—and a large one. Each year, Americans spend roughly $40 billion on diet programs, products, foods, and drinks. Despite the diets and the dollars, however, for many people, losing weight—and keeping it off—remains an elusive objective.

And yet, successful weight loss is a worthy goal for many people, especially many of those with Type 2 diabetes, of whom about 80% are overweight. Excessive weight is linked to a number of health problems, including heart disease, stroke, high blood pressure, gallbladder disease, osteoarthritis, sleep apnea, and certain types of cancer. Even moderate weight loss—losing, say, 10 or 20 pounds—can help many of these problems. For example, moderate weight loss can lower total cholesterol levels and raise HDL cholesterol (the "good" cholesterol). Losing excess weight can also help control blood sugar levels by decreasing insulin resistance, allowing glucose to enter muscle and fat cells more easily.

For those who want and need to lose weight, there are a number of sound methods to choose from. Before beginning any weight-loss program, however, consider these guidelines:

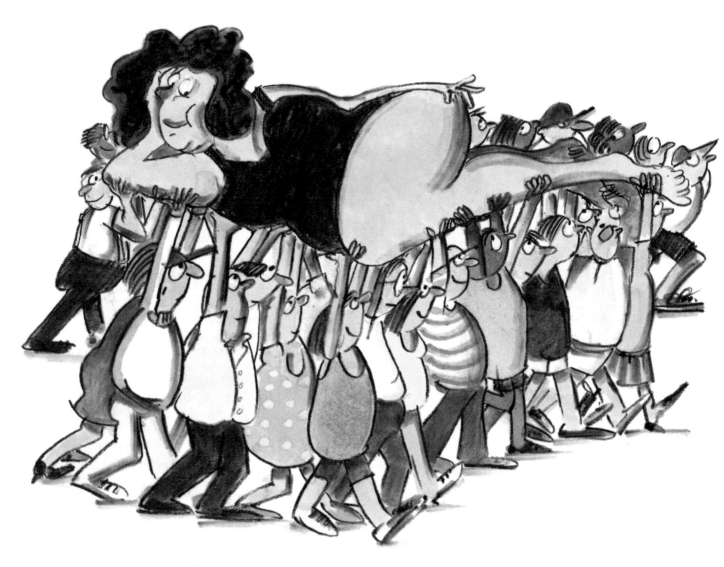

Time it right. Remember that obesity is a chronic condition that will not be solved with short-term changes or quick-fix "diets." Successful weight loss involves permanent changes in how and what you eat and in your physical activity level. Being committed to making these changes will increase your chances for success.

Set moderate goals. For most people, weight loss should be a slow, steady process. A goal of a 5% to 10% reduction in body weight at a rate of about one pound a week is reasonable. For example, a person who is 5'5" and weighs 186 pounds might aim to lose between 9 and 18 pounds and expect to spend a number of months doing it.

Look before you leap. Before you make any changes, discuss your weight-loss plans and any specific diet with your health-care provider to make sure your plans mesh with your diabetes treatment. Ditto for any major changes in your physical activity level.

One path to weight reduction that millions of Americans embark on each year is organized weight-loss programs. These programs can range from rather loosely structured groups in which no particular eating plan is followed, to those that provide a highly tailored plan and sell the food to accompany it, to tightly controlled, medically supervised, very-low-calorie diets. Before joining any organized program, it's a good idea to spend some time determining whether the program is responsible and safe, what costs are involved, and whether the particular program is right for you. (How to evaluate a program is discussed later in this article.)

Many organized weight-loss programs offer group support as part of the plan, a feature that proves useful to some people. Support groups provide an opportunity for individuals to meet with like-minded others for encouragement, reinforcement, information, and inspiration. Weight-loss support groups may be found in many locations, including local hospitals, YMCA/YWCA's, churches, and the offices of registered dietitians or social workers. Even among these groups, considerable variation exists. Overeaters Anonymous, for example, endorses no specific plan of eating, while the Weight Watchers program includes a detailed, calorie-controlled plan.

This article takes a closer look at several nationwide weight-loss programs that include support groups in their structure. (Note: Information regarding these programs was provided by the organizations themselves.) Addresses, phone numbers, and World Wide Web addresses are provided in "Getting in Touch" on page 340.

OVEREATERS ANONYMOUS

Overeaters Anonymous (OA) is a 12-step program modeled after Alcoholics Anonymous. The program is designed to help individuals who are recovering from compulsive overeating. No specific eating plan is provided or recommended, but members are encouraged to work with a professional to develop one. (Physical activity is not specifically addressed in OA.)

Group meetings led by members are held at least once a week. There are no weigh-ins. Individuals are also assigned a sponsor with whom they have daily contact.

Although members can't be counted because they are, literally, anonymous, Overeaters Anonymous currently has about 7,500 meeting groups in over 50 countries. OA is a nonprofit organization, and there are no dues or fees for members. Programs are self-supporting through member contributions.

Local branches of OA can be found in the telephone book or through the organization's main office in New Mexico.

TOPS

TOPS, which stands for Take Off Pounds Sensibly, is a nonprofit group whose mission is to provide information, motivation, encouragement, and fellowship to help members attain and maintain their weight goals. Members must have food and exercise plans as well as weight goals from their doctors. TOPS recommends an exchange-type diet and publishes a book that describes this plan and provides advice on nutrition, exercise, lifestyle, and motivation.

Group meetings are held once a week and are led by volunteer chapter leaders. Chapter leaders are chosen by group members and serve for one year. There are weekly, private, weigh-ins. Meetings may include presentations by guest speakers and recognition awards.

TOPS has approximately 250,000 members in some 11,000 chapters worldwide. Membership in TOPS in the United States costs $20 plus local dues set by each chapter (usually less than $5 per month). Members receive a monthly magazine. The first visit is free.

TOPS programs can be found by calling the organization's headquarters or by visiting its Web site. If there are no TOPS programs available locally, the organization will provide assistance in setting one up, provided there will be at least four members.

FIRST PLACE

First Place is an interdenominational, Christian-oriented health program that emphasizes weight management. Programs are held in churches of all denominations and may also be held in nonchurch locations. Meetings are based on the preset First Place program, which runs 11 to 13 weeks. Members are asked to make nine commitments, including weekly attendance, prayer, reading and studying the Bible, adherence to the First Place food plan, keeping food records, exercising, and calling one class member weekly. The food plan is an exchange plan based on the U.S. Department of Agriculture Food Guide Pyramid. Members are encouraged to obtain their doctor's approval before beginning the program.

First Place is a nationally developed plan, administered locally. Meetings are held once a week and include food planning, class discussion, Bible study, and prayer. Groups are led by members. Leaders use Instruction Guides, lesson plans, and other materials produced by the national office.

First Place has more than 100,000 members in over 12,000 churches. Members pay approximately $80 for the program, which includes a Member Manual and one of five Bible packets. Reenrolling members pay only for a new Bible packet.

Information about availability of local programs can be found by calling the organization's toll-free number. First Place will also assist individuals in setting up programs in area churches.

WEIGHT WATCHERS

Weight Watchers is a commercial program that is based on the premise that healthful weight management includes a comprehensive program encompassing a food plan, activity plan, and behavior modification provided in a supportive group environment. Weight Watchers uses its own, nationally developed eating plans and program materials. Programs are developed by health professionals and are

GETTING IN TOUCH

For more information about any of the programs mentioned in the accompanying article, use the following contact information.

OVEREATERS ANONYMOUS
P.O. Box 44020
Rio Rancho, NM 87124-4020
(505) 891-2664
E-mail: info@overeatersanonymous.org
Web site: www.overeatersanonymous.org

TOPS (Take Off Pounds Sensibly)
4575 South Fifth Street
P.O. Box 070360
Milwaukee, WI 53207-0360
(800) 932-8677
Web site: www.tops.org

FIRST PLACE
720 N. Post Oak, Suite 330
Houston, TX 77024
(800) 727-5223 or (713) 688-6788
E-mail: custservice@firstplace.org
Web site: www.firstplace.org

WEIGHT WATCHERS
Attn: Consumer Affairs Department
175 Crossways Park West
Woodbury, NY 11797
(800) 651-6000
Web site: www.weightwatchers.com

CONSUMER RESPONSE CENTER
Federal Trade Commission
600 Pennsylvania Avenue, N.W.
Washington, DC, 20580-0001
(202) FTC-HELP (382-4357)
Web site: www.ftc.gov/ftc/consumer.htm

PARTNERSHIP FOR HEALTHY WEIGHT
MANAGEMENT
www.consumer.gov/weightloss
This site contains the Voluntary Guidelines for Providers of Weight Loss Products or Services. Those who do not have access to the Web can receive the same information by contacting the Federal Trade Commission's Consumer Response Center.

SHAPE UP AMERICA!
Web site: www.shapeup.org

WEIGHT-CONTROL INFORMATION
NETWORK
1 WIN Way
Bethesda, MD 20892-3665
(877) 946-4627 or (202) 828-1025
E-mail: win@info.niddk.nih.gov
Web site:
www.niddk.nih.gov/health/nutrit/win.htm

designed to incorporate the recommendations of major health organizations. The program includes both a weight-loss and a maintenance phase. Members set a goal weight (with program assistance) that must be at least 5 pounds less than their current weight.

Meetings include a weekly weigh-in, presentations, group discussion time, and awards for weight loss. Weight Watchers food products are sold commercially and may be sold at meetings but are not a mandatory part of the program. Current members may attend meetings anywhere they are held.

Weight Watchers has approximately 1 million members and 29,000 weekly meetings in 29 countries. "Traditional" membership involves a registration fee of approximately $20 plus weekly fees of about $12 a week. Promotional offers may lower the cost. Once the weekly fee has been paid, members can attend as many meetings as they like that week. To maintain current registration, members must pay the weekly fee each week regardless of whether they attend any meetings. (Members can always reregister; this may be a less expensive option if more than one meeting is missed.) Members are provided with a variety of program materials.

Information about the availability of local programs can be found by calling the organization's toll-free number or through the Weight Watchers Web site.

Evaluating weight-loss programs

Eight million people enroll in organized weight-loss programs each year. To help these people be informed consumers, a coalition of organizations and individuals, including the Federal Trade Commission, formed the Partnership for Healthy Weight Management. The Partnership released guidelines in 1999 to suggest what sort of information providers of weight-loss products and services disclose to consumers. The guidelines also suggest how to make the information clear and easily understood. However, any disclosure is voluntary: Providers are not required to follow the guidelines, or they may decide to follow some but not all of the guidelines.

Specifically, the guidelines suggest that weight-loss providers inform consumers about the health risks associated with being overweight and about the difficulty of maintaining weight loss. In addition, each weight-loss provider is advised to clearly inform consumers about components of the program, its cost, any risks associated with a product or program, and the qualifications of program staff.

This information, if provided, is a good place to start in evaluating a program. You may also want to ask yourself the following questions:
■ Is the program nutritionally sound? Are any food groups left out or severely limited? (You can use the Diabetes Food Guide Pyramid, reprinted on page 342, as a guide.) Is a variety of foods offered within each group?
■ Does the program encourage slow, steady, weight loss?
■ Is a maintenance plan included?
■ Does the program include help in behavior modification and adopting a healthier lifestyle?
■ Is physical activity addressed?
■ Does the program fit your needs? Are meetings held in locations and at times convenient for you? Are you comfortable with the format and structure of the program?
■ Are the costs of the program affordable within your budget?
■ If you live with others, can recommended eating plans be adjusted so that the whole family eats in the same way, or will you be eating different foods or preparing multiple meals?
■ If you travel or eat out frequently, can the program be adapted to your situation?
■ Are you required or pressured to buy supplements or other products through the program?

Weight-loss resources

Even if you decide not to join an organized weight-loss program or support group, you can find support and information regarding weight loss in a variety of written materials. Publications of the Federal Trade Commission and the Weight-control Information Network can be obtained through the mail; Shape Up America! can be accessed only through the World Wide Web. (See "Getting in Touch" on page 340 for contact information.

Federal Trade Commission. The FTC has produced a brochure entitled "Setting Goals for Weight Loss." The brochure and other materials about weight loss are available on the Internet or through the FTC's Consumer Response Center.

Weight-control Information Network. WIN is a service of the National Institute of Diabetes and Digestive and Kidney Diseases. It provides consumers and health professionals with scientifically accurate information on weight control and obesity. You can call or write for an order form for WIN publications.

Shape Up America! For those with World Wide Web access, an excellent resource is the Shape Up America! site, founded by Dr. C. Everett Koop, a former U.S. Surgeon General. The Web site provides a wealth of information including a BMI center where individuals can determine their body-mass index, a health and fitness center that provides individualized information on fitness levels and recommends activities, and a support center that provides information and help with motivation and weight maintenance and access to an on-line support group. The site also includes a library of weight-loss resources, on-line publications, and current, scientifically sound information on weight issues.

Weight loss isn't easy, so getting the support you need as you pursue your goals is very important.

Although the final decision about what and how much you eat or exercise is a totally personal one, involvement in an organized support group may help some people achieve their goals. At the very least, support groups can make the path to weight loss a more companionable journey. ❏

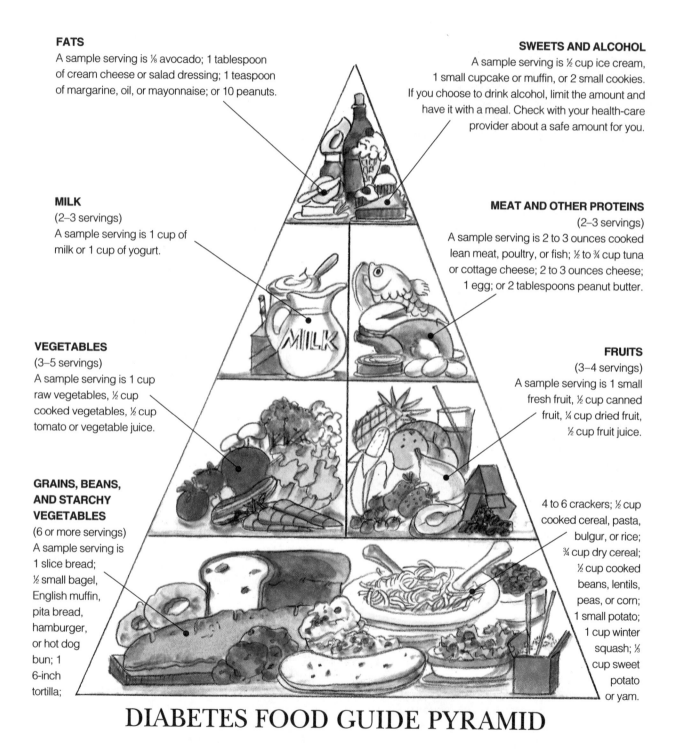

FATS
A sample serving is ⅛ avocado; 1 tablespoon of cream cheese or salad dressing; 1 teaspoon of margarine, oil, or mayonnaise; or 10 peanuts.

SWEETS AND ALCOHOL
A sample serving is ½ cup ice cream, 1 small cupcake or muffin, or 2 small cookies. If you choose to drink alcohol, limit the amount and have it with a meal. Check with your health-care provider about a safe amount for you.

MILK
(2–3 servings)
A sample serving is 1 cup of milk or 1 cup of yogurt.

MEAT AND OTHER PROTEINS
(2–3 servings)
A sample serving is 2 to 3 ounces cooked lean meat, poultry, or fish; ½ to ¾ cup tuna or cottage cheese; 2 to 3 ounces cheese; 1 egg; or 2 tablespoons peanut butter.

VEGETABLES
(3–5 servings)
A sample serving is 1 cup raw vegetables, ½ cup cooked vegetables, ½ cup tomato or vegetable juice.

FRUITS
(3–4 servings)
A sample serving is 1 small fresh fruit, ½ cup canned fruit, ¼ cup dried fruit, ½ cup fruit juice.

GRAINS, BEANS, AND STARCHY VEGETABLES
(6 or more servings)
A sample serving is 1 slice bread; ½ small bagel, English muffin, pita bread, hamburger, or hot dog bun; 1 6-inch tortilla;

4 to 6 crackers; ½ cup cooked cereal, pasta, bulgur, or rice; ¾ cup dry cereal; ½ cup cooked beans, lentils, peas, or corn; 1 small potato; 1 cup winter squash; ⅓ cup sweet potato or yam.

DIABETES FOOD GUIDE PYRAMID

PREVENTIVE HEALTH

THE BUG STOPS HERE
A GUIDE TO HOME FOOD SAFETY
by Patti Bazel Geil, M.S., R.D., L.D., C.D.E.

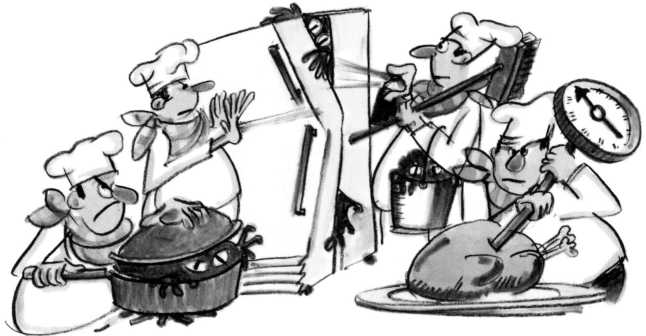

I t's a typical Wednesday evening as Jennifer stands in front of her open refrigerator, peering at its contents and trying to decide what to eat for supper. "Leftover chicken casserole? It's been in the refrigerator since the weekend; it's probably still OK to eat. What about that fried rice from last night's Chinese dinner? I left it out on the counter for a few hours before refrigerating it, but surely a brief reheating will kill any stray bacteria. Or maybe I should just grill a fish fillet. I wonder about that date on the package—is it the 'sell by' or 'use by' date?"

Is Jennifer about to have a delicious meal? Or is she more likely to develop a debilitating case of foodborne illness? Knowing the right answers to food safety questions like hers can make all the difference.

Although the United States has one of the safest food supplies in the world, it also has, according to the U.S. Centers for Disease Control and Prevention, an estimated 76 million cases of foodborne illness each year, resulting in 5,000 deaths. Many cases of foodborne illness go unreported, mistakenly attributed to the flu or a 24-hour virus. In view of alarming statistics like these, a federal program called the National Food Safety Initiative was launched in early 1997 and charged with reducing the incidence of foodborne illness in the United States to the greatest extent possible.

For a person with diabetes, the nausea, vomiting, diarrhea, and inability to eat that accompany foodborne illnesses are not only unpleasant but may also have serious consequences on blood glucose control. In this article, we show you how to reduce the likelihood of foodborne illness striking in your home.

The culprits

You can't see them or, in most cases, smell or taste them, but the bacteria that cause many cases of foodborne illness can be found everywhere in nature and the environment. (Viruses, parasites, and household chemicals can also cause foodborne illness.) Most adults are unaffected by low levels of bacteria in food (although children, elderly adults, and people with weakened immunity may become sick). Bacteria begin to pose a threat when they are given the right conditions: food, moisture, the right temperature, and time to multiply.

Who are these sneaky varmints? And where are their favorite hideouts? The predominant foodborne bacterial pathogens may have uncommon names—*Salmonella, Campylobacter,* and *Escherichia coli* 0157:H7—but they can be found in the most common places: animal protein foods such as meat, eggs, poultry, and fish.

Salmonella. These bacteria are most often found in raw or undercooked poultry and poultry products, meat and meat products, eggs, dairy products, seafood, and fresh produce. Although farmers, food manufacturers, supermarkets, and restaurants are required by law to follow strict food safety regulations, large amounts of salmonella do sometimes enter the food supply. In one incident, 224,000 people became ill from eating a batch of ice cream contaminated with salmonella.

When a food is contaminated with salmonella (or any other bacteria), it can not only make you sick but it can contaminate other foods in your kitchen. Such cross-contamination typically occurs when a raw food containing salmonella touches a cooked food that is ready to eat, a raw food that won't be cooked, or a surface that is later used to prepare or serve cooked foods. The bacteria can also hitch a free ride on sponges or dishcloths used to clean surfaces or utensils that were touched by the contaminated food.

Campylobacter. These bacteria are less well-known than some of the other bacteria that cause foodborne illness, but this bug has recently been recognized as one of the leading causes of diarrhea in the United States. *Campylobacter* is most commonly found in undercooked poultry and meats, raw (unpasteurized) milk, and untreated water. Campylobacteriosis has been known to occur in children after school outings to dairy farms where milk was tasted "straight from the cow."

Escherichia coli. An especially toxic strain of *Escherichia coli* bacteria (called *E. coli* for short) has created an emerging crisis in foodborne illness. Even a very small amount of *E. coli* O157:H7 can produce a deadly toxin that causes severe damage to the intestinal tract and kidneys, particularly in children and the elderly. This strain of *E. coli* can survive refrigerator and freezer temperatures but is killed when heated to 160°F. It is usually found in undercooked beef prod-

ucts, unpasteurized milk, contaminated water and mayonnaise, improperly processed cider, and vegetables grown in cow manure.

Because bacteria cause a substantial proportion of cases of foodborne illness, taking steps to avoid bacteria and prevent against cross-contamination reduces your overall risk of foodborne illness. (Many of the tips in this article also offer protection against viruses and parasites.) Luckily, there's a lot you can do to stop bacteria in their tracks.

Safety in numbers

Bacteria grow fastest in the temperature range known as "the danger zone," namely, from 40°F to 140°F. Your refrigerator should therefore be set to below 40°F to slow the growth of bacteria; your freezer should be set at or below 0°F. Heating foods thoroughly to temperatures above 160°F destroys bacteria. The best way to accurately measure the temperature of foods during cooking and before serving is to use a food thermometer. Such thermometers are typically used to assess doneness in roasts or whole chickens or turkeys, but they can be used in other meats, casseroles, and egg dishes, as well.

Bacteria can double in number every 20 to 30 minutes, so it's important to get food out of the temperature danger zone as soon as possible after cooking it or after removing it from the refrigerator. The longest any perishable food should be allowed to sit at room temperature is two hours. As a general rule, if a food feels comfortable to the touch, it is probably in the danger zone of 40°F to 140°F.

To market, to market

Home food safety starts even before the food reaches your kitchen. When shopping for groceries, keep these tips in mind:

■ Look for the new safe handling labels on raw meat and poultry products that summarize the guidelines for keeping food safe (see "Safe Handling Instructions" on page 348). Shop for meat, poultry, and seafood last. Place meats in separate plastic bags when possible to keep the packages from dripping on other foods in your shopping cart.

■ Pay attention to food product dating. Purchase dated packages only if the "sell by" date has not passed. "Use by" dates have been determined by the product manufacturer as the last date recommended for use of the product while at peak quality.

■ Don't buy foods in cans that are dented, cracked, or rusted or have bulging lids.

■ Be sure frozen foods are frozen solid. Put all frozen foods in the same bag to keep them colder longer.

■ Return home quickly after grocery shopping. Bring a cooler if the time from store to home will be longer

IS YOUR KITCHEN BUGGED?

A FOOD SAFETY QUIZ

Bacterial contamination causes a substantial proportion of cases of foodborne illness. Take this quick quiz to determine if your kitchen may be bugged.

1. Do you thaw frozen foods on the countertop at room temperature?

2. Do you chop fresh vegetables or salad ingredients using a knife or cutting board that was used for raw meat (without washing the board or knife first)?

3. Do you leave leftovers sitting out for more than two hours after cooking?

4. Do you prepare recipes that call for raw or partially cooked eggs?

5. Do you marinate meat in the refrigerator and then brush the same marinade on the meat while cooking it (without boiling the marinade first)?

6. Do you use the same spoon to stir and "taste test" foods?

7. Do you leave your groceries sitting in shopping bags in your car for more than 30 minutes at a time while you run errands between the grocery store and home?

8. Do you sometimes forget to wash your hands before beginning food preparation?

If you answered "no" to all of the above questions, you're taking some important steps toward preventing foodborne illness. If you answered "yes" to any of the questions, you need to think of ways to make that "yes" a "no."

than 30 minutes. Since the trunk is the hottest part of the car during the summer, keep your groceries in the passenger compartment instead.

Safe storage

Foods maintain their quality longer when stored properly. Proper storage will also slow the growth of any bacteria present or prevent it from traveling to other foods. When putting away the groceries, keep these tips in mind:

■ Store foods in clean areas, away from stoves, ovens, or other heat sources.

■ Wrap raw meat, poultry, and seafood that will be used within a few days in separate plastic bags. Set each bag on a plate on the lowest shelf of your refrigerator to keep juices from dripping onto other foods or refrigerator surfaces.

■ Use refrigerated beef steaks, roasts, deli meats, and poultry within three to four days. Ground meat, ground poultry, and fish should be used within one to two days.

■ Freeze fresh meat, poultry, and seafood immediately if you don't plan to use them within a few days.

■ Store eggs in their original cartons inside the refrigerator. Eggs don't stay fresh as long when stored in the refrigerator door, where the temperature is warmer.

■ If a food has been kept beyond its "use by" date or is moldy, discolored, or smelly, don't taste it. Just discard it. Remember, when in doubt, throw it out.

■ Freezing inactivates but does not destroy bacteria. Once thawed, bacteria become active again and capable of multiplying under the right conditions. For this reason, never thaw foods at room temperature. Thaw foods only in the refrigerator or in the microwave. Thawing in the refrigerator requires planning ahead, since it may take several hours. If you thaw in a microwave, finish cooking immediately.

Now you're cooking

How you handle food during preparation and cooking is important, too. When cooking, keep these tips in mind:

■ Wash your hands with hot soapy water for at least 20 seconds before starting any food preparation. Wash them again if you stop to do something else, particularly if you use the bathroom, change a diaper, blow your nose, or touch a pet.

■ Thoroughly rinse poultry and seafood in cold water before cooking. Rinse all fresh fruits and vegetables, including those that will be peeled or have inedible rinds, using a brush to scrub if necessary. (Don't use soaps or detergents on food.)

■ Keep raw meat, poultry, seafood, and their juices from coming into contact with other foods during preparation, especially foods that won't be cooked. Never chop fresh vegetables or salad ingredients on a cutting board that was used for raw meat without properly cleaning it first.

■ Marinate meat, poultry, or seafood in a covered, nonmetal container in the refrigerator. Throw out the leftover marinade that was in contact with the raw meat, or bring it to a rolling boil for one full minute before using it on cooked meat.

■ Do not eat raw cookie dough or taste any food that contains meat or eggs while it is raw or partially cooked.

■ Never use the same spoon for stirring and tasting a food. If you do, you may end up sharing the bacteria in your mouth with everyone who eats the food.

■ Cook eggs until the whites are completely firm and the yolks are just beginning to thicken. Throw away or modify recipes that call for uncooked or partially cooked eggs. Some examples of dishes that traditionally contain partially cooked eggs include egg-drop soup, hollandaise sauce, Caesar salad, and fried eggs cooked sunny-side up.

■ Microwave cooking is convenient and safe as long as the food is heated evenly and thoroughly. For the best results, use microwave-safe cookware, cut food into small, uniform pieces, cover foods while microwaving, and stir or rotate dishes periodically during cooking. Be sure to follow recommended standing times outside the microwave so that food completes cooking.

What's left?

If you're lucky, there are leftovers, and you won't have to cook again tomorrow. To make sure those leftovers stay safe and edible, follow these tips:

■ Refrigerate cooked foods within two hours after cooking. Freeze any leftovers that you won't eat within a few days.

■ When storing leftovers, divide large amounts into smaller amounts and place them in shallow containers to allow foods to cool more quickly.

■ When reheating leftovers, bring soups, sauces, and gravies to a boil before serving. Cover and reheat other leftovers to 165°F or until steaming hot to destroy any bacteria that may have grown.

Cleanup time

Keeping your kitchen and cooking utensils clean lowers the risk of bacterial cross-contamination. Here's how to do it:

■ Clean all kitchen surfaces routinely. A sanitizing solution for kitchen cleaning can be made from 2 teaspoons chlorine bleach in one quart of water. Wash all kitchen utensils thoroughly with hot, soapy water after each use.

■ Launder kitchen towels and dishcloths after one day's use, and allow them to dry thoroughly after washing. This is because bacteria can continue to live as long as there is moisture.

Sponges present a special problem because they don't truly dry between uses and they are hard to clean. Some experts recommend putting sponges in the dishwasher, but there is no guarantee that the hot water will kill bacteria in the interior of the sponge or that the sponge will dry completely during the dry cycle. The U.S. Department of Agriculture advises rinsing sponges in a disinfectant solution (1 teaspoon

SQUEAKY CLEAN

Still have questions about food safety? The following resources may have the answers:

CONSUMER INFORMATION CATALOG
Pueblo, CO 81009
(888) 8-PUEBLO (878-3256)
www.pueblo.gsa.gov
Many of the informative U.S. government publications in this catalog are free.

U.S. CENTERS FOR DISEASE CONTROL AND PREVENTION (CDC)
Voice and Fax Information System
(888) 232-3228
www.cdc.gov/health/foodill.htm
The CDC recommends calling your local health department to report foodborne illness.

U.S. DEPARTMENT OF AGRICULTURE
Food Safety and Inspection Service
www.fsis.usda.gov
Meat and Poultry Hotline
(800) 535-4555

U.S. FOOD AND DRUG ADMINISTRATION
Center for Food Safety and Applied Nutrition
(888) SAFEFOOD (723-3366)
http://vm.cfsan.fda.gov/list.html

disinfectant to 1 quart of water) to reduce bacteria levels. The agency also recommends changing sponges every two weeks. Another option is to buy sponges that contain substances that kill bacteria (O-Cel-O StayFresh and Scotch-Brite scrub sponges are two such varieties) and replace them every couple of weeks. Throwing your sponge in the laundry every day or two may also help keep bacterial counts down.

■ Don't worry about whether to use a wood or plastic cutting board. Either type of board is safe, as long as it's kept clean. However, a government food safety survey reported that one out of four people doesn't wash his or her cutting board with soap and water before preparing another raw food. Make sure you're one of the three who do!

■ It's been called "the dirtiest half-inch in the kitchen." Don't forget to clean your can opener blade!

Special situations

Some situations present special food safety concerns. Among those are power outages, bag lunches or picnics, and holiday meals.

Power outages. If your power goes out but you expect it to resume within a few hours, just keep your refrigerator and freezer closed until you have power again. A fully stocked freezer will usually keep food frozen for two days without power. Unopened refrigerators can keep food cold for four to six hours, depending on the temperature in the room. If, after power is restored, you are uncertain about the quality or safety of a food, play it safe and throw it out.

Bag lunches. If you prepare your lunch the night before, store it in the refrigerator to keep it cool overnight. And if your workplace has a refrigerator, take advantage of it to keep perishable foods cold until lunchtime. For hot foods, use a thermos to hold them at the proper temperature. When eating outdoors, keep picnic baskets and coolers in the shade. In hot weather, food should not sit out for longer than one hour.

Holiday meals. Holiday festivities usually involve lots of food, much of which requires special food safety attention. For example, the stuffing in the traditional stuffed turkey is an excellent spot for bacteria to grow if it is left inside the bird for any length of time. It may be safer to cook the stuffing separately in a pan and serve it on the side. When preparing for your holiday meal, don't try to save time by partially cooking an item ahead of time and completing cooking at the last minute. Incomplete cooking can promote bacterial growth. Food served from a buffet should be kept out of the danger zone. Keep cold foods on ice below a temperature of 40°F and hot foods above 140°F until they are eaten.

Just in case

Despite the best precautions, you may find yourself the victim of a foodborne illness. Most symptoms appear within four to 48 hours after eating a contaminated food. Symptoms may include severe abdominal cramps, diarrhea, vomiting and nausea, and flulike symptoms such as fever, chills, headache, and backache. You or your doctor should report serious cases of foodborne illness to your local health department.

As with any illness, use your judgment to determine whether you need to seek medical care, and be sure to follow your diabetes sick day rules. They are as follows:
1. Always take your insulin or diabetes pills, even if you cannot eat, unless your doctor tells you differently.
2. Test your blood sugar at least every four hours. If your blood sugar is over 240 mg/dl, test your urine for ketones.
3. Drink plenty of liquids. Take at least ½ cup of water or other calorie-free, caffeine-free liquid every half hour. Drink liquids in small sips to help avoid vomiting.
4. If you cannot keep solid food down, try to eat enough soft foods or liquids to take the place of the carbohydrate you usually eat. Suggested foods and amounts to replace one serving (15 grams) of carbohydrate include the following:
■ ⅓ to ½ cup fruit juice
■ ½ cup sugared soft drink
■ ½ cup regular gelatin
■ ½ cup hot cereal
■ ½ cup vanilla ice cream
■ 1 cup broth-based soup.
5. Call your doctor if you cannot keep down food, liquids, or diabetes pills; if your illness lasts more than 24 hours; if your temperature is over 101°F; or if your ketone test is moderate or high.
6. Postpone exercise until your blood sugar is stable. ❑

SAFE HANDLING INSTRUCTIONS
This label should appear on raw meat and poultry products

This product was prepared from inspected and passed meat and/or poultry. Some food products may contain bacteria that could cause illness if the product is mishandled or cooked improperly. For your protection, follow these safe handling instructions.

 Keep refrigerated or frozen. Thaw in refrigerator or microwave.

 Keep raw meat and poultry separate from other foods. Wash working surfaces (including cutting boards), utensils, and hands after touching raw meat or poultry.

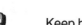 Cook thoroughly.

Keep hot foods hot. Refrigerate leftovers immediately or discard.

HOW TO FIGHT FATIGUE

by Linnea Hagberg, R.D.

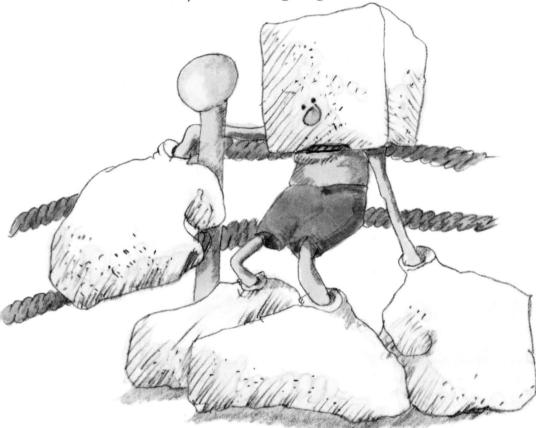

Webster's defines it as weariness or exhaustion from labor, exertion, or stress. Others call it feeling wiped out, done in, bushed, or bone tired. Under any name, fatigue is a condition with which many of us are all too familiar.

Fatigue is a very common feeling, ranking only behind pain as the most frequent cause of visits to the doctor. Fatigue can be difficult to pin down. It can arise from a number of causes, from the obvious to the obscure. Fatigue can be insidious, creeping up so slowly that you aren't even fully aware of its impact, or it can hit you like a 5-ton elephant, stopping you in your tracks.

Exhaustion can be an early symptom of a major medical problem, or it can accompany a relatively minor illness like the flu. Although its impact can be huge, fatigue is usually a symptom of another problem or condition, rather than being a medical problem in and of itself. (The one exception is chronic fatigue syndrome.) What's more, feeling perpetually tired is almost never simply a side effect of growing older! Once you discover the underlying causes of your fatigue, it is often possible to treat them or make lifestyle changes to restore your energy.

So what makes us feel so tired? Although they aren't independent of one another, the primary causes of fatigue can be grouped into lifestyle factors, medical conditions, and mood disorders.

Lifestyle factors

As a general rule, healthy lifestyle habits such as following your diabetes meal plan, managing stress, and exercising will give you energy, while unhealthy habits such as smoking, excessive drinking, and erratic eating can leave you feeling drained.

Stress. While some stress in life is necessary, too much of it can be harmful. Stress can cause fatigue by triggering what is known as the "fight-or-flight" response, which involves the release of the so-called stress hormones adrenaline and cortisol. This hormone release and the bodily changes that accompany it—including tensed muscles, increased blood pressure and heart rate, and shallow breathing—use up a lot of energy.

The fight-or-flight response allows us to respond quickly to dangerous situations. And since danger occurs only occasionally in most of our lives, the stress response shouldn't cause more than occasional episodes of tiredness. Unfortunately, our bodies respond to more common, anxiety-provoking situations, such as running late for an appointment, in the same way. And sources of chronic stress, such as a heavy workload at home or at the office, can cause the stress response to turn on and stay on for days or weeks at a time.

Chronic stress can also contribute to any number of medical problems—from migraines to infections—that can cause or aggravate fatigue. And many sources of stress, such as unresolved marital or financial problems, can keep you up at night worrying, leading to a loss of sleep and subsequent exhaustion. If chronic stress is sapping your energy, look for ways to reduce it. Regular exercise, meditation, or talking things out with a trusted friend or counselor can all help.

Nutrition. The foods we eat (or don't eat) can also contribute to fatigue. Food is our primary fuel source, and the old adage "you are what you eat" holds true. If you eat a well-balanced diet, you will probably enjoy better health.

When you eat can be as important as *what* you eat. Skipping meals and eating at irregular intervals are both known to contribute to fatigue, not to mention unstable blood sugar levels. On the other hand, eating smaller, more frequent meals has been shown to boost energy, as well as make weight management and blood glucose control easier.

Eating too few calories or following a diet that provides an inadequate amount or variety of nutrients can lead to fatigue. So can eating too many calories, especially when eating too much leads to or adds to obesity. Carrying extra pounds is extra work for the body and can make everyday activities such as doing the laundry or walking from the parking lot to your office exhausting.

Following a diabetes meal plan designed specifically for you may be your best weapon against food-related fatigue. If you do not yet have a meal plan, think about seeing a registered dietitian now to help you design one. Ask your doctor for a referral to a dietitian, or see "Help Is Out There" on the opposite page for other resources.

Dehydration. An often overlooked contributor to fatigue is dehydration. When the body doesn't get enough water, blood gets thicker and blood volume decreases. This makes the heart work harder and reduces the flow of blood—and, therefore, oxygen and glucose—to your brain. The result can be weakness, dizziness, confusion, and, of course, fatigue.

Thirst isn't always a reliable marker of dehydration. To be on the safe side, drink eight or more glasses of water or other liquids a day, whether or not you feel thirsty. Another way to gauge hydration is to look at your urine. If your fluid intake is too low, your urine will be small in volume and dark yellow in color. Having pale yellow or straw-colored urine is a sign that you are getting enough fluid. (If you take a vitamin supplement, your urine may be a bright greenish yellow because of the riboflavin most supplements contain. This is nothing to worry about.)

Exercise. While a lack of physical activity won't necessarily cause fatigue, regular exercise can help eliminate it and give you more energy. That's because exercise increases blood flow, allowing more oxygen to reach your organs and other tissues. This helps them work more efficiently. Exercise also enables you to better control your diabetes and keep your weight in check. It can help you manage stress, relieve anger or aggression, and promote a feeling of well-being. And studies in older adults have shown that exercise can help promote restful sleep.

Smoking. Among its many other health hazards, smoking contributes to fatigue in several ways. First, the carbon monoxide in cigarette smoke decreases the amount of oxygen that gets delivered to the tissues in your body, and less oxygen means less energy. Second, respiratory problems caused by smoking can make the act of breathing much harder, which uses up more energy. Finally, since nicotine is a stimulant, smoking close to bedtime can interfere with sleep.

Medical conditions

Of course, even the most health-conscious among us still occasionally get weary. One reason is that fatigue can accompany scores of diseases and other conditions, from allergies to multiple sclerosis. In some cases, fatigue is a prominent part of the condition, while in others it is less of a factor. The level of fatigue you feel is not necessarily related to the severity of the illness. The exhaustion that accompanies the flu or a foodborne illness, for example, can be surprisingly long-lived. Sometimes, fatigue is the clue that uncovers a previously unknown medical problem. It's worth noting, too, that fatigue can be a side effect of many drugs. If you're experiencing fatigue, consider reviewing your medicines with your doctor.

Although many medical conditions can cause fatigue, here are some of the most common culprits:

High blood sugar. For people with diabetes, elevated blood sugar levels can cause fatigue and sluggishness. In fact, fatigue can be a signal that your blood sugar control is slipping and needs to be adjusted and improved. Testing your blood sugar will help confirm that high blood sugar is (or is not) the problem. Taking steps to keep your blood sugar within goal limits, with your diabetes team's help, if necessary, should relieve the associated fatigue.

Infection. When an infection occurs, the body's defenses mobilize to fight it off. This process uses up a great deal of energy and can result in fatigue. Even after the acute phase of an infection is over, fatigue can linger for a considerable period of time.

Although specific symptoms will vary according to the illness, fatigue caused by infection may occur suddenly and will generally be accompanied by other symptoms such as fever, chills, swollen glands, a sore or scratchy throat, headache, nausea, vomiting, diarrhea, or loss of appetite.

Infections in which fatigue may be a prominent symptom include endocarditis (an infection of the valves or lining of the heart), hepatitis (inflammation of the liver), mononucleosis, and Lyme disease.

Hypothyroidism. Another cause of fatigue is hypothyroidism, or an underactive thyroid. The thyroid gland normally secretes a hormone that regulates metabolism. In hypothyroidism, too little thyroid hormone is released. In the United States, most cases are thought to be the result of an autoimmune reaction, in which the body develops antibodies and essentially destroys its own thyroid.

Hypothyroidism is much more common in women than in men. In addition to fatigue, other symptoms include weight gain, sensitivity to cold, muscle cramps, dry skin, constipation, anemia, coarse hair, and menstrual changes. Hypothyroidism can be detected with a simple blood test and is generally treated with pills containing synthetic thyroid hormone.

Heart disease. In the most common type of heart disease, coronary heart disease, the walls of the arteries supplying blood to the heart muscle become hardened and narrowed, forcing the heart to work harder to pump blood throughout the body. This inefficient pumping causes less oxygen to reach tissues, which causes fatigue.

In addition to fatigue, symptoms of heart disease include shortness of breath, difficult or painful breathing, a chronic cough, and angina (a feeling of pain, tightness, or pressure in the chest). Signs of heart disease can differ slightly in women. Often, one of the first warning signs of heart disease in women is profound fatigue that occurs during activities such as walking up stairs. Symptoms of heart disease should be reported to your doctor immediately.

Mitral valve prolapse. The mitral valve of the heart regulates blood flow from one chamber to another. When mitral valve prolapse occurs, this valve is floppy or loose, allowing blood to leak backwards.

The condition is often inherited and is fairly common: As many as 5% of adults may have it. In addition to fatigue, mitral valve prolapse can cause shortness of breath and an irregular heartbeat. These symptoms can disrupt sleep if they occur during the night. Symp-

HELP IS OUT THERE

Many organizations offer information packets and referral lines on different health topics. Here are three organizations that can help you take charge of your health:

To find a registered dietitian in your area, ask your doctor for a referral, call The American Dietetic Association's Nutrition Hotline at (800) 366-1655, or visit the Association's Web site, www.eatright.org. The Web site of the American Association of Diabetes Educators, www.aadenet.org, can also be of help.

For more information about chronic fatigue syndrome, contact the Chronic Fatigue and Immune Dysfunction Syndrome (CFIDS) Association of America at (800) 442-3437, or visit its Web site, www.cfids.org

To learn more about iron overload, check out the Iron Overload Diseases Web site at www.ironoverload.org or send a self-addressed, stamped envelope to Iron Overload Diseases Association, 433 Westwind Drive, North Palm Beach, FL 33408-5123.

toms often don't appear until people reach their thirties or forties. Mitral valve prolapse often does not require treatment, but in some cases, an irregular heartbeat is treated with drugs.

Cancer. Cancer occurs when cells begin to divide out of control and form tumors. Cancer has widespread effects on the body, including fatigue. Other symptoms of cancer include loss of appetite, weight loss with no apparent cause, anemia, fever, a lump or change of shape in the breasts or testes, bleeding or discharge from a nipple, a change of appearance in a mole, persistent hoarseness, a change in bowel habits, and irregular vaginal bleeding.

Fatigue, resulting from both the disease and its treatment, is extremely common. In fact, much of the current research into the nature and treatment of fatigue centers on cancer-related fatigue.

Iron-deficiency anemia. A common cause of fatigue, anemia is a condition in which the concentration of hemoglobin in the blood is lower than normal. Hemoglobin is carried in red blood cells; its function is to transport oxygen from the lungs to tissues throughout the body.

Anemia can have many causes, but the most common is iron deficiency. Dietary iron is needed to make hemoglobin, so inadequate intake of iron can lead to anemia. Anemia can also result when iron is lost through bleeding. In adults, bleeding—caused by such problems as ulcers, inflammatory bowel disease, intestinal tumors, or long-term aspirin use—accounts for most cases of iron-deficiency anemia. In women, heavy menstrual periods are a common cause of iron deficiency. In fact, a study published in *The Journal of the American Medical Association* found that between 2% and 5% of American women and girls have iron-deficiency anemia.

In early, mild stages, iron deficiency may cause people to feel cold as well as tired. If anemia becomes severe, symptoms can include a pale complexion, shortness of breath, a rapid pulse, and curved, brittle nails. Your doctor can diagnose anemia with a blood test. Treatment generally includes finding and treating any underlying causes for the anemia, taking iron supplements, and increasing your intake of iron-rich foods.

Iron overload. Just as it is possible to have too little iron, it is also possible to have too much. Hemochromatosis, or iron overload, is a genetic disease in which the body absorbs too much iron. Because iron can only be lost from the body through bleeding, the excess iron builds up in organs and joints. If left unchecked, this buildup causes widespread damage and can be deadly. One in 250 Americans may have inherited genes for this disease from both parents.

In addition to fatigue, symptoms of hemochromatosis may include extreme weakness, lethargy, joint pain, heart irregularities, and weight loss. The disease can be identified with a blood test. Treatment involves periodically removing blood from the body. This is done the same way that a regular blood donation is carried out. For more information about hemochromatosis, see "Help Is Out There" on page 351.

Sleep disorders. Many medical conditions can cause excessive tiredness by interfering with sleep. Examples include painful conditions such as diabetic neuropathy, restless legs syndrome, and arthritis, and problems that can cause frequent urination such as a urinary tract or prostate infection or poorly controlled diabetes.

Certain sleep disorders can directly affect your sleep patterns. One disorder that affects as many as one out of four people over age 60 is *obstructive sleep apnea*. This occurs when the muscles and soft tissues in the back of the throat relax too much during sleep, narrowing or constricting the airways. Although they are unaware of it, people who have sleep apnea stop breathing repeatedly during the night and wake up gasping. The continual waking prevents them from getting restful sleep. As a result, they may fall asleep easily during the day, making driving hazardous.

Obstructive sleep apnea is almost always accompanied by loud snoring. Men are more likely than women to have it. Obesity and smoking exacerbate the condition. Upper respiratory problems like a cold or flu can also make it worse. And because alcohol can relax muscles, drinking can aggravate the problem.

Obstructive sleep apnea can be diagnosed in a sleep laboratory, where doctors monitor your breathing while you sleep. Treatment may include weight loss, eliminating behaviors that exacerbate the condition, and if needed, taking medicine to clear nasal congestion. Sleeping on your side and elevating the head of your bed can also help.

If simple measures don't do the trick, your doctor may recommend the use of a continuous positive airway pressure machine at night. This device consists of a small mask (similar to an oxygen mask) that feeds air into the nose and mouth to keep airways open. Special dental plates may also help by holding the jaw in proper position so the airway doesn't close up.

Almost everyone has experienced *insomnia* at some point. Defined as the inability to fall asleep within 30 minutes of going to bed, or the inability to stay asleep, insomnia may affect as many as one in three adults in the United States. Insomnia can be transient, affecting people in short bouts. These periods often occur during stressful times, such as right after a job loss. But insomnia can also be a chronic condition that occurs night after night, impairing a person's health and well-being. Because stress is a leading cause of insomnia, techniques such as exercise or relaxation training, which reduce stress, can help restore sleep.

For some people, simply finding enough time for a decent night's sleep may be difficult. Recognizing that a lack of sleep can have consequences ranging from irritability to difficulty concentrating to a depressed immune system may help you make sleep a priority. For hints on getting a good night's sleep, see "Sleep Easy" on the opposite page.

Chronic fatigue syndrome. As many as 500,000 Americans suffer profound fatigue that is ascribed to chronic fatigue syndrome. Much is still unknown about the causes and cures of the condition. Because there are no specific laboratory tests or procedures to diagnose this illness and the symptoms are so general, a detailed procedure has been set up to diagnose the condition.

A diagnosis of chronic fatigue syndrome is considered only when symptoms have been clinically evaluated by a doctor, other potential causes of fatigue have been eliminated, and the fatigue has lasted for at least six months, is not eased by bed rest, and is severe enough to substantially reduce daily activity. In addition, at least four of the following symptoms must accompany the fatigue: sore throat; tender lymph nodes; muscle pain; multi-joint pain without swelling or redness; headaches of a new type, pattern, or severity; sleep disturbances; short-term memory or concentration impairment that is severe enough to interfere with usual activities; and fatigue that lasts for more than 24 hours after exertion.

There is currently no standard treatment or medicine for chronic fatigue syndrome other than rest and treatment of specific symptoms, when possible. A small but promising study published in *The Journal of the American Medical Association,* however, found that the condition may be linked to a certain form of low blood pressure. While results were preliminary, researchers in the study had good results treating chronic fatigue syndrome with a high-salt diet and drugs that encourage the body to retain sodium. For more information about chronic fatigue syndrome, see "Help Is Out There" on page 351.

Mood disorders

Just as physical disorders can sap our energy, mood disorders can also contribute to fatigue.

Depression. Fatigue figures prominently in major depression, which occurs in about one in 10 Americans and affects women more often than men. Depression generally results from a number of factors rather than one single, specific cause. Genetic, biological, psychological, and environmental factors can all come into play. In addition, some drugs, such as beta-blockers, may increase the risk of developing depression.

Both the symptoms of depression and their severity vary from person to person. In addition to listlessness and fatigue, symptoms can include loss of interest in life or activities that used to be enjoyable, insomnia or excessive sleeping, feelings of worthlessness, guilt, helplessness, and sadness, changes in appetite, difficulty concentrating or making decisions, unexplained bouts of crying, irritability, and thoughts of suicide. People may also experience physical symptoms such as headaches that do not respond to treatment.

Depression is generally diagnosed through a complete medical and psychiatric evaluation. Treatment can involve drug therapy and counseling.

Seasonal affective disorder. Fatigue may also accompany seasonal affective disorder (SAD), a sort of seasonal depression that affects people during the fall and winter months. SAD is believed to be caused by a lack of sunlight, which in turn decreases the brain chemical serotonin. Women are much more likely than men to experience seasonal affective disorder.

Symptoms usually begin in October or November and subside by April. In addition to fatigue, symptoms include sadness or anxiety, difficulty concentrating, withdrawal, increased appetite, food cravings, and weight gain. SAD is usually treated with light therapy, in which the person is exposed to repeated doses of artificial light. Antidepressants may also be prescribed.

Giving fatigue a rest

Often the cause of fatigue is obvious: You've been staying up late reading or watching TV for several nights in

SLEEP EASY

Adopting sound sleeping habits can help you get a good night's rest. Here are some hints for a more peaceful night:

■ Determine how much sleep you really need and then program your body by going to bed and getting up at about the same time every day. If, occasionally, you aren't able to get to bed on time, try to rise at your usual time anyway.

■ Limit nap times to about a half an hour per day. Avoid napping late in the day.

■ Get regular exercise: It has been shown to improve sleep. However, don't exercise right before bedtime because you'll be energized at the wrong time.

■ Plan activities you find relaxing such as reading a book (though maybe not the latest thriller) or doing a crossword puzzle toward bedtime. Save stimulating activities for earlier in the day.

■ Do not drink alcohol close to bedtime. It can interfere with sleep.

■ Avoid caffeine after 5 PM.

■ Adjust your meal plan to include a light snack at bedtime if low blood sugar levels are a problem at night or early in the morning.

■ Use your bedroom for sleeping, not as an extension of your office or family room.

■ Create a comfortable sleeping environment in your bedroom. Pay attention to light, noise, and temperature.

a row. You've been lying awake in bed worrying about something. Or you're getting over a bad cold. When your lifestyle is wiping you out, making rest, healthful eating, and regular exercise a priority can make a big difference. (If you're getting over an illness, follow your doctor's advice on whether or when to exercise.)

At other times you may not be sure why you're feeling so tired. Since fatigue can have so many different causes, it may help to note any other symptoms you are experiencing in addition to fatigue to pinpoint the cause of your fatigue. It may also help to identify when your exhaustion began and what else was happening in your life at the time. Sometimes, fatigue is the only sign you have that a particular event is causing psychological stress.

When fatigue lasts for more than two weeks without an obvious cause, consult your doctor. And make sure you call your doctor immediately when fatigue is sudden and severe or when it is accompanied by symptoms such as fever, shortness of breath, or chest pain. ❑

THE FLU
More Than Just a Nuisance
by Laura Hieronymus, R.N., M.S.Ed., C.D.E.

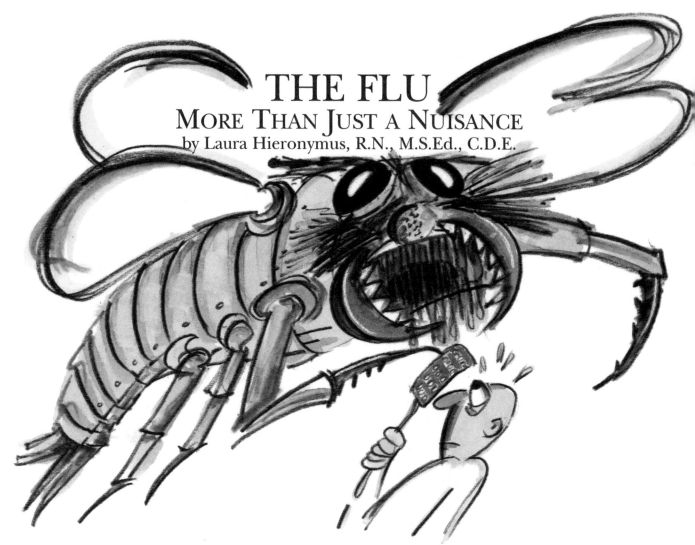

When the flu bug bites, it can be a pain in the neck for anyone. Not only do you feel terrible for days on end, but you basically have to put your life on hold until you feel better.

But the flu is not just a nuisance: In the United States, influenza (the flu) is a major cause of illness and death, causing, on average, approximately 20,000 deaths and over 110,000 hospitalizations each year. The toll among people with diabetes is particularly high: Individuals with diabetes who have the flu are six times more likely to end up in the hospital, and the death rate from complications of the flu, such as pneumonia, is three times higher in the diabetes population.

This article explains what the flu is, why it can be a big problem for people who have diabetes, and how you can avoid getting this potentially life-threatening infection.

The ABC's of influenza

Influenza is a respiratory infection caused by a virus. There are three main strains of the influenza virus: A, B, and C. The A and B strains tend to make individuals the sickest and cause flu epidemics. Infection with a C virus usually causes only mild respiratory symptoms or, in some cases, no symptoms at all. C strains do not cause epidemics.

The flu is highly contagious. It is most commonly spread from person to person when an infected person sneezes or coughs, releasing the virus into the air, where it can linger for hours. The virus is then inhaled by other persons, who may become infected. The flu can also be spread via contact with objects—such as door handles or faucets—that have been contaminated with the flu virus.

Onset of the flu happens fast, usually within 24 to 48 hours after a person has been infected. Symptoms can occur quite suddenly and usually begin with high fever and chills. Other symptoms may include feelings of fatigue, muscle or joint aches (common in the back and legs), runny nose, dry cough, and headache that worsens in bright light. Children with the flu may experience nausea, vomiting, and diarrhea; however, these symptoms are not common in adults. So-called "stomach flu" is usually not caused by the flu virus.

Flu symptoms usually begin to disappear in three to four days. However, the effects of the flu on the body may not totally disappear for one to two weeks, and the fatigue can linger for many more weeks.

The flu and diabetes

Having higher-than-normal blood sugar levels can impair the body's ability to fight off infection. So a person with diabetes who has high blood sugar is more susceptible to getting the flu. Such individuals are also likely to have a more difficult time recovering from the flu if their blood sugar is not brought down to recommended goals.

Complicating matters, however, is that the stress hormones released when a person has the flu tend to raise blood sugar. Having the flu is a physical stress, and when stress occurs, the body reacts by secreting higher-than-normal amounts of the hormones epinephrine, cortisol, and glucagon. These hormones cause extra glucose to be released from the liver to give the body extra energy to cope.

In people who don't have diabetes, the pancreas responds to the extra glucose by secreting extra insulin so that the glucose can be used by the cells. But in people who have diabetes, the pancreas either no longer produces insulin or may not produce enough to balance the effect of the stress hormones. The result is higher blood sugar levels. Taking steps such as monitoring more frequently and perhaps using supplemental insulin (based on the advice of a doctor), may be essential to assist with blood glucose control. The potential for extremely high blood sugar during an illness is greater among people whose blood sugar control was not optimal before the illness.

As the flu infection resolves, blood sugar levels should come back down, and the normal diabetes management routine reinstated. However, having sustained high blood sugar during an illness can make it more difficult to bring levels back down after the illness.

An ounce of prevention

The most effective way to avoid getting the flu is to get a flu vaccine every year. Healthy lifestyle measures, including maintaining control of blood glucose, getting enough sleep, eating right, getting moderate exercise, and washing hands frequently, help, too.

Flu vaccines are recommended annually because the viral strains change, or mutate, all the time. So the flu shot you got last year probably won't protect you this year. In the United States, the flu vaccine is made from inactivated, or "killed," influenza viruses identified as major strains for the year. The flu vaccine for the 2000–2001 season contained three virus strains: A/Panama, A/Caledonia, and B/Yamanashi.

Because the virus is inactivated, flu vaccines do not cause the flu. Some people have some soreness, redness, or swelling on the arm where the shot is given, and about 5% to 10% of people have mild side effects such as headache or a low fever for about a day after

DRUGS TO TREAT THE FLU

Four antiviral drugs have been approved to treat people who get the flu, and three can also be used for prevention. If used promptly, the drugs can shorten the duration of flu symptoms by about a day. All require a prescription from a physician. Precautions, side effects, and contraindications should be reviewed with a doctor or pharmacist before use.

■ Amantadine (brand name Symmetrel) is approved to treat symptoms caused by influenza A and to be taken for prevention of influenza A in persons age one and older. It is taken as a pill or a syrup. Amantadine can cause lightheadedness, nervousness, difficulty concentrating, and inability to sleep.

■ Oseltamivir (Tamiflu) is approved to treat symptoms of influenza A and B in persons age one and older and to be taken for prevention in persons age 13 and older. It is taken as a pill or a liquid suspension. Oseltamivir can cause nausea and vomiting if not taken with food.

■ Rimantadine (Flumadine) is approved to treat symptoms caused by influenza A in persons age 14 and older and to be taken for prevention of influenza A in persons age one and older. It is taken as a pill or a syrup. Rimantadine can cause lightheadedness, nervousness, difficulty concentrating, and inability to sleep, although it appears to do so less frequently than amantadine.

■ Zanamivir (Relenza) is approved to treat symptoms of influenza A and B in persons age seven and older. It is inhaled by mouth. Zanamivir can cause a decline in respiration rate and volume as well as spasmodic contractions of the airways, and is not generally recommended for people with chronic respiratory disease.

vaccination. For most people, the danger from getting the flu far outweighs any danger from the side effects of the vaccine.

Even with a yearly vaccine, it is difficult to provide total protection from the flu. For one thing, the flu shot is not 100% effective. The U.S. Centers for Disease Control and Prevention (CDC) reports that flu vaccines are 70% to 90% effective in preventing influenza in healthy adults. If a person is elderly or has a chronic disease, the vaccine may be less effective. However, people who get the flu after having a flu shot are likely to have a milder case than if they hadn't had the shot.

There are some other reasons a person who has had a flu shot may get the flu. There may be minor strains of the influenza virus, not covered by the vaccine, in circulation. Or one of the viruses identified as a major strain for the year may change slightly after the vaccine for the year has been made. And some people—whether they've had the flu shot or not—think they have the flu when they really have another respiratory infection with similar symptoms.

Who should get a flu shot

Most individuals would probably benefit from getting a flu shot, especially since the flu virus is easily transmitted and can quickly spread through a family, close down a school, and even disrupt corporate production when many workers are off the job simultaneously. For some people, however, the flu carries greater risks than feeling ill for a week and missing school or work. According to the CDC, the following people are at risk for serious illness from the flu and should get a flu shot every year:

■ People 65 years of age and older.
■ Residents of nursing homes and other long-term care facilities.
■ Adults and children who have chronic heart or lung diseases.
■ Adults and children with diabetes, kidney disease, or severe forms of anemia.
■ Health-care workers who come in contact with people in high-risk groups.
■ Caregivers or people who live with someone in a high-risk group.

Other candidates for the flu shot include women who will be in their second or third trimester of pregnancy during flu season, which is generally December through March in the United States.

You may be advised not to get a flu shot if any of the following apply to you:

■ You are allergic to eggs. The viruses for flu vaccines are grown in eggs and may cause severe allergic reactions in persons with egg allergies.
■ You have had Guillain–Barré syndrome, especially within six weeks of getting a flu shot. This syndrome affects the nerves and produces rapidly worsening muscle weakness, sometimes leading to paralysis.
■ You have had any past reaction attributed to the flu vaccine.
■ You are allergic to thimerosal, a preservative used in many vaccines and in contact lens solution.

If there is any reason you think you should not get a flu shot, be sure to discuss it with your diabetes-care team. If you can't get a shot (and even if you can), consider the vaccination for the rest of your family (every-

one over two years old) to reduce your risk of illness. Since flu season in the United States is primarily in the winter months, fall (late September or early October) is the prime time to get the vaccination. If you don't have a regular doctor's appointment scheduled during the fall months, it may be in your best interest to call the office and set up a time. If you get your flu shot in another setting, such as the local health department or your workplace, be sure you let the doctor's office staff know, so that the vaccination can be documented in your medical record. It takes approximately two weeks after you get the vaccine to develop protection against the flu.

Pneumonia

While you're thinking about getting a flu shot, think also about getting a pneumonia vaccination if you haven't had one already. Pneumonia is an infection of the lungs and a common complication of the flu. It can be caused by the flu virus itself or by a secondary bacterial infection that sets in when the lungs are weakened by the flu. (There are other causes of pneumonia, as well.)

Symptoms of pneumonia include chest pain (especially with breathing), shortness of breath, cough, chills, fever, and fatigue. While young, healthy people can have pneumonia and not even know it, older people and those with weakened immune systems (because of treatment for cancer, for example) can become seriously ill and even die. If you experience the symptoms of pneumonia, particularly on the heels of a bout with the flu, see your doctor.

The pneumonia vaccine protects only against pneumococcal pneumonia, the most common form of bacterial pneumonia. However, since the flu virus can also cause pneumonia, getting a flu shot will help protect against that type of viral pneumonia as well. The pneumococcal pneumonia vaccine is recommended for everyone 65 or older and for people with diabetes of any age.

A pound of cure

If you get the flu (or any other illness for that matter), being prepared is key. Even while you are coping with the illness, you need to pay extra attention to your diabetes and blood sugar control. Talk with your diabetes-care team ahead of time about guidelines for sick days. It is best to have the guidelines in writing, so that when the time comes, you will have them to refer to. As you develop your sick-day guidelines with your diabetes-care team, the following suggestions may be helpful:

Check blood sugar levels at least every four hours when you feel sick. People who use a rapid-acting insulin such as lispro (brand name Humalog) with an insulin pump may need to check every two hours. The goal is to look for patterns in your blood sugar levels. If your blood sugar goes up (or down) and stays there, you will likely need to call your doctor. Discuss with your diabetes-care team at what blood sugar level you should call.

Check your urine for ketones if your blood sugar levels are higher than 240 mg/dl or if you experience gastrointestinal symptoms such as nausea, vomiting, or stomach pain. Such symptoms can be caused by the presence of ketones in the blood. Ketones are more common with sustained high blood sugar in people with Type 1 diabetes. However, during the stress of illness, individuals with Type 2 diabetes may produce ketones as well. Having ketones present in the urine means that the body is breaking down fat stores for energy. This is abnormal and can lead to coma and death if not treated.

Most people don't feel like eating or drinking much when they are ill, but it is important to try to sip liquids to help prevent dehydration. Sugar-free soft drinks or water may be consumed at any time. If you can't eat solid foods, stick to your meal plan as well as possible by substituting soft foods or beverages that contain carbohydrate in the amounts you need. You may need to try a little at a time to be sure you can tolerate it. The following items contain approximately a serving (15 grams) of carbohydrate each:

- ⅓ to ½ cup fruit juice
- ½ cup regular (not sugar-free) soft drink
- ½ cup regular gelatin
- ½ cup vanilla ice cream
- ½ cup hot cereal (such as Cream of Wheat)
- 1 cup broth-based soup

Even if you are not eating and drinking normally, you are likely to need your diabetes medicines when ill. As you monitor your blood sugar (more frequently with illness), the results will help you or your doctor make any necessary medication adjustments.

Consult with your diabetes-care team or pharmacist when selecting over-the-counter products to treat symptoms of illness such as fever, cough, or sore throat. It is important to be aware of which products are the safest for you. You may want to avoid items that contain sugar, alcohol, or certain other ingredients such as pseudoephedrine, which may disrupt blood sugar control. Children and teens should avoid taking aspirin for flu symptoms because of the possibility of developing Reye syndrome. (For more information on drug safety, see "Over-the-Counter Drugs" on page 128.)

If you are taking any prescription drugs to treat the flu, be sure you understand exactly how to take them,

IS IT A COLD OR THE FLU?

This chart is based on advice from the U.S. National Institute of Allergy and Infectious Diseases. Use it to figure out what your symptoms are telling you and what sort of complications to look out for.

SYMPTOMS	COLD	FLU
Fever	Rare	Characteristic, high (102°F to 104°F); lasts three to four days
Headache	Rare	Prominent
General aches, pains	Slight	Usual; often severe
Fatigue, weakness	Quite mild	Can last up to 2–3 weeks
Extreme exhaustion	Never	Early and prominent
Stuffy nose	Common	Sometimes
Sneezing	Usual	Sometimes
Sore throat	Common	Sometimes
Chest discomfort, cough	Mild to moderate; hacking cough	Common; can become severe
COMPLICATIONS	Sinus congestion or earache	Bronchitis, pneumonia; can be life-threatening
PREVENTION	None	Annual vaccination; drugs—amantadine, oseltamivir, or rimantadine
TREATMENT	Only temporary relief of symptoms	Amantadine, oseltamivir, rimantadine, or zanamivir within 24 to 48 hours after onset of symptoms

and be aware of any precautions, side effects, and contraindications (reasons not to take them). Get the prescription filled as soon as possible: The drugs are most effective in treating the flu if started within 24 to 48 hours of the onset of symptoms. (See "Drugs to Treat the Flu" on page 355 for more information.)

As a general rule, antibiotics are not used to treat viral infections such as the flu. However, if you develop a bacterial infection (such as pneumonia) as a complication of the flu, you may need to take one.

Resting is probably the best thing you can do for yourself when sick, but if you are sleeping a lot during the day, don't forget about your diabetes-care routine. Set an alarm as a reminder to check blood sugar levels and take medicines on schedule.

Take care to avoid spreading the virus by washing your hands frequently and by covering your mouth and nose with a tissue when you cough or sneeze.

Take your temperature every four hours and keep a record of it. Even if you don't think you have a fever, it is useful information to determine if fever is present.

Confirm with your doctor when he or she expects you to call. Most doctors expect you to call in the following situations:
■ Your blood sugar levels (at least two consecutive checks) stay outside your sick-day management goals.
■ You have moderate to large amounts of ketones in your urine.
■ Your sickness lasts longer than 24 hours.
■ You experience nausea, vomiting, or diarrhea over several hours.
■ Your temperature stays over 101°F.
■ You have difficulty breathing or unusual pain.

Be prepared

Getting a flu shot is the best way to prevent or at least minimize your chances of getting the flu. The flu shot is covered by Medicare, most health maintenance organizations, and many private insurance plans. If you do become ill, be prepared with sick-day guidelines to avoid getting any sicker from high blood sugar levels. After all, when your health is at stake, an ounce of prevention is worth a pound of cure! ❏

MORE THAN JUST A PRETTY SMILE
ORAL HEALTH FOR PEOPLE WITH DIABETES
by Joan I. Gluch, R.D.H., Ph.D., and Susanne K. Giorgio, R.D.H.

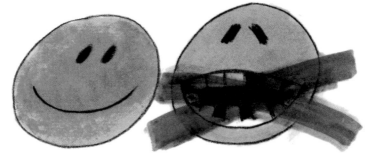

To most people, a pretty smile means white, straight teeth and fresh breath. However, a pretty smile may not always be a healthy smile, and people with diabetes face special challenges in keeping both a healthy and pretty smile. Recent research has shown a relationship between healthy gums and teeth, blood glucose levels in the normal range, and overall good health in people with diabetes. Each one is dependent on the other two. This three-way interdependence challenges people with diabetes to keep their mouths healthy as part of their diabetes care regimen.

To see how oral health and blood glucose levels affect each other, let's see what happened to one man with diabetes when he developed an apparently minor gum problem. John, age 72, had had diabetes for 20 years, and his blood sugar levels were generally in his target range. For the past month, however, he had had problems maintaining control of his blood glucose levels. Both he and his doctor were confused as to why his blood glucose levels were fluctuating.

At his routine dental cleaning visit, John mentioned the problem to the dental hygienist. A thorough evaluation of his mouth revealed that John had developed a gum pocket next to one of his molars. Although John had no discomfort or pain in this area, this pocket indicated an infection. (In a person with diabetes, any infection in the body can raise blood glucose levels.) After a thorough cleaning of the pocket and of his teeth and a review of his oral hygiene techniques, the infection was eliminated, and his blood glucose levels stabilized a short time later.

Like many people with diabetes, John was careful with his oral hygiene and kept regular appointments for preventive care with his dental hygienist. However, people with diabetes are particularly susceptible to gum infections, or periodontal diseases. Like John, everyone with diabetes must be alert to the early signs of periodontal disease (more on this later) and maintain a schedule of frequent oral evaluations and cleanings. Oral hygiene procedures are critical to maintaining not only oral health but good overall health.

Diabetes and periodontal diseases

While many people know about diabetic complications of the eyes, kidneys, nerves, blood vessels, and heart, few know much about the connection between periodontal health and diabetes. Periodontal diseases are infections in the mouth that affect the soft gum tissues and the supporting bone that holds the teeth in place. People with diabetes, particularly those with chronic high blood glucose levels, are more susceptible to bacterial infections everywhere in the body, including in the mouth. In addition to making a person susceptible to infections, high blood glucose levels also inhibit the healing of infections. When an infection in the mouth tissues is not controlled, the teeth can become loose, and chewing can become painful or difficult. An uncontrolled infection can eventually cause tooth loss.

High blood glucose levels can raise the risk of periodontal disease in another way as well: When blood glucose levels are high, the glucose levels in all body fluids, including saliva, become very high. Certain bacteria feed on sugar and grow readily in the mouth, particularly when saliva glucose levels are high. And having higher levels of these bacteria in the mouth increases the risk for both periodontal diseases and dental decay.

One early complication of diabetes—namely, changes in the blood vessel walls—can also increase the risk of developing periodontal diseases. In short, the vessel walls become thicker. Blood is necessary to bring oxygen and nutrients to all body tissues and to remove waste products made by cells in the body tissues. Thicker blood vessel walls slow down these processes and weaken resistance to infection. Without a good blood supply, the periodontal tissues become too weak to fight infections.

The impact that smoking has on the lungs and heart is widely publicized. Less well known is that smoking has a major impact on the development and severity of periodontal diseases. Scientific studies show that smokers are five times more likely than nonsmokers to have periodontal diseases and that smokers have more severe forms of periodontal diseases. The combination of smoking and diabetes even further increases the risk of periodontal diseases, especially in people with chronic high blood glucose levels.

However, periodontal disease is not inevitable for people with diabetes. Research has shown that keeping blood glucose levels in the target range lowers the risk of developing diabetic complications of the eye, nerve, kidney, and heart. This is also true for periodontal diseases. Many scientific studies show that people with chronic high blood glucose levels develop periodontal diseases more often and more severely and have a greater chance of losing teeth than people whose blood sugar stays in the target, near-nondiabetic, range. It has also been shown that people with diabetes who can maintain near-normal blood sugar levels have no more periodontal diseases than people who don't have diabetes. To ensure healthy periodontal tissues, blood glucose control (along with not smoking) is key.

If you are having difficulty with blood glucose control, consider being evaluated by an oral health-care professional to screen for periodontal diseases. Recent scientific findings suggest that severe periodontal diseases may influence the course of diabetes. A combination of antibiotic treatment and traditional periodontal therapy has been shown to be effective in reducing blood glucose levels and in helping people with diabetes to maintain blood glucose control.

How periodontal diseases develop

There are two general categories of periodontal diseases: *gingivitis* and *periodontitis*. Both are infections. Gingivitis generally occurs when a person does not brush thoroughly enough or clean well enough between the teeth. As bacterial plaque builds up, an infection develops. Signs of gingivitis include gum tissue that is redder than normal, bleeds easily, or appears swollen. Gingivitis can be reversed by proper oral hygiene and professional dental care, which includes thorough and frequent cleaning. If gingivitis continues, it can lead to a more serious type of gum disease, periodontitis, which is an infection of the bone and soft tissue surrounding the teeth.

In periodontitis, the plaque buildup that occurred at and above the gum line in gingivitis now extends underneath the tissue. The gum tissue pulls away from the tooth, allowing pockets to form, which trap more plaque bacteria and food particles. Infection continues into the pockets and starts destroying the bone surrounding the teeth. The gum tissues recede, the tooth becomes loose, and in severe cases, it can eventually be lost.

It is important to note that in the early stages of gum infections, there is no pain or warning signs to alert the person that an infection is present. Pain or discomfort may not be noticed until later stages, when abscesses (accumulations of pus) or loose teeth occur.

Professional help

Control of periodontal diseases includes both professional dental treatment and careful oral home care. Both of these treatment components are necessary; if either one is missing, periodontal diseases can progress more rapidly.

Visit the dental office at least twice a year. More frequent visits may be recommended depending on the health of your mouth tissues and your diabetes control. At each dental visit, remind your hygienist and dentist that you have diabetes. Give them a clear idea of your current state of diabetes control, including current blood glucose levels. This information is important to each dental visit: If oral problems are present, your dentist will want to consult your doctor to ensure that you get appropriate care and to avoid any emergency.

To determine whether you have periodontal disease, dental professionals conduct a periodontal examination. The exam includes measuring the spaces between the gums and teeth with a small, ruler like instrument called a periodontal probe. The exam also includes taking individual x-rays of the teeth to evaluate the supporting bone around the teeth and gums. Examinations for periodontal diseases should be done at least every six months and sometimes more frequently in people with diabetes.

How periodontal disease is treated depends on the extent of the disease and the amount of damage to the gum and bone. Treatment may include removal of soft and hard plaque above and below the gum line, treatment with antibiotics, and special antibacterial mouthrinses. If the periodontal disease is very advanced, surgical procedures may be recommended to allow access to very deep pockets, to reshape damaged bone, and to replace damaged supporting structures.

Although brushing and flossing remove most bacterial plaque on the surfaces of the teeth, oral bacteria can also hide in the spaces between the teeth and under the gum line—places most home-care products can't reach. Dental hygienists and dentists use small dental scalers to thoroughly remove all hard and soft plaque above and below the gum line. The professional term for these procedures is *debridement* or *scaling and root planing*. Periodontal debridement is more

than just a "cleaning" because these procedures thoroughly remove the major bacterial causes for periodontal diseases and help create smooth surfaces that will encourage the healing gum tissues to tighten around the teeth. For someone with periodontal disease, debridement is generally completed in segments over several visits. A series of visits allows the oral health-care professional to evaluate how well the person is healing and whether other additional therapies are needed.

In conjunction with debridement, dental professionals may also use and prescribe antibacterial products to further reduce plaque levels to promote healing of the periodontal tissues. When the spaces between the teeth and gums become too large and the supporting bone is lost around the teeth, gum surgery may be recommended.

Daily home care

Daily oral hygiene care is essential for health. But choosing which oral home-care products to use can be difficult because of the great number of products available today. Not every product is best for every person. Individuals should seek the advice of a dental hygienist or dentist to learn which products are best for them and to learn how to use these products in the best way to remove the most plaque bacteria. Experts agree that the most important factor is not the specific brand or product used but rather how frequently and effectively the individual uses the product to clean the mouth.

The American Dental Association evaluates oral hygiene products through the Council on Dental Therapeutics and designates products as "accepted" when they meet the standards set by the Association. When selecting oral-care products, you may want to access the American Dental Association Web site to check which products have been accepted.

Brushing. In the past decade or so, we have seen a tremendous change in the availability and design of toothbrushes. Toothbrushes now come in a variety of bristle and handle styles. Battery-powered toothbrushes are also available with rotating bristles, sonic vibrations, or unusual brush heads. The American Dental Association rates a number of toothbrushes, both battery-powered and manual, as acceptable and does not designate any one toothbrush type as superior. However, experts agree that a soft-textured bristle in the toothbrush is best and that people should choose a brush that they like and can use comfortably. Firm bristles in medium or hard textures are no longer recommended.

When brushing your teeth, the bristles of the toothbrush should be placed into the space between the gum and the tooth (the *sulcus*) with a small, vibrating motion. This technique, called sulcular brushing, removes the plaque bacteria that lodges in the sulcus. Soft-bristled toothbrushes are preferable because toothbrushes with medium or hard bristles, when placed in the sulcus, can tear or otherwise damage gum tissue, possibly causing the gum to recede from the tooth.

After completing sulcular brushing, use gentle strokes to clean the insides of the cheeks, the tongue, and chewing surfaces of all of the teeth in a thorough manner. Only small, gentle strokes should be used. Avoid large, scrubbing motions, which can damage the gum tissue and teeth.

The tongue should be brushed with gentle sweeping strokes to remove all the surface bacteria and debris that collects readily each day. It is best to start from the back of the tongue and use long, gentle, forward strokes to the tip of the tongue. Tongue cleaning can be done with either a soft toothbrush or a flexible tongue scraper. It is especially important for people with dry mouth—a common problem for people with diabetes—because the less saliva there is in the mouth, the more easily bacteria will collect on the tongue and mouth tissues. Regular tongue cleaning can help you avoid oral infections and bad breath.

Everyone should brush his teeth at least twice a day, and most experts recommend brushing in the morning and before bedtime at a minimum. Many people like to brush after meals to remove food particles and bacteria more frequently. However, the length of time and the thoroughness of brushing is more important than the number of times you brush during the day. Most people don't spend enough time brushing their teeth. Experts recommend brushing for at least three minutes and suggest brushing for the length of a song on the radio or using a three-minute timer to ensure adequate brushing.

Using a powered toothbrush, many of which have a built-in timer, can also help people increase their brushing time and effectiveness. Powered tooth-

PERIODONTITIS
Periodontal disease develops when a sticky film of bacteria called plaque builds up under the gum line. As the plaque hardens, the gum tissues pull away from the teeth, forming pockets of infection. Untreated periodontal disease will cause the gums to recede, and teeth may loosen or even fall out.

FLOSSING
Daily flossing removes trapped food and bacteria from between the teeth and under the gums and helps to prevent periodontal disease. To floss, first gently saw the floss down between two teeth. Then curve the floss around each tooth and scrape back and forth from below the gum to the top of the tooth.

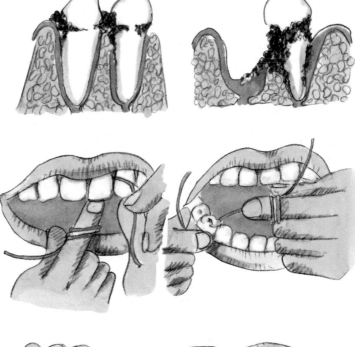

BRUSHING
Brush your teeth twice a day with a soft-bristled toothbrush and fluoride toothpaste. Use small, vibrating motions to clean along the gum line, where your gums and teeth meet. Then gently brush the chewing surfaces of all the teeth, the insides of the cheeks, and the tongue. Avoid large, scrubbing motions, which can damage the gum tissue and teeth.

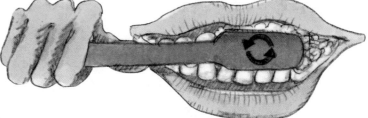

FOR MORE INFORMATION

For further information about dental products and good oral health, contact the following organizations by calling the phone numbers listed or visiting their Web sites:

AMERICAN DENTAL ASSOCIATION
(312) 440-2500
www.ada.org/public
Call or visit the Web site for information about finding a dentist and the seal of acceptance program. The seal of acceptance page of the Web site allows you to search for specific brand names of oral-care products to see if your favorite product has received the seal of acceptance.

AMERICAN DENTAL HYGIENISTS'
ASSOCIATION
(800) 243-ADHA (243-2342)
www.adha.org
This Web site offers information on oral hygiene methods and dental hygiene care. You can also call for fact sheets and other information.

AMERICAN ACADEMY OF PERIODONTOLOGY
(800) FLOSS-EM (356-7736)
www.perio.org/consumer
The consumer section of this association's Web site offers assistance in finding a periodontist and provides information about periodontal health and periodontal diseases. You can also order a free brochure about diabetes and oral health.

brushes are often easier to use and remove more plaque bacteria than traditional toothbrushes. Many older people find that it is easier to grasp the larger handle and guide the powered toothbrush in their mouths, especially if they have limited motion in their hands or arms. Powered toothbrushes must be used carefully in a gentle guiding motion, never with large scrubbing strokes. Powered toothbrushes also make it easier for caretakers to brush someone else's teeth. Since brush action is provided by the powered brush, caretakers need only guide the brush in the mouth. However, powered toothbrushes are often expensive to purchase and maintain, especially since brush heads and batteries must be replaced periodically.

You should replace your toothbrush at least every three months. Experts agree that a new toothbrush will remove more plaque than a toothbrush with frayed or missing bristles. Bacteria will grow on tooth-brush bristles, so toothbrushes should be replaced after illnesses, especially cold sores on the lips.

Flossing. Regular toothbrushing removes bacterial plaque from most tooth surfaces. However, standard toothbrush bristles cannot penetrate deeply enough to thoroughly clean between the teeth. To prevent periodontal diseases, use some type of device to clean between your teeth at least once a day.

Using dental floss is the most common way to clean between the teeth. In the past five years, several new floss products—some of which are flavored or more heavily waxed—have become available that make it easier and more convenient to floss. Waxed dental floss is much easier to use than unwaxed because it slides through the tooth contacts without shredding, and experts agree that waxed floss is equally effective in removing bacterial plaque.

To floss, break off a comfortable length of floss, usually 12 to 18 inches, and wrap it around your index and middle fingers or tie it in a circle for easier use. Flossing consists of two basic motions. First, gently saw the floss down between the tight contacting portions of the teeth. Never snap the floss down because this could injure the gum tissue. Second, gently scrape the side of each tooth with the floss, starting below the gum line. Many people only remove food particles when they floss and never do the gentle scraping motion that removes most of the bacterial plaque.

Sometimes the gum tissue may bleed slightly during flossing. This bleeding indicates early periodontal disease and a need for more thorough removal of plaque bacteria. If you see bleeding when you floss, alert your dental hygienist or dentist. And rather than avoiding that area of your mouth, floss and brush the area more thoroughly to remove the bacterial plaque that is causing the bleeding tissues.

Another method to clean between the teeth is to use small tapered (interproximal) brushes or toothpicks. These are especially useful if the gum tissue has lost its tight contour against the teeth and larger spaces are present between the teeth. Water pulsating devices can also be used with antibacterial rinses to flush out bacteria. However, water pulsating devices may not be appropriate for some people, so check with your dental hygienist or dentist for advice regarding the best products and customized instructions for your mouth.

Mouthwash. Many people use mouthwash for fresh breath, but most major brands of mouthwash contain alcohol, which tends to dry out the mouth. Since many people with diabetes already experience a dry mouth, using an alcohol-based rinse is not advisable, even though some of them do control gingivitis. Instead, people with diabetes should brush with toothpaste to control gingivitis.

Other dental problems

In addition to periodontal diseases, there are some other dental problems that people with diabetes frequently encounter. Dry mouth is a common side effect of both insulin and drugs used to treat high blood pressure and depression. The dry feeling in the mouth comes from a reduction in saliva, and it can cause soreness and ulcers. Frequent sips of water and artificial saliva products (available at most drugstores) can help reduce the dry feeling.

A dry mouth also increases the chance of developing dental cavities, because the acids that cause decay are not diluted as much as usual by saliva. In addition, people with diabetes tend to have higher glucose levels in the saliva, and this increases the risk for dental decay. Everyone with diabetes should use fluoride each day to prevent dental cavities. Fluoride is found in some toothpastes and mouthrinses. (Remember to avoid mouthrinses that contain alcohol.) Special fluoride gel treatments can be provided at the dental office and given for use at home for people who are experiencing several areas of dental decay.

Fungal infections (also called thrush) can be found in many people with diabetes due to the high glucose levels found in the saliva. People who wear dentures or partial plates are especially at risk for fungal infections in the mouth and mouth ulcers when their mouths are dry. Most fungal infections appear as white patches that easily rub away to reveal sore, red tissue, but not all fungal infections fit this pattern. If you have false teeth, keep them as clean as possible and visit the dental office as soon as possible if ulcers appear. Because false teeth can be infected with the bacteria or fungus causing the mouth infection, treatment should include using medicines both in the mouth and on the denture.

People with diabetes face special challenges in preventing periodontal diseases. Good preventive care, including both thorough oral hygiene care and frequent visits to the dental office, is essential to maintaining a healthy mouth, optimum blood glucose levels, and good overall health. Everyone deserves a pretty and a healthy smile! ❑

SHOPPING FOR EYEGLASSES

by Joseph Gustaitis

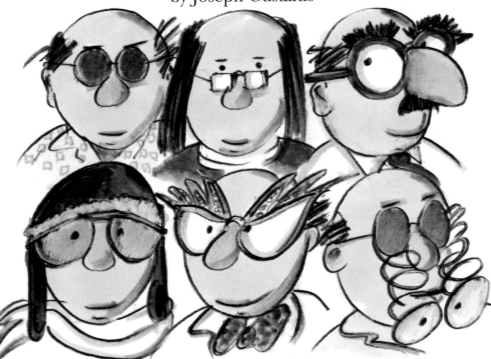

Eyeglasses, like many other things, prove that yesterday's necessity can become today's fashion statement. Glasses are now available in a dizzying range of frames, styles, colors, and shapes. And not only that—a wearer faces some fairly technical decisions that go beyond looks. Do you want (or need) high-index lenses? Progressive lenses? A keyhole bridge? UV protection? What are these things anyway? And are there any special considerations for people with diabetes?

The specialists

When buying eyeglasses, the first thing you have to consider is the kind of eye-care professional you will choose. The three specialists are the ophthalmologist, the optometrist, and the optician. An ophthalmologist is a medical doctor with an M.D. degree, which means this person will have not only a knowledge of your eyes but of the rest of your body—and how any ailments you may have can affect your eyes. Because they are physicians, ophthalmologists are able to treat disease and perform surgery (the field is becoming increasingly specialized). An optometrist is someone who has graduated from a postgraduate optometry course and has an O.D. degree. As a rule, optometrists confine themselves to prescribing glasses, giving eye exams, diagnosing eye diseases, and administering vision therapy, although recently some optometrists have been licensed to treat some eye diseases. An optician fills eyeglass prescriptions and fits lenses and other optical devices. Although opticians do not prescribe eyeglasses or conduct eye exams, because they deal with a great many people, they are usually the best source of information on frames, design, and fit. In many states, however, opticians are not required to be licensed, so the level of expertise you encounter can vary.

The eye exam

Whether your eye examination is done by an ophthalmologist or an optometrist, that person usually begins with basic questions about your general health, your history of eye problems, your family history, and your past experience with glasses. You are tested to see how well you see things at a distance and up close, how your eyes work together, and how good your peripheral vision is. The examiner also uses a process called *refraction*. This can be done with several methods; it may involve shining a light into your eye or using a computerized machine. The purpose is to determine which lens combination works best for you.

The examiner will also use special devices to look at the structures within your eyes and to measure the interior pressure. Measuring the interior pressure tests for glaucoma, a disorder that damages the optic nerve and causes vision loss. Sometimes the examiner will dilate the pupil with eyedrops in order to view the retina. If necessary, the examiner may call for tests that are not routine—tests that look at such things as visual fields, coordination, and color vision. Because some of the complications associated with diabetes take the form of eye problems (such as diabetic retinopathy, cataracts, and glaucoma), it is recommended that persons with diabetes have a glaucoma

test and a dilated-pupil exam performed at least annually by an ophthalmologist or optometrist who is knowledgeable about diabetic eye problems and their management.

The problem that glasses correct is known as *refractive error*, a condition in which the eye's lens focuses the incoming light either short of the retina (resulting in nearsightedness, or *myopia*) or beyond it (resulting in farsightedness, or *hyperopia*). When an examiner discovers either of these, that person writes a prescription for glasses (or contact lenses), enabling you to have corrected vision.

For people with diabetes, however, the procedure may not be so simple. This is due to the fact that a rise in blood sugar level can cause swelling in the lens of the eye and bring about a change in refractive error—that is, a vision change. Indeed, blurry vision is often an indication that blood sugar is high. Because this change may be temporary, the timing of a lens prescription is critical. If your glasses are prescribed at a time when your refractive error has been altered by high blood sugar, they will probably not work properly when your blood sugar level returns to normal. Consequently, experts recommend that you not be measured for glasses if you have recently changed your glucose-control regimen. And when you are measured for glasses, you should be certain that your blood sugar level has been stable for a few weeks.

The big frame-up

OK, so you've had your exam (at the proper time) and the examiner says you need glasses. You've got your prescription and you're ready to be fitted.

How much can you expect to pay? The eyeglass industry reported near the end of the 1990's that the average pair of glasses in the United States sold for about $150. According to a 1996 survey of some 50,000 *Consumer Reports* readers (published in the July 1997 issue), the figure was a bit higher. The average cost of a pair of glasses between 1994 and 1996 at a doctor's office was $171, at a small shop $166, and at a large chain it ranged from $102 to $210 per pair—a smaller difference than one might expect. Of course, it's like buying a car: Start adding extra features and the price can climb much higher. If you want the name of a trendy designer on your frames, expect to pay for it.

Everyone wants his glasses to be attractive, but not all frames suit all lens prescriptions—or faces. The lens you need may not fit properly into the frame you covet. And that frame may not fit your face, which means that the lenses won't align correctly over your eyes.

A typical eyeglass frame has several elements that you need to consider. The part that lies on each side of your head is known as the temple. Skull temples, the most common, are slightly curved to bend over and rest on top of your ears. Library temples are straight to make the glasses easy to remove, but they are also the most likely to slip. Comfort cables are U-shaped coils that wrap around the back of the ears, and they give glasses the securest hold. When trying on glasses, it's important to make sure that whatever temples you have, they don't interfere with your peripheral vision. The hinges at the corners of the frame also help keep the eyeglasses on your face; many people like spring hinges for their security. The bridge is the part above the nose. A keyhole bridge puts most of the glasses' weight on the sides, and a more rounded saddle bridge distributes the weight along the top and sides of the nose. Adjustable nose pads are a third option; they can be moved in, out, or down to get the best fit.

Looking into lenses

In addition to pondering the frame, you have to consider the lenses. In fact, the lens often determines the frame, at least in part. Some frames are too thin or too shallow to carry the kinds of lenses that are needed. But if your vision is poor, it doesn't mean you're going to have to wear "Coke-bottle" lenses in thick clunky frames. Today you have the option of high-index lenses. Because high-index lenses are made of especially dense material, they can be thinner—and more attractive. And if they're made out of plastic (rather than glass) they can be surprisingly light.

Glass versus plastic is another consideration. Traditionally, glass, although heavier, had the advantage of being more scratch-resistant than plastic. Nowadays, however, special coatings have made plastic lenses much harder to scratch. Plastic is also less likely to crack, break, or shatter than glass. If you want tinted lenses, it's worth remembering that on glass lenses, tints are applied as a coating, and that coating can wear off. Tinted plastic lenses, however, are tinted throughout. You've probably heard of lenses that darken and brighten according to the light. They're called *photochromic* lenses, and most opticians believe that this option works better in glass than in plastic. Other options are UV protection, a dye that screens out ultraviolet light that can damage the eye, anti-reflection coating, which cuts down glare, and polycarbonate lenses, which are more expensive than regular plastic lenses but are very highly impact-resistant.

Lenses also come in different configurations, depending on what you use or need them for. If you need glasses for only one thing, say driving or reading, you likely need a *single-vision* lens. If your glasses serve more than one function, you may need a *multifocal* lens. The best-known multifocal lens is the bifocal,

WHAT ABOUT CONTACT LENSES?

Some 25 million Americans wear contact lenses. Can a person with diabetes be one of them? The answer is decidedly yes—with some qualifications.

Anyone who wears contact lenses, whether that person has diabetes or not, must commit to a program of careful hygiene. Failure to clean the lenses regularly can lead to infection. But people with diabetes, because their condition makes them more susceptible to infection in general, must exercise special vigilance by washing their hands before inserting the lenses, by cleaning and disinfecting the lenses faithfully as recommended, and by watching for signs of problems, such as discomfort or redness. If you follow such a regimen, your risk will be probably no greater than anyone else's. If you have problems following such a scrupulous regimen, your risk will be greater. For these reasons, eye-care professionals do not recommend extended-wear lenses for people with diabetes (these are the lenses that can be slept in and kept in the eye for up to a week). In fact, the trend is to discourage extended-wear lenses for anyone.

Another important issue is desensitivity of the cornea (the transparent part of the eyeball that covers the pupil and the iris). Some (not all) persons with diabetes develop a desensitized cornea—one that does not feel pain. And it is pain that tells you that something is wrong with your contacts. A person with diabetes needs to be tested for cornea desensitivity as part of an eye exam. This can be as simple as brushing the cornea lightly with cotton; a person with a normal cornea will blink. If you choose contacts, make sure this test is repeated at every eye exam. The contact lenses will not cause desensitivity, but it may develop while you are wearing them.

which combines prescriptions for reading and distance, but there are also trifocal lenses that contain an additional prescription for intermediate vision. Bifocals were once obvious because of the line they had across the lens, but today they can be made without it. As the wearer, you can tell you are wearing bifocals, but others can't. Even more sophisticated are progressive addition lenses. These incorporate a transition between the reading area and the distance area, so that all distances can be viewed as the eye scans up or down.

If you need reading glasses only, you've probably wondered about those off-the-rack glasses you see in drugstores and specialty shops. They can be fine—at those prices you can afford to have many pairs lying about wherever you might need one. Keep in mind, however, that the prescription in each lens is identical—if your eyes are different from each other, then off-the-rack glasses won't work best for you. Also, these glasses are made to fit an average face; if it turns out that they don't fit you properly, you may experience headaches or double vision.

Seeing how they work

According to the *Consumer Reports* survey, about a third of eyeglass buyers needed "substantial" adjustments to their new pair of specs; about one out of 10 reported headaches or similar problems (though that can be a reaction to a new prescription, not a problem with the prescription itself). This means that you have to take your glasses for a substantial test drive to make sure they're OK.

Eye-care specialists advise it will nearly always take you a little time to get used to new glasses, and you don't need to worry unless these problems don't go away after a few days. Getting used to multifocal lenses can be frustrating for some people, but most accomplish the task in time.

But if your glasses still don't seem right, go back to the shop and have them check a couple of things. First, is the prescription the correct one? Second, lenses have something called an *optical center* where the prescription is the most precise, and this spot should be directly over your pupil (the spot at the center of your eye). If it's not, you could experience double or blurred vision, aches, or dizziness. Now is also the time to make certain that the frame is sitting properly on your face. Some people have one ear slightly higher than the other, which causes lopsided glasses. Or it could be that one lens is slightly closer to your face than the other. A frame that tilts too much (or differently than your old pair of glasses) may also create a sense of discomfort. If you have chosen a large frame because you like the way it looks, you may find that it is too big, resulting in distortion or glare.

Whatever the problems, your eye-care professional has ways of double-checking the fit and the lens so that you should soon be both looking good—and seeing well. ❑

WOMEN'S CONCERNS

EXPECTING THE BEST
DIABETES, PREGNANCY, AND BLOOD GLUCOSE CONTROL

by Laura Hieronymus, R.N., M.S.Ed., C.D.E.,
and Patti Bazel Geil, M.S., R.D., L.D., C.D.E.

Pregnancy can be a special and exciting time in a woman's life. The anticipation begins as soon as you hear the words, "You're expecting a baby." Once you've gotten used to the amazing news, you may wonder about such things as whether the baby will be a boy or girl, when the baby is due, and, perhaps most important, what you need to do in the meantime to make sure the baby stays healthy and develops normally.

All women feel a certain amount of anxiety and sometimes even fear about how pregnancy will affect them and whether their baby will be healthy and normal. Women with diabetes are no different, but they do have one more thing to be concerned about: maintaining control of blood glucose levels. This is true whether a woman has Type 1 or Type 2 diabetes before becoming pregnant or whether she is diagnosed with a condition called gestational diabetes during pregnancy. The good news is that if a woman who has diabetes (of any type) learns as much as she can about managing her blood glucose and puts that knowledge into practice, she can have a healthy pregnancy and a healthy baby.

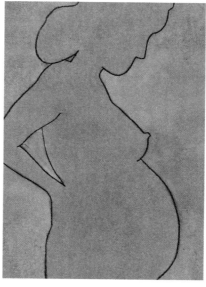

Blood glucose control essential

Optimal blood glucose control is important throughout pregnancy, both for the mother's health and the baby's. Glucose in a mother's blood crosses the *placenta* to her baby, affecting the baby's blood glucose level. (The placenta, a flat, circular organ, links the unborn baby to the mother's uterus to provide oxygen, nutrients, and elimination of wastes.) The baby begins making its own insulin around 13 weeks of ges-

tation. If the baby is constantly exposed to high levels of glucose, it is as if the baby were overeating: The baby produces more insulin to absorb the extra glucose, resulting in weight gain and an increase in size. Under these conditions, the baby can become too large, a condition known as *macrosomia.* Macrosomia is associated with difficult vaginal delivery, which can lead to birth injury and/or *asphyxia,* a condition in which the baby doesn't get enough oxygen.

Another reason that blood glucose control is important right up to the day of delivery is that if an unborn baby has high levels of insulin on a consistent basis or if the mother's blood glucose level is high during labor, the baby may experience hypoglycemia (low blood sugar) or other complications when the umbilical cord (and the maternal blood supply) is cut.

The details of managing blood glucose levels during pregnancy may be different for women who already have either Type 1 or Type 2 diabetes before pregnancy and for those who are diagnosed with diabetes during pregnancy, or gestational diabetes. (These differences are covered later in this article.) The recommended blood glucose goals, however, are the same.

It is important to note that the blood glucose goals suggested by the American Diabetes Association (ADA) for pregnant women are lower than those for the general population with diabetes. (See "Blood Glucose Goals During Pregnancy" on page 369.) In addition, the ADA suggests that pregnant women check their blood glucose levels up to eight times per day: once before each meal, again one hour after each meal, at bedtime, and once in the middle of the night. (Any woman who is taking insulin or certain kinds of blood-glucose-lowering pills would need to do additional checks before driving and if she experienced any symptoms of low blood sugar.) Your health-care team may recommend a somewhat different monitoring schedule depending on the type of diabetes you have and how you treat it. However, frequent self-monitoring is needed to ensure that blood glucose levels remain within the recommended range.

In addition to blood glucose monitoring, daily urine ketone testing is often advised for pregnant women with diabetes. Ketones are acid substances that collect in the bloodstream if the body is unable to break down glucose for energy. This can occur if there is not enough insulin to break down glucose in the bloodstream or if there is not enough glucose available to meet energy needs. In either case, the body begins to use stored fat for energy, a process that yields the acidic by-products called ketones. If the body is unable to get rid of the ketones fast enough (via the lungs and urine), they build up and can cause a potentially deadly condition called ketoacidosis.

Ketones in the blood during pregnancy are associated with decreased intelligence in the baby, and an episode of ketoacidosis during pregnancy greatly increases the risk of the fetus dying in the uterus. Diabetic ketoacidosis may develop rapidly and at lower blood glucose levels in women who are pregnant than in those who are not. The best approach for preventing this outcome is to closely monitor blood glucose levels outside the recommended range for pregnancy and to promptly treat elevated blood glucose levels, as directed by your diabetes management team. Notify your diabetes health-care team immediately if you detect ketones in your urine and have a high blood glucose level.

Ketones that occur when there isn't enough glucose in the bloodstream are called "starvation ketones." They may occur in women with gestational diabetes as well as in those with Type 1 or Type 2 diabetes. A woman with starvation ketones would typically have a blood glucose reading in the normal range or lower than normal. If you are getting starvation ketones, your medical team may advise you to increase the amount of calories and carbohydrate in your meals and snacks.

During your pregnancy, if you are not already seeing an endocrinologist, your obstetrician may refer you to one. Most likely, you would see the endocrinologist at least once monthly during the first and second trimesters (approximately the first six months of pregnancy) and every two weeks in the third trimester (the

BLOOD GLUCOSE GOALS DURING PREGNANCY

The American Diabetes Association's recommended goals for blood glucose during pregnancy are even closer to the normal, nondiabetic range than for the general population with diabetes. These goals have been set with the health of both mother and developing baby in mind.

WHEN	WHOLE BLOOD	PLASMA VALUE
Fasting	60–90 mg/dl	69–104 mg/dl
Before meals	60–105 mg/dl	69–121 mg/dl
1 hour after meals	100–120 mg/dl	115–138 mg/dl
2 AM–6 AM	60–120 mg/dl	69–138 mg/dl

Adapted from *Medical Management of Pregnancy Complicated by Diabetes* (Third Edition), American Diabetes Association, 2000.

last three months). In addition to your scheduled appointments, you should discuss specific guidelines for prompt follow-up if blood glucose levels are not staying within recommended ranges. Your obstetrician will likely evaluate the growth and condition of your baby throughout your pregnancy with tests such as ultrasound to monitor your baby's size and the nonstress test, which measures a baby's heart rate in response to his or her own movements. Additional testing to monitor your baby's health or yours may be recommended by your obstetrician or by members of your diabetes health-care team.

Insulin needs during pregnancy

During any pregnancy, a woman's insulin needs change, because the normal hormone production and weight gain that occur during pregnancy increase insulin resistance. (See "Insulin Requirements During Pregnancy" on page 373.) In women who do not have or develop diabetes, blood glucose levels remain stable because the pancreas is able to produce more insulin to accommodate the increased demand. In women who have preexisting diabetes or who develop gestational diabetes, the pancreas cannot keep up with the increased demand, so blood glucose levels rise unless steps are taken to lower them.

In women with preexisting diabetes, insulin needs during the first several weeks of pregnancy are not usually that different from those before conception. However, in the latter part of the first trimester, women with preexisting diabetes may have a higher

MORE READING ON PREGNANCY

For more information on diabetes and pregnancy, you may find the following resources helpful.

Books
Books published by the American Diabetes Association can be purchased via the Internet (http://store.diabetes.org/adabooks) or by calling toll-free (800) 232-6733.

DIABETES AND PREGNANCY
What to Expect
American Diabetes Association
Alexandria, Virginia, 2000

GESTATIONAL DIABETES
What to Expect
American Diabetes Association
Alexandria, Virginia, 2000

Brochures
These brochures can be read online or ordered by phone, using the toll-free numbers listed below.

"Diabetes and Pregnancy"
Juvenile Diabetes Research Foundation International
www.jdf.org/living_w_diabetes/pages/pregnancy.html
To order, call the JDRF at (800) 533-CURE (533-2873).

"Understanding Gestational Diabetes: A Practical Guide to a Healthy Pregnancy"
National Institute of Child Health & Human Development
www.nichd.nih.gov/publications/pubs/gesttoc.htm
To order, call the NICHD at (800) 370-2943.

risk of hypoglycemia because of an increase in sensitivity to insulin, rapid fetal growth, and a reduction in eating associated with morning sickness. Around the 16th week of pregnancy, insulin needs gradually increase due to increasing levels of hormones, including human placental lactogen (hPL), a form of "growth hormone" for the baby.

All women with Type 1 diabetes and most with Type 2 either inject or infuse insulin during pregnancy. Women with gestational diabetes also have to take steps to control their blood glucose level, but not all have to inject insulin. Some women with gestational diabetes can keep their blood glucose at recommended levels with changes in diet and moderate exercise. Many, however, must eventually use insulin.

Control before conception

In women with Type 1 or Type 2 diabetes, optimal blood glucose control is essential prior to conception, because it's hard to be absolutely certain of when conception takes place. The incidence of fetal malformations is reduced significantly in women who have near-normal glycosylated hemoglobin (HbA_{1c}) levels before they become pregnant. The rate of miscarriage in women with preexisting diabetes is also reduced by keeping blood glucose levels as close to normal as possible in the first trimester.

Ideally, you should strive for a near-normal HbA_{1c} test result at least three months prior to pregnancy. It is important to discuss any plans to become pregnant with your diabetes health-care team, particularly if you have vascular complications related to your diabetes such as eye or kidney disease. In this situation, pregnancy is a potential risk to your health. For women with no vascular complications, a thorough physical exam, good nutrition (including a folic acid supplement), and excellent blood glucose control before you become pregnant will help minimize any health risks to you and your baby. Be sure you are using a reliable method of birth control as you work toward optimal blood glucose levels.

Gestational diabetes

Gestational diabetes is a form of glucose intolerance, or difficulty metabolizing glucose, that is first recognized during pregnancy. It affects about 7% of all pregnancies. Factors that may contribute to a high risk of gestational diabetes include overweight, a strong family history of diabetes, a personal history of gestational diabetes in a prior pregnancy, glycosuria (glucose in the urine, which would be found in a routine urine test), and a strong family history of diabetes. In addition, African-Americans, Asian-Americans, Hispanics, Native Americans, and Pacific Islanders, as well as women with polycystic ovary syndrome (PCOS), have shown an increased risk for gestational diabetes. Women who are 25 or older and/or are pregnant with two or more babies are also more likely to develop gestational diabetes.

In general, screening tests are recommended between 24 and 28 weeks of gestation for any woman considered at risk for gestational diabetes by her obstetrician. However, women who are considered at high risk for gestational diabetes should be tested earlier—in fact, as early in the pregnancy as possible. The screening tests usually involve drinking a premeasured glucose solution, then having blood samples drawn and checked for glucose level to determine if the body tolerates the glucose load normally. Test levels that are out of range may indicate that the mother's blood glucose levels are likely to rise as the pregnancy progresses.

If you are diagnosed with gestational diabetes, your obstetrician may refer you to a diabetes educator or to an endocrinologist (or both) for help managing your diabetes and your pregnancy. Because blood glucose control is essential during pregnancy, weekly follow-up with the health professional managing your diabetes is usually recommended.

Most cases of gestational diabetes disappear after delivery because two of the primary factors that contribute to insulin resistance and high blood glucose levels are either diminished (the extra weight gained during pregnancy) or gone (the hormones produced by the placenta). If your blood glucose levels were normal prior to pregnancy, they will most likely return to normal after delivery. However, once you have had gestational diabetes, you are likely to develop it again in another pregnancy. You also face a higher risk for developing Type 2 diabetes later in life.

Tools for control

The tools used to maintain blood glucose control during pregnancy are the same as those used to control any case of diabetes. They include a meal plan, an exercise plan, and possibly an insulin plan.

Meal plan. Whether you have preexisting diabetes or gestational diabetes, you should work with a registered dietitian to design an individualized meal plan for your pregnancy. The plan should focus on foods that provide good nutrition for you and your baby and that help keep your blood glucose level in the desired range. Because carbohydrate has the most immediate impact on blood glucose levels, your meal plan should specify how much carbohydrate to eat and when to eat it. Carbohydrate is found mainly in foods such as breads, cereals, pasta, starchy vegetables, fruits, and sweets. Frequent blood glucose monitoring will help you determine the appropriate amount and timing of carbohydrate.

Your dietitian can also suggest how many calories you need each day based on your recommended weight gain. The amount of weight you should gain during pregnancy depends on your weight before pregnancy. In general, a woman at a healthy weight before pregnancy should gain 25 to 35 pounds during her pregnancy. Your health-care team may advise you to gain more if you are underweight or less if you are overweight. Keep in mind, however, that pregnancy is definitely not a time to try to lose weight. Most mothers require about 100 extra calories per

WEIGHT GAIN DURING PREGNANCY

Ever wonder why pregnancy usually involves gaining at least 25 pounds, when a baby weighs only 7 or 8? Here's a breakdown of what accounts for the other 17 or more pounds:

WHAT	POUNDS
Developing unborn baby	7–8
Placenta	1–2
Amniotic fluid	2
Uterus	2
Increase in blood volume	3
Breasts	1
Body fat	5 or more
Increased muscle tissue and fluid	4–7
	TOTAL: 25 or more

day during the first trimester and an additional 300 calories per day during the remainder of the pregnancy to ensure the ideal weight gain for the mother and birth weight for the baby. ("Weight Gain During Pregnancy," on this page, illustrates how pregnancy weight gain is distributed.)

In most cases, your dietitian will recommend that you eat three meals a day with two to four between-meal snacks. An evening snack is particularly important to prevent hypoglycemia during the night and urine ketones or nausea in the morning.

You may be concerned about the safety of consuming sugar substitutes during pregnancy. At this time, research shows that the four sugar substitutes most commonly used in the United States (acesulfame-K, aspartame, saccharin, and sucralose) are safe to use in moderation during pregnancy. Some of these sweeteners do cross the placenta and can reach the baby, but there is no evidence they cause ill effects. If in doubt, follow the advice of your obstetrician.

For more specifics on the components of a well-balanced diet during pregnancy, see "Eating for Two" on page 373.

Physical activity. Regular physical activity is essential to diabetes control and to general health and well-being. Your health-care team can help you determine a safe level of exercise for you during pregnancy. If you have always exercised in the past, you may be able to continue to exercise at a more moderate level while you are pregnant. If exercise was not part of your pre-pregnancy routine, check with both your obstetrician and endocrinologist before you start, and choose an activity such as brisk walking or swimming to incorporate into your daily routine. Because exercise usually lowers blood glucose, be alert to the symptoms of hypoglycemia, and check your blood glucose level before and after you exercise.

Insulin management. Insulin is the most common medicine used for blood glucose control during pregnancy. Blood-glucose-lowering pills are used much less often because of a lack of data on their safety. However, at least one recent study concluded that glyburide (brand names DiaBeta, Glynase PresTab, or Micronase), when taken by women with gestational diabetes during the last six months of pregnancy, did not change fetal outcome.

Women with Type 1 diabetes may prefer to stick with their usual insulin delivery method during pregnancy, or they may decide to try something new such as insulin pump therapy. For some, using a pump during pregnancy allows them to fine-tune their insulin requirements.

Women with Type 2 diabetes who take pills as part of their diabetes treatment plan are usually advised to switch to insulin during pregnancy. In fact, many health-care practitioners recommend that women with Type 2 diabetes switch to insulin therapy before becoming pregnant. This may help them adjust to insulin therapy and possibly allow them to bring their blood glucose levels into the ranges recommended during pregnancy before they become pregnant.

As mentioned earlier, women with gestational diabetes usually start by seeing how well dietary changes control their blood glucose levels and then add insulin if blood glucose levels do not stay within recommended ranges. Women who must learn to use insulin because of gestational diabetes may find that using an insulin pen is easier than using a syringe. Using premixed insulins, rather than mixing your own, may also simplify your diabetes management.

The most common side effect of insulin therapy is hypoglycemia. Once insulin enters the body and begins working, blood glucose levels may drop lower than recommended if you do not eat to balance the effects, or if you exercise too much. Women using insulin during pregnancy should make sure they receive information about the warning signs and treatment of hypoglycemia. In addition, they should be aware that hypoglycemia unawareness (the inability to detect early signs of low blood sugar) may be more common in pregnant women, especially those with Type 1 diabetes.

Labor and delivery

Most physicians prefer that women with diabetes deliver as close to their due date as possible. Babies delivered after their due date tend to be larger and risk more complications. If natural labor is not timely and a woman plans to deliver vaginally, a hormone called oxytocin can be given, usually intravenously, to induce labor. If a woman is scheduled for a cesarean section, oxytocin is not necessary.

Many women with diabetes are able to deliver vaginally. A cesarean delivery may be needed if a baby is too large (macrosomic), if a woman's pelvis is too small, or if a woman has vascular complications or blood pressure problems. A cesarean delivery may also be required if a baby is in the breech position (when a baby's feet or buttocks enter the birth canal first).

Labor is an intense, active process which can lower a woman's blood glucose level. A cesarean delivery, on the other hand, may raise a woman's blood glucose level because the surgical procedure is a stress on the body. If you have Type 1 or Type 2 diabetes, your doctor may have you on insulin intravenously (IV) during labor and delivery. The IV apparatus continually infuses quick-acting insulin and may allow for smoother blood glucose control since adjustments can be made as necessary. The goal is to keep blood glucose levels as normal as possible to prevent hypoglycemia in your newborn. Most women with gestational diabetes do not require any insulin during the labor and delivery process.

After delivery, continuing to maintain blood sugar levels in a near-normal range facilitates the healing process.

Recovery

If you have Type 1 or Type 2 diabetes, your insulin requirements may return to what they were before your pregnancy within a few weeks of delivery. Check your blood glucose levels frequently, and make adjustments in your insulin dosage as needed.

If you had gestational diabetes, it is likely that your blood glucose level will return to normal almost immediately after your baby is born. But since gestational diabetes puts you at increased risk for developing Type 2 diabetes in the future, you should have your blood glucose level measured at your first postpartum checkup (usually four to six weeks after delivery) and yearly thereafter. To minimize your risk of developing Type 2 diabetes, eat a balanced diet, exercise regularly, and keep your weight at a reasonable level.

Breast-feeding

Diabetes is no barrier to breast-feeding. Breast milk provides the ideal source of nutrition for babies as well as antibodies that fight certain infections. Breast-feeding also promotes weight loss in the mother, may

INSULIN REQUIREMENTS DURING PREGNANCY

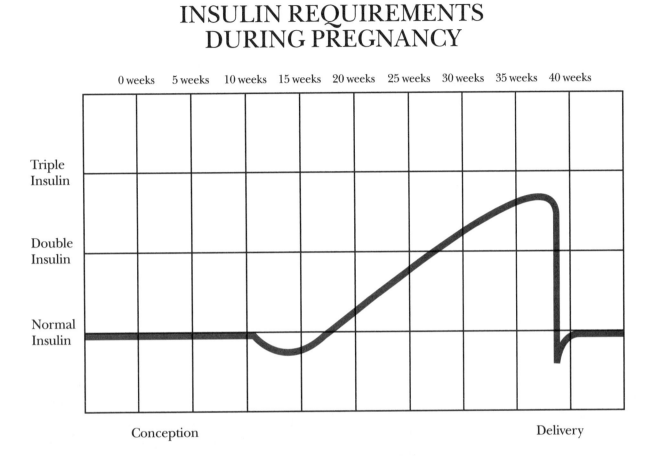

EATING FOR TWO

Eating enough of the right foods is one of the most important things you can do to ensure that your baby is healthy. Although nutrient needs increase during pregnancy, most women can meet these needs by eating a balanced diet that includes a variety of foods. However, for some women, prenatal vitamin and mineral supplements, particularly iron, may be necessary. When planning your meals during pregnancy, pay special attention to the following nutrients:

Protein. Pregnant women require an extra 10 grams of protein daily (or a total of 60 grams daily) for a healthy baby and placenta. A 3-ounce serving of meat provides approximately 20 grams of protein.

B vitamins. The requirements for B vitamins increase during pregnancy; B vitamins help to metabolize the energy from food and help protein to make new body cells. Getting adequate amounts of a B vitamin called folate, or folic acid, is particularly important in the first three months of preg-

nancy. Consuming enough folate before pregnancy and in the early stages may lower the risk of neural tube birth defect (birth defects that involve the spinal column) in the baby. Pregnant women require 600 micrograms of folate daily. A half-cup serving of boiled navy beans provides 125 micrograms of folate.

Calcium. Calcium is critical for preserving a mother's bone mass while the baby's skeleton develops. Pregnant women need 1,000 milligrams of calcium daily. An 8-ounce glass of milk provides 300 milligrams of calcium.

Iron. Iron is essential in making hemoglobin, a blood component that carries oxygen through the body to the placenta. It can be difficult to get enough iron in the diet because it is not well absorbed from food, and many women start with low iron stores. Pregnant women require 27 milligrams of iron daily. A 3-ounce serving of lean beef has almost 3 milligrams of iron.

help protect the baby from developing diabetes in the future, and may help to establish a special mother–baby bond.

If you decide to breast-feed, speak with a registered dietitian about the foods you need to eat so that you get enough calcium, fluids, and protein. Breast-feeding increases a woman's caloric needs and, because it takes energy, may increase her risk of developing hypoglycemia. Episodes of hypoglycemia are more likely to occur within an hour after breast-feeding, so this is an important time to check your blood glucose level. Napping after meals and snacks is also recommended to lower the risk of hypoglycemia. You may need to adjust your insulin dosage, particularly overnight, to prevent your blood glucose level from dropping during late-night feedings.

Women with Type 2 diabetes who switched from oral pills to insulin during pregnancy are generally encouraged to stay on insulin for at least a month after delivery. For many of the newer diabetes drugs, little or no research has been done on their use in breast-feeding women.

Tough job, big rewards

Managing your diabetes during pregnancy means paying extra attention to your lifestyle during these important months. Though you may feel overwhelmed at times, your health-care team is available to answer your questions and help you attain excellent blood glucose control. The commitment you make now will pay off with the best results in the future: a healthy, happy baby, and a healthy you! ❑

CONTRACEPTION
PART OF PLANNING A HEALTHY BABY
by Rita Revak-Lutz, A.R.N.P., M.S.N., C.D.E.

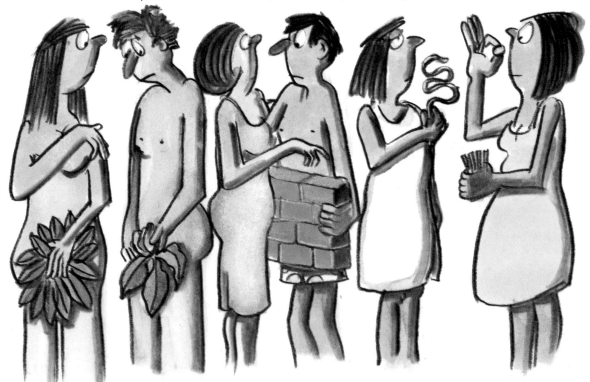

E very sexually active person should know about contraceptive methods and their correct use. This is true for men and women alike, regardless of their desire to have or not have children. Contraceptives are essential in preventing an undesired pregnancy and in delaying a desired pregnancy until the best time. They also play a role in preventing the spread of sexually transmitted infections.

For women with diabetes and their partners, using birth control while planning a pregnancy can help achieve the goal of a healthy baby by allowing a woman the time she needs to get her blood sugar in

NATURAL CONTRACEPTION

Other than abstinence, natural methods of birth control have a high failure rate with typical use. That's why most sex educators recommend using a more reliable method unless pregnancy is desired.

METHOD	PROS	CONS	UNINTENDED PREGNANCY RATE FOR FIRST YEAR OF USE
No method	■ No cost	■ No protection against pregnancy or sexually transmitted diseases	85%
Abstinence	■ No cost	■ No protection from sexually transmitted diseases if bodily fluids are exchanged	0% if there is no sexual intercourse or ejaculation near the opening of the vagina
Coitus interruptus	■ No cost ■ Always available	■ No protection from sexually transmitted diseases (the virus that causes AIDS is present in pre-ejaculatory fluid) ■ Effectiveness dependent on male partner to determine when ejaculation will take place	19% (typical); 4% (when used perfectly)
Fertility awareness	■ No cost or low cost (price of thermometer) ■ Always available	■ No protection from sexually transmitted diseases ■ Fertile times vary from woman to woman and cycle to cycle ■ Cervical secretions may vary because of factors other than ovulation	25% (typical); 1% to 9% (when used perfectly, depending on method)

the best control possible. It can also help maintain a woman's general health, particularly if she has any long-term complications of diabetes.

Risks to the baby

One of the most important reasons for women with diabetes to use a reliable method of birth control is the role it plays in decreasing the risk of birth defects. It has long been recognized that women with diabetes have an increased risk of giving birth to a baby with a birth defect. This risk increases as a woman's average blood glucose level, as indicated by her glycosylated hemoglobin (HbA_{1c}) test results, increases. The HbA_{1c} test gives an indication of a person's overall blood sugar control over the previous two to three months. The American Diabetes Association recommends that most people with diabetes attempt to keep their HbA_{1c} result under 7%. Any result over 8% should prompt a review of a person's diabetes man-

agement routine. Women intending to become pregnant are advised to aim for a "near-normal" HbA_{1c} of about 6%.

One study has suggested that the risk of having a baby with a birth defect is as much as 22% when a woman's HbA_{1c} result is higher than 8.5%. However, by tightening her blood glucose control and taking a daily folic acid supplement before attempting to get pregnant, a woman with diabetes can bring her risk of birth defects down to that of a woman who doesn't have diabetes.

Bringing blood glucose into goal range before trying to conceive is one step in what is called "preconception planning." For a woman with diabetes, other steps include getting a full medical evaluation, perhaps switching from oral diabetes medicine to insulin, and starting a folic acid supplement. All these steps are aimed at raising the chances of giving birth to a healthy baby. Using a reliable method of birth

BARRIER CONTRACEPTIVES

Of all contraceptive methods currently on the market, male condoms may offer the best protection against sexually transmitted infections, including HIV. To improve protection against pregnancy, they can easily be combined with another contraceptive method. In fact, when used as birth control, condoms should always be used with a spermicide.

TYPE	PROS	CONS	UNINTENDED PREGNANCY RATE FOR FIRST YEAR OF USE
Cervical cap	■ Can be worn for up to 48 hours at a time	■ Made of latex, so not suitable for someone with a latex allergy ■ May be difficult to find a practitioner experienced in fitting cervical caps	20% (typical); 9% (when used perfectly)
Diaphragm	■ Can be inserted six hours before intercourse	■ Increased risk of urinary tract infection ■ Risk of pregnancy increases with the frequency of sexual intercourse	20% (typical); 6% (when used perfectly)
Male condom	■ Can be purchased over the counter ■ Offers excellent protection against sexually transmitted diseases	■ Condoms made of latex are not suitable for someone with a latex allergy, but polyurethane condoms are available	14% (typical); 3% (when used perfectly)
Female condom	■ Available over the counter ■ Offers protection against sexually transmitted diseases ■ Made of polyurethane so it can be used with oil-based or water-based lubricant	■ May initially be difficult to insert ■ May be difficult to locate in retail stores	21% (typical); 5% (when used perfectly)

control prevents conception before these steps are completed.

Risks to the mother

In some cases, pregnancy may pose a risk to a woman's health. For example, pregnancy may accelerate the progression of diabetic retinopathy (eye disease). Kidney disease (diabetic nephropathy), too, may worsen temporarily during pregnancy, increasing the risk of high blood pressure, which may place the pregnancy at risk.

However, these risks do not mean that a woman with either diabetic retinopathy or nephropathy cannot have a baby. If the condition is stabilized prior to

pregnancy, the risk to the woman can be minimized. Here again, using birth control can prevent pregnancy until treatment can take place.

Women with diabetes who have heart disease may be advised not to become pregnant, because pregnancy may actually place their lives at risk. For these women, birth control may be a life-saving necessity.

Myths and realities

Despite these powerful reasons for using birth control, the unplanned pregnancy rate for women with diabetes is an astonishing 76%. Myths and misconceptions about diabetes, pregnancy, and birth control

INTRAUTERINE DEVICES

While not widely used in the United States, IUD's are very effective at preventing pregnancy and are considered safe, even for women with diabetes. However, they do not protect against sexually transmitted infections.

TYPE	PROS	CONS	UNINTENDED PREGNANCY RATE FOR FIRST YEAR OF USE
Progesterone T (Progestasert)	■ Easy to use ■ May decrease blood loss during menstruation ■ May decrease menstrual discomfort ■ Provides contraception for one year	■ No protection against sexually transmitted diseases	2.0% (typical use); 1.5% (perfect use)
Copper T-380A (ParaGard)	■ Can be left in place for 10 years ■ Cost-effective ■ Easy to use	■ May increase menstrual discomfort ■ No protection against sexually transmitted diseases	0.8% (typical use); 0.6% (perfect use)
Mirena	■ Easy to use ■ May decrease blood loss during menstruation ■ May decrease menstrual discomfort ■ Provides contraception for 5 years	■ No protection against sexually transmitted diseases	0.1% (typical use); 0.1% (perfect use)

undoubtedly have influenced this high rate of unintended pregnancy.

One often-heard myth is that women with diabetes can't get pregnant. The intended meaning of this statement is not known for sure: It could mean that it is physically impossible for women with diabetes to get pregnant, or it could mean that women with diabetes shouldn't get pregnant. The 1989 movie *Steel Magnolias,* in which Julia Roberts played a woman with diabetes who gets pregnant and subsequently dies, has likely fueled this myth.

Regardless of the statement's intended meaning, it is incorrect. Women with diabetes generally don't have any problems getting pregnant, and with correct planning, there is no reason why a woman with diabetes shouldn't have a child (unless she has heart disease and pregnancy would put her life in danger).

Another common myth is that women with diabetes can't use birth control. This, too, is incorrect.

And when you consider that birth control can help decrease the incidence of birth defects and preserve the health and perhaps even the life of a woman with diabetes, it is easy to see that the benefits of using birth control are far-reaching.

These days, all women and their partners have a range of birth control options. Those options can be divided into two broad categories: nonhormonal methods and hormonal methods. None of the contraceptive methods described in this article are off-limits to a woman with diabetes just because she has diabetes. However, it's always a good idea to talk with your health-care provider about other medical conditions or habits (such as smoking) that might affect your choice of contraceptive.

Some endocrinologists may be comfortable prescribing contraception, while others may prefer to refer you to a women's health-care provider. Family-planning clinics are also a good source of information about birth control and other sexuality issues. In addition, they can sometimes offer contraceptives at reduced prices. It's also a good idea to check your health insurance plan benefits to see what sort of contraceptive services, if any, are covered.

When deciding on a method of birth control, be sure to discuss it not only with your health-care provider but also with your sexual partner to make sure you are in agreement about what to use and how to use it. Inconsistent or incorrect use of contraceptives accounts for over a million unintended pregnancies in the United States each year.

No discussion about birth control would be complete without also discussing protection against sexually transmitted diseases (STD's), so each of the following descriptions includes comments on the method's effectiveness at minimizing disease transmission.

Nonhormonal contraception

Nonhormonal birth control methods used in the United States include "natural" methods, barrier methods, and one type of intrauterine device (IUD). With the exception of the IUD, the effectiveness of nonhormonal contraception is highly dependent on the user to control each sexual encounter in a specific way to prevent sperm from reaching the egg.

Natural methods

The oldest forms of birth control—abstinence, coitus interruptus, and fertility awareness—require no special tools, but with the exception of abstinence, they may require a great deal of effort and in some cases luck on the part of the user. In addition, and again with the exception of abstinence, natural birth control methods are not very effective at preventing pregnancy for most people, and they do not protect against disease transmission.

The term abstinence means different things to different people. For some it means strict avoidance of all sexual contact, while for others it may mean elimination of intercourse from the sexual act. Either way, it prevents pregnancy (as long as no ejaculation takes place near the opening of the vagina) but may not prevent the transmission of infections if bodily fluids are exchanged by some other route.

Coitus interruptus (also known as withdrawal or onanism) is documented in the Bible, with Onan using withdrawal as a birth control method when having intercourse with his brother's widow. With coitus interruptus, vaginal intercourse takes place until the nearing of male ejaculation, when the penis is withdrawn from the vagina. A man must take care to ejaculate away from the opening of the vagina, because any sperm that makes its way into the vagina can continue on up through the woman's reproductive tract

and fertilize an egg. Some studies suggest that the failure rate of the withdrawal method can be lowered if a man urinates before intercourse; this washes out any sperm left in the urethra from a recent previous ejaculation.

Fertility awareness methods of contraception require a woman to assess her menstrual cycle, cervical mucus, or basal body temperature to determine when she is likely to be fertile. During this time, she must abstain from sex or use a barrier method of birth control to prevent pregnancy.

As stated earlier, coitus interruptus and fertility awareness have low efficacy rates in preventing pregnancy. For a woman with diabetes, the health-related risks of pregnancy typically outweigh any benefit provided by these natural methods.

Diaphragms and cervical caps

Forerunners of the diaphragm—a dome-shaped cup with a flexible rim that fits over the cervix, blocking the entrance to the uterus—have been used as birth control for centuries. Innovative women placed wool soaked in acidic nut and fruit concoctions or a lemon half over their cervix. Not only did these homemade contraceptives provide a physical barrier, but the acidic juice worked as a spermicide to increase effectiveness.

Modern diaphragms are made of latex or another synthetic material, and chemicals such as nonoxynol-9 provide spermicidal action, but the mechanism of action remains the same. Diaphragms offer some protection against certain sexually transmitted infections, but for more complete protection, using a latex or polyurethane condom in addition to a diaphragm is recommended.

In the 1940's, the diaphragm was the most popular contraceptive in the United States, with one-third of American couples using the method. The introduction of oral contraceptives and IUD's diminished diaphragm popularity, and it is estimated that fewer than 2% of American couples use it today.

Before being inserted into the vagina, the rim of a diaphragm should be coated and the dome partially filled with spermicidal jelly or cream. (Completely filling the dome with spermicide can interfere with the suction needed to keep the diaphragm in place.) A diaphragm can be inserted up to six hours before intercourse. If more time elapses or intercourse is repeated, an applicator of spermicide should be inserted into the vagina (without removing the diaphragm).

The diaphragm should be left in place for at least six hours after intercourse, but no longer than 24 hours because of an increased risk of toxic shock syndrome. (Toxic shock syndrome is a rare staphylococcal infection in which the staphylococci bacteria produce poisons that enter the bloodstream.)

HORMONAL METHODS OF BIRTH CONTROL

Listed here are hormonal methods of birth control for which detailed effectiveness data are available. In general, hormonal methods are very effective at preventing pregnancy. However, none of them offers any protection against sexually transmitted infections. To prevent against STD's, a male condom should be used.

METHOD	UNINTENDED PREGNANCY RATE FOR FIRST YEAR OF USE
Progestin-only pills	5.0% (typical); 0.5% (when used perfectly)
Combination pills (estrogen and progestin)	5.0% (typical); 0.1% (when used perfectly)
DMPA (Depo-Provera)	0.3% (typical); 0.3% (when used perfectly)
Levonorgestrel implants (Norplant)	0.05% (typical); 0.05% (when used perfectly)

In the late 1980's, the cervical cap was added to the menu of female barrier methods of contraception. The cervical cap is smaller than the diaphragm, is shaped essentially like a thimble, and fits directly over the cervix; it adheres to the cervix through suction. Like the diaphragm, the cervical cap should be partially filled with spermicidal jelly or cream and the rim coated before insertion. It can be kept in place for up to 48 hours with no need for additional spermicide. The cervical cap also offers some protection against certain sexually transmitted infections, but not as much as a latex or polyurethane condom does.

Diaphragms and cervical caps require a pelvic exam by a health-care provider who is experienced in determining the size needed for a good fit.

Condoms, male and female

Just as women of yore used homemade diaphragms, men of yore used "penis protectors" made of animal membranes and linen—forerunners of the modern condom. Rather than contraception, however, their original intent was to prevent against sexually transmitted disease.

Vulcanized rubber and latex revolutionized the manufacturing of condoms, and concern over the AIDS epidemic greatly increased the popularity of condoms in the 1980's. Using a latex or polyurethane condom with each act of intercourse provides the best protection (short of abstinence) against the transmission of HIV, the virus that causes AIDS. (Make sure the condoms you buy have the words "disease prevention" on the label to be sure they meet U.S. Food and Drug Administration [FDA] standards.) Natural membrane condoms (often called lambskin, although they are actually made of sheep's intestines), while they do prevent pregnancy, do not effectively prevent the spread of STD's.

Female condoms were introduced in the early 1990's. Only one brand, the Reality Female Condom, has come on the U.S. market. Designed as a loose-fitting polyurethane sheath, an internal ring is placed in the vagina near the cervix, while an external ring covers the vulva and acts as an anchor. While the female condom offers protection against sexually transmitted infections, it is not as effective as the male condom. However, the two methods should not be used simultaneously because they may slip out of place. Male and female condoms are available without a prescription and are sold in most drugstores.

Barrier methods of birth control are effective, but only if they're used. Condoms used perfectly will provide the best contraceptive benefit. Perfect condom use includes using one with every act of intercourse, putting the condom on before any contact between penis and vagina takes place, pinching the tip of the condom to create a reservoir while unrolling it onto the penis, and holding the rim of the condom while withdrawing the penis from the vagina to prevent spills.

However, even with perfect use, condoms have a 3% rate of unintended pregnancy for the first year of use. If you are a woman with cardiovascular disease or progressive retinopathy, this pregnancy risk may not be acceptable. To retain the protection against STD's that condoms provide and lower your risk of an unintended pregnancy, you may want to use both condoms and a birth control method with a lower failure rate, such as a hormonal method.

Intrauterine devices

There are three intrauterine devices (IUD's) currently sold in the United States, one of which is a nonhormonal device, and the other two of which are hormonal devices. All three are small, T-shaped pieces of plastic that are inserted in the uterus. Two threads attached to the device protrude through the cervical opening, allowing a woman to make sure the device is in place.

The nonhormonal IUD has a different mechanism of action than other nonhormonal birth control options. It was previously believed that the main contraceptive action of an IUD was to prevent implantation of a fertilized egg in the uterus. However, current research indicates that the IUD prohibits fertilization of the egg.

The nonhormonal IUD currently available in the United States is sold under the brand name ParaGard. It is covered with copper, which it releases into the uterus, changing the chemical makeup of fluids in the uterus and fallopian tubes. This chemical change hampers the ability of sperm to swim and may actually damage the sperm. In addition, the copper released by the IUD thickens cervical mucus, making it more difficult for the sperm to enter the uterus.

Of the two hormonal IUDs approved for use in the United States, one contains the female sex hormone progesterone and is sold under the brand name Progestasert; the other contains the related hormone levonorgestrel and is marketed under the brand name Mirena. Progestasert releases enough progesterone daily to thicken cervical mucus, interfere with ovulation (the release of an egg from the ovary), alter the uterine lining, and impair the uterine and fallopian tube movement that help move the egg from ovary to uterus. Fertilization is impaired by preventing the sperm from reaching the egg. Mirena seems to work in similar ways.

Although IUD's are widely used in other parts of the world, less than 1% of all married women in the United States currently use them for birth control. This low rate is probably related to fears generated by the Dalkon Shield IUD, which was linked to an increased risk of pelvic inflammatory disease in the 1970's. The infection risk was attributed to the wicking effect of the Dalkon Shield's multifilamented string. Even though the Dalkon Shield was removed from the market more than two decades ago, the public's perception of the safety of IUD's was so altered by the negative publicity that all but one company ceased to promote IUD's in the United States.

Results of large studies indicate that the risk of pelvic inflammatory disease related to IUD's is very low. If a woman and her partner are mutually monogamous, there is no significant increase in risk. Some clinicians hesitate to place IUD's in women with diabetes because of a concern of an increased risk of pelvic inflammatory disease related to diabetes. But again, studies have failed to demonstrate an increased risk of pelvic inflammatory disease in women with diabetes who use an IUD.

While they are effective at preventing pregnancy, IUD's offer no protection from sexually transmitted infections. They are recommended only for couples in monogamous relationships.

Hormonal contraception

The hormones estrogen and progestin (of which progesterone and levonorgestrel are two types) are the active ingredients in contraceptive implants, injections, and pills, along with the recently introduced contraceptive skin patch and vaginal ring. Emergency contraceptive pills, which are intended for use after unprotected intercourse, also contain these hormones. Contraception occurs mainly as a result of preventing ovulation, the release of the egg from the ovary. In addition, cervical mucus may be thickened and the uterine lining altered, enhancing contraception. Contraceptive implants, hormonal IUD's, one type of contraceptive injection, and a few oral contraceptives contain only progestin, while other hormonal contraceptives available in the United States contain both estrogen and progestin.

Some women are concerned that hormonal contraception may affect future fertility. However, none of the hormonal contraceptives permanently affect fertility. With one type of currently available injection, ovulation may be delayed for up to six to 12 months after the last injection, but it is possible to become pregnant sooner than that if an injection is missed. With the other type, women may start ovulating within two to four months following their last injection. There is also a rapid return to fertility when oral contraceptives are discontinued, implants are removed, or other hormonal devices are discontinued.

All hormonal contraception methods have similar risks and benefits. They all have excellent rates of pregnancy prevention. Because injections and implants do not depend on the user remembering to take a daily pill, they have the best pregnancy prevention rates. However, no hormonal method provides protection against STD's, so it is recommended that condoms be used in conjunction with hormonal methods in order to decrease the risk of disease transmission.

The pill

The original FDA approval for the oral estrogen–progestin combination, in 1957, was not for birth control, but rather "gynecologic disorders." Three years later, in 1960, the indication of birth control was approved. The estrogen content of these initial oral contraceptives was over 50 micrograms per pill and was associated with certain health risks. Today the estrogen content is in the range of 20 to 35 micrograms and carries significantly lower risks.

MORE ON CONTRACEPTION

To read more about contraceptive choices, have a look at the following resources. Some articles can be read only on the Internet; others are available in booklet format and can be ordered by phone.

FEDERAL CONSUMER INFORMATION CENTER
(888) 878-3256
www.pueblo.gsa.gov
The FCIC distributes useful information published by federal agencies, including the booklet "Guide to Contraceptive Choices." Based on an article originally published in *FDA Consumer* (a publication of the U.S. Food and Drug Administration), the booklet compares 13 methods of birth control according to convenience, health risks, and how well they protect users from sexually transmitted diseases. To order this free booklet (#543F), visit the Web site or call the toll-free number.

OBGYN.NET
www.obgyn.net/women/contraception/contraception.htm
A compilation of links to information on all different types of contraception and on sexually transmitted infection prevention.

PLANNED PARENTHOOD
(800) 669-0156
www.plannedparenthood.org
Planned Parenthood provides sexuality education and medical services for millions of men, women, and teenagers each year. Its publications relating to contraception include "Facts About Birth Control," a 40-page booklet that describes the effectiveness, cost, and safety of 14 contraceptive methods, including hormonal implants and injections, the condom, and the pill. To order, call the toll-free number or visit the Web site. "Facts About Birth Control" can also be read online at www.plannedparenthood.org/bc/bcfacts1.html.

U.S. FOOD AND DRUG ADMINISTRATION
www.fda.gov
The Web site of the FDA offers "Protecting Against Unintended Pregnancy," an article highlighting contraceptives. The article can be reached directly at www.fda.gov/fdac/features/1997/397_baby.html. The site also has guidelines for using condoms, spermicides, and lubricants, which can be reached at www.fda.gov/oashi/aids/condom.html.

In fact, it is now recognized that hormonal contraceptives offer many noncontraceptive health benefits, including a decreased risk of ovarian and endometrial cancer and diminished blood loss during menstrual periods. Oral contraceptives that contain estrogen also provide protection against osteoporosis.

The effects of estrogen and progestin are not limited to pregnancy prevention, however. Both affect blood cholesterol levels, and progestins have an effect on carbohydrate metabolism. In the past, there was concern that these effects would not be beneficial for women with diabetes. Luckily, hormonal contraception is one of the most studied topics in drug therapy. There is growing evidence that for most women with diabetes, the benefits of hormonal contraception far outweigh the risks. Numerous studies involving both women with and without diabetes have indicated that progestin in low-dose oral contraceptives does not increase the risk of developing diabetes or worsen blood glucose control in women with diabetes.

Estrogen has a positive effect on lipid metabolism by increasing the level of beneficial high-density lipoprotein (HDL) cholesterol and decreasing the level of low-density lipoprotein (LDL) cholesterol. Some progestins can have the opposite effect—lowering HDL cholesterol and raising LDL cholesterol—but most medical professionals agree that the risk of an unplanned pregnancy in a woman with diabetes is greater than the risk posed by the effect of progestin on lipids. The newer, third-generation progestins (desogestrel and norgestimate) may actually provide a health benefit by increasing HDL's and decreasing LDL's.

Some oral contraceptive pills contain only progestin, and some contain both progestin and estrogen. Those containing both progestin and estrogen, called combination pills, may deliver a constant amount of progestin throughout the menstrual cycle (monophasic) or have two or three different progestin doses during the cycle (biphasic or triphasic). The estrogen content stays constant throughout the cycle in all combination pills. Progestin-only pills have a constant amount of hormone throughout the cycle.

For most women with diabetes who do not smoke, the contraceptive and noncontraceptive benefits of the pill seem to outweigh potential risks. Experts are mixed on the use of oral contraceptives for women with retinopathy and nephropathy. The World Health Organization suggests that the theoretical risks of oral contraceptives in the presence of these complications outweigh benefits. But others in the medical profession believe that with close medical supervision, oral contraceptives are appropriate. Because oral contraceptives do present a slight increase in the risk of blood clots, experts agree that they should not be prescribed to women with peripheral vascular disease (narrowed arteries in the legs or arms).

As with barrier methods, the main determinant in the effectiveness of oral contraceptives is correct use. They must be taken daily for consistent suppression of ovulation. It is very important that progestin-only pills be taken at the same time every day. The risk of pregnancy goes up significantly if a progestin-only pill is not taken within 24 hours of the previous pill. A few more hours of leeway are provided with combination pills. However, in the event of missed pills, a backup method of contraception should be used. The health-care provider who prescribes the pills should provide written guidance on pill use, including guidelines on what to do if one or more pills are missed.

Emergency contraceptive pills should be taken only after known or suspected contraceptive failure or unprotected intercourse; they should not be used as routine contraception. The first dose must be taken within 72 hours of intercourse and the second dose 12 hours later. The pills are not effective if a woman is already pregnant.

Implants and injections

Contraceptive implants and injections do away with the need to take a daily pill. A medroxyprogesterone acetate (DMPA) injection (brand name Depo-Provera) has a 14-week contraceptive effect but is typically scheduled at 12-week intervals to minimize the chance for a lapse in contraception. An estrogen–progestin injection (brand name Lunelle) has a one-month duration. Levonorgestrel implants (Norplant) have a five-year period of contraception. Like oral contraceptives, both methods prevent pregnancy primarily by preventing ovulation. They also alter cervical mucus and the uterine lining, further improving contraceptive action.

Both DMPA injections and implants may cause a change in the menstrual cycle. Levonorgestrel implants may cause irregular bleeding. During the first three-month cycle of DMPA use, women may experience irregular spotting. Irregular bleeding typically diminishes with each additional injection. After a year of taking DMPA, 50% of all users do not have a menstrual period (a condition called amenorrhea). This may concern some women, but there is no health

risk associated with amenorrhea caused by DMPA. The estrogen–progestin injection offers less menstrual disruption and a more rapid return to fertility compared to DMPA. The addition of estrogen provides the noncontraceptive benefit of protection against osteoporosis.

New hormonal approaches

Two new hormonal contraceptive methods were approved by the FDA in late 2001; both were expected to become available in the United States in 2002. One, bearing the brand name Ortho Evra, is a seven-day contraceptive skin patch that slowly releases a combination of the progestin norelgestromin and the estrogen ethinyl estradiol through the skin and into the bloodstream. The other, produced under the brand name NuvaRing, is a plastic vaginal device about 2 inches in diameter that releases a combination of the progestin etonogestrel and ethinyl estradiol. It is used on a monthly cycle: a woman places it in her vagina, where it remains for three weeks, after which she removes it and goes one week without a ring. Like the injection and implant methods, both Ortho Evra and NuvaRing offer the advantage of a high rate of effectiveness without the need to remember a daily pill. Ortho Evra, however, seems to be a bit less effective in women weighing more than 198 pounds. Some women who use NuvaRing may experience infection or irritation of the vagina or a vaginal discharge. Women with diabetes who have complications of the kidneys, eyes, nerves, or blood vessels are advised not to use NuvaRing or Ortho Evra.

Planning a pregnancy

Eventually you may want to start a family. Planning a pregnancy is the best insurance for an ideal outcome: a desired, healthy baby whose parents are physically and emotionally prepared to offer the love and nurturing every baby needs and deserves.

Every baby also deserves the healthiest start possible, and this means that parents, and especially mothers, may need to make some lifestyle changes before discontinuing contraception. Women with diabetes need to pay special attention to blood glucose control. In addition, all women and their partners should stop smoking before conception to prevent both pregnancy complications and health problems for the baby. Women should stop drinking alcohol and start taking a folic acid supplement prior to attempting pregnancy. **Folic acid.** Taking 400 micrograms of folic acid (a B vitamin) each day for at least a month prior to conceiving, and continuing it during the pregnancy has been proven to decrease the risk of a type of birth defect called a neural tube defect. One of the most common neural tube defects is called spina bifida. In this birth defect, an area of the spine does not form correctly, and the spinal cord may be exposed and damaged. Spina bifida varies in severity but can result in paralysis, mental retardation, or even death of the baby.

A pharmacist can help you choose a nonprescription vitamin supplement that contains 400 micrograms of folic acid. Folic acid is also found in orange juice, green leafy vegetables, peanuts, and enriched grain products.

Alcohol. No amount of alcohol consumption is safe during pregnancy. It has long been recognized that heavy drinking can cause fetal alcohol syndrome, which may cause birth defects and mental retardation. However, even light or moderate maternal consumption of alcohol can cause fetal alcohol effect, which can result in heart defects, lowered intelligence, and behavior problems.

Since brain development begins very early in pregnancy—within two weeks of conception, even before many women realize that they're pregnant—it is important that a woman refrain from drinking alcohol from the moment she and her partner decide to get pregnant.

Men may also benefit from refraining from alcohol when trying to start or add to a family. Heavy alcohol consumption by men may decrease testosterone production, which in turn may decrease the sperm count.

Smoking. Smoking during and after pregnancy is unwise for either partner for a variety of reasons. Women who smoke have an increased risk of an ectopic pregnancy (in which an embryo develops outside the uterus), miscarriage, and a decrease in placental function that could result in stillbirth or a low-birth-weight baby. Low-birth-weight babies are at a greater risk for chronic health concerns, as well as mental retardation. Babies and children who are exposed to cigarette smoke have an increased incidence of upper-respiratory infections, asthma, and behavioral problems.

Getting help

If you are thinking about having a baby, talk to your endocrinologist (or the doctor who provides most of your diabetes care) and your obstetrician–gynecologist about planning for pregnancy before you start trying to conceive. Don't wait for your health-care providers to bring up the subject of preconception care, though. One study found that only half of women with diabetes seeking pregnancy care recalled their health-care providers discussing preconception care.

For more help in preparing for a healthy pregnancy, the March of Dimes is an excellent source of information. Look on the organization's Web site, www.MODimes.org, or call (800) 367-6630 to request free materials on pregnancy planning and having a healthy pregnancy.

Don't let the discussion of contraception and planning for a pregnancy stop with your health-care providers and your partner. Talk over these topics with your friends—both those who have diabetes and those who don't. Do them a favor by letting them know the important role birth control plays not only in reaching their family-planning goals, but also in managing their diabetes and in helping to have healthy babies. ❑

MYSTERIES OF THE MENSTRUAL CYCLE

by Helen L. Ross, M.D.

Just about all women and girls past puberty are familiar with at least some parts of the menstrual cycle: the bleeding, the bloating, and the general blahs. While few women or girls would describe menstruation as a pleasant experience, most manage to muddle through somehow, armed with a supply of tampons, pads, and pain relievers.

For women with diabetes, however, the muddling may involve one more thing: paying closer attention to blood sugar levels and possibly making some adjustments in insulin regimen or meal plan. That's because high levels of the female hormones estrogen and progesterone can interfere with the action of insulin, causing high blood sugar levels just before the start of a woman's period and in some cases during the period.

While many of the effects of the menstrual cycle may be familiar, what's going on behind the scenes to produce these effects is often not well understood. Let's have a look at what happens inside the body over the course of the menstrual cycle.

The mystery unveiled

Menstruation is the usual end of the body's continual, cyclical way of preparing itself for pregnancy. Once an egg is released near the middle of this cycle, there exists the potential for a woman to become pregnant. If, however, the egg is not fertilized, the body drops its production of certain hormones, resulting in menstruation, and readies itself to do it all over again.

The average menstrual cycle spans 28 days, although a "normal" cycle can last anywhere from 24 to 38 days. The start of bleeding, or menses, is considered day 1 of the cycle; the last day of the cycle, day 28 in a 28-day cycle, is the same as day 1 of the next cycle.

Hormone fluctuations. The start of the menstrual cycle involves a gradual rise in estrogen (see "Hormone Levels During the Menstrual Cycle" on the opposite page.) A hormone known as follicle-stimulating hormone (FSH), secreted by the pituitary gland, influences the increase in estrogen levels. FSH stimulates several follicles, or potential future eggs and their neighboring cells, in the ovaries. Somehow the body later decides which one of these stimulated follicles will reach full maturity while the rest degenerate. FSH stimulates the egg's neighboring cells to produce estrogen.

When the level of estrogen reaches a critical, or "threshold," value (which is different for different women), there is a surge in luteinizing hormone (LH). The LH surge is what is detected in ovulation kits. Approximately 24–36 hours after the LH surge, ovulation, the release of an egg from an ovary into a fallopian tube, takes place (on day 14 of a 28-day cycle). The egg will gradually wend its way down the fallopian tube and into the uterus. The estrogen level gradually decreases following ovulation until menses begin, and then rises again with the start of the next cycle.

After ovulation, LH causes some of the remaining cells in the follicle to form what is called the *corpus luteum*. The corpus luteum produces progesterone, which keeps the uterine lining primed for the implantation of a fertilized egg. The progesterone is present for 14 days and then falls (if a woman does not become pregnant) with the degeneration of the corpus luteum, and this is what results in the withdrawal bleed, or menses. If fertilization does occur, the early placenta produces a hormone (HCG) that maintains the corpus luteum and thus maintains progesterone production.

Progesterone causes a slight temperature rise, thickening of the cervical mucus, and some of the symptoms of premenstrual syndrome (PMS, discussed later). In general, progesterone is present in all women for 14 days; this is considered the "constant phase" of the menstrual cycle. Therefore, women who do not have the textbook 28-day menstrual cycle do not ovulate on day 14 of the cycle. A woman with a 30-day cycle ovulates on day 16; a woman with a 26-day cycle ovulates on day 12.

Endometrial changes. These changing hormone levels have effects on many areas of the body, particularly the endometrium, or lining of the uterus. As the estrogen level increases, the lining of the uterus grows. Following ovulation and progesterone availability, the lining stops growing and "stabilizes."

If a woman has had unprotected intercourse around the time of ovulation, the egg and a sperm may unite, optimally in a fallopian tube. The newly fertilized egg, or zygote, then travels to the uterus and implants itself in the endometrium. The building up and stabilizing of the endometrium has all been to prepare a suitable landing place for the zygote and eventually to serve as the site for nutrient transfer between mother and child once the placenta develops.

If fertilization does not occur, progesterone levels fall, which causes part of the endometrial lining to shed, resulting in menses. The menstrual flow lasts, on average, three to five days. The average blood loss with menses is 8 tablespoons, and about 50% of this occurs on the first day.

Fertile period

One common reason women track their menstrual cycles is to know when they are likely to be fertile, or able to become pregnant. If pregnancy is desired, the best time to have intercourse is around the time of ovulation.

Some women get a pain, or *mittelschmerz*, when they ovulate. Other signs of ovulation include changes in the cervical mucus. Just before ovulation, the cervical mucus becomes clear, thin, and stretchy. Some women also experience breast tenderness close to ovulation. An ovulation kit, which detects the LH surge 24–36 hours prior to ovulation, can be used to predict the timing of ovulation.

For approximately 24 hours following ovulation, an egg is able to be fertilized. Sperm, on the other hand, are viable for approximately 72 hours. The sperm need certain chemicals and environmental conditions that the female reproductive tract provides to mature fully. Once mature, the sperm are ready to attempt to penetrate the coat surrounding the egg to fertilize it.

Blood sugar control

Women with diabetes have another reason to keep track of their menstrual cycles: anticipating (and possibly taking steps to prevent) higher blood glucose levels during the premenstrual period as well as during the menses. Blood sugar level changes around the time of menstruation appear to be quite common. One study of women with Type 1 diabetes found that 61% had premenstrual rises in blood glucose and that 36% of these women adjusted their insulin doses because of these rises. The study also found that 67% of the women who took constant-dose oral contraceptives had premenstrual blood glucose changes.

Although the exact reason for changes in blood glucose control with the menstrual cycle phases is unknown, it has been hypothesized that the rise in blood glucose is due to the increase in female hormones during this period. Women who do not have diabetes have also been shown to have changes in insulin resistance during the premenstrual and menstrual phases of their cycle, and this supports the idea that changes in hormone levels may affect insulin resistance in women with diabetes.

Another possible reason for changes in blood glucose control is that some women have an increase in carbohydrate consumption during the premenstrual phase, especially if they have food cravings associated with PMS. It has also been suggested that a decrease in activity just before and during the menses may affect blood glucose control in some women.

Women with diabetes should be aware of the possible need for changes in their diabetes care plan during certain phases of the menstrual cycle. To determine if changes are necessary, what they might be, and when to make them, it helps to track blood sugar levels, insulin doses (if any), activity level, and diet on a calendar for two to three cycles.

Severe problems with blood glucose control during the premenstrual and menstrual phases are rare. However, diabetic ketoacidosis may occur in women more often premenstrually. One study of women admitted to hospitals for ketoacidosis showed that 50% were premenstrual or menstruating.

If symptoms involving blood glucose control are severe and recurrent during the premenstrual or menstrual phases of the cycle, one can consider medical menopause, in which menopause is induced with drugs. In extreme cases, hysterectomy and removal of

HORMONE LEVELS DURING THE MENSTRUAL CYCLE

These illustrations show the relative levels of estrogen, progesterone, follicle-stimulating hormone (FSH), and luteinizing hormone (LH) over the course of a 28-day menstrual cycle.

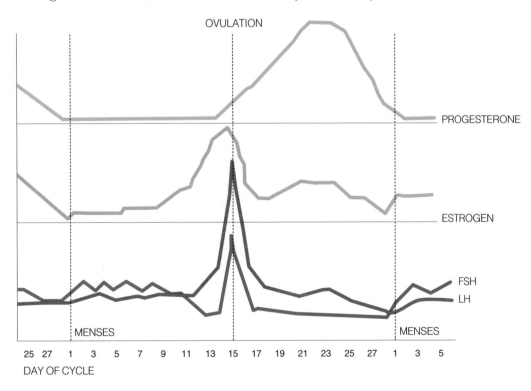

FEMALE REPRODUCTIVE ORGANS

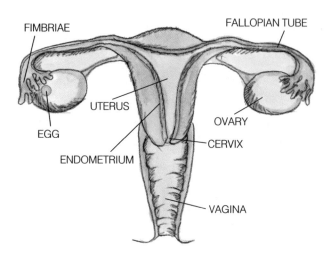

FIMBRIAE
FALLOPIAN TUBE
UTERUS
OVARY
EGG
CERVIX
ENDOMETRIUM
VAGINA

the ovaries has been performed to prevent the monthly hormone fluctuations.

Premenstrual syndrome

Of course, blood sugar control is not the only problem associated with the menstrual cycle. Many women (an estimated 85%) experience physical and emotional changes during the period between ovulation and the first few days of menstrual flow. These physical and emotional changes, or premenstrual symptoms, are considered both common and normal. However, some women (5% to 10%) experience symptoms severe enough to interfere with their daily activities or personal interactions.

The term PMS is used by most people to describe any physical or emotional symptoms that precede menstruation. Medical professionals use the term premenstrual dysphoric disorder (PMDD) for the 3% to 8% of women with severe symptoms. Women with PMS or PMDD generally have a cyclic pattern to their symptoms, with a symptom-free interval from their menses until ovulation. Physical symptoms include abdominal bloating, breast tenderness, acne, appetite changes, food cravings, swelling of the hands, feet, or legs, headaches, and gastrointestinal problems. Emotional symptoms may include fatigue, irritability, emotional lability, depression, and oversensitivity.

Exercise and stress reduction may help with the symptoms of PMS. Medical treatments include oral contraceptives and a class of antidepressants called selective serotonin reuptake inhibitors (SSRI's), which

includes such well known drugs as fluoxetine (brand names Prozac and Sarafem). Occasionally, diuretics are prescribed to relieve swelling.

Menstrual pain

Another common complaint related to menstruation is pain or cramping with the menses, usually lasting one to two days. If the pain is severe enough to interfere with daily activities, it is called *dysmenorrhea.*

For many women, over-the-counter products such as ibuprofen, and home remedies such as exercise, getting plenty of sleep, and heat (from a heating pad or warm soaks) are adequate to ease the pain of dysmenorrhea. (For safety, check bath water temperature with a hand or thermometer before stepping into the bathtub, and keep soaking times short.) Taking oral contraceptives can also help.

When dysmenorrhea has an identifiable, underlying cause, such as infection, adhesions (scar tissue), leiomyoma (fibroid tumors of the uterus), or endometriosis (a condition in which endometrial tissue grows in places other than the uterus), treating the pain may depend on treating the underlying cause.

Feminine hygiene products

While menstrual hygiene remains in many ways a taboo topic, spoken of only in euphemism, the market for feminine sanitary products is enormous. However, the choice still basically boils down to pads or tampons, and the most important factor in making that choice is personal preference.

Sanitary pads, or napkins, come in a variety of absorbency strengths, sizes, and thicknesses and with or without deodorant. Some even have "wings" that wrap around the underwear to prevent staining. Most pads have an adhesive on one side that allows for attachment to the underwear. However, reusable sanitary napkins that are washed between uses are also available.

Tampons sold in the United States are made of cotton, rayon, or a blend of the two. Some tampons are inserted into the vagina with a plastic or cardboard applicator; some with the fingers. A string attached to the tampon allows for removal.

Tampons come in four, standardized absorbencies: junior, regular, super, and super plus. Women should select a tampon absorbency based on the amount of menstrual flow. Normally, a woman should change her tampon every four to six hours. If she needs to change the tampon more frequently, she may want to switch to a more absorbent tampon. If a tampon is difficult to remove, a less absorbent one should be used.

Tampons are generally considered safe to use. However, in the 1980's they were associated with toxic shock syndrome (TSS), a sometimes-fatal disease caused by a bacterial toxin. Although the exact cause of TSS is still unclear, the risk appears to be connected to use of high-absorbency tampons. (Certain high-absorbency products and materials were taken off the market after this association was discovered.) Today, the number of reported cases of TSS that can be associated with tampon use is very small. Nonetheless, to prevent TSS, women are advised to use the least absorptive tampon possible. Any woman who develops symptoms of TSS, which include fever, chills, a rash, nausea and vomiting, diarrhea, dizziness, and fainting, should seek medical help immediately.

A lesser-known option for menstrual hygiene is the menstrual cup, which was first introduced in the 1930's. Various models have come and gone over the years. A reusable menstrual cup, the Keeper, has been on the market since the 1980's. It is made of rubber and is inserted into the vagina like a diaphragm. It collects the menstrual flow and can be removed, rinsed, and reinserted as needed, but it must be rinsed at least every 12 hours. The Keeper is available in two sizes, one for women who have had a vaginal birth, and another for those who have not delivered vaginally. It's environmentally friendly and saves money on the cost of disposable sanitary products.

A disposable menstrual cup, the Instead, is also available. It works the same way as the Keeper but is discarded when removed. It is constructed of a non-latex plastic derivative and should be discarded in the trash, not flushed down the toilet.

A relatively new product designed to handle light menstrual flow is the inSync miniform. The inSync is a 2-inch-long pad that is placed lengthwise between the labia (vaginal lips), which hold it in place. It can also be used for added protection with a tampon or to absorb small urine leaks. The miniform is dislodged with urination and is flushable.

When to see your gynecologist

In the United States, the average age at which girls begin menstruating is 12 years. (Any girl who has not begun menstruating by age 16 should see a doctor about it.) At the other end of the spectrum, menopause, or the cessation of menstrual cycles, occurs, on average, at age 51.

It is generally recommended that girls first see a gynecologist at age 18 or when they become sexually active, whichever happens first. Most women should have an annual gynecologic examination for routine health screening and to screen for cancers of the breast and reproductive system.

Your annual exam is an excellent time to ask any questions you might have about your menstrual cycle. However, it's a good idea to schedule an interim

FOR FURTHER READING

You can never know too much about your body and how it works. These books and Web sites can help inform you and answer your questions.

Books
ENCYCLOPEDIA OF WOMEN'S HEALTH AND WELLNESS
American College of Obstetricians and Gynecologists
Washington DC, 2000

OUR BODIES, OURSELVES FOR THE NEW CENTURY
A Book by and for Women
The Boston Women's Health Book Collective
Simon and Schuster Trade
Paperbacks
New York, 1998

Web sites
www.medem.com
Click on "Medical Library" then "Women's Health" for information sponsored and provided by the American College of Obstetricians and Gynecologists.

www.teenshealth.org
Click on "Sexual Health" for information about menstruation and other topics of teen interest.

appointment if you experience any of the following:
■ You miss a period.
■ Your period is not regular or you are bleeding or spotting between periods.
■ Your period is more frequent than every 21 days or less frequent than every 38 days.
■ You are having to change a pad or tampon at least once an hour or you are having symptoms of anemia, including light-headedness and fatigue.
■ Your menstrual cramps are interfering with your daily activities.
■ You have premenstrual symptoms that are interfering with your daily activities or relationships.

Menstruation is a perfectly normal part of life, but there's no denying it can be a pain in the neck. If over-the-counter and home remedies aren't enough to ease your pain or discomfort, ask your gynecologist for help. Likewise, if you're having trouble with blood glucose control around the time of your period and aren't able to resolve it on your own, ask your gynecologist or diabetes team for help. That's what they're there for! ❑

HORMONE REPLACEMENT
MORE THAN JUST ESTROGEN

by Julia V. Johnson, M.D.

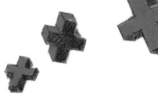

I n recent years, the normal bodily changes that accompany menopause, and the medical problems that often follow menopause, have generated increased interest among both the public and the medical community. Such growing interest stands to reason since women who have gone through menopause make up an ever-larger segment of our society: There are currently more than 40 million women over the age of 50 in the United States.

At the beginning of the 20th century, women generally lived less than 10 years after their last menstrual period, so the cessation of production of the hormones estrogen and progesterone from the ovaries at menopause was not considered important. Today, the average woman lives for 35 years after her last period. This increasing longevity makes the study of these hormonal changes and their effects on the body crucial to maintaining women's health.

New research on menopause and particularly on the role of estrogen in the body has given women much information on how to maintain their health during their midlife years and later. Research has shown that estrogen, in addition to its role in the reproductive cycle, influences many bodily systems, including the brain, bladder, bones, and heart. The slowdown in the body's production of estrogen that occurs at menopause greatly increases a woman's risk of developing conditions such as osteoporosis (bone loss) and heart disease. Hormone replacement therapy can lower the risk of osteoporosis and relieve menopausal symptoms.

The consequences of hormone replacement therapy for heart disease risk are more complicated. For women with diabetes, who already have an increased risk of heart disease, it is important to consider the effect of estrogen therapy on heart attack risk when deciding whether or not to take hormones. In this article, we describe the normal bodily changes that occur during menopause, the potential benefits and risks of hormone replacement therapy, and the available choices for hormone replacement and its alternatives.

Normal changes during menopause

At an average age of 51, women stop their menstrual cycles as the ovaries cease production of estrogen and progesterone. Typically, women begin to experience signs of approaching menopause for several years prior to their last period, as the hormone levels begin to decrease. Because the lining of the uterus is very responsive to changes in estrogen and progesterone levels, the first sign of approaching menopause may be *irregular periods*. Women may find that their menstrual cycles run closer together, or they may skip periods. Menstrual bleeding may become lighter, although occasionally a heavier period may occur, especially if the previous period was missed. However, very heavy periods or unexpected episodes of spotting can be a sign of a uterus problem and should be evaluated by a doctor.

In addition to irregular periods, women may experience *hot flashes* as an early sign of menopause. The temperature regulation center in the brain is very sensitive to estrogen levels, and a drop in estrogen can lead to an increase in skin temperature accompanied by increased heart rate, flushing of the neck and face, sweating, mild nausea, and headache.

Ninety percent of American women experience hot flashes during menopause. Hot flashes that occur during the night, known as *night sweats,* can disrupt sleep, leading to mood changes and irritability during the day. For most women, hot flashes are tolerable, but for about 10%, they can interfere with normal activities. Estrogen replacement therapy can decrease hot flashes and thereby improve sleep. Fortunately, hot flashes usually decrease over time: Most women report only minimal hot flashes by five years after their last menstrual period.

The drop in estrogen that comes with menopause can also weaken the muscles and tissues of the vagina. After menopause, some women experience dryness and thinning of the vagina and vulva, which can lead to discomfort during intercourse and vaginal irritation. Newly developed vaginal lubricants can help relieve dryness. In addition, estrogen therapy can strengthen these tissues and increase moisture.

Another problem for some women after menopause is urinary leakage. The loss of estrogen can compound the effect of other risk factors for incontinence, such as childbirth. Typically, loss of urine occurs when a physical stress such as laughing or sneezing puts pressure on the bladder. This type of leakage is called *stress incontinence*. After menopause, the muscles at the base of the bladder weaken, which can worsen urinary incontinence. There are a number of treatments for stress incontinence. Both estrogen therapy and special exercises for the pelvic floor muscles (called Kegel exercises) can help. Surgery that tightens the muscles that control the bladder can also stop urinary leakage.

Potential benefits

Research has found considerable evidence that hormone replacement therapy can have substantial health benefits. In addition to alleviating hot flashes and vaginal and bladder changes, estrogen protects the bones and may possibly also benefit the cardiovascular system. There is also some evidence suggesting that estrogen may protect memory and brain function in older women.

Osteoporosis. The condition called *osteoporosis*, in which the bones become porous and less dense, is related to the loss of estrogen. Normally, bone is constantly being broken down and rebuilt. Estrogen regulates this bone turnover. When the level of estrogen drops, bone is lost more quickly than it is rebuilt, leading to a net decrease in bone density.

Both men and women lose bone as they age, but after menopause, women who do not take estrogen experience an accelerated loss of 1% to 2% of their bone mass each year. By age 80, women who are not taking hormones can lose over half of their total bone thickness. This thinning leads to fragile bones that can break or fracture easily. By age 60, one-quarter of women have fractures in their vertebrae (spinal bones), a site that is very sensitive to the lack of estrogen. These fractures cause a loss in height, possible back pain, and curvature of the upper spine. By age 90, 20% of women experience a hip fracture, which is life-threatening at that age.

All women are at risk for osteoporosis after menopause. Women who are Caucasian, slender, smokers, or who have a family history of women with fractures have a particularly high risk. Fortunately, special x-rays, called *bone density studies,* can measure bone thickness, predict the risk of fractures, and help women keep tabs on their bone loss. These studies are easy to perform and give very accurate results. New blood tests can be useful in showing increased bone breakdown. Finding osteoporosis early is critical—the disease can be prevented or slowed down but cannot be reversed once the damage has occurred.

In studies that have followed women for up to 20 years, estrogen therapy has been shown to prevent bone thinning and fractures. Although good diet, adequate calcium (at least 1,200 milligrams per day for women over 50), and exercise will slow bone loss, women should still monitor their bone health after menopause to assess their need for treatment.

There also are nonhormonal drugs available for the prevention and treatment of osteoporosis, among them alendronate sodium (brand name Fosamax).

Heart disease. Premenopausal women who do not have diabetes have a much lower risk of developing heart disease than men. After menopause, as estrogen production drops off, their risk increases. Premenopausal women who have diabetes, on the other hand, have as high a risk of developing heart disease as men with diabetes at the same age, and that risk rises even further after menopause. Some studies suggest that the use of hormone replacement therapy after menopause may generally reduce the risk of heart disease in women. Research also suggests, however, that hormone replacement therapy may lead to an increased risk of heart disease in women who already have heart problems.

The effect of estrogen on the heart and blood vessels is being actively researched. It is known that estrogen taken by mouth lowers total cholesterol levels and raises levels of "good" high-density lipoprotein (HDL) cholesterol. These blood lipid changes are associated with reduced risk of heart disease. (Some women, however, may see their triglyceride levels rise.) In addition, estrogen is thought to have a direct effect on the blood vessels, preventing the buildup of plaque, or hard deposits, along blood vessel walls, although some evidence indicates this may not apply to women who already have heart disease. Research also suggests that women without a history of stroke who use hormone replacement therapy may have a reduced risk of stroke.

Brain function. Recent studies have suggested that estrogen may have an effect on brain function. Although studies testing memory and general intellectual function have found some improvement in

FOR MORE INFORMATION

For more information about menopause and the pros and cons of hormone replacement therapy, contact the following organizations, or look for the books listed below at your local bookstore or library:

Organizations

AMERICAN SOCIETY FOR REPRODUCTIVE MEDICINE
1209 Montgomery Highway
Birmingham, AL 35216-2809
(205) 978-5000
Web site: http://www.asrm.com

THE NORTH AMERICAN MENOPAUSE SOCIETY
P.O. Box 94527
Cleveland, OH 44101
(800) 774-5342, (440) 442-7550
Web site: http://www.menopause.org
This society offers a series of booklets that provide current information on the health and emotional issues surrounding menopause.

Books

MENOPAUSE
Isaac Schiff, with Ann B. Parson
Times Books
New York, 1996

PERIMENOPAUSE
Preparing for the Change: A Guide to the Early Stages of Menopause and Beyond
Nancy Lee Teaff and Kim Wright Wiley
Prima Publishing
Rocklin, California, 1999

WHAT EVERY WOMAN SHOULD KNOW
Staying Healthy After 40
Lila E. Nachtigall, Robert D. Nachtigall, and Joan Rattner Heilman
Warner Books
New York, 1996

women taking estrogen replacement, the change is minimal and is not consistent between studies. More exciting is the evidence that memory disorders may be affected by hormones. Menopausal women have a higher risk for Alzheimer disease, and some researchers have proposed that this risk may be related to the loss of estrogen. If this is true, it is possible that women who take estrogen may have a reduced chance of developing Alzheimer disease and that women with the disease may function better mentally when on hormone therapy. Although studies are promising, it is too early to encourage women to take hormone therapy for this reason.

Potential concerns

While hormone replacement therapy offers benefits to women, it also raises some concerns.

Blood glucose control. In the past, there was some concern that taking estrogen and progesterone could adversely affect blood glucose control. However, studies have found that this is not the case. It is true that the higher levels of hormones found in oral contraceptives can minimally increase fasting blood glucose levels and decrease glucose tolerance. But the small doses of hormones used after menopause do not impair blood glucose control. Some studies even suggest a small improvement in glucose control, and in animal studies, estrogen has been found to decrease insulin resistance.

The most commonly used progesterone, medroxyprogesterone acetate, has no effect on blood sugar. Other progesterone drugs, although rarely used for hormone replacement, may slightly diminish the body's ability to process glucose. As with any new therapy, it is important to monitor blood glucose levels closely when starting hormone replacement. However, it is unusual for women to have to alter their insulin dose or oral diabetes medicines while taking hormone replacement therapy.

Blood pressure. In spite of earlier concerns, neither estrogen nor progesterone appears to have any significant effect on blood pressure. And since women with high blood pressure are at increased risk for heart disease, some of them may derive benefit from estrogen therapy.

Blood clots. For most women, taking hormones raises the risk of developing a blood clot minimally, if at all. Studies have suggested that a woman's risk of getting a blood clot may increase slightly when she first starts taking hormones. Women with a history of developing blood clots should watch closely for signs of blood clots, such as pain, when taking hormones.

Other problems. With some medical problems, hormone therapy may not be recommended. Women with active gallbladder or liver problems may not be able to take hormone replacement and should discuss the issue with their doctor.

Cancer. For many women considering hormone therapy, perhaps the most significant issue is the risk of developing estrogen-related cancers. It is important to realize that estrogen is not associated with most cancers. No increases in cancers of the lung, skin, or bowel are seen in women taking hormone therapy. Early studies even suggest a reduced risk of colon cancer in women who take long-term hormone therapy. The concerns about hormones and cancer involve a few specific diseases: *ovarian cancer, endometrial cancer,* and *breast cancer.*

A recent study suggested that women who used hormone replacement for more than 10 years doubled their risk of dying of ovarian cancer.

Estrogen taken alone increases the risk of endometrial cancer (cancer of the lining of the uterus). Taking progesterone along with estrogen, however, eliminates this increased risk. This would seem to indicate that unless you have had a hysterectomy, you may want to consider taking a combination of estrogen and progesterone.

There are some data suggesting, however, that using a combination of the two hormones is associated with a higher risk of breast cancer than is estrogen when taken alone. In general, the effect of hormone therapy on breast cancer remains under study. Although it is known that estrogen and progesterone stimulate breast cells to divide, the effect of these hormones on breast cancer risk is not entirely clear. Some studies have found that estrogen does not increase, and may even decrease, the risk of developing breast cancer. On the other hand, some studies have shown an increased risk in women who take hormones, especially for periods of 10 years or longer. For this reason, some healthcare providers suggest that women only take hormone therapy for fewer than 10 years.

Making your choice

Women who are going through menopause need to consider the risks and benefits of hormone therapy in light of their own health history. It is important to discuss the different therapy options with your healthcare provider.

For those who decide to start hormone therapy, there are several different preparations to choose from. Estrogen comes in three forms: pills, skin patches, and vaginal creams. Each type can fulfill different needs. To relieve vaginal symptoms, women may choose to use an estrogen cream. Estrogen pills have the greatest effect on lowering cholesterol levels, as well as treating hot flashes and vaginal symptoms and preventing bone loss. Some women prefer a skin patch, which is placed on the abdomen or buttocks and gives a steady release of estrogen.

Progesterone therapy is necessary to prevent overgrowth of the uterine lining. It can be given in two ways: cyclic or continuous. The cyclic method, which involves taking progesterone pills for 10 to 12 days out of the month, triggers a light menstrual period once a month. Women who want to avoid bleeding may pre-

fer continuous progesterone therapy, in which a smaller dose of progesterone is taken every day. Although some women have spotting for the first 6 to 12 months, 80% of women have no bleeding after one year if they take progesterone pills every day.

Mild side effects such as headache, breast tenderness, fluid retention, and mood changes can occur with hormone replacement therapy. Fortunately, these side effects can often be eliminated by changing the type or dose of medicine. It is important to call your doctor if you have any concerns after starting hormone therapy.

Some people have touted the use of herbal products or "natural" hormones to ease menopausal symptoms. Unfortunately, since these products are out of the jurisdiction of the U.S. Food and Drug Administration, their potency and purity is poorly controlled. Many of these products have little hormonal effect, and they can be very costly. In addition, no studies have been done to determine whether they benefit the bones or heart. For women who choose to use hormone replacement therapy, it makes sense to use only agents that have been thoroughly tested.

The good news for women who prefer not to take estrogen and progesterone is that several new drugs that address some of the same health concerns are becoming available. The first of these drugs, raloxifene (brand name Evista), was approved for use in preventing osteoporosis and limiting bone loss in December 1997. Raloxifene is one of a very promising group of drugs called *selective estrogen receptor modulators.* These so-called "designer estrogens" act like estrogen but only in some tissues. In other tissues, such as the breast, these drugs actually oppose the effect of estrogen. These agents may improve blood cholesterol levels in a manner similar to estrogen. Unfortunately, they do not prevent hot flashes or treat vaginal symptoms, and little is known about their ability to prevent heart disease.

Hormones and your health

It is important for women to consider the potential benefits and risks of using estrogen and progesterone. Treatment of symptoms such as hot flashes and vaginal or bladder changes and prevention of osteoporosis and, perhaps, heart disease should be balanced against such concerns as a possible increased risk of certain types of cancer. While research suggests that some women who are at risk for heart disease may lead longer and healthier lives if they choose to take hormones, the picture is more complicated for others, among them women with diabetes. It is important to talk to a doctor about the pros and cons of hormone replacement therapy. Once you have all the information, the choice is yours. ❑

CUTTING YOUR RISK OF OSTEOPOROSIS

by Linda Pachucki-Hyde, R.N., M.S., C.D.E.

When you look at old family pictures, does your mother look taller and stand straighter in the photos than she does now? Does she look a little shorter and more hunched over each time you see her?

Or maybe your son seems taller every time you see him, and you have to stretch up that much further to give him a kiss. "How is that possible?" you ask yourself. "He's an adult now. Surely he stopped growing years ago."

It's unlikely that your adult son is still growing. But it's entirely possible that your mother—and you—are getting shorter. Loss of height and spinal curvature (a "dowager's hump") are common among older women, and they are almost always signs of osteoporosis, a progressive condition in which the bones lose mass, become weak and brittle, and, often, fracture.

Osteoporosis is a common disorder; it currently affects or threatens more than 28 million Americans, including 10 million who have the disease and another 18 million with low bone mass that places them at an increased risk of developing it. While men can get osteoporosis, it is much more common among women, especially postmenopausal women. Having Type 1 diabetes places a woman at higher risk of developing osteoporosis. Having Type 2 diabetes, on the other hand, appears to lower the risk, although it is not entirely clear why this is so. (Of course, a lower risk does not guarantee that a person will not develop a given condition.)

Because osteoporosis is much more easily prevented than treated, it makes sense for everyone to take some common-sense preventive measures long before any signs of osteoporosis would be expected to show up. Among other things, such measures include consuming adequate amounts of calcium and vitamin D and exercising regularly.

Bone growth and loss

In spite of its permanent appearance, bone is living, growing tissue that is constantly being broken down and rebuilt (a process doctors call "resorption and formation"). In children, more bone is built than is broken down. However, as a person ages, the balance shifts, and bone begins breaking down faster than it is rebuilt. Bone loss generally begins around age 35 at a rate of about 0.25% to 1% per year. At menopause,

the rate of bone loss can accelerate to 2% to 3% per year for three to seven years or longer among women who do not take hormone replacements. Later, the rate of bone loss slows down again.

In osteoporosis, so much bone is lost that the inner structure of the bones actually looks porous when compared with healthy bones under a microscope. In many cases, osteoporosis leaves bones so fragile that fractures result not from serious trauma (like getting in a car accident or falling out of a tree) but from everyday movements such as lifting something heavy, twisting around to reach for something, or stepping off a curb.

It is estimated that one in every two women will sustain an osteoporotic fracture in her lifetime. The most vulnerable sites are the hip, spine, and wrist, but any bone other than the skull is at risk.

There are two main factors that influence your risk of osteoporosis: the maximum amount of bone you ever have, called your *peak bone mass*, and how much bone you lose as you age. The strongest predictor of peak bone mass, which occurs between ages 20 and 30, is heredity. Other factors, such as childhood nutrition and anything that delays or interrupts normal menstruation, can also affect bone formation.

Heredity is the strongest predictor of developing osteoporosis. If you have family members who have had hip or spine fractures, your risk of developing osteoporosis is probably higher. Caucasians, especially those of European ancestry, and Asians have an increased risk of osteoporosis. However, many other factors affect bone loss. You can control some of these risk factors, but not all of them.

Diet and lifestyle. Calcium is the primary mineral component of bone. However, your body uses calcium for many things besides building bone. Therefore, if you don't get enough calcium from your diet, your body leaches calcium from your bones for its other needs, making your bones weaker. (To find out how much calcium you need to consume on a daily basis, see "Calcium Counts" on page 395.)

Getting adequate amounts of vitamin D, which aids in calcium absorption, is another important part of the picture. The main food source of vitamin D is fortified milk. Some vitamin D is also available in egg yolks and oily fish. Your body also manufactures vitamin D when skin is exposed to sunlight. However, in

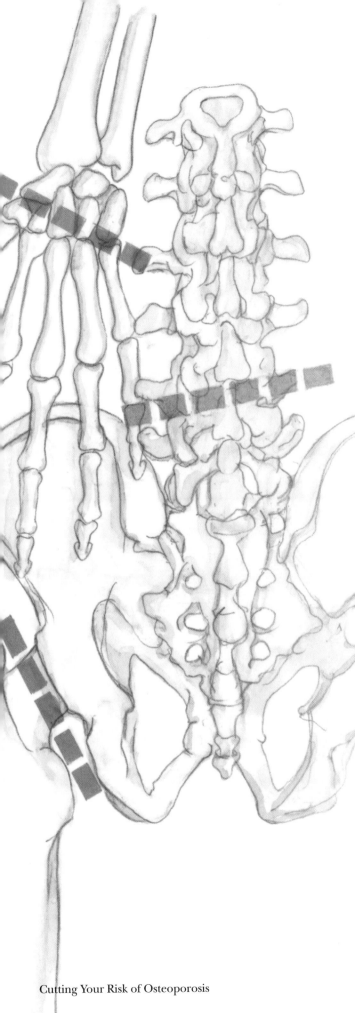

the northern part of the United States and in Canada, the sun is not bright enough during the winter to produce any vitamin D.

Excessive alcohol intake (usually defined as more than one drink per day for women and more than two drinks per day for men) is thought to decrease bone formation and to reduce the body's ability to absorb calcium. Smoking increases bone loss and is considered a major risk factor for osteoporosis. Excessive caffeine intake has also been suspected of contributing to osteoporosis, but no one can say just how much is too much.

Exercise, especially weight-bearing exercises such as walking, jogging, and dancing, helps to strengthen bones, while a sedentary lifestyle raises the risk for osteoporosis. Being tall and thin is also a risk factor for osteoporosis, so having a little extra weight on your bones if you're tall is actually protective.

Medical conditions. In addition to Type 1 diabetes, certain medical conditions, including thyroid disorders, rheumatoid arthritis, asthma, and organ transplantation, are all associated with increased risk of osteoporosis, chiefly because of the medicines used to treat them. Conditions that interfere with your body's ability to absorb nutrients, such as stomach surgery or celiac disease (an allergic intolerance to gluten, a protein in wheat, rye, and other grains), will limit the amount of calcium you can absorb from your diet.

Drugs used to control seizures interfere with vitamin D metabolism, thereby decreasing the absorption of calcium. Steroids such as prednisone and cortisone accelerate bone loss, impede bone formation, and reduce calcium absorption. If you must take one of these drugs, talk to your doctor about monitoring your bone density and taking precautions to help prevent bone loss.

Diabetes and osteoporosis

The relationship between diabetes and osteoporosis is complex. Because insulin is necessary for bone growth, having too little insulin leads to increased calcium loss through urine, decreased absorption of calcium from food, decreased levels of active vitamin D, and fewer bone-building cells, known as *osteoblasts*. All of these factors interfere with bone growth. The effects of inadequate insulin are most apparent at the onset of Type 1 diabetes. At the time of diagnosis, people with Type 1 diabetes have about a 10% lower bone density than people of the same age and sex who do not have diabetes. Once insulin and glucose levels are controlled, however, bone loss can be stabilized.

People with Type 2 diabetes, who usually get diabetes after they have reached their peak bone mass, may actually have a lower rate of bone loss than the average person without diabetes. One reason for this may be that people with Type 2 diabetes have, on aver-

RISK FACTORS

The following characteristics increase a person's risk of developing osteoporosis:

PHYSICAL RISKS
Female sex
Over age 65
Family history of osteoporosis
Caucasian or Asian ancestry
Postmenopausal (surgical or natural; risk even higher if menopause occurs before age 40)
Any prolonged absence of menstruation after puberty

LIFESTYLE FACTORS
Smoking
High alcohol intake
Low calcium intake
Sedentary lifestyle
Prolonged periods of bed rest or immobility

MEDICAL CONDITIONS
Asthma
Celiac disease
Cushing syndrome
Hyperparathyroidism
Hyperthyroidism
Multiple myeloma
Organ transplantation
Rheumatoid arthritis
Seizure disorder drugs
Stomach or intestinal surgery

age, a higher body-mass index, which seems to offer some protection. Studies also suggest that people with Type 2 diabetes experience less bone turnover than people who don't have diabetes, which reduces their net bone loss even if they start out with a lower peak bone mass.

Diagnosing osteoporosis

Often, the first sign of osteoporosis is a bone fracture. Fractures of the bones of the spine (the vertebrae) can cause painful backaches, but can also go unnoticed. This is probably because the vertebrae are often crushed, or squashed, rather than broken. Such crushing fractures are what lead to loss of height and curvature of the spine. Repeated spinal fractures can also lead to breathing and digestive problems. Other fractures, such as those of the hip and wrist, are much more obvious when they occur. Hip fractures lead to death in 15% of cases and loss of independence in more than 50% of cases.

Luckily, you don't have to wait for a fracture to find out if you have osteoporosis. Instead, you can have a bone-density test. There are many ways to measure your bone density, but the most reliable test is called *dual energy x-ray absorptiometry (DEXA)*. At one time, this test could only be done at large medical centers, but now you may find it at clinics and even in some doctors' offices. The test takes only 10 to 15 minutes to perform, and the radiation used is lower than that used to take a chest x-ray. (Regular x-rays cannot detect osteoporosis until you have lost 30% or more of your bone density.) If a DEXA test shows a low bone density, blood tests that measure calcium levels and other components may be used to monitor the progress of treatment. (Such blood tests cannot be used to diagnose osteoporosis.)

Treatment

Treatment and prevention of osteoporosis have a lot in common. The first step for both is to ensure that you are getting an adequate supply of calcium and vitamin D. No form of therapy will be effective if you are not getting enough of these nutrients.

If you are unable to take in enough calcium in food to meet your daily needs, you may want to think about taking a supplement. Many forms of calcium are sold as supplements. The two most common forms are *calcium carbonate* and *calcium citrate*. Calcium carbonate, often called oyster shell calcium, is the least expensive type of calcium supplement. (This is the kind of calcium found in Tums.) The only drawback is that it may cause constipation. It works best when taken with meals. Calcium citrate, while more expensive, does not cause constipation and is absorbed very easily. It does not have to be taken with meals. Whichever type of supplement you take, keep in mind that your body can only absorb about 500 to 600 milligrams (mg) of calcium at one time. So be sure to take no more than that at one time and to wait three to four hours before taking another calcium supplement.

Vitamin D can also be taken as a supplement, if necessary. The U.S. National Academy of Sciences recommends that people aged 51 to 70 should have 400 international units (IU) of vitamin D a day, with a target of 600 IU a day for people over 70. However, many osteoporosis experts believe these levels may be too low and recommend taking 700 to 800 IU each day. Most multivitamins contain 400 IU of vitamin D per pill. Many calcium supplements also contain some vitamin D, but the amount varies widely. You can also buy individual vitamin D supplements. But be careful not to take too much: Taking more than 2,000 IU daily of vitamin D can be harmful.

Exercise is as important for treatment as it is for prevention. Since your back muscles help hold you erect and can help lessen the load on your spine, keeping them strong helps keep your spine strong. Back exercises known as *extension exercises* are good for your upper spine. If you have osteoporosis, ask your doctor for a referral to a physical therapist who can teach you how to do extension exercises and other back strengtheners safely at home.

Drugs. While calcium, vitamin D, and exercise are essential to treating osteoporosis, they may not be enough. Fortunately, new drug therapies have been developed to prevent bone loss or slow its progression. These include estrogen replacement therapy for women and therapies using bisphosphonates, calcitonin, and, most recently, selective estrogen receptor modulators.

Estrogen replacement therapy is recommended as the first line of defense for the prevention of postmenopausal osteoporosis. The chief reason for accelerated bone loss after menopause is the loss of estrogen. Studies show that women who replace the estrogen their ovaries no longer make experience much slower bone loss than postmenopausal women who do not take estrogen. Both estrogen pills and estrogen patches have beneficial effects on bone health. However, estrogen replacement therapy may increase the risk of certain types of cancer. In addition, oral estrogen can raise triglyceride levels in susceptible individuals. Since many women with Type 2 diabetes already have or are predisposed to having elevated triglyceride levels, those who decide to try estrogen replacement therapy may be better off using a patch. (For a full discussion of the pros and cons of estrogen replacement, see "Hormone Replacement Therapy: Not Just Estrogen" on page 388.)

In December 1997 a drug called raloxifene (brand name Evista) was approved for the prevention of postmenopausal osteoporosis; more recently it was approved for treatment as well. Raloxifene belongs to a class of drugs called *selective estrogen receptor modulators (SERMS)*, nicknamed "designer estrogens." These drugs offer some of the benefits of estrogen, including protecting the bones and lowering cholesterol levels (although not as well as estrogen), without the same risks. SERMS do not stimulate breast or uterine tissue and therefore do not increase the risk of breast or uterine cancer or cause menstrual bleeding.

The osteoporosis drugs alendronate sodium (brand name Fosamax) and risedronate sodium (Actonel) belong to a class of drugs called *bisphosphonates,* which work by slowing the rate of bone loss. They are used both to prevent and treat osteoporosis. Studies have shown that they reduce the risk of fractures. When used correctly, they cause very few side

CALCIUM COUNTS

Most Americans get far less calcium than they should each day. Recommendations made in 1994 by the U.S. National Institutes of Health regarding daily calcium intake are as follows:

Birth to 6 months . . . . 400 mg

6 months to 1 year . . . . 600 mg

1 to 10 years . . . . 800–1200 mg

11 to 24 years . . . . 1200–1500 mg

25 to 50 years. . . . . 1000 mg

51 to 64 years. . . . . 1000 mg
   (men, and women on hormone
   replacement therapy)

51 years or older . . . . 1500 mg
   (women not on hormone
   replacement therapy)

65 years or older . . . . 1500 mg
   (all men and women)

Pregnant or
breast-feeding women . . . . 1200–1500 mg

The U.S. Academy of Sciences in 1997 issued the following estimated daily requirements for calcium:

Birth to 6 months . . . . 210 mg

6 months to 1 year . . . . 270 mg

1 to 3 years . . . . 500 mg

4 to 8 years . . . . 800 mg

9 to 18 years . . . . 1300 mg

19 to 50 years. . . . . 1000 mg

51 years or older . . . . 1200 mg

Pregnant or breast-feeding
women 18 years or less . . . . 1300 mg

Pregnant or breast-feeding
women 19 to 50 years. . . . . 1000 mg

effects. However, it is important to follow the directions for taking them exactly: Alendronate and risedronate must be taken on an empty stomach first thing in the morning. Always take the drugs with a full, 8-ounce glass of water. Studies show that any other beverage severely limits their absorption. After taking the drug, wait at least half an hour before eating or drinking anything besides water, and don't lie down for at least 30 minutes. If you do not take these drugs according to the instructions, they may not be absorbed and may cause heartburn and inflammation of the esophagus.

RESOURCES

To learn more about osteoporosis, contact these organizations:

NATIONAL OSTEOPOROSIS FOUNDATION
1232 22nd Street, N.W.
Washington, DC 20037-1292
(202) 223-2226
www.nof.org

OLDER WOMEN'S LEAGUE
666 11th Street, N.W., Suite 700
Washington, DC 20001
(202) 783-6686
(800) TAKE-OWL (825-3695)
www.owl-national.org

THE CALCIUM INFORMATION CENTER
(800) 321-2681
This hotline, a cooperative venture of the New York Hospital–Cornell Medical Center and the Oregon Health Sciences University, offers information about calcium and a question-and-answer service.

CALCIUMINFO.COM
A Web site with calcium information, sponsored by GlaxoSmithKline, the maker of Tums:
www.calciuminfo.com

Calcitonin, a hormone normally produced in the thyroid gland, also decreases the rate of bone loss. It is sold under the brand name Miacalcin. Until recently, calcitonin could only be taken by injection, but now Miacalcin is also available in a nasal spray. Like the other osteoporosis drugs, calcitonin has minimal side effects as long as you take it correctly. However, the nasal spray has been known to cause nasal irritation in some people.

Avoiding fractures

Drug therapy can slow the progression of osteoporosis, but if the damage has started, you will have a higher risk for fractures. That's why it is important to safeguard your home against any hazards that might trip you up.

Most hip fractures result from falls. While it is impossible to eliminate every hazard from your life, you can take steps to "fallproof" your home. Start by keeping floors and stairways clear of clutter. Throw rugs can be dangerous when they slide or bunch up, so avoid using them. Do not wax your floors to the point that they become slippery. Make your bathroom safer by using adhesive grip pads or a mat inside the tub, and install grab bars to help you steady yourself.

Having good lighting in your home is another important safety measure. Plug your lamps into outlets that are controlled by a wall switch so you don't have to lean over a table or walk through a dark room to reach them. Use night-lights, and place reflective strips on steps and doorways to make sure you see them.

To keep yourself steady on your feet, wear supportive, flat shoes that have good traction. Use a cane or walker if you need the extra support. Get up slowly from sitting or lying positions to avoid dizzy spells, and consider purchasing a cordless phone to keep by your side so you won't lunge for the phone when it rings.

Spinal fractures are more likely to occur after any bending, twisting, or jarring motion. To avoid these movements, try not to bend at the waist; bend your knees instead if you need to lower your body. This may mean doing some exercises to strengthen your thigh muscles. Avoid lifting anything heavy, especially if you have to bend to do it. Walk around tables and furniture rather than reaching over them. And place frequently used kitchen items in cabinets where you can reach them without bending or stretching. You might also want to consider investing in tools and gadgets that can help you avoid bending. For instance, you can buy a "reacher," or metal claw on a pole, to retrieve items from high shelves, and elastic shoelaces that allow you to slip your feet into and out of your shoes without untying them.

Certain drugs can disrupt your balance or make you dizzy. Be careful with strong pain relievers, especially narcotics, since these can make you dizzy. Blood pressure medicine and some antidepressants may also cause dizzy spells, especially when you get up from a chair or bed. Alcohol, too, can disturb your sense of balance.

Certain diabetic complications increase your risk of falling. Retinopathy that is serious enough to affect vision, and nerve damage of the hands or feet that is serious enough to cause numbness can lead to falls. If you have either of these conditions and also osteoporosis, you will want to use extra caution in order to prevent falls.

Pain control

Osteoporotic fractures of the spine can cause significant and chronic pain. One of the best treatments to minimize pain and prevent future fractures is exercise. Visit a physical therapist as soon as possible after a fracture to learn proper posture and back-strengthening exercises. While exercise may seem like the last thing you would want to do, you may find it is the most helpful. Your physical therapist or doctor may also recommend supports and braces that can help you. To relieve pain, sitting against an ice pack often has the best pain-numbing effect.

Standing up to bone loss

Osteoporosis is known for being a sneaky disease, but you don't have to let it sneak up on you. Regardless of your age, make sure you consume at least the minimum recommended daily amount of calcium and vitamin D. Remember to take that daily walk: Exercise is key to keeping bones healthy. And if you are approaching or have already passed menopause but haven't yet talked with your doctor about bone-density studies, hormone replacement therapy, and other therapies to slow bone loss after menopause, do it now. Just as good diabetes self-management lowers your risk of developing diabetic complications, taking steps to lower your risk of osteoporosis and to treat it if you have it also improves your chances of living a longer, healthier life. ❏

PREVENTING HEART DISEASE

by Charles A. Reasner, M.D.

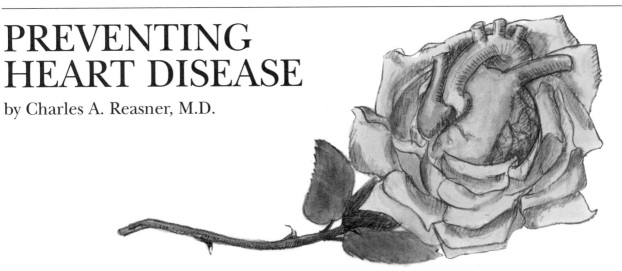

Coronary heart disease is the leading cause of death in men and women in the United States. Each year an estimated 500,000 women die as a result of some form of cardiovascular disease, a mortality rate that exceeds all cancer deaths combined. While men and women have similar risks of having a heart attack, women typically have their first heart attack 15 to 20 years later than men. This is because premenopausal women secrete estrogen, which is known to protect them from cardiac disease. After menopause, however, the risk of a woman developing coronary heart disease increases rapidly. The bad news is that the "protection" from coronary heart disease most premenopausal women enjoy is lost if a woman develops diabetes.

The largest study to examine risk factors for developing heart disease was carried out in Framingham, Massachusetts. The results of this landmark study clearly showed that while men between 35 and 64 years of age who don't have diabetes were two or three times more likely to develop coronary heart disease than their female counterparts, women with diabetes were just as likely to have heart disease as men with diabetes *at the same age*. Put another way, diabetes doubles the risk of a man dying from coronary heart dis-

ease while it increases a woman's risk of dying of a heart attack fivefold.

Several studies have shown that doctors are less likely to investigate complaints of coronary ischemia (an insufficient supply of blood to the heart) in women than in men. In one large study, angina (chest pain), a symptom of ischemia, was experienced at least once a week by three-fourths of men and women documented to have coronary heart disease. Similar degrees of physical activity caused chest pain in both sexes, with 40% of men and women reporting angina even at rest. Although the prevalence, frequency, and severity of angina was similar in men and women in this study, only half as many women as men were referred for cardiac catheterization (a procedure used to detect narrowed or blocked arteries) or coronary bypass surgery.

I suspect that many doctors still feel coronary heart disease is uncommon in women. But since coronary heart disease occurs at the same age and with the same frequency in women with diabetes as men with diabetes, it is important that women with diabetes find doctors who appreciate their risks of having a heart attack and who will work with them to limit the development and progression of this devastating disease.

Syndrome X

Syndrome X, also known as the insulin-resistance syndrome, is responsible for the dramatic increase in coronary heart disease seen in people with Type 2 diabetes (see "Syndrome X and Heart Disease" on the opposite page). Syndrome X has a hereditary component: Researchers have measured insulin levels in children of two parents with diabetes and found that they need to make twice as much insulin to keep their blood sugar normal as children of parents who don't have diabetes. Because these individuals require such high levels of insulin to control their blood sugar, doctors say they are *insulin resistant.*

Weight gain is also associated with insulin resistance. Therefore, if a person with insulin resistance gains weight, the amount of insulin required to keep the blood sugar under control will increase even further. If the person's pancreas cannot produce enough insulin to keep up with the high demand, the person's blood sugar will increase, and he or she will develop Type 2 diabetes.

Unfortunately, insulin resistance and the resulting high levels of insulin in the blood (called *hyperinsulinemia*) cause other metabolic abnormalities: High insulin levels are associated with high blood pressure and high levels of cholesterol and triglycerides (abnormal lipids) in the bloodstream. The combination of insulin resistance, hyperinsulinemia, abnormal blood lipids, high blood pressure, and obesity lead to the development of atherosclerosis, the formation of plaques in the inner lining of the arteries. And atherosclerosis dramatically increases the risk of coronary heart disease.

Prevention strategies

Many steps can and should be taken by women to prevent or delay the onset of cardiovascular disease. The two most important reversible risk factors for coronary heart disease are elevated blood lipid levels and cigarette smoking. In this article, we also look at the roles of estrogen, high blood pressure, obesity, some diabetes pills, and folic acid in the development and prevention of coronary heart disease.

Blood lipids

The most important risk factor for heart disease in men and women is abnormal blood lipids (cholesterol and triglycerides). While many more studies have been done in men than in women with high cholesterol levels, available evidence suggests that women may respond better to lipid-lowering therapy than men.

In the Arteriosclerosis Specialized Center of Research trial, people with very high cholesterol levels were treated with either modest or aggressive cholesterol-lowering therapies. After two years, aggressively treated women showed significant shrinkage of atherosclerotic blockages in their blood vessels. However, only modest improvement was seen in men.

In the Canadian Coronary Atherosclerosis Interventions Trial, only 4% of women who had their cholesterol lowered with the drug lovastatin developed new blood vessel blockages, compared with 45% of women given a placebo pill. Again, women responded better than men: In this trial, 18% of men treated with lovastatin developed new blockages.

In the Scandinavian Simvastatin Survival Study, 827 women with documented coronary artery disease were studied. The women who had their cholesterol lowered with the drug simvastatin experienced 35% fewer major coronary heart events than women given a placebo.

More recently, the Cholesterol and Recurrent Events study compared people with heart disease and mildly elevated cholesterol levels who were treated with either the cholesterol-lowering drug pravastatin or a placebo. Men in this study had a 20% reduction in coronary heart disease events, whereas women had a 46% reduction.

The results of all of these studies underscore the importance of women achieving the lipid levels recommended by the American Diabetes Association for all people with diabetes (see "Recommended Lipid Levels" on page 400). Unfortunately, few people (men or women) are reaching these goals. A recent survey of 2,763 postmenopausal women with heart disease showed that while 47% of participants were taking a cholesterol-lowering drug, only 9% had met rational guidelines for low-density lipoprotein (LDL) cholesterol (the "bad" cholesterol).

Cigarette smoking

Cigarette smoking is the number one preventable cause of premature death in the United States. Smokers have about twice the risk of developing coronary heart disease as do nonsmokers. When an individual stops smoking, his or her risk of having a heart attack gradually diminishes until it reaches that of a nonsmoker in about two years.

Many of the effects of cigarette smoking have been implicated in the development of coronary heart disease. Cigarette smoking causes a decrease in the level of high-density lipoprotein (HDL) cholesterol (the "good" cholesterol). It raises the levels of LDL cholesterol and triglycerides. Smoking also makes blood clot more easily by activating blood platelets and raising the level of fibrinogen (a blood component involved in clotting). This may increase the risk that a blood clot will block a coronary artery and cause a heart attack. Finally, cigarette smoking may damage the lining of the coronary arteries, which makes them more likely to constrict (become smaller) rather than dilate (become larger) in response to stress.

Unfortunately, in spite of compelling data detailing the health risks of cigarette smoking, approximately 3,000 Americans start smoking each day. They often continue to smoke until they experience their first heart attack or undergo coronary artery bypass surgery.

Estrogen

Estrogen has been in the news a lot lately, and its popular reputation seems to almost seesaw between that of savior and villain. That makes it all the harder to decide whether taking estrogen is right for you. However, a number of studies have helped spell out the benefits and risks of taking estrogen, either for birth control or for hormone replacement after menopause.

Oral contraceptives. These synthetic drugs contain estrogen and progestin in doses high enough to prevent a woman from ovulating, or releasing an egg. Several studies have shown an increased risk of coronary heart disease in women who take oral contraceptives. However, the increased risk seems to be seen primarily in women who smoke cigarettes.

In a study published in 1981 by the Royal College of General Practitioners, women who took oral contraceptives and smoked heavily had a 21-fold increase in heart attacks. Women who took oral contraceptives and did not smoke had no increased risk of heart attacks. Because the oral contraceptives commonly used today contain less estrogen than those used when this study was conducted, the risk of coronary heart disease may be lower now for women who smoke.

Estrogen replacement. Numerous studies have examined the impact of postmenopausal estrogen use on coronary heart disease. A number of studies suggest that a woman can expect a reduction in the risk of coronary heart disease if she takes estrogen after menopause. In particular, they point to an apparent improvement in a woman's blood lipid levels, with a decrease in LDL cholesterol and an increase in HDL cholesterol. Additionally, estrogen use in postmenopausal women has been associated with lowering blood pressure, blood glucose, and plasma insulin levels. Some evidence, however, points to a possible association between estrogen replacement therapy and an increased risk of heart problems in women who already have heart disease. In addition, estrogen use may slightly increase the risk of developing certain kinds of cancer. Any postmenopausal woman with diabetes who does not have a medical condition that makes using estrogen unwise should discuss with her doctor the likely benefits and risks of taking estrogen for the purpose of reducing her chances of developing coronary heart disease.

Blood pressure

Controlling high blood pressure will reduce the risk of coronary artery disease by 15% and will reduce the risk of stroke by 40%. While many classes of antihypertensive drugs are effective in lowering blood pressure, I use angiotensin-converting enzyme

SYNDROME X AND HEART DISEASE

This illustration shows the relationship of the insulin-resistance syndrome (Syndrome X) to the development of coronary heart disease. Insulin resistance gives rise to unhealthy conditions, which, in combination, increase the risk of coronary heart disease.

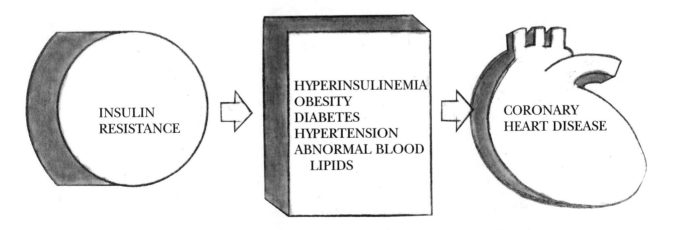

INSULIN RESISTANCE

HYPERINSULINEMIA
OBESITY
DIABETES
HYPERTENSION
ABNORMAL BLOOD
LIPIDS

CORONARY
HEART DISEASE

RECOMMENDED LIPID LEVELS

These are the American Diabetes Association recommendations for lipid levels in people with diabetes:

LDL Cholesterol:	below 100 mg/dl
Triglycerides:	below 200* mg/dl

*Triglyceride levels below 150 are desirable.

(ACE) inhibitors as first-line therapy for hypertension in people with diabetes. ACE inhibitors not only reduce the risk of coronary heart disease, but will protect the kidneys, as well. In fact, the ACE inhibitor ramipril has been shown to prevent heart disease in women with diabetes who have normal blood pressure.

Weight loss

Obesity decreases the quantity and quality of life. But weight alone is not the only important measure. The distribution of fat on a person's body predicts the risk of coronary heart disease in men and women. Accumulation of fat around the waist increases the risk of heart disease to a much greater extent than weight gained in the hips.

You can tell if your fat distribution places you at increased risk for developing coronary heart disease by measuring your waist and hips. Divide your waist measurement by your hip measurement. For example, if your waist measures 25 inches and your hips measure 35 inches, divide 25 by 35 for an answer of 0.7. Ideally, the answer you get should be less than 0.8. If it is higher, you may need to lose some weight.

A reduced-calorie, low-fat, high-fiber diet combined with a sensible exercise program is one of the most effective ways to reduce the risk of coronary disease in individuals with diabetes.

Diet pills or appetite-suppressant drugs have drawn considerable interest. While most of these drugs have been proven to help some people lose weight, none are without significant side effects. A frank discussion with your doctor regarding the potential risks as well as the benefits of these drugs is mandatory to allow you to make an informed decision regarding their use.

Diabetes pills

People with Type 2 diabetes who take pills to lower their blood glucose levels because they have been unable to control their blood glucose with diet and exercise alone should note that certain "insulin sensitizers"—drugs that make insulin work better—may also have beneficial effects for the heart in some individuals. An insulin-sensitizing drug such as metformin (brand name Glucophage; generic versions were approved for marketing in the United States in 2002) not only lowers blood sugar but helps to reverse metabolic abnormalities associated with the insulin-resistance syndrome. In addition to lowering blood sugar levels, metformin reduces triglyceride levels about 15% and causes an average weight loss of 8 to 10 pounds during the first six months of use. Other examples are pioglitazone (Actos) and rosiglitazone (Avandia), which in addition to lowering glucose also nudge triglyceride levels down; pioglitazone and rosiglitazone, however, may promote weight gain. When used alone to control blood glucose, none of these drugs will reduce blood glucose to lower than normal levels.

Homocysteine

There is a high incidence of coronary heart disease in adolescents with a rare metabolic disease called *homocystinuria*. This disease results in extremely high blood levels of homocysteine, an amino acid. (Amino acids are the basic structural units of all proteins.) It is believed that these high levels of homocysteine damage the lining of the blood vessels.

Recently, higher than average levels of homocysteine have also been found in individuals who smoke, have high cholesterol levels, and have high blood pressure. It is not known what role modest increases in homocysteine play in the development of coronary heart disease. Folic acid, a vitamin, appears to be able to effectively lower homocysteine levels with no side effects, and so some doctors suggest that their patients supplement their diet with folate (the active form of folic acid). The daily intake of folate recommended for healthy adults by the U.S. Institute of Medicine is 400 micrograms (abbreviated either μg or mcg on most labels), with higher intakes recommended for pregnant women (600 μg) and lactating women (500 μg). Adults should not consume more than 1 milligram daily unless specifically instructed to do so by their doctor. More data will be necessary for scientists to determine if taking folate will reduce the risk of coronary heart disease.

One step at a time

As you can see, there are many steps you and your doctor can take to lower your risk of coronary heart disease. Some of the steps we describe in this article, such as stopping smoking, losing weight, and maintaining a healthy diet and exercise program, may require some hard work on your part. Others, such as using estrogen replacement therapy or cholesterol-lowering drug therapy or taking an insulin-sensitizing diabetes pill, require a discussion with (and a prescription from) your doctor.

Whichever step you choose to take first, enlist your doctor's help in coming up with a coronary heart disease prevention plan that's right for you. Keep in mind that you're taking these steps for a longer, more active life. ❏

STRATEGIES FOR HANDLING STRESS
Guidelines for Women
by Ivy D. Marcus, Ph.D., C.D.E

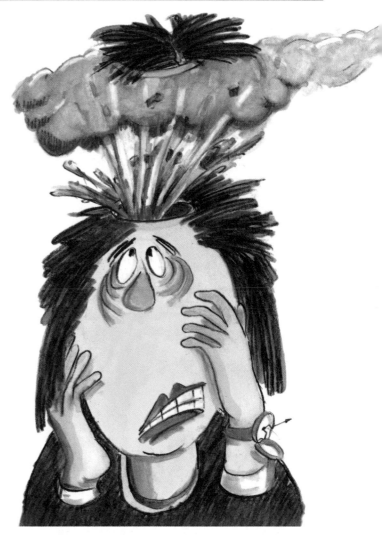

I f you're about to read this article, chances are good that you believe you have too much stress in your life and would like to eliminate it. Well, the bad news is that everyone has stress, and no one will ever get rid of it.

The good news, though, is that most people can learn how to manage the stress in their lives more effectively, and that can help them feel much less burdened. In fact, there are many benefits to effectively managing stress, ranging from more stable blood glucose control to an increased sense of well-being.

Understanding stress

It is important to understand just what we mean when we talk about stress, and theoretical definitions of stress abound. Probably the best definition was offered by the renowned Austrian-born Canadian stress researcher Hans Selye, who summarized stress as "...any bodily change produced as a response to a perceived demand being placed upon the individual." This definition highlights the notion that there are two important facets to stress: the psychological (or mental) and the physiological (or physical).

Stress can be typically negative events, called "distress," as well as the more positive happenings in life that nonetheless demand change and adjustment. After a demand is perceived, bodily or physical changes occur as a reaction. These biological responses typically include increased heart rate, respiration rate, blood pressure, and muscular tension, shallow (rather than deep) breathing, and the increased release of certain so-called stress hormones such as adrenaline and cortisol.

Such bodily changes occur for what is commonly known as the "fight-or-flight" response. The fight-or-flight response served a purpose ages ago, when acute, sudden stressors such as animal predators immediately threatened a person's existence. Successfully fighting off or fleeing from the threat greatly increased one's chance of survival. And, as with other creatures, our fight-or-flight stress reaction became "wired in" as a protective mechanism.

Stress continues to serve us today, as mild to moderate levels of stress can sharpen our alertness and motivate positive growth, spur the need to accept challenges, and promote change in our lives. Stress becomes a problem only when you consider the nature of some of our stressors. Unlike the saber-toothed tigers of long ago, today's stressors tend to be more chronic in nature. Most people struggle with the demands of health problems, interpersonal difficulties, financial worries, and negative or critical self-imaging, to name just a few. These concerns have a propensity to stick around. When you begin to experience any one of them, your body reacts with predictable changes. However, because these stressors usually stay around and dominate parts of our existence for long stretches of time, the bodily changes that get "turned on," stay "turned on," which can cause or influence numerous undesirable consequences.

Chronic stress can contribute to such physical problems as migraine headaches, lower back pain, ulcers, digestive disorders, TMJ (temporomandibular joint) syndrome, suppressed immunity, and, of particular concern to people with diabetes, difficulty controlling blood sugar. There is even some evidence that cardiovascular disease, high blood pressure, and certain types of cancer can be adversely affected by stress. Chronic stress also appears to contribute to many psychological and behavioral disorders such as depression, anxiety disorders, and low self-esteem.

Everyone attempts to cope with the stress in their lives, whether they do so consciously and deliberately or not. Unfortunately, many of the strategies people use to deal with stress actually produce additional sources of stress. Overeating, excessive alcohol consumption, cigarette smoking, and drug use are examples of stress management attempts gone awry.

Any effective strategy of stress management needs to do more than just distract you from that which is causing the stress. It needs to address both the physical and the psychological aspects of stress. To efficiently deal with stress, you must first get to know yourself and observe how stress tends to affect you.

Diabetes and stress

You may already have some idea how stress affects your blood glucose level. In the past, it was thought that increased levels of stress contributed only to elevated blood glucose and that people with diabetes needed to compensate for this rise in blood sugar with less food, added insulin, or increased activity. Now, however, we also know that many people develop hypoglycemia (low blood sugar) in reaction to stress. This is particularly true for people practicing tight blood glucose control.

In addition to individual differences in blood sugar responses to stress, a number of other factors can influence the effects of stress on blood glucose levels. These factors include a person's coping style, personality, health beliefs, attitude toward diabetes and dia-

betic complications, and degree of perceived social support. In addition, the nature of the stressor itself, and how well-controlled a person's blood glucose levels were before the stressful event, can have an influence on blood sugar response to stress.

The mechanism through which blood sugar is affected by stress is thought to be a hormonal reaction. However, equally possible is a behavioral element, whereby a person under chronic stress changes actions and routines. If the person's adherence to healthy habits weakens, blood sugar will be affected. For example, for some people, stress on the job could lead to binge eating or less consistent exercising.

It seems probable that both hormonal and behavioral influences play a role in the reaction of blood glucose to stress. To find out how stress affects your blood sugar, test and keep an ongoing log of your blood glucose levels and observe any changes following stressful events. Once you are familiar with the impact that stress has on your glucose levels, you can take preventive measures when stress occurs.

Women and stress

Women have a special reason to take an interest in stress management. Research shows that women and girls are at least two to three times more likely to experience anxiety and mood disorders than men and boys. The reasons for this are many, ranging from biology to socialization. Luckily, women are also more likely to talk about and seek out help for distress.

The types of stressors that girls and women typically encounter change throughout the life cycle. Throughout childhood and adolescence, most girls struggle with issues of peer acceptance, as well as issues of independence and autonomy from their families. Growing up with diabetes adds a layer of pressures that girls and their families must learn to overcome.

Young adulthood brings with it the challenges of career choices, intimacy, partnership, and sexuality, and possibly choices about becoming a mother. Body image concerns can also become paramount for young women.

Middle adulthood, sometimes called the "sandwich years" because women are generationally sandwiched between their children and their parents, presents challenges of balancing and redefining roles, financial pressures, aging, and health-related concerns.

The elder years generally bring additional health concerns, the loss of significant others, and the opportunity to reflect upon—and, one hopes, not regret—the way one has lived one's life.

Regardless of the stage of life you are in and the types of stress you are facing, you can benefit from learning to manage stress. And, given the ever-changing roles for women and the lack of a variety of female role models, helping yourself through stress management training can be a real gift.

Management techniques

Any strategy you use to deal with stress must focus on both the physical and the psychological aspects of stress. The techniques themselves can be divided into two broad categories:

■ Those that specifically target the physical changes that occur in reaction to stress and that bring those changes back to normal, and

■ Those that target the perceptual or cognitive component of stress and help to change unproductive or destructive thoughts into rational, productive, and beneficial perspectives on living.

Physical strategies

Deep-breathing exercises, relaxation training, yoga, meditation, biofeedback training, massage, and prayer are all examples of coping techniques that target the bodily changes that occur as a result of stress. Each of these strategies involves learning skills that focus on regulating your breathing so that it becomes deep and abdominal, rather than shallow and centered in your chest, and so that your respiration rate slows. All of these approaches tend to relax and loosen muscle tension. And, with consistent training, they can readjust and regulate heart and pulse rate, blood pressure, and body chemistry, bringing them in line with healthy levels.

Physical exercise such as walking or aerobics is often recommended for stress reduction. The benefits of regular physical exercise cannot be overestimated, and exercise has long-term effects in reducing stress. However, in the immediate sense, physical exercise does not lower heart and respiration rates. Instead, it increases most of the physical manifestations of stress. So, although exercise is an important resource for stress management and can be an acceptable way to blow off steam, other methods of stress management are still necessary to bring the fight-or-flight changes back to normal.

All stress-management techniques involve learning new skills, and that can take time. They also must be performed consistently and seriously to get long-term benefits. Here's an exercise to get you started practicing deep relaxation breathing:

1. While sitting or lying down, place one hand on your abdomen and the other hand on your chest.
2. Close your eyes.
3. Breathe in through your nose to a count of three, and breathe out through your mouth to a count of five. Continue for several minutes.

If you're performing deep relaxation breathing correctly, you should feel the hand on your abdomen move out and in, while the hand on your chest stays relatively still. This exercise can be useful in combating acute stress: It can be performed almost anywhere and is immediately available. Practicing deep relaxation breathing for one to five minutes each time you feel yourself becoming stressed can help you calm down enough to address the stressor directly.

Psychological strategies

There are a number of psychological or cognitive-behavioral approaches to stress reduction. What they all have in common is a focus on helping you change your perceptions and attitudes toward stressful events.

It is important to accept the idea that stress will be ever-present in your life before you can unburden yourself from it. Like it or not, for every stressful situation that resolves or affects you less over time, a new one will eventually crop up. Once you can embrace the inevitability of stress in your life, you can proceed with dealing with the particular stressors that exist in your life.

Following is a list of steps you can take that may help in problem-solving your way through stress. Keep in mind as you read, though, that each step may be a lot easier said than done. After all, change doesn't happen overnight; it can take weeks, months, or even years of hard work.

Remember, too, that you may need help at some steps along the way. Sometimes talking with friends or family members can help you see things from a new perspective. If you have a mentor, you might also want to talk with him or her about some issues. For problems that just seem to stick around or that repeat over and over no matter what you do, you might consider talking with a licensed professional such as a psychologist, psychiatrist, or social worker.

Ten steps toward reducing stress

The following ten steps form a logical way to confront that which is stressful for you.

1. Identify just what it is that is causing you stress. Seems obvious, doesn't it? Well, it isn't always. Oftentimes, people who are feeling overwhelmed by stress incorrectly assume that *everything* in their lives is going wrong. There may be many stressors in your life, but rarely does everything go wrong at once. It is important to clearly and specifically define just what your stressors are.
2. Identify exactly what portions of the stressor are beyond your control. There is always a part of any situation that is outside your influence.
3. Make peace with that which is beyond your control. It's not easy, but it's necessary. Acceptance of your limitations is an important step toward mental health and contentment.

4. Identify exactly what portions of the stressor are within your control. One portion that is always within your influence is your outlook and perspective. Ultimately, we are in charge of how we choose to perceive the world. However, long-held beliefs based on past experiences can sometimes cloud our interpretations of events. That's why getting a second opinion—preferably from someone uninvolved with the stressful situation—can sometimes serve as a sort of "reality check." Besides your perspective, it is important to identify any other aspects of the stressful situation at hand that are under your control.

5. Decide on the way you would realistically and practically want things to be. Specify how you'd like things to change, and establish short-term and long-term goals to bring about those changes. Make sure your goals are not unrealistically high and impossible to attain.

6. Identify the steps you need to take to achieve those goals.

7. Anticipate obstacles to achieving those goals. There will almost always be obstacles along the road to change.

8. Generate possible solutions to break through obstacles and setbacks.

9. Learn from your mistakes, and reward yourself for your achievements.

10. Never give up.

How they work

To see how these steps might be applied to an actual stressful situation, let's take being diagnosed with diabetes as our example of a stressor and go through the ten steps:

1. Identify the fact that being diagnosed with diabetes is a stressful event in your life.

2. Portions of this stressor that are outside your control include the fact that diabetes, at present, has no cure, and you cannot undo the diagnosis, nor can you control exactly how events unfold.

3. Accepting the diagnosis and the full range of possible emotional reactions to being diagnosed with diabetes is something to be made peace with. Resisting denial and embracing the feelings of having a chronic illness are important aspects to managing the course of this stressor. Oftentimes, people do benefit from professional help with these issues.

4. There are many portions of this stressor that are within your control. Following a healthy and appropriate meal plan, taking medications regularly and on schedule, testing your blood glucose consistently, exercising, visiting your endocrinologist regularly, and taking responsibility for a major part of your prognosis are all within your influence. Additionally, it is crucial to modify your attitude and outlook on having a chronic illness so that you see the illness as a challenge rather than as a threat.

5. Given the nature of the stressor, your goals are likely to include developing a specific meal plan, insulin (or other drug) regime, and exercise schedule, and determining acceptable blood sugar ranges.

6. To meet your goals, you might decide on such matters as when you will do your grocery shopping, as well as what kind of exercise you will do and when you will do it. You might also decide to learn proper blood glucose testing procedures and insulin administration and, perhaps, to collect information and data on diabetes so that you stay well-informed.

7. Some possible obstacles to meeting these goals might include your tendency to forget to test your blood sugar, your weakness for ice cream, or your general dislike of exercise.

8. To break through these obstacles, you might set alarm timers to prompt you to test your blood sugar at appropriate times, and you might add an additional walk to your schedule so that you can occasionally have ice cream. To make exercise more enjoyable, you might ask your spouse or a friend to join you for daily walks. In addition, considering who you will talk to about your concerns and issues related to diabetes is an important step in avoiding and overcoming obstacles.

9. When you achieve a goal successfully, try reinforcing yourself with a special something. When you have difficulty achieving a goal, examine your difficulties with curiosity and a willingness to learn preventive measures in the future, rather than looking at them with a punitive, critical eye.

10. Never give up. You may need to try out several solutions to a problem until you find the right one. Seek out help when you need it. None of us can do it all by ourselves.

Sticking with it

Keep in mind that learning to cope with stress involves learning skills that take time to master. Be patient with yourself, and don't forget that stress management should be a nurturing and nourishing process, not a punishing one.

You don't need to work constantly. Give yourself a break now and then. We all need to occasionally distract ourselves from stress, by reading, watching TV, listening to music, or doing whatever strikes our fancy.

But remember that we all need to ultimately confront and deal directly with the stress in our lives if we are going to reduce it. The complex demands of being a woman, combined with maintaining tight glycemic control over diabetes, can be quite taxing. Stress management can be a real asset in handling these challenges. ❏

LEARNING TO TAKE CARE OF YOU, TOO

by Robert Taibbi, L.C.S.W.

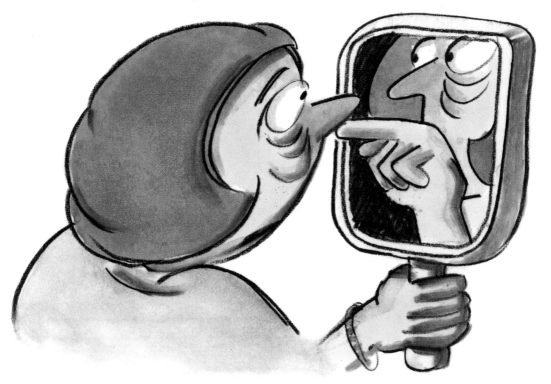

Susan's mother just called. "Could you go with me to the doctor on Wednesday afternoon?" she asked. "Oh, of course," Susan said, without even thinking. She looked at her desk calendar. It was going to be another tough day. Not only did she have a busy day at work, but she also had to drive her 13-year-old son, Scott, to soccer practice after school, then come home, make dinner, do a quick blood glucose check, and eat before running off to the finance committee meeting at church that evening. Now she would have to take some time off work to take her mother to the doctor as well.

A lot of women could easily stack their own jam-packed to-do list alongside Susan's. In spite of the woman's movement and the ever-growing majority of women holding down jobs outside the home, women continue to be the primary caregivers in our society. Whether it's raising children, helping parents, tending to sick friends, supporting grandchildren, looking out for younger siblings, serving in soup kitchens, or welcoming new neighbors, it's women, rather than men, who more often step up and extend their time, rearrange their busy schedules,

and reach out a caring hand to the people who are around them.

Their willingness and ability to seemingly "do it all" is an obvious testimonial to the inherent strength, capability, and compassion of women, but too much caregiving is not without its price. When you always put others first, you thereby always put yourself second. The ongoing stress of additional responsibilities, as well as the frequent juggling of your time and attention, can not only leave you feeling tired, or irritable, or depressed, it can easily undermine the healthy habits that are of crucial importance to your diabetes management.

The world of girls and boys

So why does caring for others so easily fall into the laps of women? Why do women seem to have such a hard time putting their needs first? For a clue, you only have to visit any elementary school playground during recess. What you'll probably notice first are the boys running around in large groups engaged in king-of-the-mountain-type games, whirlwind battles of football or soccer, and fantasy dramas with imaginary swords or guns, supplemented with lots of pushing, jostling, wrestling, and generous amounts of name-calling and verbal put-downs. Then, as your eyes drift across the field, you'll notice the girls clustered in smaller groups of twos and threes scattered about the edges. Compared to the boys, their play seems much less rambunctious: hopscotch, jumping rope, galloping about each other pretending they're a herd of horses. It's quieter, less physical, and usually merely the backdrop for a steady stream of conversation.

Anthropologists tell us what we're seeing here on the playground is one of the fundamental differences between the sexes. Both in their play and in their relationships with each other, the social world of boys tends to revolve around who's in charge, who's the best, who's on top—basic issues of dominance, competition, and control enacted through their bodies. Girls, on the other hand, seem to gravitate toward something different—namely, equality, connection, and intimacy, generated and sustained through the medium of conversation. While the running packs of boys are developing the physical and emotional skills they will need to compete and achieve in the larger world, the smaller groups of girls are learning the subtleties of listening, soothing, and nurturing vital to creating and maintaining close relationships. As the boys push themselves to stand out and stay ahead, the girls practice holding back and holding on, so both they and their friends can feel supported and cared for.

Once back home, girls see the patterns of the playground mirrored and reinforced. Mothers, aunts, and grandmothers, backed up by a steady stream of nurturing images from television, movies, and books, serve as walking demonstrations of adult support and caretaking. If a girl is the firstborn or only child in the family, her close contact with the adults makes it especially easy for her to adopt a junior-parent role and develop a strong sense of responsibility. Similarly, should her home environment push her to be a protector of her siblings, as is common in families with alcoholic, addicted, or emotionally absent parents, it takes little time for these caretaking skills to become ingrained.

The expectations and praise of others help to nourish and maintain these skills once they have become established. So does the girl's own sense of feeling important, having control, or finding herself in the socially accepted role of the silent martyr, asking little for herself while continually sacrificing for others.

By the time the woman-to-be is a teenager, the path to her own internal life can become overgrown and lost by neglect. Rather than using her unique needs and wants as the starting point for setting goals and choosing her behavior, she instead gets pushed along by a head full of rules. These are the "shoulds" and "oughts," the first of which is that others *should* come

first. And so the pattern is set in motion in which the caregiver cares for everyone except herself.

Periodically, the adult caregiver burns out, physically or psychologically. Her diabetes may get out of control, she may be overcome by depression, or suddenly and unexplainably she may explode with anger as a realization of the imbalance and unfairness in her relationships, and the neglect of her own needs, rises to the surface. But this insight never stays there long enough to stimulate change, because guilt—the Great Enforcer of "shoulds"—quickly moves in to push it back down. Her wants and needs go underground once more, setting the stage for a repeat of the cycle.

Breaking out

It doesn't have to be this way. It is possible to care for others without undermining your own physical and psychological needs. In fact, by reducing your stress and making more time to take better care of yourself, you actually will be healthier and be able to contribute more. Even if the quantity of your help may be less, the quality, namely of yourself and what you can give to others, will in the long run be enhanced. Here are some guidelines for starting to put yourself first:

Handling guilt. Psychologists tell us that guilt is not only normal, it is deeply ingrained within us. It originates from our fear as young children that our parents will stop loving us and may even abandon us if we say no or refuse to do what they want. Saying no as an adult can trigger that same infantile fear, although now we call it guilt. If you normally take care of others' needs before your own, you can expect to feel guilty anytime you say no or put yourself first, and you may find others doing their best to help you feel that way. If Susan, for example, were to tell her mother that she really didn't have time to take her to the doctor, her mother might remind her of all the things she did for her when she was growing up, lament about how miserable she feels and how no one apparently cares, or get angry about how she asks for so little but her daughter can't even do this small favor. Even if her mother were to say nothing at all, or offer to find someone else to take her to the doctor, Susan is still apt to get that heavy feeling in the pit of her stomach.

Under this kind of motherly plaint or her own self-scolding, it's easy for Susan to cave in. But Susan's feelings of guilt don't mean that her mother is right, or that Susan has to respond as she did when she was younger and automatically do what her mother wants. Rather than giving in to the guilt, it would be better for Susan to think of it as an opportunity for choice, a chance to take one small step away from the automatic pilot she normally runs on.

Learning to help. Realize the difference between helping and being responsible for. Often, much of the weight of helping is the result of heaping on the additional load of responsibility. Helping is exactly that—supporting someone in doing something that he or she needs or wants to do. Being responsible for means taking over and making the problem your own. Helping her mother find ways of getting to the doctor would feel very different to Susan than believing that she is the one ultimately responsible for ensuring that her mother gets there. It's best to keep the problem in the other person's lap where it belongs, rather than transferring it to yours.

Cutting back on obligations. Look over both your activities and your time and then brainstorm a plan. Susan may decide to ask her brother to help with her mother's medical needs or ask her husband to take Scott to practice. Similarly, she might decide that it's OK to cut back on some of her church activities until her children are older.

Where can you cut back on your responsibilities or the time you spend attending to the needs of others? Are there some daily or weekly duties or tasks that you can put aside, perhaps to another time in the future, or pass along to others who can step in and take them on? Are there ways you can make time to nurture yourself—by taking a warm bath, perhaps, while your husband puts the kids in bed, or claiming an hour of quiet in the late afternoon for meditation or rest before everyone gets home for the day?

How can you take better care of your diabetes needs? Can you make time to pack a healthier lunch to eat at work, rather than go to the fast-food drive-through on most days? How about reserving an evening twice a month to attend a diabetes support group? Ultimately, deciding where to start is less important than realizing that your needs are important and starting somewhere.

Reshaping your family

Saying yes to your own needs will obviously mean learning to say no to others who have become accustomed to your availability and accommodation. The hardest place to do this will be with close family members who have come to see your caregiving as simply "who you are," who may have grown dependent on your help, and where change on your part will stir your strongest feelings of guilt.

But there's much you can do to help your family change as you do. Begin by talking, without anger, about the ways you've felt pulled, or drained, or overwhelmed by all the demands that you feel. Educate them about your diabetes self-care needs, the way stress can make it more difficult to maintain your healthy habits and keep your blood sugar under control, and how by spending so much time caring for them you are neglecting to care for yourself.

Family members often want to find ways to "give back" and help the helper, but they feel stymied and put off by the helper's seeming self-sufficiency and "Don't worry about me" message. Once they understand how you've been feeling, you open the door to their help. Make specific suggestions: Tell your kids that you will show them how to use the washing machine so they can do their own laundry, work out a weekly schedule with your partner that gives you time for yourself, ask your older teenager to drive your younger child to gymnastics after school, ask a sibling who lives nearby to baby-sit your kids a couple of times a month so you and your husband can go out. By letting them know that you too have needs, that you too need help, you not only help create a more balanced relationship, but you give them an opportunity to feel important and valued. And the advantage of your being specific is that they will know exactly what you have in mind.

As they begin to make changes, however small, be sure to notice and thank them. This is not only courteous but will encourage them to keep it up. Expect that you may not think they do things the same or as well as you might, but realize that these thoughts are normal reactions to your learning to give up some of your far-reaching sense of control, and resist the urge to correct and coach. This would only discourage them and quickly lead you back to doing everything all by yourself.

What do you do if they don't follow through, start to complain, or backslide after a couple of weeks? Again, keep in mind that change is hard. Everyone's natural instincts, including your own, are to keep things as they were. Expect some grumbling, sloppiness, and forgetfulness on your family's end and hold to your stance. If you stay the course, focus on the positive, and try to ignore the negative, the old rigid patterns and roles will sooner or later be broken. Everyone, including you, will find themselves developing new psychological muscles and plowing new emotional ground.

Mastering the art of caring

As a sensitive, caring person, you already demonstrate a tremendous inner strength that enables you to do a lot for others. It is this same strength that can serve as the foundation for making the shift from being a caretaker who takes on too much to becoming a caring person who is there to help. By learning to put your needs alongside those of others, you are not only showing a healthy respect for yourself, you are, through your example, teaching your daughters, nieces, and granddaughters how they can learn to do the same. What a wonderful gift and a wonderful way of showing just how much you care. ❏

WHAT YOU SHOULD KNOW ABOUT EATING DISORDERS

by Ivy D. Marcus, Ph.D., C.D.E.

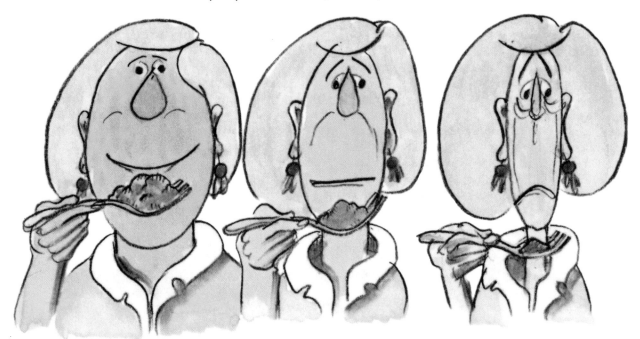

Since the early 1980's there has been a rapidly growing awareness of the prevalence and consequences of eating disorders. It is only more recently, however, that the interaction of disordered eating and diabetes, especially Type 1 diabetes, has become a focus and concern. If you or a loved one has an eating disorder, it is important—and possible—to get help. This article describes eating disorders, their connection to diabetes, and what types of help are available.

Types of eating disorders

The three main eating disorders are bulimia nervosa, anorexia nervosa, and binge eating disorder. *Bulimia nervosa* is characterized by recurrent episodes of binge eating, or eating in a relatively short time period (usually two hours) an amount of food that is larger than most people would eat in similar circumstances. Other features of bulimia include feeling a lack of control over one's eating during bingeing episodes, and repeatedly engaging in behavior to prevent weight gain after binges. Example of such behavior include self-induced vomiting; abuse or misuse of enemas, laxatives, diuretics (drugs that increase urine production), or other drugs (including insulin); fasting; severely restrictive dieting; and excessive exercise. Persistent overconcern with and self-evaluation based on weight and body shape are typical, as well. A depressed mood and self-deprecating thoughts often follow binges.

Two types of bulimia exist: One is the purging type, in which self-induced vomiting or laxatives, diuretics, or enemas are used to prevent weight gain following binges. The other is the nonpurging type, in which other behaviors are used to prevent weight gain following binges. The misuse, omission, or alteration in dosage of insulin falls into this category. A diagnosis of bulimia is made when the bingeing and the unhealthy behaviors to prevent weight gain both occur, on average, at least twice weekly for at least three months. In spite of their eating habits, people with bulimia usually maintain a normal body weight, although some may be slightly overweight or underweight.

Anorexia nervosa is defined as a refusal to maintain one's body weight at or above minimal normal standards for age and height, accompanied by an intense fear of gaining weight or becoming fat, a disturbance or distortion in body image, and (in girls and women) amenorrhea, or the absence of at least three consecutive menstrual periods. Two types of anorexia exist: the restricting type, in which no regular bingeing or purging behavior occurs, and the bingeing/purging type, in which regular bingeing or purging occurs.

Binge eating disorder is characterized by recurrent episodes of binge eating. Usually, the bingeing episodes involve rapid eating, eating until one feels uncomfortably full, eating large amounts of food despite not feeling physically hungry, eating in solitude to avoid embarrassment over the amounts eaten, and feeling disgusted with oneself, depressed, or guilty after overeating. People who binge do not enjoy their food during a binge; instead, they tend to experience marked distress. No regular use of behaviors to avoid weight gain occurs in binge eating disorder, and the frequency of the binges is lower than in cases of bulimia. While bulimia and anorexia affect more people with Type 1 diabetes than people with Type 2 diabetes, binge eating disorder may affect both groups equally. But so far, little formal research has been conducted on binge eating disorder.

Eating disorders are becoming quite common in American society. It is estimated that up to 1% of teenage girls have anorexia. The rate of bulimia is reportedly as high as 19% in the female population. And the rate of binge eating appears to be very high, especially among young women. In some studies of certain populations, up to 86% of the group studied has been found to binge. Although binge eating has certainly been around for a long time, it has been officially recognized by the medical community as an eating disorder only since 1994. More research is needed on binge eating disorder to understand its causes and prevalence in the general population and among people with diabetes.

It is currently understood that eating disorders are the end result of a variety of developmental factors. Psychological, societal, biological, and familial factors all contribute in varying degrees to the development of an eating disorder.

Although many people have mild eating disturbances, a full-fledged eating disorder is a serious and potentially life-threatening condition that needs to be treated. Both medical and psychological consequences can result. Some of the possible medical consequences of an untreated eating disorder include amenorrhea (cessation of menstruation, indicating a shutdown of hormonal regulating systems in the body), osteoporosis, dehydration, irregular heart rhythms, tears in the lining of the esophagus and stomach, constipation, tooth cavities, swollen parotid glands (a type of salivary gland), chemical imbalances possibly leading to cardiovascular problems, and obesity. Possible psychological consequences include depression, anxiety, loss of concentration, low self-esteem, and social isolation. These serious issues become further complicated when a person also has diabetes.

Why women?

People of all ages, races, and ethnicities and of both genders can struggle with eating disorders, but women are affected on a much more frequent basis. Let's take a look at why this is the case.

Social factors. Despite the multifaceted nature of the development of eating disorders, it is generally believed that dieting or attempts at dieting are associated with the evolution of these disorders. Is it any wonder, then, that women appear to suffer from eating disorders to the degree that they do?

In any society where the pursuit of slimness becomes a way of life, eating disorders become widespread. Rigid dieting and severe restriction of calories inevitably lead to a preoccupation with weight, shape, and size, and also to increased hunger. This magnified hunger almost always results in an episode of overeating or bingeing, which in turn prompts some sort of behavior to prevent weight gain and to quell the emotional distress accompanying the deviation from the diet. A cycle is easily created, in which the person alternates between strict dieting and compensation for deviations from that diet. In cultures that believe that women can never be too thin, it is easy to understand how a full eating disorder can develop.

Family issues. Familial issues also play a role in the development of eating disorders. The methods family members (especially parents and siblings) use to express feelings—and the way they teach children to express feelings—become key in how individuals learn to experience, communicate, and cope with difficult emotions. For example, if a family teaches a young girl—either directly through words or indirectly through body language—that it is unacceptable to feel or express anger, that girl will not learn to express herself assertively and may instead learn to "stuff" her anger down with food. She will also learn to feel bad about herself and to believe in the inappropriateness of her negative feelings. However, appropriate assertive behavior is crucial for a person's well-being, self-esteem, and ability to negotiate relationships in life.

Family issues can also arise around expectations for achievement, especially if those expectations are unrealistic and perfectionist in nature. For example, it is unrealistic to expect children to get straight A's throughout their entire academic career; this expectation sets up a rigid and virtually impossible goal. It is realistic, on the other hand, to expect children to strive for the best grades they can get; this expectation focuses on effort and leaves room for normal human variation.

Family dynamics can also come into play. In some families, relationship alliances, or unhealthy partnerships in which some family members band together and leave others out, arise. For example, Mom may be the disciplinarian when it comes to food choices, while Dad and daughter Susie ally and sneak off together to eat "forbidden" foods. Although Susie may initially enjoy these secret snacks, ultimately this system works well for no one, and certainly not for Susie's eating habits.

Struggles for control in families, and the ways in which parents foster independence and autonomy in their children can also be related to the development of eating disorders. Modeling, or the learning of a behavior through the observation of others, enters into the equation, too. For example, by watching their mother or father eat when confronted with stressful situations, children may learn to do the same to anesthetize the pain of stress. Or they may learn to diet at a very young age, just as they observe a parent doing. Many people learn to eat as a coping strategy simply because they never learned other, more productive tools for coping.

Children also may learn to be critical of their bodies or to judge and/or value themselves based upon their appearances rather than on their internal, inherent self-worth. This unfortunate "lesson" is usually the net result of many different variables in a child's life, but parents can encourage a more positive self-image in their children by praising, rewarding, or focusing on valued *behaviors* and *intentions* rather than *appearances*. Girls in particular are vulnerable to absorbing the notion that their worth or value is tied into their appearance, specifically to their body weight, size, and shape. In addition, the belief that men are only interested in women if their appearance is "adequate" is oftentimes embedded in cultures and families.

Psychology and biology. Psychological issues stem from a combination of the above-mentioned social and familial influences. Many people with eating disorders, because of their propensity toward perfectionism and nonassertiveness, become depressed, anxious, and preoccupied and suffer from low self-esteem. They may also have a biological weight "set point" (a genetically determined range for body weight) that is above their liking, thereby contributing to disdain for their bodies.

The diabetes connection

Women with diabetes seem to be at particular risk for developing an eating disorder, perhaps because of the central roles that weight and food take on in the life of almost anyone with diabetes. Oftentimes, one of the first symptoms of Type 1 diabetes is weight loss—something a girl in our society may welcome with open arms. However, once the diagnosis of diabetes is made and a person begins taking insulin, he or she usually regains the weight that was lost, a development that may cause dismay in some girls.

Developing a preoccupation with food, calories, carbohydrates, and controlled eating habits can be a natural by-product of learning to manage one's diabetes. But such a mindset can prepare the stage for an eating disorder to emerge. If an adolescent girl or young woman tries to compensate for even minor episodes of overeating with excessive or unhealthy behaviors and succeeds in her attempt, she may be seduced into believing that she has found a method to eat whatever she wants and still not gain weight. Unfortunately, this can rapidly evolve into a vicious cycle, propelling the girl into emotional quicksand.

Contributing to the problem is the fact that weight loss for a person with diabetes is usually viewed as a positive event and is assumed to be the result of tight diabetes management or control. However, this is not always the case. In fact, one of the physical changes observed among those practicing "tight control" in the landmark Diabetes Control and Complications Trial was weight *gain*, not loss. Therefore, friends, family members, and even health-care providers need to be wary of the effect that their questions and compliments about weight loss may have on a person. It is better to comment on healthy behaviors, rather than on resulting weight loss. For example, you might compliment a friend's efforts to exercise regularly. A doctor, rather than praising weight loss, might compliment a person's efforts to keep thorough blood sugar or food records. Or a concerned friend or doctor might ask a person who has lost weight how he or she feels about it, rather than declaring the weight loss either bad or good. As we all know, listening to how a friend or child feels is often a more powerful tool than talking to that person.

People with diabetes may also discover an uncanny "trick": that decreasing or completely omitting their insulin doses, particularly after overeating or bingeing, not only prevents weight gain but promotes weight loss. Unfortunately, there are seriously dangerous side effects to this practice: extremely high blood glucose levels and a dramatically higher risk of complications. Recent studies have documented some of the risks inherent in the toxic blend of diabetes and eating disorders: poorer diabetes control, the increased likelihood of the presence of the protein albumin in the urine (a predictor of the risk of diabetic kidney disease), and a greatly increased risk of microvascular complications such as retinopathy, which can lead to blindness.

Another important risk factor for the development of an eating disorder in a person with diabetes is the sense of loss of control many people with diabetes experience as a result of having a chronic, high-maintenance disease. The illusion of being in total control of one's food can appear to be a panacea for such feelings. But the type of "control" wielded by a person with an eating disorder is indeed illusory. Allowing an eating disorder to dominate one's life is actually akin to giving up control and responsibility for one's food intake and well-being. Treatment for an eating disorder involves taking back that responsibility and control over food and health.

The families of girls with diabetes are often (understandably) very involved in their food intake and their lives in general. However, such involvement may increase these girls' risk of developing eating disorders. An eating disorder may be a girl's attempt at securing her separation and independence from her family. Parents of a child with diabetes have a difficult and unique challenge in that they must assess when and how to allow their child to take more responsibility for his or her diabetes while simultaneously balancing this independence with some degree of supervision and guidance.

In summary, when eating disorders and diabetes coexist, they do indeed appear to feed on each other. This interaction typically results in a worsening of both conditions. More frequent hospitalizations for diabetes-related complications and an increased resistance to resolving the eating disorder are not uncommonly seen.

Despite the apparent gloominess of the situation, treatment is available, and there are ways for individuals to get help.

Treatment

If you or someone you know has diabetes and is struggling with an eating disorder, it is a good idea to get some professional treatment as soon as possible. Eating disorders tend not to go away on their own.

A variety of psychological therapies are used for the treatment of eating disorders. One of these, cognitive–behavioral psychotherapy, is a well-researched type of treatment that has had a great deal of success in helping people change disordered eating and regain emotional well-being. This type of psychotherapy focuses on building new coping strategies to handle difficult emotions and situations. It helps to change eating habits and ways of thinking about food, weight, and body image, and it addresses the multitude of issues related to body image, weight, food, and gender in our culture. It also helps to impart an understanding of why one thinks, feels, and behaves the way one does, based on one's own individual personal history and experience. Ultimately, this therapy seeks to impart a sense of empowerment and control, as well as responsibility for one's eating behavior and related issues.

FOR MORE INFORMATION

If you think that you or someone you know may have an eating disorder, the following organizations can provide invaluable information.

ANOREXIA NERVOSA AND RELATED EATING DISORDERS, INC.
e-mail: jarinor@rio.com
www.anred.com
Provides literature on eating disorders.

MERCY CENTER FOR EATING DISORDERS
(410) 332-9800
Provides literature on eating disorders; professional counseling and support groups are available on-site. A service of Mercy Hospital, Baltimore, Maryland.

NATIONAL ASSOCIATION OF ANOREXIA NERVOSA AND ASSOCIATED DISORDERS
P.O. Box 7
Highland Park, IL 60035
(847) 831-3438
www.anad.org
Offers fact sheets, information packets, referrals to professional help, and counseling.

NATIONAL EATING DISORDERS ASSOCIATION
603 Stewart Street, Suite 803
Seattle, WA 98101
(800) 931-2237
www.nationaleatingdisorders.org
Offers a toll-free information and referral line as well as printed literature. Access to the referral list is also available on the association's Web site.

Psychotherapy can take place either individually or in a group setting. What's important is to find a mental health professional who is experienced in treating eating disorders and who is also trained and experienced in working with diabetes. Treating an eating disorder when diabetes is present is more complex than treating an eating disorder alone. To find such a therapist, try asking your endocrinologist for a referral. You can also try getting in touch with your local American Diabetes Association chapter or such organizations as the National Eating Disorders Association and the National Association of Anorexia Nervosa and Associated Disorders, which provide information and help with referrals. (See "For More Information" on this page.)

If you have an eating disorder and have not already worked with a certified diabetes educator and dietitian, it might be a good idea to do so now. But keep in mind that all members of your health-care team need to work with one another so that their efforts are coordinated properly. For example, it is essential that the eating disorder be treated first before ideal blood sugar control can be attained. Therefore, you and your dietitian may need to wait until you have made some progress in therapy before focusing on your nutrition needs. If you are experiencing severe depression, your mental health professional may feel that a course of antidepressant drugs are appropriate at this time. If this is the case, all the members of your diabetes team need to know what drugs you are taking since some of them can have an effect on blood sugar, insulin dose, and/or appetite. Communication among all team members is vital for the most successful outcome.

If someone you know appears to be caught in the tangled web of an eating disorder, you can certainly encourage him or her to seek help. In doing so, how-ever, be careful not to bring up the issue at emotionally sensitive times. Wait for a calm moment instead. It's also important not to be judgmental or critical in your approach, but rather to offer information on why it's a good idea to seek treatment and where to find it. For example, if you know that someone has been bingeing, you might say at a quiet, private moment, "It seems to me that you're struggling with some issues, perhaps related to food. Would you like to talk about it? Maybe I can help." You might want to have some brochures or other written information on hand when you broach the subject. Ask if there's any way you can help, and leave the door open for future communication.

There's help out there, and the more quickly it is sought, and the more involved a person can become in conquering an eating disorder, the better chance that person has in avoiding serious medical complications caused by compromised diabetes self-care. If you need help, don't be afraid to reach out and ask questions. You deserve to get the best and most appropriate treatment. ❏

FOR PARENTS

TALKING TO YOUR KIDS ABOUT DIABETES

by Robert Taibbi, L.C.S.W.

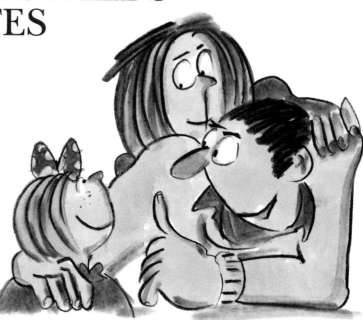

When Ellen started testing her blood sugar and taking insulin injections for her diabetes, she was prepared for all the questions her adult children asked about her treatment plan. It was the reaction of her grandson that surprised her. Six-year-old Matthew seemed both horrified and curious when he overheard her talking about giving herself shots every day. Ellen wanted to explain to him what she was doing and why, but she didn't know what to say without scaring him or talking over his head.

Whether you're a grandparent or parent, uncle or aunt, or just someone who's around kids a lot, you know that if you stick around long enough, they're bound to ask you questions, with no topic, including your diabetes, off-limits. And when they ask about sensitive or complex subjects, it's easy to feel put on the spot. Like Ellen, you may wonder not only what to say, but how to say it.

As we all know, talking to kids isn't quite the same as talking to adults. Children's ability to understand, their curiosities and concerns, and the way they ask questions are different; and all of these are constantly changing as they grow. Just as you start having wonderful conversations with your three-year-old granddaughter, you find yourself getting tongue-tied trying to talk with your 11-year-old grandson.

But talking is only half of any conversation; listening is the other. Wrapped inside children's questions and comments are their feelings, including their worries and confusions. By talking with you, they hope to sort out their feelings; by your response, they know whether they're being understood and accepted. How you say something—that is, the tone of voice you use and the emotions you express—often turns out to be more important than what you say. And how well you listen is probably most important of all.

Developmental psychologists tend to sort children into four different groups: infants, ages 0–2; preschoolers, ages 2–6; school-age children, ages 6–12; and adolescents, ages 12–18. While each child's personality and talents are unique, children within a particular age group are similar in the way they think about themselves and the world, in their interests, and in their ability to communicate with others. Knowing the basic characteristics of each group can help you know how to talk and listen to the kids in your life. And that's important when you need to discuss a difficult subject like diabetes.

"Da-da!" (Infants)

Children under two years old aren't terribly interested in your diabetes. What they do care about, however, is you. They especially need to know that you care about them and that you're able to provide for their needs. Because words are still largely incomprehensible, infants understand and react to sensations, moods, and feelings—their own and those of their caretakers. One-year-olds, for example, can sense when their mother is having a hard day and will often react with cranky behavior, crying, and having trouble sleeping.

If your infant seems chronically cranky or tense, and your efforts at soothing don't seem to work, take a look at your own life. Are you under a lot of stress? Have you been feeling overwhelmed by all of the obligations in your life? To take good care of your baby, you first need to take good care of yourself, and that means finding ways to reduce your stress level. If your diabetes management is part of the problem, it may be time to visit your diabetes educator to discuss ways of adjusting your self-care routine so that it is less of a burden. You may also want to consider joining a parenting support group if there is one in your area. Another option is to make an appointment with a mental health professional who specializes in parent–infant interaction. Such a professional will be able to show you ways to relate to your child that make both of you happier and more satisfied.

"What's dat?" (Preschoolers)

As children get older and begin to speak, they use language to organize the world around them. People and things are given names, feelings are identified as sad or happy, and the behaviors and words of adults are imitated in play. Preschoolers flit around from one activity to another, pushed along by curiosity and the attraction of loud noises, colors, and interesting textures. For them, the lines between reality and imagination are fuzzy: Dreams are real, clocks can talk, and unicorns live in a forest on a magical island in the middle of the ocean. At this age, animals, plants, and things are always more interesting than people. In addition, preschoolers typically believe that if they think something or wish it, they can cause it to happen.

Preschoolers are naturally self-centered and assume that everyone feels and reacts like they do. They think that most everything that happens within a family is connected to them in some way.

Because preschoolers still can't match many words with ideas, they learn best by looking at something, rather than talking about it. Even though their memory isn't very good (which is why they always forget their mittens), they can easily recognize things they've seen in the past. They think in terms of pictures, like to draw them, and, of course, frequently ask, "What's that?" and "Why?" However, these questions usually aren't exactly what they seem. Unlike older children, who are actually looking for a label or an explanation, preschoolers use such questions more to signal their own amazement and curiosity.

What does all this mean in terms of talking to young children about diabetes? First of all, you can skip the long, abstract, explanations—their brains simply can't handle them. When they ask a question, answer in short sentences. Show them things—your

pills, for example, or your glucose meter—and give them simple names. Relate your experiences to their own: Tell them that you have to go to the doctor sometimes just like they do, that your shots are like shots they may have had, that eating snacks keeps you from feeling hungry, and that exercise helps you stay strong.

Most of all, talk about your feelings and listen to theirs. Preschoolers associate injections with pain and fear; talking about how shots sting a little or how you don't like them but know they're good for you both confirms a child's own experience and helps him or her see that you're taking care of yourself. Let preschoolers tell you about how they feel when they go to the doctor or get sick. Ask them if they worry about you. And let them know that they can't catch diabetes from you the way they can catch a cold from another person. Because preschoolers often link illness with punishment, let them know that having diabetes has nothing to do with being bad or with something you have done. Tell them you have diabetes because of the way your body was made and that you'll be able to take care of it.

Don't be surprised if a child quickly gets bored and wants to move onto something else: It's a sign that he or she is filled up with information for now. Don't be surprised either if preschoolers ask the same questions again later. Remember, their memory isn't all that strong. Repeating a question may also be a sign that they didn't understand something you said the first time around, or that they need more reassurance that everything is going to be OK. It can also indicate that they want additional information but don't know how to formulate a question that addresses their specific query.

You may see the child later imitating in play what you talked about. He or she may pretend to give shots to a doll or pretend to take medicine or go to the doctor. It's the nature of young children to imitate (a good reason to keep pills, syringes, and other diabetes self-care items away from them), and play is their normal and healthy way to intellectually and emotionally integrate and understand new information.

Above all, be honest: Make sure your verbal and nonverbal behavior match. Young children understand more by how you sound and look than by what you say. If you talk calmly about medicine or injections, they'll believe what you are saying and be reassured that you'll be all right.

"How does it work?" (School-age kids)

As children get older, they shift from the world of imagination and fantasy to a world of reality and logical thinking. By the age of six or seven, most children know that mice really can't talk (although Santa Claus might still exist) and that if you're a boy, you can't grow up and become a girl.

School-age children generally believe what they're told and become fascinated by how things work. This is the age of taking apart clocks (though not necessarily trying to put them back together), being able to recognize and name 87 different types of dinosaurs, or collecting innumerable Barbie dolls simply for the sake of collecting them. Unlike their younger siblings, these children are more interested in people and how they think, are less self-centered and less likely to assume that everything revolves around them, and can differentiate among a wider range of emotions. Rules are important, questions are requests for real information, attention spans are longer, and memory is good.

What the school-age brain can't yet do is think abstractly. Like younger children, school-age children learn best by seeing and touching. When talking about diabetes, showing them pictures or the equipment itself makes the information more comprehensible. Long explanations about physiology or the biochemistry of insulin put them to sleep.

Children at this age want to understand, but they don't always know how to ask the right questions. Good pacing is the key to helping them out. When a child shows curiosity about what you are doing or asks a question, give a couple of sentences of information, then wait for the child to ask something else. The child's response lets you fine-tune what he or she really wants to know about. Encourage children to say what they are thinking by posing questions like, "How come you're asking about that?" or "Are you wondering why I have to be so fussy about when I eat?" Such questions will also help you zero in on the child's interest or concern.

As you would with younger children, relate your feelings and experiences to theirs when possible. For example, you could admit that you don't always feel like exercising or monitoring your blood sugar, just like they don't always feel like going to school on Monday mornings or studying for a spelling test. Both of you know, however, that you just need to do it.

While infants and preschoolers are extremely sensitive to the way you feel and how well you're doing, school-age children can often feel responsible for doing something about it. It's not uncommon for the oldest child in a family not only to look out for his or her younger brothers and sisters, but to feel worried and protective of a parent or grandparent who's not feeling well.

This is especially true in single-parent homes where an older child can easily fall into a second-in-command role. It's not unusual for such children to

READING TOGETHER

IT'S TIME TO LEARN ABOUT DIABETES
Jean Betschart
John Wiley & Sons
New York, 1995

This workbook, written by Jean Betschart Roemer especially for kids with diabetes, is also useful for teaching kids about diabetes when someone else in the family has it. The book, as well as an accompanying video, can be ordered on Ms. Roemer's Web site, www.diabetes.fyi.net.

remind a parent to take his or her medication, to worry about a visit to the doctor, or to make sure the other kids stay out of the way whenever they sense that their mom or dad is not feeling well.

If you see this happening, it's helpful to take the time to talk, and more important listen, to your child about these concerns. Your child needs to be reassured that you as a parent can manage, that if you need help you'll ask for it, and that he or she doesn't need to take over or take care of you. Give enough information to allay worries, but resist the temptation to confide in your oldest child as though you were talking to an adult.

What's important for preschoolers is important here, as well: Match your words with your feelings, and encourage school-age children to talk about theirs. Children this age can understand the subtleties of emotions better and are curious about how others feel and think. Look at questions not only as opportunities to share information, but also as chances to understand what is happening within them.

"Yeah, whatever" (The world of teens)

Teenage years are in some ways a mix of the previous two stages. Like preschoolers, teens can easily get preoccupied with themselves and what's happening in their own world. Like school-age kids, they like learning about new things and are sensitive to their role in the family.

The great learning leap of the teenage years is the ability to think abstractly. This is the time a child can really understand what diabetes is about—how the physical process works and why you have to do the self-care tasks you do. Because teens have had more life experience and are acutely sensitive to their own emotions, it's fairly easy for them to hear and empathize with the mix of good and bad feelings that you may have. The problem is that they're not always ready to listen, at times they don't seem to care, and they can quickly tune you out or even seem annoyed when your needs get in the way of their own.

The key to talking to teens is finding those windows of opportunity—often cloaked in an offhanded, out-of-the-blue remark—when they express interest or concern about you and when they're not preoccupied and can really listen. As with kids of all ages, pacing is important. If you talk too long, teens hear "lecture" and hit the off switch in their brains. If you wait around for them to ask questions like their eight-year-old sister, they'll assume you don't really care about what they think.

So bring things up, but don't beat them into the ground. Talk at dinner about your checkup at the doctor, ask your teen during a quiet moment whether he or she ever gets worried about you, or ask what your teen means when wondering aloud why you have to go to the podiatrist *again*. Then see what happens. If the response is short or snappy, back off and come back to it another time. If the teen responds with questions, answer them honestly. When teens (gasp!) talk about how they feel, take a deep breath, shut up, and listen. Whenever a good conversation starts, do your best to keep it going.

What teens need is information that can help them understand how diabetes can affect them, both in terms of the family and in terms of their own physical health. They also need good modeling, or learning how to face life's challenges by watching and listening to you. And they need someone to listen to them, so that they can begin to sort out and make sense of their feelings, and so that they can begin to define who they are and develop a sense of place in the world.

What teens don't need to do is take care of you. An older teen is even more likely than a school-age child to feel overresponsible or overprotective of a parent or grandparent. They'll need help from you in drawing the line between supporting you and feeling responsible for you. They need to know, even more so than younger kids, that you're in charge of both yourself and the family.

Keeping the door open

It's easy for all of us to close the door on difficult topics as a way of keeping awkward, anxious feelings away. But silence is deadly. In the absence of clear and accurate information about diabetes and your feelings about it, everyone around you—children and adults alike—is forced to fill in the blanks on his or her own, making up their own explanations for what is happening and why.

What children usually wind up doing is linking your diabetes to themselves in some way, or they come up with wild theories based on their limited understanding of the world that are absolutely wrong. They need some basic information so they don't fill in the knowledge void with junk. They also need to know that they can come to you for information and that they can talk to you about diabetes at any time. Communication with children can only start with communication from you.

If you need help educating your children about your diabetes or talking with them about it, consider contacting your diabetes educator or your doctor or seeking help from a counselor. Keep the door open. ❏

NAVIGATING DAY CARE

by Jean Betschart Roemer, R.N., M.N., C.P.N.P., C.D.E.

W hen their daughter Katie turned three, Sandi and John decided to enroll her in day care or preschool. They had been getting by on just John's income since Katie's birth, but things were a bit stretched, and both parents and child seemed ready to make the transition. As Sandi explored the day-care options in their area, however, she began to realize this was not a simple decision.

She wanted to find just the right place for her daughter, but nowhere seemed just right. One day care had a nurturing environment, but the rooms were small and crowded and not air-conditioned. Another had a great play area, but

PUTTING TOGETHER A DIABETES-CARE PLAN

When your child goes to day care or preschool, it's important for the teacher or care providers to understand the basics about diabetes. The teacher doesn't need to be an expert but should know enough to help your child follow the daily care routine and to respond appropriately if there are any problems.

The American Diabetes Association puts out a brochure called "Children With Diabetes" that can help your child's teacher learn the basics about caring for kids with diabetes. It's free, and you can get a copy from your local ADA affiliate.

Or you can check out the offerings on the Web site www.childrenwithdiabetes.com for some helpful tips on what to tell the teacher.

The teacher should understand or recognize the following: the basic definition of diabetes; signs of high or low blood glucose; your child's target blood glucose levels; the meaning of ketones and how to do a urine ketone test; and how to balance insulin, food, and activity.

A written care plan can be very helpful to the teacher. Below are examples of the kinds of things it could contain.

INFORMATION ABOUT YOUR CHILD

Child's name: _____

Child's age: _____

Here is my child's daily schedule, including times for blood glucose checks, injections, meals, and snacks. Please record each blood glucose reading in my child's logbook. I will review the logbook regularly. (<u>Note to parents:</u> Make sure to include specifics. If your child needs an insulin injection before lunch, write down what kind of insulin and how many units.)

Daily schedule:

TIME	ACTIVITY
7 AM	*Check blood glucose, take 10 units of Regular insulin.*
7:15	*Breakfast*

SPECIAL CIRCUMSTANCES

High or low blood sugar:

If my child displays symptoms of high or low blood sugar, please do a blood sugar check, even if one is not scheduled at the time. For treatment of low blood sugar (hypoglycemia), see the special instructions on my child's Hypoglycemia Action Plan. If blood sugar is over _____ mg/dl, call a parent or doctor.

Symptoms of high blood sugar include:
- Acting lethargic or sleepy
- Excessive thirst
- Frequent need to urinate

EMERGENCY INFORMATION:

Parent's name _____

Home phone _____

Work phone _____

Parent's name _____

Home phone _____

Work phone _____

Emergency contacts (if parent cannot be reached):

_____

_____

_____

PARTIES AND OTHER SPECIAL OCCASIONS

If my child eats extra food, such as candy or cake, an adjustment in insulin dose may be needed. Please notify me ahead of time about special occasions that involve food, such as Halloween parties and birthday celebrations. Here are specific instructions for these events:

_____

_____

_____

_____

_____

LUNCHTIME ACTION PLAN

Your child's diabetes-care plan probably includes a blood sugar check every day before lunch. To help your child's teacher or day-care provider know how to respond to the lunchtime reading, write out some instructions like those in the following chart. You will need to adapt this example to reflect your child's target blood glucose range and preferred treatment for low blood sugar, as well as your doctor's instructions.

SYMPTOMS	ACTION
Blood glucose below 70 mg/dl or child has symptoms of low blood sugar (hypoglycemia).	Provide 4 to 6 ounces of juice or 2 to 3 glucose tablets and four crackers. Recheck blood in 10 to 15 minutes.
Blood glucose between 70 mg/dl and 300 mg/dl.	Provide food and/or insulin as usual.
Blood glucose higher than 300 mg/dl.	Check urine for ketones.
Ketones present in urine.	Call parent. Child may require additional insulin.

the playground equipment was on asphalt instead of grass or sand, and Sandi could imagine all the skinned knees and elbows that Katie might endure. Another day care seemed spacious, clean, and bright, but the snacks consisted of candy, cupcakes, and doughnuts—foods Sandi didn't encourage at home. Another day care seemed to have little structure in the day, and the children Sandi observed seemed to hit each other a lot. She also wondered about hygiene and individual attention.

In the course of this exploration, Sandi was surprised at her own reluctance to "let go." Although she visited several day-care centers that seemed OK, none of them seemed quite good enough. She always found something she didn't like: either the sick-day policy, or the snacks provided, or the number of staff members, or the ability of the staff to communicate with parents, or the staff's attitude toward visiting parents. And then there were the little things that tugged at her conscience, such as who would read Katie's favorite story before naptime or make sure that her coat was zipped up when they went outside. Would her day-care providers discipline her harshly, gently, or at not all? How would Katie respond to all of these changes?

Just as Sandi and John were getting a handle on their priorities for a day care and on their feelings about leaving Katie in the care of others, Katie suddenly started to lose weight, become dehydrated and thirsty, and vomit. She was diagnosed with diabetes. From one day to the next, Sandi's and John's lives changed as both of them reeled from the impact of having a child with diabetes. They worried more, slept less, laughed less, and were far less optimistic about their freedom and spontaneity as a family.

But for the mental health of the family and to be able to afford Katie's added medical expenses, both of them felt it was a good idea for Sandi to return to work as planned. So she was back on the trail of finding a day care, but this time with a whole new list of diabetes-related concerns on top of her previous list of the usual parenting concerns. One of Sandi and John's main concerns was whether any day-care center would be willing to accept Katie, now that she had a complex medical condition.

Antidiscrimination laws

Sandi and John were happy to learn that there are federal laws that prohibit discrimination against people with disabilities, including children with diabetes. Laws such as the Rehabilitation Act of 1973, section 504, the Individuals with Disabilities Education Act of 1991, and the Americans With Disabilities Act of 1992 make it illegal for any federally funded group to refuse service to someone just because of a disability. This means that any day-care center receiving funds from the federal government must accommodate children with diabetes.

However, most day-care centers and preschools are privately owned and operated. But the Americans With Disabilities Act declared that schools and day-care centers provide a public service, so they must abide by the law even if they are privately owned. In fact, in 1996 a woman in Ohio sued a nationwide day-care chain, KinderCare, for refusing to enroll her three-year-old grandson, who has diabetes. The day-care company had a policy of refusing to administer the blood glucose checks the boy needed. After the U.S. Justice Department was notified of the case, KinderCare agreed to modify its policy. Now, the cen-

HYPOGLYCEMIA ACTION PLAN

Episodes of low blood sugar (hypoglycemia) require a quick response. The information on this page will help you recognize and treat low blood sugar.

Child's name: _____

Child's usual signs of low blood sugar: _____

_____

Other signs might include crying, irritability, sweating, shaking, twitching, or clammy skin. Child might be hungry, sleepy, uncoordinated, restless, or tired.

POSSIBLE REASONS FOR HYPOGLYCEMIA:

Not enough food	Delayed meal or snack
Too much insulin	Extra physical activity

TREATMENT FOR HYPOGLYCEMIA:

Step 1: Give food or drink containing sugar. Parent and child preferences:

FOOD	AMOUNT
(Example) Apple juice	*4 ounces*
(Example) Saltines	*4 crackers*

Alternative choices (for example, syrup, icing, candy, or regular soda): _____

_____

Please note: Water and diet soda will not help hypoglycemia. Chocolate and ice cream may not be the best choices, because the fat they contain can prevent sugar from being quickly absorbed from the stomach.

Step 2: In extreme cases, the child may be unable to eat, drink, or swallow. If this happens, inject glucagon, a hormone that raises blood sugar. The dose is 0.5 milligrams for children under six years.

The following staff member is trained to inject glucagon: _____

The glucagon kit is kept here: _____

_____

Step 3: If the child does not regain consciousness within 15 minutes of the glucagon injection, call 911.

Step 4: After an episode of hypoglycemia that requires a glucagon injection, the child's doctor or medical team should be informed.

ter will conduct daily blood glucose checks for its children with diabetes, and it will not ask if a child has diabetes before granting admission. Under the agreement, KinderCare is not obligated to administer insulin shots, and parents are responsible for providing any special food items or equipment their child may require.

The upshot is that it is illegal for most day-care centers to refuse to admit your child just because the child has diabetes. (An exception is day-care centers controlled by religious organizations, which are exempt under the law.) The center must also make accommodations that your child needs, such as allowing blood glucose checks or access to snacks even when it isn't snacktime. The best way to make sure this happens is to communicate with the teachers and care givers at your child's center.

Safety issues

All parents of children who attend preschool or day care are concerned with such safety issues as hygiene and the environment in the classroom and play areas. As parents of a child with diabetes, Sandi and John also needed to know that the day-care staff would keep Katie safe and healthy by following her diabetes-care plan. That included following her daily schedule and making sure she had meals and snacks on time. It also meant allowing for blood glucose checks and possibly insulin injections. In addition, it meant learning the signs and symptoms of low and high blood sugar and learning how to respond to them.

Each parent–provider arrangement is different and depends on the needs of the individuals involved. Some parents may prefer to visit the center during the day to perform a blood glucose check, even if a staff member has been trained to do it. A center that has cared for a child with diabetes before will probably need less education than one that has not. Discussion and ongoing communication is the best way to make sure everyone's needs are met.

To find a day-care provider that would meet their needs, Sandi met with the director and staff of several centers to determine whether they were cooperative and willing to work out an individualized plan of care for Katie. She also talked to parents of children who attended the centers to hear their level of satisfaction. And she asked if there were other children with diabetes or other chronic illnesses who attended the centers and, if so, how they were managed. Sandi looked for a staff that was eager to help. She asked detailed questions about parental visits, both spontaneous and planned. She wanted to feel welcomed by the staff for her interest and support.

The day-care center directors that Sandi interviewed had some questions too. They wanted to know how monitoring and injections could be done in a safe way so that others were not put at risk of being stuck with a used needle. They wanted to know how to safely dispose of used lancets, needles, and bloody wipes. And they needed information on how to respond to Katie's blood glucose levels when checks were done. For example, what is the level at which action must be taken to treat low blood glucose? At what high level should ketones be checked or a parent called?

Sandi realized that even the most helpful day-care providers couldn't be expected to memorize all the details of Katie's diabetes-care regimen. So she and John drew up a written care plan with the help of their diabetes educator. Their plan of care included Katie's daily routine, including the times at which she needed meals, snacks, blood glucose checks, and shots; information about what to do in an emergency and when to call for help; and the names and phone numbers of both parents and Katie's doctor. They made the plan as specific as possible so that everyone involved would have an understanding of who does what. (See page 418 for an example of a written plan of care.)

Planning for your child

When it is time to choose a day-care provider for your child, it is a good idea to prepare a list of questions and expectations to discuss when meeting the day-care director. Set up an appointment rather than just popping in. Once you've decided on a center, arrange to talk to the staff about diabetes so that they have some understanding of it and of your child's needs. Be prepared to answer questions. (Remember, most people know nothing about diabetes.)

Even with the best education, it will take time for staff to be comfortable with diabetes tasks. Helping the day-care or preschool staff to understand what the issues are is usually the first step in addressing any problems. Ultimately, staff education will go a long way to relieve anxiety. Although in most situations you will be the one to provide this education, your diabetes educator may have the resources or time to assist you.

The most important consideration for all involved is the recognition and treatment of hypoglycemia. Will there be a responsible adult present at all times who is knowledgeable about the signs, symptoms, and treatment of hypoglycemia? Who treats emergencies, and how far away is help? Can someone inject glucagon if necessary?

In addition, you will need to explore questions regarding blood glucose monitoring, the communication of results, and other aspects of your child's routine. Will meals and snacks be properly provided and on time? Staff should be made aware that changes in food, schedule, or activity can cause blood glucose levels to go too high or too low. An individualized plan of care must be worked out between parents and staff. If it is essential to provide an injection of insulin during school hours, who will do it? How will communication occur between the school and parent when there are changes in daily routines?

Any parent of a child with diabetes knows how overwhelming following a diabetes-care regimen can seem at first—and how routine it can become over time. The staff at your child's day care will need to go through this same adjustment process if they have never before cared for a child with diabetes. But if both parents and staff are aware of what needs to be done and why, most diabetes-related issues can be worked out to everyone's satisfaction in a reasonable way. ❑

SETTING BLOOD GLUCOSE GOALS FOR CHILDREN

by David E. Goldstein, M.D.

In 1993, the long-awaited results of the Diabetes Control and Complications Trial (DCCT) were announced. The study monitored blood sugar control for up to nine years in 1,441 people with Type 1 diabetes who were between the ages of 13 and 39 when they entered the study. Researchers used periodic measurements of glycosylated hemoglobin (HbA_{1c}) to evaluate overall control. HbA_{1c} test results indicate average blood sugar control during the preceding two to three months.

The DCCT conclusively proved that in people with Type 1 diabetes, degree of blood sugar control is directly related to the risk of developing diabetic complications or experiencing progression of existing complications. Keeping blood glucose levels near the non-diabetic range reduced the risk of developing retinopathy by 76%, the risk of progression of existing retinopathy by 51%, and the risk of needing surgery to treat retinopathy by 50%. Such blood sugar control also reduced the risk of early kidney damage by 42%, the risk of more severe kidney damage by 51%, and the risk of neuropathy by 60%.

Based on the study results, the researchers recommended that most people with diabetes strive to maintain blood sugar levels as close to the nondiabetic range as possible. They cautioned, however, that the closer to normal one keeps blood sugar levels, the greater the risk of severe hypoglycemia (low blood sugar). The researchers also cautioned that the results might not apply to some groups, such as children, since they were not included in the study.

Practice guidelines

Shortly after the DCCT reported its results, the American Diabetes Association (ADA) published a series of treatment goals for blood sugar control based on those results. (The association's recommendations are summarized in "ADA Guidelines for Blood Sugar Control" on the opposite page.)

These treatment goals are widely used today by adults with diabetes. However, it remains unclear whether they should also be used by children with diabetes. This subject is hotly debated among pediatric diabetes specialists. Some experts say that treatment goals for children should be the same as those for adults, while others recommend less aggressive goals, such as HbA_{1c} levels greater than 8% or 9%.

Why is there such a difference of opinion among the experts? To answer this important question, we need to consider the pros and cons of achieving near-normal blood glucose levels in anyone with diabetes and specifically in children.

Hypoglycemia

Hypoglycemia—blood sugar lower than 60 mg/dl—is a potentially serious, acute complication of diabetes. Anyone who takes insulin is at risk of developing it. Hypoglycemia impairs mental function and—if blood sugar sinks low enough—can lead to coma and even death. The dangers of hypoglycemia are heightened if a person is involved in an activity, such as driving a car or riding a bicycle, during which mental impairment could cause a crash or an injury.

Studies in young children, particularly children whose diabetes was diagnosed before age five, have uncovered another possible danger of hypoglycemia. These children have a slightly increased incidence of learning disabilities later in childhood. It has been suggested that these developmental problems, which are generally quite mild and do not occur in all children diagnosed at an early age, may be the result of repeated episodes of hypoglycemia. There is some evidence from animal studies that young brains may be particularly susceptible to damage from hypoglycemia. So one argument for maintaining higher blood sugar levels in children is to avoid hypoglycemia and the risk of developing brain damage.

Do the preteen years count?

Chronic complications of the eyes, kidneys, and nerves rarely, if ever, occur before the onset of puberty (about age 11 in girls and age 12 in boys), regardless of blood sugar control during the childhood years. It has been argued that because complications do not occur until puberty, there's no reason to maintain blood sugar levels as close to normal as possible during childhood and increase a child's risk of serious episodes of hypoglycemia.

However, recent investigations have demonstrated that the development of diabetic eye and kidney diseases is related to both level of blood sugar control during childhood and total duration of diabetes, not just duration after puberty. Thus, the "clock" for the development of diabetic complications begins ticking at diagnosis, and lower blood sugar levels during childhood can reduce the risk of developing complications later in life.

Developing a plan

So how do children with diabetes and their families figure out what to do? There are no easy answers, and each family and its health-care providers must examine these issues and decide on their own course of action. I will share my approach with you, although I do not have a secret formula for success.

I do not believe that hypoglycemia is more or less dangerous for children with diabetes than for adults. For example, driving a car during an episode of hypoglycemia is potentially dangerous, but so is an episode of hypoglycemia while playing on the school playground, where a fall could result in an injury. I do believe, however, that every effort should be made to minimize the risk of hypoglycemia in children, particularly very young ones who cannot verbalize how they feel.

The aim of blood sugar control is to achieve blood sugar levels similar to levels in a person without diabetes: A person who doesn't have diabetes has an average HbA_{1c} level of less than 6%. There's no single correct way to maintain near-normal blood sugar levels, nor is there any guarantee that one who follows one's diabetes care plan "perfectly" will always have blood sugar levels in the desired range. For this reason, the terms "good control" and "bad control" should be avoided, because they imply a link between a person's behavior and blood sugar control, which is not necessarily the case.

In seeking realistic goals for blood sugar control in children, the ADA guidelines are an excellent place to start. Goals must be individualized, though, because

ADA GUIDELINES FOR BLOOD SUGAR CONTROL

The American Diabetes Association suggests target ranges for blood glucose control, which appear below. These are only guidelines, however. Everyone needs individualized goals for blood glucose control, so your child's target range may be different from the ones given here. The blood glucose goals are listed for whole blood readings and for the equivalent plasma readings. All home meters test whole blood, but some give a reading in plasma values.

BLOOD GLUCOSE GOALS	WHOLE BLOOD	PLASMA
Before meals	80–120 mg/dl	90–130 mg/dl
Bedtime	100–140 mg/dl	110–150 mg/dl

HEMOGLOBIN A_{1c} Goal: less than 7%
Additional action recommended if higher than 8%

every child is different. For example, during the "honeymoon" phase, early in the course of childhood diabetes, insulin requirements are low, and the risk of hypoglycemia is low. At that time, it's realistic to shoot for HbA_{1c} levels less than 7%.

After the honeymoon phase, insulin requirements increase, and risk of hypoglycemia is higher. Many children are not able to maintain HbA_{1c} levels less than 7% during this time, so for them, keeping HbA_{1c} levels below 8% is an appropriate goal. For most children with diabetes, this degree of blood sugar control will achieve the right balance between the ideal goal of normal blood sugar levels and the realities of day-to-day life with diabetes, including the risk of hypoglycemia.

What if a child with diabetes can readily maintain HbA_{1c} levels in the 5%–7% range without many episodes of hypoglycemia? I would not attempt to "loosen" the blood sugar control to raise the HbA_{1c} level. I would, however, frequently review the child's management plan and discuss ways to minimize the risk of hypoglycemia since, over time, maintaining a low HbA_{1c} level may become more difficult, and hypoglycemia may become more of a problem.

If HbA_{1c} levels are consistently above 8%, a change should be made to the diabetes care plan, whether or not the child has frequent episodes of hypoglycemia. This situation is difficult and requires a meeting between the child's health-care providers and family to figure out which parts of the treatment plan are working and which are not. Perhaps the treatment plan is a good one but is not being followed exactly. Or perhaps the plan is not working and needs to be altered. For example, switching from Regular insulin to lispro (brand name Humalog), changing the injection schedule, or working out a new meal plan might make all the difference.

The best solution to the problem will be different for each child and family.

For many years at the University of Missouri Children's Hospital Diabetes Program, we have tracked HbA_{1c} levels in the children we see. We have found a steady fall in the average HbA_{1c} level, beginning about the time the DCCT results were announced in 1993 and continuing until the present. The average HbA_{1c} level of all our patients under 18 fell from about 8.5% to 7.7%. We have not noted any increase in the frequency of hypoglycemia. I believe (but cannot prove) that the lower blood glucose levels are mostly related to having specific blood sugar control goals based on DCCT results.

Tips for preventing hypoglycemia

There are a few steps you can take with your child to help prevent hypoglycemia without giving up blood glucose levels near the normal range. I will pass along the excellent recommendations of Dr. Julio Santiago, a noted diabetes specialist from Washington University in St. Louis, who passed away in 1997. Hypoglycemia frequently occurs at night, when it may go unnoticed. This is serious, because if hypoglycemia is not noticed and treated right away, blood glucose can continue to drop. To prevent nighttime hypoglycemia, Dr. Santiago recommended the following:

■ Check your child's blood sugar level at bedtime (or have the child do it). The child should eat a snack if the result is below 120 mg/dl (or the level specified by the doctor).

■ Nighttime hypoglycemia should be suspected if morning blood sugar levels are frequently below 80 mg/dl.

■ Regimens that give high insulin levels overnight should be avoided. For example, large doses of intermediate-acting insulin (such as NPH and

Lente) should not be given at supper, and large doses of short-acting insulin should not be given at bedtime.

■ Glucagon should be available in the home of every child with diabetes, and its proper use should be well understood by family members and other caregivers alike.

Other diabetes experts suggest doing a blood glucose check in the middle of the night (at 3 AM) once a week to monitor for nighttime hypoglycemia. Monitoring at 3 AM is also recommended if a child was more active than usual during the day, hasn't eaten well, or had low blood sugar at bedtime.

A few products on the market may help prevent hypoglycemia during the night. Special snack bars that contain "resistant starch," which is broken down slowly and absorbed slowly from the digestive tract, have been shown to lower the risk of nighttime low blood sugar.

Other products in development, such as continuous blood glucose monitoring devices, are just beginning to become available. They promise more effective protection against hypoglycemia in the future, but we won't know how well they work until people have a lot more experience with them. Meanwhile, there's no substitute for regular blood glucose monitoring.

Hard work pays off

We know much more about the management of childhood diabetes today than we did before the results of DCCT were announced. However, treatment remains a constant challenge for children with diabetes, their families, and their health-care providers. Achieving the proper balance between the best possible blood sugar control and the risk of hypoglycemia requires hard work, and it's a team effort. Now that the DCCT results are in, families can put in the work knowing that their efforts will pay off. ❏

GETTING ACCURATE INSULIN DOSES

by Karen Kelly, R.N., B.S.N., C.D.E.

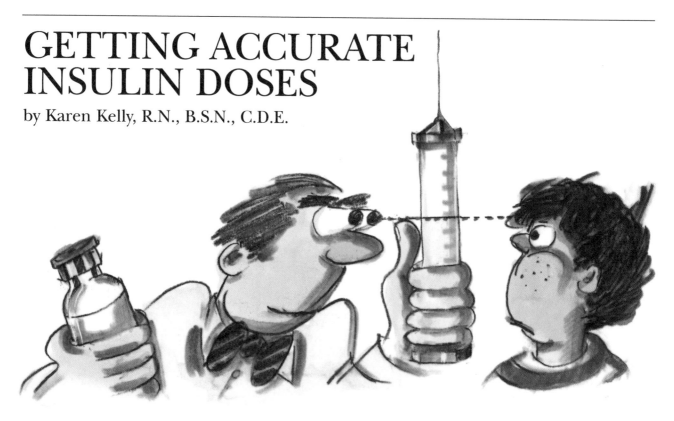

If you're like most parents, you work hard to make sure your child's blood glucose level stays within the recommended range. You test the blood glucose level several times a day, follow the insulin dosing schedule prescribed by the doctor, plan healthy meals, and pay attention to how much your child exercises. But sometimes, in spite of your best efforts, your child's blood sugar level is higher or lower than expected. Why does this happen?

Any number of things can affect blood glucose levels, but if everything about your child's diabetes-care plan seems to be in order, you may want to recheck the accuracy of the insulin doses your child is receiving. This is especially true if your child receives very small doses of insulin (less than 30 units per shot), or if more than one parent or caregiver delivers your child's insulin shots. Studies show that either of these circumstances raises the likelihood of inaccurate doses. You may also want to double-check the accuracy of the doses if the child does the injecting.

If you use syringes for insulin administration, refining your insulin measurement technique—with the help of a doctor or diabetes educator, if necessary—will almost certainly ensure a more accurate insulin dose. You may also want to investigate some of the newer insulin-delivery devices currently on the market such as syringes with shorter needles, insulin pens, and needleless jet injectors. In this article we look at some of the available options and discuss how they could help your child get the right insulin dose. Remember, however, that before you try any new way of giving insulin, you should always contact your child's doctor or diabetes team to discuss the best choices for your child's particular needs.

Syringes

A syringe is the most common way of giving insulin. Syringes come in a variety of sizes, with different sizes appropriate for different people. For younger children, who generally need relatively small amounts of insulin (mostly because of their small body size), a 25-unit or 30-unit syringe often works best. The unit markings on these low-dose syringes are spaced a little further apart than on larger syringes, making the measurement of smaller doses a little easier. And in children on a small dose of insulin, a half-unit difference can be important.

Unfortunately, even with a smaller syringe, measuring half a unit of insulin can be tricky. Some studies show that when measuring out a smaller dose of insulin, both parents and professionals tend to draw up a little more rather than a little less than the desired amount, a practice that could lead to low blood glucose levels. In addition, each person draws up insulin a little differently. If Dad gives the morning dose and always moves the syringe a "hair" past the line, and Mom gives the evening dose and habitually goes on the "light" side, a child's blood glucose readings are likely to fluctuate depending on who gives the shot. It may be easier to achieve control, therefore, if one person consistently draws up and gives all the insulin shots.

Children on doses of 30 to 50 units of insulin can use a 50-unit syringe. Each line on these syringes is a one-unit measure. (As doses of insulin become larger, half-unit measurements are used less frequently.) As children continue into adolescence, rapid growth and development and the hormones of puberty often increase a child's insulin requirements. Adolescents who take more than 50 units of insulin with one injection often do well using a 100-unit syringe. When

changing to a 100-unit syringe, be careful to note that each line on the syringe represents two units, not one unit. While 200-unit syringes are available, they are rarely used. If by chance you come across one, be aware that each line on these syringes measures five units of insulin.

The length of the needle can also play a role in the absorption—and therefore the accuracy—of the insulin dose. The newer, shorter needles often work well in smaller children because they usually have less fat on their bodies. A shorter needle may also make having shots a little less scary and reduce the chance of having a child pull away from the shot. If you change from longer to shorter needles, keep a close eye on blood glucose levels during the transition.

Shorter needles may not be suitable for older children and adolescents who have more body fat because the shorter needles may not deliver a deep enough injection. (Needles should generally be inserted at a 90-degree angle, regardless of a child's age or size.) If the insulin does not go deep enough, you may see a bubble on top of the skin or you may see the insulin leak out. If your child's blood glucose readings are too high when using a shorter needle, you may do better with a longer needle.

Insulin leaks are a common problem among children and adolescents. When a drop leaks out of the injection site, the child is not getting the correct dose of insulin. To make sure all the insulin you are giving your child stays in, try keeping the needle in place for a count of five and then pulling it out. Another way to prevent a leak is to let go of the pinch of skin as you are injecting the insulin. Make sure you do not keep the skin pinched up after you take the needle out.

As children get older and begin to assume more responsibility for their diabetes care, it is likely they will begin giving their own insulin shots. Even if you feel confident that your child can draw up a dose of insulin correctly, you should keep working together as a team to make sure the correct amount of insulin is being given. This is especially important during stressful times such as final exams or team tryouts when other concerns may seem more important than diabetes care. While some teens would prefer that their parents not be involved in their diabetes care at all, most are willing to recognize that taking total responsibility for their diabetes is a big, hard job for which they may not be quite ready.

Tim, for example, was a 16-year-old who had taken complete responsibility for his insulin injections. However, he was having trouble keeping his blood glucose in his goal range. Tim's diabetes team suggested that having his mother watch him draw up and give his shot might improve his control. When she did, she saw that Tim was rushing through the injection process and not always giving himself the right amount of insulin. Tim and his mother discussed this, and Tim admitted that he felt rushed because of school pressures and his other activities. They decided to work together to make sure he got the correct insulin dose. With more supervision, Tim was able to bring his blood glucose level back into his goal range and keep it there much more successfully.

Pros and cons. As an insulin-delivery device, syringes have stood the test of time. They are portable and easy to use, come in a variety of sizes and needle lengths, and are relatively inexpensive. Since each person tends to measure a little differently, however, accuracy is best insured if one person consistently administers all insulin shots.

Insulin pens

As more people with diabetes have begun using multiple daily injections, insulin pen use has grown in popularity. Each pen holds a single cartridge of insulin and has a pen needle attached to it. In some pens the cartridge is removable. Other pens come prefitted with a cartridge and are disposable. Types of insulin available in pen cartridges or disposable pens include NPH, Regular, and lispro, as well as premixed 70/30 and 75/25 insulin. The pen needle should be changed with every dose of insulin given.

Some pens deliver insulin in half-unit increments, some in one-unit increments, and some in two-unit increments. "Drawing up" the insulin with the pen is done by dialing in the dose. Before giving a dose, you should always dial one unit (or two units if that is the smallest increment available), press the plunger, and look for a drop of insulin at the end of the needle. This will ensure that the pen is working before you give the injection.

The convenience of having both insulin and syringe in one device, and the ease of the dial-in method for drawing up the dose, makes the insulin pen a good choice for many children and adolescents. These features may also leave less room for dosing error.

Before you can use an insulin pen, it must be prescribed by your doctor, and you and your child must be shown how to use it by a diabetes educator who can answer your questions and concerns and teach you the mechanics of the pen.

Pros and cons. Insulin pens are portable and generally easy to use. They are very convenient for people on multiple daily injections and for people with busy lifestyles. The dial-in dosing method may increase dose accuracy. However, for some children, the pen may feel too heavy, and its length may be difficult to adjust to. Since you cannot give combinations of insulin with the pen, it is unlikely to work well for children who take only two injections daily.

Insulin jet injectors

Insulin jet injectors have been available for several years and are marketed as needle-free or needleless injectors. They come in child and adult sizes. The injectors can deliver a dose anywhere between half a unit to 50 units of insulin. Dose adjustments can be made in half-unit increments. A single kind of insulin may be given, or the insulin can be mixed. The pressure with which insulin enters the skin can be adjusted to accommodate each individual's comfort level. Jet injectors may be useful for children who have a fear of needles or injections.

Some studies have suggested that needle-free injectors deliver more accurate doses of insulin than standard syringes. This seems particularly true when it comes to measuring small insulin doses. When changing from syringes to a jet injector, there is an adjustment period. It can take some time to get the correct depth of injection with a jet injector. Special attention needs to be paid to blood sugar levels during this transition period.

Pros and cons. While jet injectors may be more effective than syringes in delivering small amounts of insulin accurately, they tend to be heavy and not highly portable. If you want to try one, most manufacturers have a 30-day trial period, during which you can test an injector and return it if it does not meet your needs.

A good start on good control

The case for good blood glucose control has never been stronger. The Diabetes Control and Complications Trial, a major study of Type 1 diabetes conducted from 1983 to 1993, showed that keeping blood sugar levels as close as possible to normal significantly lowers the chances of developing diabetic complications. Making sure your child gets the correct insulin dose is a vital step toward achieving that goal.

Picking the right device and using correct technique are equally important parts of the picture. To offset problems before they arise, review your technique with your child's doctor or diabetes educator periodically. Before investing in any new insulin-delivery products, do some homework. Ask your child's diabetes educator about any device you want to try. He or she can help you and your child to make an educated, safe, and appropriate choice. In addition, write or call the companies that make the products; they are usually more than happy to send you information. Before using any new device, make sure you have been completely instructed on its use. You will have a considerably better chance of measuring doses accurately if you understand how to use the product the right way. ❏

INSULIN PUMP THERAPY FOR KIDS

by Jo Ann Ahern, A.P.R.N., M.S.N., C.D.E.

There's no doubt that interest in insulin pumps is up among people with diabetes. In fact, the most commonly asked question of the staff at the Yale Program for Children With Diabetes in New Haven, Connecticut, is, "Am I a candidate for the pump?" or "Is my child a candidate for the pump?" In many cases, the answer is yes.

Let's have a look at what makes a child a good candidate for a pump and what's involved in getting started using one. As you read, keep in mind that this article describes primarily how the Yale Program for Children with Diabetes operates. As in all aspects of diabetes care, there are many "right" ways of doing things, and the diabetes center in your area may do things differently. If you are interested in any of the methods or products mentioned in this article, please check with your health-care team before making changes in your child's diabetes-care routine.

Who's a pump candidate?

The children who are most likely to be offered a pump at Yale are those who are working very hard to maintain normal blood glucose levels, those who are not meeting goals, those who ask about pump treatment and how it might help them, those whose episodes of hypoglycemia or high blood glucose are affecting their school work, sports performance, and normal, day-to-day living, and those who know carbohydrate counting.

However, pump treatment will succeed only if both child and parents are motivated and have reasonable expectations of what a pump can and can't achieve. They must understand that a pump is only as good as the person operating it. In addition, parents need to be reliable, and a child must be willing to check the blood glucose level at least four times a day. In fact, a child or teen wouldn't be considered for pump treatment at the Yale Program if this minimum requirement were not already being met.

Since many children are afraid of any change, a little persuasion is sometimes in order for a child to try a pump. It's important to let children know that pump treatment can help them feel better, have more normal blood glucose levels, perform better in school and sports, and have fewer episodes of hypoglycemia. They will also have much more flexibility in terms of mealtimes and food choices. And, if more normal blood glucose levels are achieved, the incidence of long-term complications of diabetes will be greatly decreased or eliminated.

Youth no object

The age of a child is a consideration for pump candidacy, but no age rules out the possibility of using a pump. I recently put Maggie, age 18 months, on an insulin pump. She was having difficulty with both high blood glucose and hypoglycemia at all times of day and night. Her blood glucose level would frequently drop overnight, even with no insulin in the evening. Her mother was checking her blood glucose levels eight to 10 times a day and was becoming very discouraged. Clearly, it was time to try other treatment options.

Presently, there are 44 children under the age of seven on pump therapy in the Yale Program. Their reasons for starting on pump therapy have varied. Sometimes a child in this age group is doing well with insulin shots, but the parents would like the flexibility that the pump offers. Many parents would like to make mealtimes more pleasant and to not have arguments over food. (Even at their best, children in this age group tend to be finicky eaters.) They would also like to smooth out the blood glucose swings that are so common in a young child.

Children of age three or four are able to deliver an insulin bolus (the dose taken before meals) themselves, but they need someone to verify the amount before activating it. When children younger than seven are started on the pump, we usually use the block feature on the particular pump we use, which keeps the children from activating the buttons on their own. This feature is usually used only for the first week or so; after that, the novelty usually wears off, and the children don't tend to play with their pump.

School-age kids (seven to 12 years old) are great pump candidates. They tend to be excited about the pump and want to help as much as possible. They also tend to be very successful at keeping their blood glucose level in the normal range most of the time. They can give bolus doses themselves but need some help deciding how much to bolus. They can begin counting carbohydrates and are able to use their insulin-to-carbohydrate ratio, as determined by their health-care provider, to tell how much insulin they require per carbohydrate exchange. (A carbohydrate exchange is approximately 15 grams of carbohydrate.) In general,

MORE ON PUMPS

To read more about pumps, have a look at these Web sites or call the pump manufacturers at the following numbers:

ANIMAS CORPORATION
www.animascorp.com
(877) YES-PUMP (937-7867)
Maker of the R-1000 insulin pump.

DISETRONIC MEDICAL SYSTEMS, INC.
www.disetronic-usa.com
(800) 280-7801
Maker of the D-TRON, H-TRONplus, and Dahedi insulin pumps and Tender infusion set, among others.

INSULIN INFUSION SPECIALTIES
www.insulininfusion.com
(800) 838-PUMP (838-7867)
Seller of pumps and supplies. Web site also provides practical information about using a pump.

INSULIN PUMPERS WEB SITE
www.insulin-pumpers.org
Offers information, tips, and reader exchanges.

MINIMED, INC.
www.minimed.com
(800) 933-3322
Maker of the 508 insulin pump, Sof-set, Quick-set, and Silhouette infusion sets, among others, and Sof-serter and Quick-serter automatic insertion devices. MiniMed also publishes the booklets "Teens Pumping It Up!" which can be ordered online, and "Pumper in the School!" for school nurses, teachers, and parents, which can be ordered by calling (800) 826-2099.

kids this age are proud to show off the pump to their friends and think it's quite cool to wear.

Teens are probably the least reliable group to start on the pump. Even though they easily learn how to use it and quickly pick up the mechanics, they are typically preoccupied with many other things, and the pump quickly goes down on the priority list. Teens frequently forget to bolus. They do better on the pump than they do with shots, but they don't do as well as younger children.

Getting started

If child and parent agree on the idea of pump treatment, the next step is to explain a little more about what the pump will and will not do. The child and par-

ents are shown an insulin pump and how it works. This provides the opportunity to clear up any misconceptions about what pump treatment entails and to address any fears.

An insulin pump is a beeper-size device that contains a cartridge filled with fast-acting insulin such as Regular or lispro (brand name Humalog). Intermediate-acting and long-acting insulins are never used in a pump. Furthermore, since the pump delivers insulin continually, intermediate-acting and long-acting insulins are no longer needed in the insulin regimen.

In addition to the insulin cartridge, the pump also contains a tiny computer, which allows it to be programmed, a motor, which pushes insulin out of the cartridge and into the body, and a battery, which must be changed periodically. The pump is worn outside the body and is generally clipped to a belt or carried in a pocket or special pump pouch.

Attached to the pump is a length of tubing, through which the insulin flows from pump to body, and the infusion set: a small insulin needle or Teflon cannula that is inserted just below the skin and taped securely in place. The infusion set must be changed every second or third day to prevent infection. The new set is inserted into a different site on the body.

The pump is intended to be used 24 hours a day. A small amount of insulin is given continually (the "basal rate"), according to a programmed plan unique to each pump user. This insulin keeps blood glucose in the desired range between meals and overnight. When food is eaten, the user programs the pump to deliver a "bolus" of insulin that is matched to the amount of food that will be consumed. It's important for prospective pump users to realize that the pump does not measure blood glucose levels, nor does it program itself. The user must do these tasks.

Children sometimes worry that the pump will fall out if they hang upside down on the monkey bars or during active sports. Parents tend to worry about their ability to learn something new, about having to inform their child's school about something new, about hurting their child, and about the pump getting disconnected during sports. These and any other fears must be addressed in an adequate way to alleviate these concerns. Children and their families are told that they can still do anything they did before and that the diabetes team will be there to address any issues that arise once pump therapy is started.

All of the children who receive care at the Yale Program are started on the pump in the office during a one-hour visit scheduled on a Tuesday morning. The child's total daily insulin dose is calculated and divided in half. One of those halves is further divided by 24, and this becomes the basal rate in units per hour. The other half is divided among the meals and snacks as bolus doses, with the larger proportion being given for breakfast, less for lunch, and more for supper.

After the pump start, the child goes to school as usual. The child or parents are instructed to test blood glucose levels at the usual times (before meals and at bedtime) and, in addition, at 12 AM and 3 AM. They phone in the blood glucose readings the following day and return on Thursday to do the infusion set change on their own with diabetes team members to coach.

During the first few weeks of pump use, the Yale Program social worker is available to discuss any adjustment problems that the child or family might be having. After approximately three to four weeks, the diabetes team (child, parents, and care providers) generally feel quite comfortable with pump treatment, and the initial trials and worries subside.

Nuts and bolts

There are now several insulin pumps on the market as well as a variety of styles of infusion sets and other accessories. Different diabetes programs favor different products; here's how we do it at Yale:

Infusion sets. After much experience with children under seven years, it became apparent that the Silhouette infusion set (made by MiniMed, Inc.) or the Tender infusion set (a Disetronic product) is the cannula of choice when initiating treatment in this age group. These sets are also good choices for very thin children, since they are inserted on an angle and therefore don't hit a muscle. They have the disadvantage of having to be inserted manually.

Most of the older pump users in the Yale Program use the Sof-set Micro QR or Quick-set infusion set (made by MiniMed, Inc.) with the Sof-serter or Quick-serter automatic insertion device (also MiniMed products), which allows them to "shoot" the cannula through the skin, decreasing the chance of crimping and pain. However, the Sof-set Micro QR tends to crimp in very young children and very thin children.

Children at Yale are instructed to insert the cannula into the upper, outer buttocks. This is the least painful site and has the most subcutaneous tissue. For very young children, Emla or Ela-Max 4% cream, a topical anesthetic, may be used. (Emla cream is not sold over the counter; it requires a prescription to purchase. Ela-Max 4% is available over the counter.) We don't recommend this for long-term use, however, since we don't know what the effects are of using it as frequently as every other day. Ice may also be used to numb the insertion area.

Insulin dosing. Once a person has begun using a pump, the basal rates and bolus doses can be fine-tuned. We have found that most children require a higher basal rate from 9 PM to 3 AM than at any other time of day. The 3 AM basal rate is the lowest. So a typical child on a total daily dose of 12 units would be on basal rate profiles similar to this: 12 AM, 0.3 unit/hour; 3 AM, 0.1 unit/hour; 7 AM, 0.2 unit/hour; 9 PM, 0.4 unit/hour. It's possible that the 9 PM basal rate would need to be increased even further. We feel that this need for more insulin during the night is a result of growth hormone secretion during sleep. Typical bolus doses for this child would be 2.5 units for breakfast, 1.0 unit for lunch, 0.5 unit for snacks, and 2 units for dinner.

After the initial adjustment to the child's usual routine, insulin-to-carbohydrate ratios can be investigated with the child, parent, and dietitian. Whatever the insulin-to-carbohydrate ratio is, this is usually the correction bolus to bring blood glucose down 100 mg/dl in the event of high blood glucose. For example, if a child has an insulin-to-carbohydrate ratio of 0.5 unit to 15 grams of carbohydrate, 0.5 unit of insulin would drop this child's blood glucose level 100 mg/dl. If the ratio were 1 unit to 15 grams carbohydrate, 1 unit of insulin would usually lower the blood glucose level by 100 mg/dl.

Our rule of thumb for finding a child's insulin-to-carbohydrate ratio is this: for children under 7 years old, use 0.5 unit to 15 grams of carbohydrate. For children 7 to 12 years old, use 0.7 unit to 15 grams of carbohydrate. For teens, use 1 unit to 15 grams of carbohydrate. These figures are just starting points, however. Insulin-to-carbohydrate ratios need to be individualized for each child.

School, sports, and vacation

What happens when a child who uses a pump goes to preschool, day care, or primary school? Like any child with diabetes, a child using a pump needs to have an individualized plan of care that is agreed on by parents, teachers, and school administrators. The plan should cover both daily care and emergency care and specify who is responsible for what diabetes-care tasks.

Getting to specifics, most children do not need a bolus of insulin for a midmorning snack that contains 15 grams of carbohydrate. However, if a child who eats a midmorning snack consistently has high blood sugar at lunch, we program a basal rate increase for one hour before snacktime. For example, if the usual basal rate is 0.2 unit/hour in the morning, we would make it 0.7 unit/hour at 9 AM and set the basal rate back to 0.2 unit/hour at 10 AM. By covering the snack this way, neither the child nor the teacher has to worry about a bolus dose. We do the same thing in school-age kids if coverage of a snack is necessary.

For young school-age children, the parent generally tells the school nurse or teacher what dose the child needs for lunch based on blood glucose level, food intake, and activity. The dose may be different if lunch is followed by gym or recess rather than an academic class. Most children, even three-year-olds, can program their own boluses with adult supervision.

For organized sports, the pump is usually removed. If the pump contains lispro, we recommend disconnecting for no longer than two hours without bolusing. A child who is at the beach may hook up and bolus every two hours or take a lunch shot of Regular insulin, which will usually last for four to five hours.

If a child lives at the beach in the summer, we can substitute Regular for lispro in the pump for the whole summer. It means a few days of re-regulating the child, but it isn't usually a big problem and it allows the child to go for four to five hours without having to hook up to the pump. (Note: If you currently use a pump, do not attempt to make this change on your own. Work with a health-care provider experienced in pump therapy.)

Good results

The Yale Program presently has 300 children on the insulin pump—close to half of all the children we see.

We initiate treatment with at least two children per week. The mean glycosylated hemoglobin (HbA_{1c}) level for all children on pumps at our center is 7.2%. (The HbA_{1c} test gives an indication of overall blood glucose control over the previous two to three months.) While a person who does not have diabetes generally has an HbA_{1c} of 4.2% to 6.3% in our lab, research has shown that an HbA_{1c} of 7.2% or lower in people with diabetes is associated with a much lower risk of long-term diabetes complications.

Our philosophy is that intensive management of blood glucose levels is essential right from diagnosis, so all of our children with diabetes are intensively managed regardless of their treatment method. The mean HbA_{1c} for all of them is 7.7%. The 0.5% decrease—without hypoglycemia—seen in those using a pump is a significant improvement.

Our hope is that all pediatric diabetes programs will offer the pump option. To quote many of the parents we see, "It gave us our life back." What an inspiration for us to continue our pump program! ❑

SAFELY SHIFTING DIABETES RESPONSIBILITIES TO YOUR CHILD

by Tim Wysocki, Ph.D.

All parents have one basic task: to help their children become healthy adults who can make it on their own. Your child's diabetes may complicate or magnify this basic responsibility, but it doesn't change it.

When it comes to diabetes self-care, parents are faced with some difficult questions about how and when to shift responsibility for self-care to their children. Giving too little responsibility could make your child feel inadequate and fearful about taking on responsibilities

430

later. But giving your child too much responsibility too soon could lead to dangerous treatment errors and failure in early self-care efforts. This could be discouraging and could cause both you and your child to feel that it is useless to try to keep diabetes in good control.

Do you think your child currently has about the right amount of responsibility for his or her diabetes self-care? Have you been able to balance your child's safety with your child's need to eventually become an independent diabetes self-manager?

If you answered, "I don't know," to either of the questions above, you're not alone. Transferring diabetes duties from parents to their children is a complicated process. However, several research studies have examined the division of diabetes responsibilities between parents and children and have produced some useful results. In this article we look at some of that research and how you can make the results work for you.

Diabetes skills and age

One way to evaluate your child's diabetes self-care skills is to find out what skills children typically acquire at what age. To help parents compare their children to the average, my research team and I surveyed 648 parents of youngsters with diabetes between the ages of 3 and 18. We asked the parents if their children were able to do 38 specific diabetes-related tasks correctly without receiving any help or prompting from others.

Here's what we found for nine common diabetes skills. The lower end of the age range (in parentheses) is the age at which 50% of children had mastered each task, while the upper end of the range is the age at which 75% of children had mastered the task.

■ Pricks finger with lancet (5–6)
■ Performs blood glucose test with a meter (6–7)
■ States symptoms of high blood glucose (7–9)
■ Gives injection to self (8–10)
■ Draws up mixture of two types of insulin (10–11)
■ States reasons for need to change insulin dose (8–12)
■ Performs urine ketone test (8–14)
■ Can adjust food intake according to blood glucose level (9–14)
■ Can adjust insulin dose according to blood glucose level (13–18)

You may notice that for many skills the age range is quite large. This suggests that there are many factors other than age that determine how much responsibility a child can handle, especially when it comes to some of the more complex skills. But these ranges show when most children become able to perform these diabetes skills.

If your child has had diabetes for at least six months, you may want to examine where he or she stands in comparison to the children whose parents participated in this study. If your child has had diabetes for less than six months, be patient: It's not appropriate to expect that children who have had diabetes for less than six months will be doing the same tasks as those who have had diabetes for longer.

The survey used in this study, with instructions on how to fill it out, score it, and interpret the results, is included in my book, *The Ten Keys to Helping Your Child Grow Up with Diabetes,* which is obtainable from the American Diabetes Association through the Web site http://store.diabetes.org or by calling (800) 232-6733. You can use the survey to get an idea of how your son or daughter compares overall or on specific tasks. The survey may help you identify some skills you and your child need to work on.

As children mature, they're able to handle more and more complex diabetes skills. But they may forget skills that they don't use often, and they may also come up with "creative" ways of doing things that differ from what they were taught. It's important that your child's diabetes management skills be examined by a diabetes professional once every year or so. I think having your child attend a diabetes summer camp is the best and most enjoyable way to do this.

Psychological maturity

Comparing your child to others of the same age is one way to judge whether he or she is progressing normally, but we all know that children at the same age vary in learning ability, social skills, and emotional maturity. This leads us to a harder question to answer: Is your child's level of diabetes self-care responsibility appropriate to your child's level of psychological maturity? I can't give you a simple answer to that one. Instead, I'm going to tell you about another study that addresses this issue.

The study was designed to explore what happens to diabetes control and treatment adherence (how well the child with diabetes follows the treatment plan) when children have just enough, too much, or too little responsibility for diabetes treatment and monitoring tasks. One hundred children with diabetes between 5 and 17 years old took tests of psychological maturity and answered questionnaires about diabetes self-care responsibility. My research team and I calculated a ratio between each child's level of diabetes self-care responsibility and that same child's psychological maturity level. That gave us a measure of whether each child's diabetes responsibility was appropriate for that child's level of psychological maturity. We divided the children into three groups based on this score: those with too much, too little, and just enough diabetes responsibility compared with their psychological maturity.

We then examined whether the children in each group differed in their diabetes control. We found that children with too much self-care responsibility for their level of maturity had all kinds of problems: less diabetes knowledge, poorer treatment adherence, more hospitalizations, and poorer control of diabetes. But the children with either too little or just enough self-care responsibility were better off on all counts. There was no evidence that children with less responsibility than they were capable of had any different diabetes outcomes than those who had just the right amount of responsibility.

These findings challenge the common belief that more diabetes responsibility is always better. They suggest that you should be careful not to push too much diabetes responsibility on your child too soon. Since it's not easy for parents (or professionals, either) to match their children's self-care responsibility to their maturity perfectly, it's probably best to err on the side of too much parental responsibility rather than too little. It gets harder to do this as your child becomes a teenager, but try to make sure that you're shifting responsibilities to your child because he or she has grown into them, not just because you're at the end of your rope.

Keys to a successful transfer

Now that you know the potential hazards of giving too much diabetes self-care freedom too soon, how do you go about transferring responsibility to your child in safe and productive ways? How can you stay involved in your teenager's diabetes management in ways that are helpful and constructive, rather than annoying or insulting?

There are three main factors that determine whether the transfer of diabetes responsibilities is smooth, comfortable, and satisfying or whether it is frustrating, conflict-ridden, and ineffective. These are the following:
■ The reaction of the parents and health-care team to the child's mistakes and failures in diabetes self-care
■ The effectiveness of communication between the child, the parents, and the health-care team about self-care responsibilities
■ The degree to which parents are effective teachers and skills trainers

How parents respond when their child makes mistakes or is irresponsible is very important. Parents who can find something positive to say about their child's

efforts and who can view errors as a painful but natural part of the learning process are more likely to find that their children accept diabetes self-management responsibilities more smoothly.

Transferring responsibility for any diabetes task from parent to child requires a partnership consisting of the parent, the child, and the diabetes health-care team. To make this partnership work, frequent, clear communication is necessary between all three parties about who is responsible for each aspect of diabetes self-care. Ideally, this communication would include the following:
■ Goal setting *with*, rather than *for*, the child
■ Occasional reviews of the child's skills by the diabetes team
■ A specific short-term plan for increasing and refining the child's skills, perhaps involving parent–child sharing of responsibility for specific tasks
■ Making sure that the parents and the diabetes team have the same ideas about the proper technique for each task

The third determining factor for success is the parents' effectiveness as teachers. Children and adults learn in very different ways. Compared with adult learners, children depend more on having hands-on experience, seeing many examples of the concepts being taught, breaking down complex skills into their components, and receiving immediate rewards for their efforts.

Adults often overlook the fact that many of the tasks that are expected of children and adolescents with diabetes are complicated. For example, correctly drawing up an insulin injection consisting of a mixture of two insulins requires about two dozen distinct steps that must be completed in a particular order.

Combining several teaching methods when instructing your child on a specific skill can help your child learn it more efficiently. For example, after demonstrating the skill several times, ask your child to talk you through each step in performing the skill. You might also play a "game" in which your child's task is to identify errors in your technique as you draw up an insulin injection or perform a blood glucose test.

The most complex skills can be broken down into parts and taught separately. For instance, you could draw up the first type of insulin and then ask your child to draw up the second type of insulin.

The amount of physical and verbal guidance that you give can be withdrawn gradually until your child masters the skill being taught. For example, when teaching a young child to self-inject insulin, you could insert the needle and hold the barrel of the syringe in place while your child pushes down the plunger. You

TIPS FOR A SUCCESSFUL TRANSFER

Helping your child take on more diabetes responsibilities takes time, repetition,
and a lot of patience. As you go through the process, keeping the following tips in mind
may help make it all less frustrating.

TRY TO:

ASK your child how to solve diabetes problems instead of solving them yourself.

BREAK DOWN complicated tasks into a sequence of steps.

PRAISE and reward your child's effort.

ASSUME some responsibility for your child's self-management errors.

STEP IN when needed to make sure your child is safe and to stop recurring mistakes.

TEACH diabetes skills by gradually withdrawing physical and verbal guidance and supervision.

MAKE SURE that you and your child's diabetes team have the same definition of acceptable performance of each diabetes task.

VIEW your child's failures and errors as a natural part of learning.

ASK your child how you can be helpful.

COMMUNICATE clearly and often with your family about who is responsible for each diabetes task.

SET specific short-term goals with your child to gradually increase the child's skills and independence.

TRY NOT TO:

QUICKLY ANSWER every question that your child asks about diabetes.

EXPECT perfect performance of complicated tasks.

CRITICIZE your child for failing.

BLAME your child for all errors in diabetes self-care.

ACCEPT the same self-care errors over and over again.

EXPECT your child to perform a new task well just by being told how to do it or by watching you do it.

ASSUME that everyone has the same standards for correct performance of each skill.

GET ANGRY when your child makes a mistake.

ASSUME that you know how to help your child.

ASSUME that everyone agrees about who does what.

PLOD ALONG with no specific short-term goals.

---

could then gradually reduce the amount of help you give until your child is both holding the syringe and pushing down the plunger. Then it might be time to teach your child to insert the needle.

For additional suggestions to help you through the process of transferring diabetes responsibilities from parents to children, see "Tips for a Successful Transfer" on this page.

Raising your child with diabetes requires you to keep a delicate balance between protecting your child's safety and preparing your child to live with diabetes without your guidance. I hope this article has given you some practical ideas on how you can help your child become an independent diabetes self-manager in the safest and most positive way possible. ❏

EQUAL TIME FOR SIBLINGS

by Ivy D. Marcus, Ph.D., C.D.E.

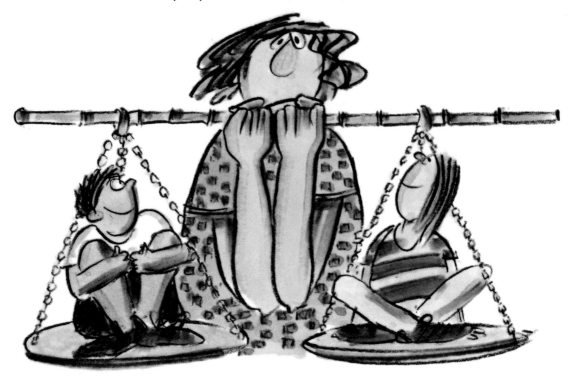

The fields of child psychology, behavioral pediatrics, and pediatric endocrinology all have populations of dedicated professionals who are devoted to the understanding and care of children with diabetes. Children with chronic illnesses, such as diabetes, provide health practitioners and parents with incredible challenges. These children are usually the focus of intense attention, both medically and behaviorally. For health-care professionals, children with diabetes present additional concerns not typically involved in the care of adults with diabetes. Parents of children with diabetes—in addition to their usual parenting tasks—are called upon to monitor their children's blood sugar levels, insulin dosages, food intake, and moods on a daily basis.

One of the effects of such intense attention on a child with diabetes is a dramatic shift in family dynamics. Such shifts in family systems can have a tremendous impact on the siblings of the children with diabetes. Yet the psyche of the sibling can easily get lost in the shuffle and chaos of caring for a chronically ill child. To preserve good parent–child relations and good sibling relations, however, it is extremely important for families and professionals alike to address the issues of siblings of children with diabetes.

Sibling relationships

In general, the significance of sibling relationships on peoples' lives is ignored or, at best, downplayed. Yet relationships with siblings can and often do have powerful and profound influences on our lives. Experiences with siblings can produce intense positive and negative feelings, both during early childhood years and throughout adult lives as well. Such feelings have the potential for shaping behaviors, thinking patterns or styles, and emotions for life.

In a sense, sibling interactions provide the first experiences in peer relationships. They may therefore form the mold from which future peer or intimate relationships emerge. Relations with brothers and sisters can teach children to love and act lovingly even when they are not feeling love in the immediate moment. They can teach the attitudes and skills necessary for all caring and enduring bonds between people. Sibling relations provide opportunities to learn about conflict resolution and can show children how to respect differences between people and even celebrate them. They can encourage kids to truly listen to one another. These relationships can also provide the most significant lessons they learn about sharing, whether it be sharing parental love and attention or sharing tangible resources, such as toys or books.

Sibling interactions can teach children to delay gratification and to negotiate with and respect others. They may also illustrate the benefits of having different strengths. Additionally, sibling relationships can shape children's views on competition and rivalry, as well as on closeness and trust versus distance and mistrust. They certainly can teach children about friendship, and they may help form their views on appropriate roles for individuals, both in families and in society. Brother and sister relations can also give children models of acceptance or rejection and thereby influence self-image, self-approval, and self-acceptance.

Given the breadth and depth of influence that siblings can have on our lives, it seems worth the effort to devote some thought to sibling relationships. When one sibling has diabetes and the other does not, even more complex issues can arise within the sibling relationship, making examination of it even more important.

Taking on roles

Typically, the siblings of children with any kind of chronic condition—diabetes, juvenile rheumatoid arthritis, asthma, cancer, mental illness, or anything else—are given a secondary role in their families. When it comes to the total amount of time allotted to each child, the so-called "healthy, less needy" child usually receives proportionally less time.

Because these children are not the focus of intense, daily attention the way their siblings are, they may feel ignored and unimportant. In response to these feelings, such children will often take on specific roles in their families. For example, some siblings take on the role of the "helper" or "aid." These children typically both protect and help their sibling and parents with the routines of medical regimes and with other household duties. Other children become "ghosts," and basically remain silent, never cause trouble to the parents or family unit, and seem to live a quiet life separate from the concerns of the sibling with the chronic illness. Another possible role is that of the "rescuer," in which a sibling acts to always be there to "save" the child with the chronic condition from harm or danger.

There are also children who become "distracters" and operate in such a way as to gain attention from their parents and significant others through unique behaviors and needs of their own. Such behaviors may be positive or negative in nature. For instance, a child may excel in a sport and draw attention and time through competitive games, while another child may develop a behavioral problem that requires ongoing attention from parents and teachers.

Still other children take on the role of the "police officer" and vigilantly monitor their sibling's management of diabetes self-care regimes. Such siblings may offer genuinely helpful and tactful bits of advice, or they may "tattle" or "rat" on their siblings for eating an unplanned piece of cake or for forgetting to take an insulin injection.

There are also those kids who play the role of "partner in crime." These siblings may encourage their brother or sister with diabetes to binge with them or to keep important information about their diabetes care from parents or doctors.

Some siblings of children with diabetes don't take on specific roles at all and just function as regular family members, often reacting in a variety of ways and playing different roles at different times.

The most significant issue to consider about role-taking on the part of children is that it inevitably short-changes all children involved. When children experience themselves as existing in a specified role, they cease to appreciate the full complexity of who they are, what they can accomplish, and what they might enjoy trying. Although we live in a society where roles are highly valued and provide us with a lot of comfort, it is important to continually attempt to encourage all children—both those with and without chronic conditions—to explore all possibilities and potentials and to discourage the limitations of one or two specific roles.

The consequences of role-taking are that children become imprisoned or locked in to their roles. They are then cut off from experiencing the freedom of limitless possibilities and change. But life demands that we be able to take on many roles if we are to function fully and effectively. As much as possible, therefore, taking on roles should be discouraged, and no child should be labeled into any role, be it a positive or a negative one.

The emotional consequences of labeling or role-taking are far-reaching. Children often feel resentful or angry at having to play out their part of the family drama. Or they may feel guilty or sad about deviating from their prescribed role. Some kids may experience a sense of being unimportant, while others may feel an unfortunate sense of relief at not having to take risks and be happy to avoid trying out new opportunities.

It is important to stay attuned to the needs and issues confronting all children and not to ignore or minimize the needs of the so-called healthy child. Siblings of children with a chronic illness need, as all children do, the encouragement to explore their whole selves. Allowing each child in the family to be a complex, multifaceted, changeable human being will help prevent the antagonism that often results between siblings when role casting is adhered to rigidly.

Challenges for siblings

The siblings of children with diabetes face some interesting challenges. At the time of initial diagnosis of diabetes, the family system typically undergoes sweeping changes. Usually, the routines of daily life are temporarily put on hold while the parents struggle to adjust to the reality of the diagnosis and to the many new tasks that they are required to learn and master.

The sibling of the child with diabetes, at least in the beginning, typically gets lost in the ebb and flow of the new adjustments. It cannot be stressed enough just how important it is for this sibling to be included as part of the process of family adjustment, as well as for the needs of this child to be attended to in some way, even at this most difficult time.

As life settles into the new routines involving care of the child with diabetes, siblings run the risk of continuing to feel ignored or less important. Tremendous care and attention needs to be given to this still very significant family member.

As time passes, the issues for the sibling will probably change. There are a number of problem areas that often arise within families, and they warrant addressing. However, the following discussion of potential problem areas is not meant to be an exhaustive list of the difficulties that can arise in families in which one child has diabetes and at least one other child doesn't.

Labeling. The first problem area is related to the previous discussion of role-taking and involves the child with diabetes taking on the role of the "identified patient." Such an identification renders the "patient's" sibling as being less in need of resources and attention. Potential consequences are cheating the sibling out of a full exploration of self and of decreasing the amount of nurturing that every child rightfully deserves.

Parents are best off avoiding the label of "patient" and treating each child as a unique individual, rather than thinking of the child with diabetes as requiring more from them. This sends a healthy, adaptive message to each child that no one person's needs are any more important than the others. The needs and desires may be different, but they are equally and distinctly important.

In a family with two children, one with diabetes and one without, for example, parents can, while attending to the medical needs of the child with diabetes, otherwise treat both these children in as normal and as similar a way as possible. Specifically, this means disciplining both children in the same way for the same issues, giving equivalent amounts of parental time and attention to each child's particular celebrations and difficulties, and focusing on the strengths of each child rather than the shortcomings.

Sibling fights. When the issue of fighting, arguing, or disagreeing between siblings arises, most parents cringe with dismay and intervene less than is perhaps ideal. Certainly, when the disagreement appears to be benign, and no physical or emotional harm is threatened or inflicted, it is best for parents to stay out of things and allow children to negotiate their own issues. However, when physical or emotional harm enters into the picture, it is important for parents to intervene.

When intervening, it is important not to favor or protect the child who has diabetes; such treatment is unfair to both children. For example, statements such as, "Don't upset your brother; just give him your toy. After all, he has diabetes, and his blood sugar may go up too high if he gets very upset," discriminate against both children. In this scenario, neither sibling learns to share, take turns, or otherwise negotiate the situation. Let the kids work out the issue of sharing toys for themselves, unless the situation begins to get too heated or volatile. For instance, if one child says, "You can't have this toy because you're not as good as I am; you're diseased with diabetes," it is certainly appropriate for a parent to intervene and to put an immediate stop to this verbal abusiveness.

Comparing siblings. Another problem area involves comparing children and their attributes. Comparisons between children should always be avoided at all costs. No two children are identical, and to compare and contrast them accomplishes nothing more than generating self-consciousness about what is lacking in comparison to the sibling.

Children (and adults alike) tend not to hear what their assets are when their strengths are compared to those of a sibling or any other person. So rather than saying, "You are so outgoing and social, and your sister is so studious and intelligent," make efforts to praise each child separately and at different times. In situations where more than one child is present, focus on describing the behaviors you observe rather than evaluating or judging them.

Recognizing the individual. Staying focused on the uniqueness of each child is crucial in building self-esteem and in fostering positive sibling relations. Many people confuse the individualized, unique treatment of children with the equal treatment of children. Children are not equal; they are unique and special in their own magnificent ways. So treating each child in unique and special ways can never lead to adverse consequences. When parents manage to interact with the siblings of the child with diabetes in a way that communicates that these children are uniquely important and special, such children then come to experience themselves as valid and special in their own right, and relationships between parent and child and between siblings are maximized and may flourish.

It is impossible to treat each child in exactly the same way. So why even try? Instead, try to interact with each of your children in an individualized, personally tailored style. The child with diabetes clearly requires specific, personalized care and attention. The child without diabetes also requires unique, personalized care and attention. Different, unique, special, and important—but definitely not equal or equivalent.

Allowing free expression. One last problem area to be discussed involves the expression of feelings on the part of siblings. Often, the siblings of children with diabetes are stifled by parents, significant others, or themselves when it comes to expressing their feelings about having a sibling with a chronic condition. But such expression needs to be encouraged rather than discouraged or punished. Having a wide variety of feelings, including some negative ones, is part of being human and is completely normal. Families are best off giving permission to the sibling of the child with diabetes to fully, respectfully, and tactfully communicate their emotions.

Children need to have an environment they perceive as "safe," nurturing, understanding, and receptive to the full range of human emotions. So when a child tells you of his or her jealousy, resentment, anger, guilt, worry, or any other feeling, even if pertains to the child with diabetes, welcome the openness of this child. Try to provide a constant and consistent environment in which all private communications about one's feelings and thoughts are received with love and understanding.

Each one is special

The siblings of the children with diabetes are children with unique needs, desires, and hopes that need to be nourished and nurtured. Remember that all children are significant and require time and attention. This is particularly important when one child in a family has a chronic illness. When raising the sibling of a child with diabetes, an awareness and devotion to the issues covered in this article can greatly influence the course of the parent–child and sibling relationships. Basically, when children, with or without diabetes, are treated fairly, with love, respect, and as distinct, important individuals, healthy relationships are much more likely to ensue, and healthy senses of self are more likely to result. ❏

FITTING IN EXERCISE

by Marilyn M. Clougherty, R.N., M.S.N., C.D.E.

Exercise is a major ingredient in anyone's recipe for diabetes management, and children are no exception. However, fitting sports and exercise into the daily schedule of a child who uses insulin can be a challenge. When to eat, when to check blood sugar, and when to take insulin are concerns that must be addressed when a child is active. These concerns should not prevent a child from participating in an activity, however. All sports are manageable, and the benefits of regular exercise outweigh the difficulties that may arise while your child tries out different activities or focuses more intensively on one sport.

Research clearly shows that regular physical activity helps prevent heart disease and enhances one's general health. Exercise is known to improve strength, self-esteem, and body image. Children who exercise often develop a lifelong commitment to physical fitness. For a child with diabetes, sports and athletics are also an opportunity to feel a part of a group.

Like many things, managing diabetes while participating in sports or other vigorous activities is easier when you plan ahead. Such planning includes not only figuring out the right time to eat dinner and the right amount of insulin to take, but also making sure someone on the team or in the class knows about your child's diabetes. It includes discussing any concerns with your health-care team. And it includes evaluating your child's management routine with frequent blood glucose checks. Here are some ideas to help make your child's exercise adjustments go smoothly.

Safety suggestions

If your child would like to join a team or try a new sport, there are several safety precautions to take before the first day of practice, as well as some to keep in mind once the season is under way.

Get the doctor's consent. To play on a school sports team, children are generally required to have a physical and get a signed consent form from their doctor giving them permission to play. Your child's regular diabetes care visits can satisfy most of the requirements for a physical, and it's a good idea to get your doctor's OK before your child begins an exercise program even if the class or team doesn't require it. Many schools provide sports physicals for team members, which should be adequate, as long as your child already has a diabetes care plan in place.

Talk to your diabetes team. Once you receive your child's practice and game schedule (or class schedule in the case of, say, swimming or dance lessons), discuss it with your health-care team. This way, your child's diabetes-care needs can be addressed individually and specific advice obtained.

Educate the coach. It is important for both parent and child to meet with the coach (or teacher) before the first day of practice. Coaches must have a basic understanding of diabetes and of their resulting responsibilities when there is a child with diabetes on the team.

Educate the coach about the signs of and treatment for hypoglycemia. Let the coach know that your child may need a snack or drink during practice or a game to prevent hypoglycemia. Show the coach the supplies your child may need to carry along, such as a meter, insulin pen, pump, or vial and syringe, and glucose tablets. Explain what glucagon is and why and how it's used. Find out if the coach is willing to learn to administer glucagon. If the answer is no, let the coach know to call the paramedics if your child loses consciousness from low blood sugar.

Educate teammates. It is best if teammates know about your child's diabetes and about the signs and symptoms of hypoglycemia. This can be accomplished by having the coach give a brief explanation. If your child objects to having the whole team know, make sure that at least a few friends on the team know so they can alert the coach to any behavior changes.

Carry medical ID. Even though wearing jewelry is prohibited while practicing or playing in a game, children should be encouraged to wear their ID at least up until game time, particularly if it's an away game. They may be able to wear a nylon ID bracelet while playing. And you may want your child to carry a wallet ID card as an extra safety measure.

Be prepared for low blood sugar. Children with diabetes should always carry a fast-acting carbohydrate such as glucose tablets or juice, along with a snack such as crackers or pretzels, in case of low blood sugar. It's a good idea for your child to carry additional snacks if it's a sport that lasts more than half an hour.

Be prepared for a delayed meal. If a game involves a long bus ride or is likely to go into overtime, be prepared for a delayed meal. Do not expect your child to always be able to get a snack at school, the ballfield, or the recreation center. Vending machines break, children lose money, and appropriate snacks are not always readily available at these venues. Make sure your child carries some food along.

Look out for postexercise low blood sugar. Body cells continue to take up glucose at a faster rate after exercise as the muscles replenish their energy stores. This can cause a drop in blood sugar up to 30 hours after your child's activity. For this reason, on active days, your child's dinner or bedtime dose of long-acting insulin may need to be reduced to prevent low blood sugar during the night.

Do extra blood sugar checking. It's a good idea to check blood sugar before, during, and directly after a new sport to determine your child's need for adjustments in food or insulin. Frequent checking can also reassure children that it is safe to fully exert themselves, instead of holding back for fear of low blood sugar.

Testing in the middle of the night can also be helpful to see whether blood sugar is dropping during sleep. You will want to test in the middle of the night when your child is beginning a new exercise, if blood sugar is low at bedtime, or if it tends to be low in the morning. Middle-of-the-night testing should be done weekly for children practicing "tight" control.

Choose the right site. When giving an insulin injection shortly before exercise, avoid injecting into a body part that will be used extensively during the exercise. For example, before a softball game, a pitcher would not want to inject into the throwing arm—a site on the legs or abdomen would be a better choice. A runner, on the other hand, would not want to inject into a leg because the insulin might be absorbed too quickly, causing low blood sugar. A swimmer, who uses legs and arms alike, might choose to inject into the abdomen to reduce the chances of developing low blood sugar in the pool.

Check for ketones. If your child's blood sugar is above 250 mg/dl before exercise, a urine check should be carried out for ketones. The presence of ketones in the urine is a sign that the body lacks insulin and is breaking down fats for energy, and exercise will speed up this process. Large amounts of ketones in the blood, combined with high blood sugar and dehydration, are a medical emergency.

Sports scheduling

Now that you know the general safety issues that need to be addressed when your child participates in sports or other exercise, here are some tips on how to handle particular exercise schedules. Children's sports take place anytime from 5 AM until well into the night, and each scenario requires different adjustments. Since no one solution works for all children, discuss changes in insulin or meal schedules with your health-care team before trying these strategies.

Early-morning practice

Some children have to be at the pool for swim practice, on the ice for hockey practice, or at the boathouse for crew practice at the break of dawn. Being active this early in the morning may require changes in the usual timing of morning insulin and breakfast. One solution is to have a snack before practice, then take the morning insulin and have breakfast after practice. This depends on the previous evening's insulin providing adequate insulin during exercise, and it allows the morning insulin to be taken on schedule, which may prevent fluctuations later in the day. However, the morning dose of insulin may need to be lowered on exercise days to prevent low blood sugar at school.

A second solution is to take the usual morning insulin dose and eat breakfast before sports practice begins. Sometimes a snack may also be necessary after practice. With this approach, a lunchtime injection of Regular or a rapid-acting insulin such as lispro (brand name Humalog) is often necessary to keep blood sugar levels within goal range because the insulin taken before 6 AM—whether fast-acting or intermediate-acting—may not last long enough to prevent high blood sugar by dinnertime.

Many children find that their blood sugar rises during morning exercise, even when they don't eat before practice. This happens because the body releases stored sugar from the liver in response to exercise. If someone with diabetes does not have enough insulin available for this extra glucose, the blood sugar level will rise. Children whose blood sugar rises with exercise may want to take a small amount of Regular or rapid-acting insulin and eat part of their breakfast before exercising. They will need to remember to take more insulin to cover food after practice.

After-school sports

Kids who participate in after-school sports probably need an afternoon snack to prevent low blood sugar during practice or a game. Some children like to have a sports drink or juice before or during exercise. However, this is not always enough for an activity that lasts longer than an hour. Carbohydrate snacks with protein, such as peanut butter crackers or pretzels and a cheese stick, are nutritious alternatives that may do a better job at preventing low blood sugar.

The best way to determine whether a snack is needed (and how big a snack is needed), of course, is for your child to check blood sugar before and after activity. Just as a child can eat too little before or during exercise, it is also possible to eat too much, which can lead to high blood sugar and excessive calories consumed. Some kids may only need to drink water to remain adequately hydrated and to decrease their morning dose of NPH or lunchtime dose of Regular or rapid-acting insulin to keep blood sugar in range during after-school activity.

Dinnertime games

As annoying as it may be to parents, many kids' sports games are scheduled to start at 5 PM—just in time to disrupt the family's usual dinnertime. A child's diabetes control doesn't have to suffer, however. Here are several options for keeping things in balance:

■ Your child can eat the usual dinner food exchanges or carbohydrate allowances for the afternoon snack, and the snack exchanges for dinner after the game.

■ If your child's insulin regimen permits only fast-acting insulin (such as lispro or Regular) before dinner, the meal can be eaten before the game at an early hour, then the long-acting insulin can be taken with additional short-acting insulin as needed before a bedtime snack. Adjust doses on exercise days based on blood sugar readings.

If your child has dinner early, it may be necessary to eat a small carbohydrate snack halfway through the game if more than four hours will pass between dinner and bedtime snack.

■ Children who use an insulin pump may be able to use a temporary basal rate or temporarily disconnect from the pump to compensate for both the exercise and the change in meal schedule. Discuss these options with your health-care team.

■ If your child takes two insulin injections per day, it may be necessary to eat a snack before and during the sport and to hold off on insulin injection until later, when dinner will be eaten. (If timing adjustments alone don't keep blood sugar in control, you may want to try a three-shot regimen.) If your child takes NPH or Regular insulin, the dose may need to be reduced to compensate for the late hour it is being given. If your child takes lispro, the dose should not be changed.

■ Even if your child's blood sugar is elevated at bedtime, a portion of the usual bedtime snack should still be eaten to prevent hypoglycemia during the night. Your child's muscles will still be replenishing their energy stores after exercise, lowering blood sugar levels, so it is recommended that at least a protein exchange (such as a cheese stick or peanut butter) be eaten before bed. You may want to check your child's blood sugar around 3 AM to be on the safe side.

After-dinner games

To determine whether any food or insulin adjustments need to be made for sports that take place after dinner, your child should check blood sugar halfway through the activity. A common mistake is to automatically cut back on insulin and increase food before an after-dinner practice or game. If your child is not extremely active, however, this can lead to high blood sugar and thirst during the game. For example, if your child plays baseball, a game that can involve a lot of sitting on the bench, blood sugar could rise.

If you find that your child's blood sugar drops below 70 mg/dl during an after-dinner event, there are several possible corrective measures you can take. One approach is to decrease the dose of fast-acting insulin taken before dinner. The long-acting insulin taken at dinner or bedtime may also need to be decreased to prevent low blood sugar during the night. A second solution is eat more food at dinner and to have a small snack available during the game in case a delay or overtime pushes your child's bedtime snack to a later hour than usual.

Away games

Dinnertime (and the dinner menu) can be unpredictable when children leave straight from school to an away event. Here are several suggestions to help maintain diabetes control in this situation:
■ Pack enough food to cover dinner and extra carbohydrate snacks for each hour of exercise.
■ Instruct your child to check blood sugar before eating or taking insulin to determine how much fast-acting insulin is needed according to the scale developed by your child's health-care team.
■ Use an insulin pen to make dosing more convenient and discreet. A pen also makes it easier to draw an accurate dose of insulin on a poorly lit bus.
■ If your child's usual insulin schedule can be maintained, there is less of a chance of blood sugar fluctuations overnight and the next day. If it cannot, and the bedtime dose is taken hours later than usual, the bedtime insulin will overlap the next morning's insulin, causing midmorning low blood sugar. Therefore, the bedtime dose of NPH should be decreased by 10% to 20% if it is taken more than two hours later than its scheduled time. If your child uses something other than NPH at bedtime, check with your health-care provider to see if adjustments need to be made.

All-night events

Most kids stay up all night at some point of their lives—for bowling, basketball, a pajama party, or the prom. This can be a nightmare for a parent whose child has diabetes, but it doesn't have to be. Both food intake and insulin can be adjusted as needed.

Since the body burns more calories while awake than while asleep, your child should eat something every two to three hours while awake to prevent low blood sugar.

How much should be eaten will depend on how active your child is and on the blood sugar level. If your child is still awake at the time, blood sugar should be checked at midnight and 3 AM. The bedtime insulin dose can be lowered to account for the extra nighttime activity.

Once they come home from their all-night excursions, children are usually ready to hit the sack. Before they do, it is important for them to eat something to prevent low blood sugar. Your child's morning long-acting insulin dose may need to be reduced and the fast-acting dose possibly eliminated to keep blood sugar in goal range during sleep. Because your child's body will still be burning energy at a higher rate from the extra activity, a blood sugar check should be carried out after four hours of sleep to make sure the level is still above 70 mg/dl.

Weekend sports

Some sports take place only on the weekends. After sitting in classes all week, this is your child's opportunity to get up and get moving. It is not unusual to need to make adjustments in food and insulin to accommodate the change in schedule.

If your child will be active between breakfast and lunch, the fast-acting insulin usually taken before breakfast should be decreased or eliminated. It may be necessary to eat a morning snack if more than four hours will pass between breakfast and lunch or if the exercise lasts for more than one hour. Check blood sugar halfway through the sport and after any new activity to determine whether your changes are sufficient or whether you should try something different next time.

If your child's activity takes place in the afternoon, reduce the long-acting insulin taken in the morning. However, if your child tends to snack while in-line skating or bowling with friends, particularly on high-fat or high-calorie foods such as pizza or chips, the insulin reduction may not be necessary. Again, checking blood sugar will indicate what adjustments need to be made.

Perpetual motion

All children with diabetes can benefit from exercise, both physically and psychologically. Kids who feel good physically are more likely to put forth their best effort, and that can help boost their self-esteem. Feeling good physically depends in part on keeping blood sugar in goal range, and the best way to figure out how to do that is to work with your diabetes-care team and use your child's blood sugar readings to fine-tune food and insulin adjustments. Be sure to include your child in the decision-making process as much as possible. The process of learning to keep their blood sugar in goal range helps children to understand their body better and become more independent in their diabetes management. ❏

QUIZZES

HOW MUCH DO YOU KNOW ABOUT SKIN CARE?

by Janice L. Woodrum, R.N., B.S.N.

Knowing how to care properly for your skin is important when you have diabetes. Your skin is your body's first and most effective protection against infection. However, problems related to diabetes such as peripheral neuropathy (nerve damage), impaired circulation, and high blood sugar levels can weaken your body's defenses, including your skin. Neuropathy can cause you not to notice small wounds on your feet. Once the skin is broken,

impaired circulation and high blood sugar slow wound healing, leaving your body vulnerable to infection. And infection, which is more common when blood sugar is high, can lead to serious complications, including amputation. The good news is that there's a lot you can do to care for your skin and to keep your whole body safe and healthy. Do you know how to care for your skin? Take this short quiz and find out.

1. Dry, itchy skin can be a sign of which of the following?
   A. Athlete's foot.
   B. Low blood sugar.
   C. High blood sugar.

2. To care for your skin, you should use skin creams or lotions designed especially for people with diabetes.

   TRUE　　　　　**FALSE**

3. What is the best way to care for a minor wound on your foot, such as a scrape or broken blister?
   A. Remove the skin from the broken blister and leave it open to dry out.
   B. Wash it with mild soap and cover it with a sterile dressing.
   C. Keep it dry and call your doctor in a week if it hasn't healed or if it shows signs of infection.

4. You should soak your feet in water at least once a week to help keep the skin moist.

   TRUE　　　　　**FALSE**

5. What are the best ways to avoid athlete's foot?
   A. Use athlete's foot ointment on your feet every day.
   B. Dry carefully between your toes after bathing.
   C. Wear water shoes in public showers and swimming areas.

6. Why are people with neuropathy in their feet more prone to skin problems? (More than one answer may be correct.)
   A. Skin sweats less than it used to and becomes dry.
   B. Skin may become less sensitive to pain, heat, cold, or pressure.
   C. Neuropathy can result in foot deformities.
   D. Neuropathy may cause swollen feet.

7. Which of the following products should you *not* use on your skin? (More than one answer may be correct.)
   A. Iodine, Mercurochrome, and similar antiseptics.
   B. Athlete's foot powder or cream.
   C. Medicated corn pads or drops.
   D. Mild antibiotic ointment such as Neosporin.

8. Signs of a skin infection can include which of the following? (More than one answer may be correct.)
   A. Coolness to the touch.
   B. Redness.
   C. Warmth.
   D. Swelling.
   E. Drainage of blood, pus, or other fluid.

442

1. C. Dry, itchy skin can be a sign of high blood sugar. When blood sugar is very high, the body excretes some of the extra sugar in the urine, and more urine is produced. Mild dehydration may result, and the skin loses some of its natural mois-ture. To avoid this problem or to correct it, keep close track of your blood sugar levels with self-monitoring, drink plenty of fluids, and apply a moisturizing lotion once or twice a day. Consult your doctor if the condition doesn't improve, because there are other causes of itching, including yeast infections and poor circulation. Although athlete's foot may also cause itching, the skin is usually moist.

2. FALSE. You don't need to buy expensive creams marketed to people with diabetes to keep your skin moist and in good condition. They're fine if you want to buy them, but less expensive skin creams can do the job, too. You may need to try several to see what works best for you. Even vegetable oil or shortening can be used if that is all you have.

3. B. Wash minor wounds with mild soap and luke-warm water. Cover them with sterile gauze, taping the gauze to itself, not to the skin. (Sticking adhe-sives such as Band-Aids to the skin can damage frag-ile skin.) After cleaning and dressing a wound, call your doctor to ask if he wants to take a look at it. Don't wait a week to call, because the wound could be seriously infected by then. Never pull the excess skin off a blister that has popped; the skin protects the wound from germs and prevents infection.

4. FALSE. While it may sound helpful, soaking your feet in water tends to leave them dryer than they were before. During the cold, dry months you may even want to bathe a little less often, and when you do bathe, use a mild, moisturizing soap. If dry skin is a problem for you, an oil-in-water skin cream such as Lubriderm or Alpha-Keri (or similar generics) may help.

5. B, C. Drying your feet carefully, especially between the toes, is an excellent way to prevent ath-lete's foot. And because the fungus that causes it thrives in warm, moist places, you should avoid put-ting any lotion between your toes, too. Wearing water shoes in public showers and swimming areas can also protect against athlete's foot. (Of course, going barefoot is never recommended, even at home.)

If you have athlete's foot often, you may want to sprinkle athlete's foot powder between your toes.

However, don't use athlete's foot ointment on a daily basis; save it for when you are actually treating an athlete's foot infection.

6. A, B, C. Neuropathy in the feet can raise a per-son's risk of skin problems in a number of ways. If it affects the nerves that control sweating, the skin on the feet can become dry and cracked, since normal sweating helps keep skin moist and supple. If the feet cannot sense pain, heat, cold, and pressure because of neuropathy, they are more prone to cuts, burns, and blisters. And if the muscles in the feet don't get proper nerve stimulation, they may change shape. This can put pressure on parts of the foot that don't usually bear weight, causing calluses and sores.

You can help prevent such problems by examin-ing your feet daily, applying moisturizing lotion to the tops and bottoms of your feet once or twice a day, testing the temperature of bath water with your hand or elbow before putting your feet in, and feel-ing inside your shoes before putting them on to check for worn spots or objects that could irritate your feet or cause injury. If the shape of your foot changes in any way, therapeutic shoes may be neces-sary. Speak to your doctor or foot-care specialist.

7. A, C. Strong chemicals such as iodine and Mer-curochrome can damage the skin and should be avoided. Medicated corn pads or corn removal chemicals should never be used, because they can penetrate too deeply into the tissues of the foot, causing very serious foot injury and infection. Ath-lete's foot preparations and mild antibiotic oint-ments are usually fine to use if needed, but check with your doctor to be sure.

8. B, C, D, E. Redness, warmth, swelling, and drainage of blood, pus, or other fluid are all signs of an infection of the skin and possibly the tissue beneath the skin. It is very important to look for these signs, especially on your feet. If you can't see your feet well, use a mirror or ask someone to help you. Any change in skin color—to red, blue, or black—can be a serious warning. Since a color change may not be easy to see, you should also feel your feet for changes in skin texture and tempera-ture. The backs of your hands or forearms may be more sensitive to heat and cold than your palms. Report any signs of infection to your doctor imme-diately. Cool skin is not a sign of infection, but it can be a sign of poor circulation. □

HOW MUCH DO YOU KNOW ABOUT WEIGHT LOSS?

by Janice L. Woodrum, R.N., B.S.N.

The hype used to promote rapid weight-loss products advertised on TV and in magazines and newspapers promises to make excess pounds melt away. They make losing weight look easy! If only it were. But quick-weight-loss schemes rarely lead to long-term weight loss. And when you have diabetes, there is another concern: Diets that cut back too drastically on calories or certain nutrients can upset your diabetes control and be a risk to your health. The secret to losing weight and keeping it off is to change your eating and activity habits for good. How much do you know about safe weight loss? This quick quiz can give you some important pointers to help you lose weight safely and maintain your weight loss.

1. On February 28, Mrs. Jones was diagnosed with diabetes. At that time, she weighed 210 pounds. She set a goal of weighing 150 pounds by Christmas. This is a realistic goal.

   TRUE   **FALSE**

2. Bill is 5′10″, follows the 1800-calorie per day meal plan designed for him by his dietitian, and walks 20 minutes twice a week. He had been losing weight steadily, but he has lost none for two weeks. What should he do?
   A. Cut back to 1400 calories a day.
   B. Just continue what he has been doing a little longer.
   C. Increase the number of walks he takes to four or five a week and the duration of each to 30 minutes or more.

3. About how many calories must you burn to lose a pound of body weight?
   A. 4,000 calories.
   B. 3,500 calories.
   C. 1,800 calories.
   D. 1,200 calories.

4. Why is losing excess weight almost always recommended for people with Type 2 diabetes?
   A. Losing excess weight decreases insulin resistance in body tissues.
   B. Losing excess weight makes you feel better about yourself.
   C. A smaller body requires less insulin.

5. Which of the following are good tips for safe weight loss?
   (More than one answer may be correct.)
   A. Get regular exercise.
   B. Eat at least three meals a day.
   C. Drink 8 glasses of water a day.
   D. Eat a variety of healthful foods.
   E. Cut down on the amount of fat you eat.

6. Jamie is a college freshman with Type 1 diabetes. Lately, she has noticed she is losing weight without trying. She has been too busy to test her blood sugar regularly. Which of the following are likely reasons for her weight loss?
   (More than one answer may be correct.)
   A. She isn't eating enough.
   B. She has a digestive disorder.
   C. Her diabetes is out of control.

7. Crash diets that cause very fast weight loss can make you fatter than you were before.

   TRUE   **FALSE**

8. Why are people rarely successful at losing weight by consuming only liquid supplements?
   (More than one answer may be correct.)
   A. This type of diet is too boring and you can't stay with it for very long.
   B. New, healthy eating habits are not learned.
   C. You can't limit calories enough to lose much weight.

1. **TRUE.** Mrs. Jones wants to lose 60 pounds in 10 months, or approximately 1½ pounds per week. Losing 1 to 2 pounds per week is both realistic and safe.

2. **C.** It's not unusual to reach a plateau after some weight loss. Because moving a heavier body requires more energy (or calories) than moving a smaller body, exercise burns fewer calories after a person has lost weight than it did before the weight loss. By increasing the frequency and length of his walks, Bill will burn more calories and speed up his metabolism somewhat. Cutting back on his food intake is probably not a good idea. A 5'10" man usually needs at least 1800 calories a day; a 1400-calorie per day diet would be too restrictive to follow for a long period of time.

3. **B.** You need to burn about 3,500 more calories than you consume to lose 1 pound of body weight. But don't try to do this all in one day. It is much easier and safer to achieve a small calorie imbalance every day and let the results accumulate. For example, if you burn 2,000 calories per day but eat only 1,500 calories, you will have a calorie deficit of 500 each day. In one week, you will have accumulated a calorie deficit of 3,500, and you will have lost 1 pound. To make sure you are losing fat, not muscle, it's advisable to make exercise part of your gradual weight-loss plan. Exercise burns calories and builds muscle at the same time.

4. **A.** Part of the reason for elevated blood glucose levels in Type 2 diabetes is a condition called *insulin resistance*, where the body tissues are not as sensitive to insulin as they should be, and glucose isn't moved from the bloodstream into body tissues efficiently. Because the main cause of insulin resistance is excess weight, losing weight helps to decrease insulin resistance and normalize blood glucose levels. Even a loss of 10 to 20 pounds can make a difference in your blood glucose levels.

5. **A, B, C, D, E.** These are all good tips for safe and effective weight loss. Regular exercise is the most accurate predictor of who will maintain weight loss and who won't. Eating regular meals is important, because when you skip one or more meals, you are more likely to get hungry later and eat more than you should. Drinking plenty of water can help you feel full and helps your body get rid of extra fluid. Eating a variety of foods will help you get enough of essential vitamins and minerals. And cutting down on the amount of fat you eat can help lower cholesterol levels and aid in weight loss, as long as you also cut down on the total amount of calories you consume.

6. **A, C.** It is possible that Jamie isn't used to planning her meals or cooking for herself, and with a busy schedule, she may not be getting enough to eat. But a more likely reason for unexplained weight loss is that her diabetes is out of control. When glucose levels are above about 180 mg/dl, excess glucose "spills over" into the urine, causing many calories to be wasted. Or, if Jamie's insulin dose doesn't match the amount she is eating, her body may be burning some body fat for energy, which can also cause weight loss. Burning too much fat can result in *ketoacidosis*, which is a life-threatening condition, so Jamie needs to begin testing her blood sugar regularly to prevent an emergency from developing, as well as to prevent long-term complications that can result from prolonged high blood glucose levels.

7. **TRUE.** It's very tempting to try crash diets, because they can cause fast weight loss. But people who lose weight very quickly on a crash diet tend to gain it back when they stop the diet. That's because they have not learned healthier eating habits. Also, rapid weight loss can cause a person to lose muscle as well as fat. So when the weight comes back, the percentage of body fat is greater than it was before. It's much healthier to lose weight gradually, at a rate of 1 to 2 pounds a week with a sensible, balanced diet. Most insurance plans will pay for you to meet with a registered dietitian to help you set up a meal plan that allows you to meet your goals.

8. **A, B.** Although you can limit calories easily with a liquid diet, it's hard to stay on such a diet for any length of time because it gets very boring, and most people miss chewing. Following a liquid diet also doesn't help you learn new eating habits that will help you keep off the weight you have lost. While occasionally substituting a liquid diet supplement for a daily meal is sometimes all right for a person with diabetes, it's a good idea to ask your dietitian how to work a liquid supplement into your meal plan. □

HOW MUCH DO YOU KNOW ABOUT ALCOHOL?

by Robert S. Dinsmoor

In the past few years, there have been many reports in the media about studies that show the health benefits of moderate alcohol consumption. Most health agencies agree that it is OK for most people with diabetes to consume alcohol in moderation as long as they check with their doctor and fit the drinks into their meal plan. But what's considered moderate drinking? Which alcoholic beverages are the best choices for people with diabetes? Are there any special precautions for people with diabetes? Take this simple quiz to see how much you know about alcohol and its effects on people with diabetes.

1. Which of the following benefits has been scientifically linked to moderate alcohol consumption? (More than one answer may be correct.)
   A. Decreased risk of heart disease.
   B. Decreased risk of stroke.
   C. Improved concentration.
   D. Decreased cancer risk.
   E. Longer life.

2. Which one of the following alcoholic beverages is likely to raise blood glucose levels the least?
   A. 4 ounces of sweet wine.
   B. 4 ounces of dry white wine.
   C. 12 ounces of a wine cooler.
   D. 12 ounces of regular beer.
   E. 12 ounces of light beer.

3. A given amount of alcohol will have the same effect on a woman as it does on a man who weighs the same amount.

   TRUE   **FALSE**

4. Alcohol can cause severe low blood sugar in people with diabetes.

   TRUE   **FALSE**

5. Alcohol can interact with some prescription and over-the-counter medicines, including some diabetes drugs.

   TRUE   **FALSE**

6. A 1½-ounce shot of whiskey is equivalent to which of the following food exchange values? (Hint: It contains 105 calories.)
   A. 2 meats.
   B. 3 starches.
   C. 1 starch, 2 fats.
   D. 2 fats.
   E. 3 fats.

7. How many 12-ounce bottles of beer would a 150-pound man have to drink in an hour to reach a blood alcohol concentration of 0.08% (the level at which you can be convicted of driving while intoxicated in many states)?
   A. One.
   B. Two.
   C. Four.
   D. Six.
   E. Eight.

8. Which of the following health problems have been linked to heavy alcohol use? (More than one answer may be correct.)
   A. Cirrhosis (hardening of the liver).
   B. High blood pressure, heart disease, and stroke.
   C. Psychiatric problems such as depression.
   D. Accidents.
   E. Cancer of the stomach, throat, and colon.

1. A, B, E. Moderate alcohol consumption (on the order of one to two drinks a day) has been shown to decrease the risk of heart attacks in middle-age people by one-third to one-half. Alcohol appears to work primarily by raising the levels of HDL ("good") cholesterol in the blood, keeping the blood from clotting as easily, and, in people with diabetes, decreasing insulin resistance. Recent research has also shown that alcohol can reduce the risk of ischemic stroke, the most common form of stroke. In a recent large study, a drink a day starting in middle age decreased the risk of premature death by 20%.

2. B. As far as blood glucose levels are concerned, the dry white wine is your best choice. The highest carbohydrate choice is the wine cooler, with 190 calories and 22 grams of carbohydrate. The sweet wine weighs in at 180 calories and 13 grams of carbohydrate. The regular beer has 150 calories and 14 grams of carbohydrate. Light beer is a pretty good choice at 100 calories and 6 grams of carbohydrate. But the uncontested winner from a blood sugar standpoint is dry white wine at only 80 calories and a scant 0.4 grams of carbohydrate.

3. FALSE. It is true that a smaller body weight makes a person more sensitive to the effects of alcohol because there is less fluid to dilute it. But there's another important difference between men and women: Women's bodies produce less of an enzyme that breaks down alcohol in the gastrointestinal tract. Because women generally weigh less and have less of the enzyme, the average woman needs only half the alcohol that the average man needs to reach the same blood alcohol concentration and level of intoxication.

4. TRUE. When consumed on an empty stomach, alcohol goes straight into the bloodstream and is broken down by the liver. When the liver is handling alcohol, it is unable to produce the normal amount of glucose, and this can cause blood sugar levels to plummet in people who take insulin or oral diabetes drugs. Making matters worse, with alcohol on your breath, you and those around you may mistakenly attribute your erratic symptoms to inebriation, keeping you from getting the help you need. For these reasons, you should never drink on an empty stomach.

5. TRUE. Alcohol can produce dangerous interactions with a number of drugs, including tranquilizers, sleeping pills, antihistamines, and pain relievers. It can also interact with the sulfonylurea drugs to produce symptoms such as headache, flushing and tingling in the face, nausea, and lightheadedness. This interaction, sometimes called the "chlorpropamide-alcohol flush," most commonly occurs with the older sulfonylureas chlorpropamide and tolbutamide, but it may also occur to a lesser extent with the second-generation sulfonylureas glyburide, glipizide, and glimepiride. Be sure to read the labels on all prescription and over-the-counter drugs you're taking, and ask your doctor and pharmacist about any possible interactions these medicines have with alcohol.

6. D. In terms of the exchange lists, alcohol is considered a fat. Always remember to fit any alcoholic beverages you drink into your meal plan. Each fat exchange is equivalent to 5 grams of fat, which, at 9 calories per gram, contain 45 calories. The shot of whiskey, at 105 calories, translates into roughly 2 fat exchanges.

7. C. Though the effects of alcohol consumption vary according to a number of factors, it takes about four typical alcoholic beverages (such as a 12-ounce beer) per hour for a 150-pound man to reach a blood alcohol concentration (BAC) of 0.08%. At levels below this, a person may still be considered to be "driving under the influence." For comparison, a BAC of 0.03% may cause only a slight change in feeling. A BAC of 0.06% may create feelings of warmth and mental relaxation—as well as a slight decrease in fine motor skills. At a BAC of 0.12%, a person becomes clumsy and unsteady in standing or walking. At 0.15%, the person becomes badly intoxicated and stuporous. At a BAC of 0.3% to 0.4%, the person may lapse into a coma, and at a BAC of 0.4% to 0.5%, he or she may die of alcohol poisoning.

8. A, B, C, D, E. Excessive alcohol consumption has the potential to harm virtually every organ system in the body, including those that are already affected by diabetes. In addition to these problems, alcohol consumption can harm the fetus in pregnant women, disrupt sleep, promote osteoporosis (bone loss), and worsen diabetic neuropathy (nerve damage). Most health agencies recommend that no one consume more than one to two alcoholic drinks a day—and for women and individuals over the age of 65, no more than one drink a day. ☐

HOW MUCH DO YOU KNOW ABOUT PHYSICAL EXAMS AND LAB TESTS?

by Janice L. Woodrum, R.N., B.S.N.

It's time for your regular diabetes checkup, and once again your doctor is brandishing a blood pressure cuff, ready to get started. You've already filled the obligatory cup with urine, donned the flimsy paper gown, and taken off your shoes and socks for a foot inspection. The nurse is standing by with blood collection paraphernalia, and several HMO referral forms for appointments with specialists are stacked on the counter, waiting for the doctor's signature. Why do you need all these tests and exams? What do they show about your health and diabetes control that blood glucose self-monitoring doesn't? Take this quiz to see if you know which medical tests and exams you should be having, why, and how often.

1. What laboratory test will detect kidney disease in its very early stages?
   A. Glycosylated hemoglobin.
   B. Cholesterol.
   C. Microalbumin.
   D. Serum creatinine.

2. After regular medical care, diabetes education is next in importance for controlling diabetes.

       TRUE   **FALSE**

3. Which of the following should be checked every time you go to the doctor? (More than one answer may be correct.)
   A. Your blood pressure.
   B. Your feet.
   C. Your cholesterol level.
   D. Your weight.
   E. Your blood glucose self-monitoring records.
   F. Your eyes.

4. Which test should be done two to four times a year to assess overall blood glucose control?
   A. Fasting plasma glucose.
   B. Glucosamine.
   C. Glycosylated hemoglobin.
   D. Oral glucose tolerance.

5. Which of the following tests or exams should be done once a year? (More than one answer may be correct.)
   A. Foot examination.
   B. Fasting cholesterol and triglycerides.
   C. Dilated eye examination.
   D. Serum creatinine.
   E. Routine urinalysis and microalbumin.

6. Why are yearly dilated eye examinations recommended for all adults diagnosed with diabetes after age 30 and anyone between the ages of 10 and 30 who has had diabetes for three to five years? (More than one answer may be correct.)
   A. It is necessary to dilate the eyes to properly see and examine the retina.
   B. It is important to discover any eye problems early so they can be treated before they threaten vision.
   C. People with diabetes may need frequent changes in their eyeglasses or contact lens prescriptions.
   D. Retinopathy is a long-term complication of diabetes.

1. C. Testing urine for microalbumin is the best way to detect early diabetes-related kidney problems. The kidneys filter the blood and pass wastes into the urine. The tiny blood vessels that make up the kidney filter don't usually allow albumin (a type of protein) to pass through. But if the blood vessels are damaged, tiny amounts of protein can escape, and the microalbumin test detects this. It is important to do this test at least once a year. A routine urinalysis will not detect such small amounts of protein.

2. TRUE. Regular visits to your doctor are of utmost importance, but getting a good education about diabetes and how to control it is your next step. That's because so much of your diabetes care is provided by you. At the very least you'll want to see a registered dietitian and a diabetes nurse educator, preferably with a certified diabetes educator credential. You may also want to take diabetes education classes, which are offered at many hospitals. Such classes often bring in health professionals such as pharmacists and podiatrists, who can give specialized information and advice. Ask your doctor about diabetes classes and resources in your area, and plan to make diabetes education an ongoing project for life.

3. A, B, D, E. All people with diabetes should see their doctor at least twice a year, and for some, more frequent visits are recommended. Since high blood pressure can hasten the onset of most diabetes complications, your doctor should check your blood pressure at every visit. Foot problems can pose serious difficulties for people with diabetes, so get in the habit of taking your shoes and socks off at each visit. This is especially important if you have thick calluses, corns, bunions, or ingrown toenails or if you have nerve or circulatory problems. (If your doctor doesn't inspect your feet, remind him!) Changes in weight can be an indicator of how well you're doing on your meal plan or, in a person with certain kidney or heart conditions, a sign of water retention. Unanticipated weight loss, particularly in a person with Type 1 diabetes, may indicate a problem with the insulin regimen. Your blood glucose self-monitoring records can also show whether you need any changes in your dietary plan, medication, or exercise routine.

For most people, a cholesterol test and eye exam can be done once a year. However, people taking cholesterol-lowering drugs and people with existing eye problems may need more frequent tests or exams.

4. C. The glycosylated hemoglobin test (also known as the hemoglobin A_{1c}, or HbA_{1c}, test) is a blood test that indicates your average blood glucose level over the past two to three months. The test measures the percentage of hemoglobin, a pigment in red blood cells, that is bonded to glucose. When glucose levels are high, more sticks; when they are low, less sticks. For most people with diabetes, the desired test result is less than 7%; a test result over 8% means that action should be taken to lower it. If you aren't sure when you last had an HbA_{1c} test, ask your doctor. If it has been more than six months, request that one be done.

The fasting plasma glucose test is used to screen for diabetes. Some doctors also use it to monitor diabetes therapy. The oral glucose tolerance test is used to confirm a diagnosis of diabetes. Glucosamine is not a lab test; it is a dietary supplement taken to relieve symptoms of osteoarthritis. Of interest to people with diabetes, however, is that glucosamine may cause increased insulin resistance, which can lead to higher blood glucose levels.

5. B, C, D, E. High cholesterol or triglyceride levels can contribute to blood vessel damage (atherosclerosis) that can lead to eye or kidney disease, strokes, heart attack, or circulatory problems in the limbs and feet. Most adults should have an annual test, although those with normal levels may need tests only every two years. More frequent tests are necessary if you are taking a drug to lower your blood cholesterol or triglycerides. Children with diabetes should have a cholesterol test upon diagnosis of diabetes and periodically thereafter.

A dilated eye exam is done to detect any blood vessel changes that could threaten your vision, as well as other eye problems such as glaucoma (which occurs more often in people with diabetes). The serum creatinine, or blood creatinine, test is used to assess kidney function. Routine urinalysis can detect numerous problems, including urinary tract infections. And the microalbumin test detects early kidney problems.

6. A, B, D. Yearly dilated eye exams are recommended so that diabetes-related eye disease can be detected and treated early. The eye problem most commonly associated with diabetes is retinopathy, in which the small blood vessels that feed the retina, the layer of tissue lining the back of the eye, are damaged. To do a thorough examination of the retina, an eye doctor must dilate the eyes with special eye drops. □

HOW MUCH DO YOU KNOW ABOUT PUMPING?

by Janice L. Woodrum, R.N., B.S.N.

Insulin pumps have been on the market for over 15 years now, but only in recent years have they become very popular. It used to be that an insulin pump was considered only when all other insulin dosing programs had failed to keep blood glucose levels in desirable range. Now, however, more people are choosing to use an insulin pump both for the flexibility it offers and for the intensive diabetes management it enables. If you are curious about pumping and would like a little more information, take this quiz to see what you already know and what questions you may want to ask your doctor.

1. Insulin pumps are appropriate for which of the following people? (More than one answer may be correct.)
   A. People with Type 1 diabetes who have widely varying blood sugar levels.
   B. Women with diabetes who are pregnant.
   C. Children with Type 1 diabetes.
   D. People with Type 2 diabetes who require insulin.

2. What is the basal insulin dose?
   A. A dose of several units of insulin taken right before eating.
   B. A temporarily slowed insulin infusion rate used during exercise.
   C. A steady, continuous, 24-hour insulin delivery.

3. Pump users need to carry urine check strips to detect which possible emergency?
   A. Unusually high blood glucose levels.
   B. Impending ketoacidosis.
   C. Hypoglycemia.

4. An insulin pump lets you vary your insulin dose so you can eat whatever you want.
   TRUE   FALSE

5. How often should a person check his blood sugar when using an insulin pump?
   A. 1 to 2 times a day.
   B. 2 to 3 times a day.
   C. 3 to 4 times a day.
   D. At least 4 to 6 times a day.

6. Insulin delivery from a pump can mimic the body's own insulin production more closely than insulin injections.
   TRUE   FALSE

7. What will do the most to help prevent infection of the tissues at the needle or catheter site?
   A. Daily bathing to cleanse bacteria from the skin.
   B. Changing the tubing and needle or catheter every second or third day.
   C. Using an antibiotic ointment at the insertion site.

1. A, B, C, D. Insulin pumps are most commonly used by people with Type 1 diabetes. Those who have widely fluctuating blood sugar levels with injections can often achieve better control with a pump. The pump is also a time-proven tool for helping control blood glucose levels during pregnancy. Some kids do great with pumps, particularly when they are motivated and their parents are trained to program the pump and watch for problems. Even people with Type 2 diabetes can benefit from the pump if they can't control their diabetes with oral medicines alone and need several injections of insulin a day.

2. C. A small amount of insulin delivered continuously, all day and all night, is called the basal rate. It can differ from person to person, so each individual must program his pump to deliver the correct amount of basal insulin. Some people use different basal rates at different times of day. For example, more insulin may be needed in the early morning hours and less during the night or during exercise. Before meals, pump users program the pump to give a *bolus* of insulin, or several units at once, to cover what they are going to eat. A person might also take a bolus if his blood sugar is too high and he needs extra insulin.

3. B. Ketoacidosis is a serious emergency that develops when there is too little insulin in the body to burn glucose normally. When that happens, the body starts burning fat or muscle instead, leaving behind toxic chemicals called ketones. All insulin users need to watch for this if blood glucose levels are above 240 mg/dl, but pump users need to be even more careful. That's because insulin pumps use rapid- or short-acting insulin only, so if insulin delivery is interrupted by a problem such as clogged tubing, blood glucose levels can rise rapidly. (People who take shots generally have some longer-acting insulin in their system to fall back on.) Pump users are advised to have urine ketone check strips on hand at all times and to learn how to troubleshoot the pump if there's a problem.

4. FALSE. Although an insulin pump can give you lots more flexibility in your meals, you still need to do some planning and make good food choices to control your blood sugar and get the nutrients you need for good health. Most people who use pumps use carbohydrate counting to plan their meals. With this system, you calculate how much carbohydrate is in each meal and take the right amount of insulin to match it, usually 1 unit of insulin per 10 to 15 grams of carbohydrate. You still need to pay attention to protein and fat and make sure your diet contains the necessary vitamins and minerals. And you need to keep an eye on total calories to avoid unwanted weight loss or gain.

5. D. Although insulin pumps do an awesome job of delivering precise insulin doses at the right times, you still need information about your blood glucose levels throughout the day. That's the only way you'll know how to program your pump to give you the right bolus and basal doses. Therefore, four to six blood glucose checks per day is a minimum, and many people like to do more.

6. TRUE. Many people who are on the pump have already tried standard injections in a wide variety of combinations and dosage schedules but haven't gotten the control they want. One reason for this is that virtually all insulins have some kind of peak action, even Ultralente, which is very-slow-acting insulin with not much peak action. (The new long-acting insulin analog called glargine is reported to have essentially no peak.) These peaks can produce unavoidable blood glucose ups and downs. With the pump, these ups and downs are largely avoided. The pump uses only short-acting insulin (Regular) or a very-short-acting insulin analog such as lispro. Because the insulin is being delivered constantly, it mimics the body's continuous basal insulin production. The bolus dose is like the burst of insulin the body puts out when you eat something.

7. B. An insulin pump is about the size of a beeper. It is connected to a small insulin needle or Teflon catheter by a length of clear tubing. The needle or catheter is inserted into fatty tissue, usually on the abdomen, and taped in place. While changing the infusion set, which comprises the tubing and needle or catheter, it's important not to touch the needle or catheter, which is sterile. Neither daily bathing nor cleansing the skin with alcohol or another germicidal solution will remove all bacteria, and if an infusion set is left in place too long, germs will grow where the needle or catheter goes into the skin, causing a skin or tissue infection. Antibiotic ointment could inhibit the growth of some germs, but it would prevent the tape that holds the needle in place from sticking to the skin and protecting the insertion site. ☐

HOW MUCH DO YOU KNOW ABOUT NEPHROPATHY?

by Janice L. Woodrum, R.N., B.S.N.

Diabetic nephropathy, or kidney disease, is associated with long-standing diabetes and blood glucose that has not been kept within the near-normal range. It is the leading cause of kidney failure in the United States. In addition, showing signs of nephropathy has been linked to an increased risk of heart disease in people with diabetes. But the news isn't all bad:

Recent studies have shown that you can work with your doctor to dramatically reduce your risk of ever developing nephropathy, and, with early detection, you can greatly slow its progression. Take this quiz to find out how much you already know about diabetic nephropathy and to familiarize yourself with steps you can take to prevent it or keep it from progressing.

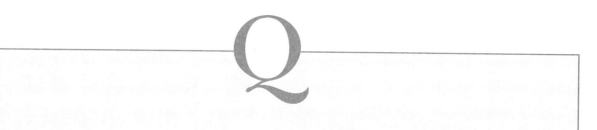

1. Diabetic nephropathy is damage to what part of the kidneys?
   A. The nerves.
   B. The blood vessels.
   C. The collecting ducts.

2. More than 50% of people with diabetes show some signs of nephropathy.

   TRUE   **FALSE**

3. Which test can catch diabetic nephropathy in its early stages?
   A. Routine urinalysis.
   B. Blood urea nitrogen (BUN) and creatinine.
   C. Serum protein.
   D. Microalbuminuria.

4. Once diabetic nephropathy is discovered, what can be done to treat it? (More than one answer may be correct.)
   A. Lowering blood pressure.
   B. Keeping blood glucose in the normal range.
   C. Eating less protein.

5. What is the most common treatment for end-stage renal disease?
   A. Hemodialysis.
   B. Kidney transplant.
   C. Peritoneal dialysis.
   D. Nephrectomy.

6. Keeping blood pressure in the normal range has been shown to prevent or delay the progression of diabetic nephropathy. Which of the following measures can help control your blood pressure? (More than one answer may be correct.)
   A. Losing excess weight and exercising.
   B. Avoiding tobacco and too much alcohol.
   C. Eating a low-sodium diet.
   D. Increasing the amount of protein in your diet.
   E. Checking your blood pressure frequently.
   F. Taking blood-pressure-lowering drugs.

1. **B.** Diabetic nephropathy is damage to the tiny blood vessels, called *nephrons*, that make up the filter system of the kidneys. Normally, nephrons act like a sieve, retaining the large components of the blood, such as blood cells and protein, while letting smaller toxins, such as urea and creatinine, pass into the urine. High blood glucose and high blood pressure can damage the blood vessel walls, allowing protein to leak into the urine. If nothing is done to prevent further damage, the problem can progress, and more protein passes from the blood into the urine. The loss of protein from the blood lets fluid seep out of the bloodstream, sometimes causing *edema*, or swelling in the body tissues. Low levels of protein and fluid in the blood hamper the kidneys' ability to remove wastes.

2. **FALSE.** According to the American Diabetes Association, 20% to 30% of people with diabetes develop nephropathy, usually after having diabetes for a long time. Nephropathy is more common in people with Type 1 diabetes than in those with Type 2 diabetes, and it progresses to kidney failure more often in people with Type 1 diabetes. Being African-American, Latino, or Native American is another risk factor associated with nephropathy.

3. **D.** The microalbuminuria test is the most sensitive test for nephropathy. It detects traces of protein that have leaked into the urine. Early stages of nephropathy cause no dramatic symptoms; protein in the urine is the first detectable sign. Routine urinalysis also checks for protein, but it is less sensitive than the microalbuminuria test. Later stages of nephropathy can be detected by other tests, as well. As the kidneys become less effective at filtering waste, the blood urea nitrogen (BUN) and creatinine tests measure higher levels of these toxins in the blood, and the serum protein test detects lower levels of protein in the blood.

Early diagnosis of nephropathy is important because appropriate treatment can greatly reduce the progression of this disease. People with Type 2 diabetes should have a microalbuminuria test when diabetes is first diagnosed and annually thereafter. People with Type 1 diabetes should first have the test at puberty or after having diabetes for five years, whichever comes second, then annually thereafter. Check with your doctor to see when you last had this test.

4. **A, B, C.** There are several ways to slow the progression of nephropathy, including maintaining normal blood pressure and blood glucose levels.

Aim for a glycosylated hemoglobin (HbA1c) level under 7%. (The HbA1c test indicates your level of blood sugar control over the past two to three months.) Have it checked every three to six months.

The American Diabetes Association recommends keeping your blood pressure below 130/80 mm Hg. Blood pressure pills called *angiotensin-converting enzyme (ACE) inhibitors* often help prevent further kidney damage, even in people who don't have high blood pressure. Your doctor may also recommend sticking to a low-protein diet, which can help in more advanced cases.

5. **A.** When the kidneys are severely damaged and filter wastes less than 10% as effectively as healthy kidneys, the condition is called end-stage renal disease, or kidney failure. This is a serious condition and will result in death if not treated promptly by removing toxins from the blood some other way. The most common treatment is *hemodialysis*. During hemodialysis, blood is drawn from the body and sent through a machine that removes wastes. It is then returned to the body. This procedure lasts three to four hours and must be performed two to three times a week. Another type of dialysis, *peritoneal dialysis*, works slightly differently. A solution is put into the abdomen through a catheter. The solution absorbs wastes for several hours, after which it is removed, discarded, and replaced with fresh solution. Peritoneal dialysis is often done at home. Kidney transplantation is an alternative to dialysis. It is more complicated and costly, and it is used less often, but it gives recipients a much more normal life routine. Nephrectomy is removal of a kidney, which is not done to treat kidney failure.

6. **A, B, C, E, F.** Following a diet relatively low in sodium (about 2400 milligrams daily), exercising regularly, and reducing your weight if you are overweight are three important steps to take to bring down your blood pressure. Nicotine constricts blood vessels, which causes blood pressure to go up, so smoking is best avoided. If you have high blood pressure, you should discuss your alcohol intake with your doctor and keep it moderate, at most. Consider getting a home blood pressure monitor to check on your progress several times a week. If these steps don't control your blood pressure, you may need a blood pressure drug. Talk to your doctor about which drug or combination of drugs is best for you. Eating more protein will not help your blood pressure or your kidneys. ❑

HOW MUCH DO YOU KNOW ABOUT STROKE?

by Robert S. Dinsmoor

Strokes, sometimes called "brain attacks," are caused by a disruption of the blood supply to the brain. Strokes affect roughly 600,000 Americans each year, killing 160,000 of them (making stroke the third leading cause of death in the United States) and disabling hundreds of thousands more. Having diabetes places a person at higher risk of having a stroke. Yet, a 1996 survey showed that the American public knows very little about what strokes are, how serious they are, how to avoid them, how to recognize them when they occur, or what to do about them. How much do you know about stroke? Take this simple test and find out. Knowing the answers to these questions, especially the symptoms of stroke, could save your life.

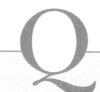

1. Which of the following is NOT a typical warning sign of a stroke?
   A. Sudden weakness or numbness of the face, arm, or leg on one side of the body.
   B. Sudden dimness or loss of vision, particularly in only one eye.
   C. Loss of speech, or trouble talking or understanding speech.
   D. Chest pain that spreads to the shoulders, neck, or arms.
   E. Sudden severe headaches with no apparent cause.
   F. Unexplained dizziness, unsteadiness, or sudden falls.

2. Strokes kill about as many American women each year as breast cancer does.

   TRUE   **FALSE**

3. If you're having a stroke, there's not much doctors can do for you except let it run its course and then begin rehabilitation.

   TRUE   **FALSE**

4. If you're disabled right after a stroke, you'll always be disabled.

   TRUE   **FALSE**

5. Which of the following does NOT increase your risk of stroke?
   A. Smoking.
   B. High blood pressure.
   C. Diabetes.
   D. Old age.
   E. Being a woman.

6. Which of the following are possible long-term complications of a stroke? (More than one answer may be correct.)
   A. Problems with balance and coordination.
   B. Trouble swallowing.
   C. Problems with memory, thinking, attention, and learning.
   D. Getting tired quickly.
   E. Depression.

7. There is more than one type of stroke.

   TRUE   **FALSE**

8. Which of the following can decrease your risk of a stroke? (More than one answer may be correct.)
   A. Controlling blood sugar.
   B. Controlling blood pressure.
   C. Controlling blood cholesterol.
   D. Exercising.
   E. Stopping smoking.

1. D. Chest pain is a symptom of a heart attack, but not a stroke. A stroke can produce sudden weakness or numbness of the face, arm, or leg on one side of the body; sudden dimness or loss of vision, particularly in only one eye; trouble talking or understanding speech; sudden severe headaches with no apparent cause; and unexplained dizziness, unsteadiness, or sudden falls. If you experience any of these symptoms, don't wait for them to go away. Seek medical help immediately!

2. **FALSE.** Despite the public's heightened awareness about the threat of breast cancer, more than twice as many American women die from stroke as from breast cancer each year.

3. **FALSE.** Only a few years ago, strokes were viewed fatalistically: Little could be done to change their course, and stroke victims were not given top priority by ambulance services and emergency rooms. Now, with better diagnosis and treatment, much of a person's brain function can be saved if he is treated in time. In some cases, doctors can inject thrombolytic (or "clot-busting") drugs such as tissue plasminogen activator (TPA), which can break up blood clots and restore the blood supply to the brain. Studies have shown that if these drugs are given within a few hours of the onset of a stroke, people are more likely to escape serious disability. For this reason, stroke should be viewed as a medical emergency and treated immediately.

4. **FALSE.** Most people experience some degree of spontaneous recovery within the first few weeks following a stroke. In other words, some of the abilities they have lost may improve or return completely. Scientists believe this happens because while some brain cells are killed and cannot recover, others are only injured. According to the National Stroke Association, 10% of stroke survivors recover almost completely, and another 25% recover with only minor impairments. Furthermore, people who are severely disabled following strokes may enroll in rehabilitation programs that may train them to accomplish essential tasks such as eating, walking, driving, and clothing themselves.

5. **E.** All of these factors except for female gender can increase your risk of stroke. (Men are more likely than women to have strokes.) Smoking raises blood pressure and increases the likelihood of clots by causing blood platelets to stick together more readily. Smokers are estimated to be twice as likely to have strokes as nonsmokers. High blood pressure makes a person four to six times more likely to have a stroke, and diabetes doubles or triples your risk of having an ischemic stroke. In addition, the risk of stroke increases with age.

Other stroke risk factors include race (African-Americans are at increased risk), heart disease, high blood cholesterol levels, heavy drinking, obesity, a sedentary lifestyle, previous strokes or transient ischemic attacks (also called "mini-strokes"), a family history of stroke, and a specific type of abnormal heart rhythm called atrial fibrillation, which increases the risk of blood clots.

6. **A, B, C, D, E.** Depending on how the brain is affected, a stroke can cause a person a wide variety of permanent problems. Stroke survivors may also have problems performing or understanding speech or writing, have pain or numbness throughout the body, or have problems with bowel or bladder control.

7. **TRUE.** There are two main types of stroke. Ischemic strokes, accounting for the majority of strokes, are caused by obstructed blood flow to the brain. The blockage can be caused by the narrowing of a blood vessel in the neck or brain or by a blood clot that gets lodged in one of these arteries. When blood flow to part of the brain is interrupted, brain cells in that region die from lack of oxygen. In hemorrhagic strokes, blood vessels in the brain burst, flooding an area of the brain with blood and causing damage.

Doctors must diagnose the type of stroke a person is having before treatment, because the proper treatment depends on the type of stroke. For instance, thrombolytic drugs are often helpful in treating ischemic strokes, but they may make a hemorrhagic stroke even worse.

8. **A, B, C, D, E.** Controlling blood sugar, controlling blood pressure, controlling cholesterol, exercising, and stopping smoking have all been shown to reduce a person's risk of stroke. □

INDEX

Cholesterol, 17, 126, 170
  effect of garlic, 151
  effect of red yeast, 152
  explained, 287
  food selection, 291, 294
  heart attack and, 160, 287
  reducing, 287-291
  in women, 397
Cholestin (red yeast), 152
Classification of diabetes. *See* Type 1
    diabetes and Type 2 diabetes
Claudication, 216
Complications
  advanced glycosylation endproducts
    (AGE), 210
  amputation. *See* Amputation
  attitude toward, 179
  causes, 211
  in children, 421
  coping strategies, 178-179
  dealing with fears, 176, 178
  emotional issues, 176-177
  exercising with, 258-262
  gastropathy. *See* Gastropathy
  impotence. *See* Impotence
  macrovascular complications.
    See Heart disease
  microvascular complications, 125
  neuropathy. *See* Neuropathy
  postprandial hyperglycemia and, 93
  prevention, 150
  retinopathy. *See* Retinopathy
  treatment, 151
Constipation, 131, 201
Contraception
  barrier contraceptives, 376, 378-379
  birth defects and, 375
  condoms, 376, 379
  hormonal methods
    compared, 379, 380
    heart attack and, 399
  information sources, 381
  intrauterine devices compared,
    377, 379
  natural methods, 375, 378
  need for, 376
Counseling
  for amputees, 230
  by clergy, 44
  treatment for depression, 53
  for impotence, 200
  marital, 70
  by social worker, 44
  for visual impairment, 184

D

DCCT. *See* Diabetes Control and
    Complications Trial (DCCT)
Dehydration, 127, 156, 186
  as cause of fatigue, 350
Denial, 48, 177
Depression, 48, 51, 163, 164
  alcohol and, 54
  drug therapy, 54

exercise and, 54, 238
  fatigue due to, 353
  information sources, 53
  symptoms, 52
  treatment, 53
Dermagraft, 217
Diabetes Control and Complications
    Trial (DCCT), 17
  blood glucose levels and, 74
  hypoglycemia and, 189
  results, 23
  retinopathy and, 182
Diabetic ketoacidosis (DKA), 186
Diagnosis
  arteriography, 218
  effect on mental health, 48
  of gastropathy, 203
  importance of, 15
  of impotence, 197
  need for accuracy, 17
  of osteoporosis, 394
Dialysis, 207
Diarrhea, 131, 201
Diet and nutrition
  alcohol
    nutrient values, 306, 307
    use guidelines, 305
  carbohydrates. *See* Carbohydrates
  effect on disease development, 336
  epidemiological studies, 330
  evaluating information, 337
  experimental studies, 332
  fatigue and, 350
  fats. *See* Fat and saturated fat
  foods that cause flatulence, 13
  gastropathy and, 204
  heart disease and, 161
  herbal supplements. *See* Herbal
    remedies
  during hospital stay, 35
  hypertension and, 167
  information sources, 335
  kidney disease and, 207
  meal planning. *See* Meal planning
  meats, nutrient values, 301
  minerals. *See* Minerals
  nighttime eating, 321-325
  osteoporosis and, 392
  during pregnancy, 373
  Recommended Dietary Allowances
    (RDA), 134
  research, 329-337
  role of dietitian, 39, 42
  senior citizens and, 276-281
  snack bars, 311-315
  travel and, 32
  triglycerides and, 172
  vegetarian diet, 308-311
  vitamins. *See* Vitamins
Dietary Approaches to Stop
    Hypertension (DASH), 167
Dietitian, 39, 42, 86
  developing a meal plan, 320
  evaluation process, 317
  frequency of appointments, 317

need for, 116
  qualifications, 316
  setting goals, 318
Diuretics (herbal), 156
Drinks. *See* Alcohol
Drugs and medications
  Actos (pioglitazone), 14, 28
  antidepressants, 54
  aspirin, 122-124
  Avandia (rosiglitazone), 14, 28
  capsaicin, 153
  carbamazepine, 193
  fibrates, 174
  flu, 355
  gabapentin, 193
  gastropathy, 203
  Glucophage (metformin), 24, 28, 89,
    124-128
  hormonal contraception, 380
  hospital stay, 34
  hypertension, 168, 169
  impotence, 197, 199
  insulin. *See* Insulin
  kidney disease, 206
  neuropathy, 193
  osteoporosis, 395, 396
  over-the-counter drugs, 128-133
  postprandial hyperglycemia, 94
  statins, 173
  United Kingdom Prospective Diabetes
    Study (UKPDS) and, 23-25

E

Eating disorders
  diabetes as risk factor, 410
  gender as factor, 409
  information sources, 411
  treatment, 411
  types, 408
Elderly. *See* Senior citizens
Emergencies, 36, 40
  hyperglycemia, 188
Emotional issues
  family support, 58
  feeling overwhelmed, 55-58
  impact of diagnosis, 48
  literature on, 49, 57
  marital relationships, 68-71
  problems in doctor–patient
    relationship, 65-67
  resolving negative feelings, 324
  self-evaluation, 63
  self-image, 61-65
  spiritual ties, 50
  threat of complications, 176, 177
Ephedra, 156
Epinephrine (adrenaline), 190
Escherichia coli, 345
Evening primrose oil, 153
Evista (raloxifene), 391, 395
Exercise
  attitude toward, 235-238
  benefits, 87, 237
  for children. *See* Children

Kidney disease, continued
  dialysis explained, 207–208
  dietary guidelines, 207, 328
  drug treatment, 206–207
  exercise guidelines, 260–261
  prevention, 206–207
  stages, 205–206
  transplant, 208

L

Lactic acidosis, 127, 188
Lancets and lancing devices, 76–78
  tips on using, 78
Lantus (glargine), 108–111
  advantages, 108, 117
  described, 109
  regimen using, 118
  research findings, 109–110
  safety, 110
  switching to, 111
Latent Autoimmune Diabetes
  of Adults (LADA), 15
Laxatives, 131, 156
Lente, 109, 117
Licorice, 154
Lispro. *See* Humalog (lispro)
Liver, 26, 116–117
Lower Extremity Amputation Prevention
  Program (LEAP), 221

M

Marriage
  challenges, 68, 70
  communication, 69
  impotence and, 201
  literature on, 71
  sexual relationships, 71
  spiritual issues, 71
Massage therapy, 44
Meal planning,
    See also Diet and nutrition.
  beef, 299–300, 301
  carbohydrate counting, 268–276
  chicken, 301, 302–303
  dietitian and, 315–320
  information sources, 271, 285
  lamb, 301, 302
  pork, 300, 301
  portion size, 264–268
  pregnancy and, 371
  recordkeeping, 286
  saturated fat, 281–286
    calculating, 286
  turkey, 301, 303
Medicare, 209
Medications. *See* Drugs and medications
Meglitinides, 94–95
Mental health, 163
  depression. *See* Depression
  psychotherapy, 44, 58–61
  stress and anxiety. *See* Stress and anxiety

Meters
  accuracy, 78–83
  adequate blood sample, 81
  cleaning, 81
  home results compared to laboratory,
    82
  precision, 79, 81
  strip problems, 81
  types, 80
  using readings, 83
Metformin.
    See Glucophage (metformin)
Miacalcin (calcitonin), 396
Microalbuminia, 206
Minerals, 133–137
  calcium, 137, 310, 392, 394, 395
  chromium, 137
  iron, 309–310
  magnesium, 137
  vegetarian diet and, 310
  zinc, 310
Mood disorder. *See* Depression *and*
    Stress and anxiety
Motion sickness, 130

N

National Federation of the Blind (NFB),
  183, 185
National Glycohemoglobin
  Standardization Program (NGSP), 75
Nephrologist, 44
Nephropathy. *See* Kidney disease
Neurologist, 44
Neurontin (gabapentin), 193
Neuropathy
  advanced glycosylation endproducts
    (AGE) and, 212
  autonomic neuropathy, 192, 203, 259
  drug treatment, 193
  effects, 193
  exercise guidelines, 259
  feet, effect on, 216
  focal neuropathy, 193
  gastrointestinal tract. *See* Gastropathy
  information sources, 194
  peripheral neuropathy, 152, 192, 197
  research, 19
Niacin (nicotinic acid), 173
Non-insulin-dependent diabetes.
    See Type 2 diabetes
Nonsulfonylurea pills, 90
Nopal cactus, 148
Novolin N (NPH insulin), 109, 110, 117
Novolog (aspart)
  as bolus, 117
  exercise guidelines, 242
Nurse educator, 38, 42
Nutrition. *See* Diet and nutrition

O

Obesity
  controlling overeating, 323–325

effect of Glucophage, 126
effect of insulin, 127, 188
fat distribution, 400
herbal remedies, 154
hypertension and, 166
information sources, 341
low-carbohydrate diet, 325–329
over-the-counter drugs, 132
support groups, 338–342
United Kingdom Prospective Diabetes
  Study (UKPDS), 24
weight-loss tips, 444–445
Occupational therapist, 44
Onion, 148
Ophthalmologist, 39, 44, 364
Oral health
  brushing, 360
  cold sore remedies, 130
  dental exam, 360–362
  dentist as part of diabetes team, 42
  dry mouth, 363
  flossing, 361, 362
  fungal infections, 363
  information sources, 362
  mouthwash, 362
  periodontal diseases, 359–360
Osteoporosis, 251
  benefits of exercise, 394–395
  calcium and, 394
  diagnosis, 394
  drug therapy, 389, 395
  information sources, 396
  insulin and, 393
  preventing fractures, 396
  risk factors, 392, 394
  vitamin D and, 394
Over-the-counter (OTC) drugs, 128–133
  safety considerations, 133
Overweight. *See* Obesity

P

Pancreas, 92
  basal secretion explained, 104
  bolus explained, 104
  transplant, 208
Pens, 99, 102, 426
Periodontitis, 359
Peripheral neuropathy. *See* Neuropathy
Peripheral vascular disease, 221, 261–262
Pharmacist, 39, 42
Physical therapist, 44
Pioglitazone, 14, 28
Pneumonia, 356
Podiatrist, 39, 44, 218
Polycystic ovary syndrome, 27, 128
Postprandial hyperglycemia
  and complications, 93
  described, 92
  resistant starch and, 312–313
  treatment, 93–95
Pregnancy
  alcohol consumption, 383
  birth defects, 375